	CVB	Chorionic vill...
	CVS	Chorionic vil...
	CXR	Chest x-ray
D	D&C	Dilation and curettage
	DEXA	Dual-energy x-ray absorptiometry
	DHEA	Dehydroepiandrosterone
	DIC	Disseminated intravascular coagulation
	DPA	Dual-photon absorptiometry
	DSA	Digital subtraction angiography
	DSMA	Disodium monomethane arsonate
	DST	Dexamethasone suppression test
E	EBV	Epstein-Barr virus
	ECG, EKG	Electrocardiography
	ECHO	Echocardiography
	EEG	Electroencephalogram
	EGD	Esophagogastroduodenoscopy
	EIA	Enzyme immunoassay
	ELISA	Enzyme-linked immunosorbent assay
	EMG	Electromyography
	ENG	Electroneurography
	EP	Evoked potential
	EPO	Erythropoietin
	EPS	Electrophysiologic study
	ER	Estrogen receptor
	ERCP	Endoscopic retrograde cholangiopancreatography
	ESR	Erythrocyte sedimentation rate
	EUG	Excretory urography
F	FBS	Fasting blood sugar
	FDPs	Fibrin degradation products
	%FPSA	Percent free PSA
	FSH	Follicle-stimulating hormone
	FSPs	Fibrin split products
	FT_4	Thyroxin, free
	FTA-ABS	Fluorescent treponemal antibody absorption test
	FTI	Free thyroxine index
G	G–6-PD	Glucose-6-phosphate dehydrogenase
	GB series	Gallbladder series
	GE reflux	Gastroesophageal reflux scan
	GGT	Gamma-glutamyl transferase
	GGTP	Gamma-glutamyl transpeptidase
	GH	Growth hormone
	GHb, GHB	Glycosylated hemoglobin
	GI series	Gastrointestinal series
	GTT	Glucose tolerance test
H	HAA	Hepatitis-associated antigen
	HAI	Hemagglutination inhibition
	Hb, Hgb	Hemoglobin
	HCG	Human chorionic gonadotropin
	HCO_3^-	Bicarbonate
	Hct	Hematocrit

Continued on inside back cover

Mosby's
Diagnostic
and Laboratory
Test Reference

Mosby's Diagnostic and Laboratory Test Reference

Seventh Edition

Kathleen Deska Pagana, PhD, RN

Professor Emeritus
Department of Nursing
Lycoming College
Williamsport, Pennsylvania
President, Pagana Seminars and Presentations

Timothy J. Pagana, MD, FACS

Medical Director
The Kathryn Candor Lundy Breast Health Center and
The SurgiCenter
Susquehanna Health System
Williamsport, Pennsylvania

Illustrated

ELSEVIER
MOSBY

ELSEVIER
MOSBY

11830 Westline Industrial Drive
St. Louis, Missouri 63146

MOSBY'S DIAGNOSTIC AND LABORATORY
TEST REFERENCE, 7TH ED.
Copyright © 2005, Elsevier Inc.

NOTICE

Health care is an ever-changing field. Standard safety precautions must
be followed, but as new research and clinical experience broaden our
knowledge, changes in treatment and drug therapy may become
necessary or appropriate. Readers are advised to check the most current
product information provided by the manufacturer of each drug to be
administered to verify the recommended dose, the method and duration
of administration, and contraindications. It is the responsibility of the
licensed prescriber, relying on experience and knowledge of the patient,
to determine dosages and the best treatment for each individual patient.
Neither the publisher nor the author assumes any liability for any injury
and/or damage to persons or property arising from this publication.

Previous editions copyrighted 1992, 1995, 1997, 1999, 2001, 2003.

ISBN-13: 978-0-323-03021-2
ISBN-10: 0-323-03021-1

Executive Publisher: Darlene Como
Managing Editor: Brian Dennison
Associate Developmental Editor: Betsy Stream
Publishing Services Manager: Catherine Jackson
Project Manager: Anne Konopka
Senior Designer: Kathi Gosche

Printed in the United States.

Last digit is the print number: 9   8   7   6   5   4   3   2

We lovingly dedicate this book to our daughters

Jocelyn Pagana Gaul

Denise Kathleen Pagana

Theresa Noel Pagana

Mosby's Diagnostic and Laboratory Test Reference provides the user with an up-to-date, essential reference that allows easy access to clinically relevant laboratory and diagnostic tests. A unique feature of this handbook is its consistent format, which allows for quick reference without sacrificing the depth of detail necessary for a thorough understanding of diagnostic and laboratory testing. All tests begin on a new page and are listed in alphabetical order by their complete name. The alphabetical format is a strong feature of the book; it allows the user to locate tests quickly without first having to place them in an appropriate category or body system. The User's Guide to Test Preparation and Procedures outlines the responsibilities for health care providers to ensure that the tests are accurately and safely performed. This guide should eliminate test repetition resulting from problems with patient preparation, test procedures, or collection techniques. Every feature of this book is designed to provide pertinent information in a sequence that best simulates priorities in the clinical setting.

The following information is provided, wherever applicable, for effective diagnostic and laboratory testing.

Name of test. Tests are listed by their complete name. A complete list of abbreviations and alternate test names follows each main entry.

Type of test. This section identifies whether the test is, for example, an x-ray procedure, ultrasound, nuclear scan, blood test, urine test, sputum test, or microscopic examination of tissue. This section helps the reader identify the source of the laboratory specimen or location of the diagnostic procedure.

Normal findings. Where applicable, normal values are listed for the infant, child, adult, and elderly person. Also, where appropriate, values are separated into male and female. It is important to realize that normal ranges of laboratory tests vary from institution to institution. This variability is even more obvious among the various laboratory textbooks. For this reason, we have deliberately chosen *not* to add a table of normal values as an appendix, and we encourage the user to check the normal values at the institution where the test is performed. This should be relatively easy because most laboratory reports include normal values. Results are given in both conventional units and the International System of Units (SI units) where possible.

Possible critical values. These values give an indication of results that are well outside the usual range of normal. These results generally require immediate intervention.

Test explanation and related physiology. This section provides a concise, yet comprehensive description of each test. It includes fundamental information about the test itself, specific indications for the test, how the test is performed, what disease or disorder the various results may show, how it will affect the patient or client, and relevant pathophysiology that will enhance understanding of the test.

Contraindications. These data are crucial because they alert the user to patients who should not have the test. Patients frequently highlighted in this section include those who are pregnant, are allergic to iodinated or contrast dyes, or have bleeding disorders.

Potential complications. This section alerts the user to potential problems that will necessitate astute assessments and interventions. For example, if a potential complication is renal failure, the implication may be to hydrate the patient before the test and force fluids after the test. A typical potential complication for many x-ray procedures is allergy to iodinated dye. Patient symptoms and appropriate interventions are described in detail.

Interfering factors. This section contains pertinent information because many factors can invalidate the test or make the test results unreliable. An important feature is the inclusion of drugs that can interfere with test results. Drugs that increase or decrease test values are always listed at the end of this section for consistency and quick access. A drug symbol (✗) is used to emphasize these drug interferences.

Procedure and patient care. This section emphasizes the role of nurses and other health care providers in diagnostic and laboratory testing by addressing psychosocial and physiologic interventions. Patient teaching priorities are noted with a special icon (**PT**) to highlight information to be communicated to patients. For quick access to essential information, this section is divided into *before, during,* and *after* time sequences.

Before. This section addresses the need to explain the procedure and to allay patient concerns or anxieties. If a consent is usually required, this is listed as a bulleted item. Other important features include requirements such as fasting, obtaining baseline values, and performing bowel preparations.

During. This section gives specific directions for clinical specimen studies (e.g., urine and blood studies). An estimate of the
approximate amount of a specimen is sometimes given; however,
this amount may vary from institution to institution. Diagnostic
procedures and their variations are described in a numbered,
usually step-by-step format. Important information such as who
performs the test, where the study is performed, patient sensation, and duration of the procedure is bulleted for emphasis.
The duration of the procedure is very helpful for patient teaching because it indicates the time generally allotted for each study.

After. This section includes vital information that the nurse or
other health care provider should heed or convey after the test.
Examples include factors such as maintaining bed rest, comparing pulses with baseline values, encouraging fluids, and observing for signs and symptoms of sepsis.

Home care responsibilities. These boxes are important
because of increasing emphasis on early discharge and outpatient
testing. As a result, patients and their families have the responsibility for detecting potential test-related problems in the home
setting. The boxes emphasize key areas for assessment and provide instructions for what to do when problems are detected.

Abnormal findings. As the name implies, this section lists
the abnormal findings for each study. Increased or decreased values are listed where appropriate.

Notes. This blank space at the end of the tests facilitates individualizing the studies according to the institution performing
the test. Variations in any area of the test (e.g., patient preparation, test procedure, normal values, or postprocedural care) can
be noted.

This logical format emphasizes clinically relevant information.
The clarity of this format allows quick understanding of content
essential to both students and health care providers. Color
has been used to help locate tests and highlight critical information (e.g., possible critical values). Color is also used in the
illustrations to enhance the reader's understanding of many
diagnostic procedures (e.g., bronchoscopy, fetoscopy, ERCP,
pericardiocentesis, TEE). Many tables are used to simplify
complex material on topics such as bioterrorism infectious
agents, blood collection tubes, hepatitis testing, and protein
electrophoresis. Extensive cross-referencing exists throughout
the book, which permits full understanding and helps the user
tie together or locate related studies such as hemoglobin and
hematocrit.

For easy access, a list of abbreviations for test names is included on the book's endpapers. Appendix A includes a list of studies according to *body systems*. This list may familiarize the user with other related studies the patient or client may need or the user may want to review. This should be especially useful for students and health care providers working in specialized areas. Appendix B provides a list of studies according to *test type*. This list may help the user read and learn about similarly performed tests and procedures (e.g., barium enema and barium swallow). Appendix C provides a list of blood tests used for disease and organ panels. Appendix D provides a list of symbols and units of measurement. Finally, a comprehensive index includes the names of all tests, their synonyms and abbreviations, and any other relevant terms found within the tests.

Many new studies such as bioterrorism infectious agents, bladder cancer markers, breast ductal lavage, lipoprotein electrophoresis, SARS, and sexual assault testing have been added. All other studies have been revised and updated. Outdated studies have been eliminated.

We sincerely thank our editors for their enthusiasm and continued support. We are most grateful to the many nurses and other health care providers who made the first six editions of this book so successful. This success validated the need for a user-friendly and quick-reference approach to laboratory and diagnostic testing.

We invite additional comments from current users of this book so that we may continue to provide useful, relevant diagnostic and laboratory test information to users of future editions.

contents

List of figures, xii

User's guide to test preparation and procedures, xiii

Diagnostic and laboratory tests, 1

Appendices

    Appendix A: List of tests by body system, 1006

    Appendix B: List of tests by type, 1016

    Appendix C: Disease and organ panels, 1025

    Appendix D: Symbols and units of measurement, 1029

Bibliography, 1031

Index, 1035

list of figures

Figure 1   Ultrasound of the abdomen, 2
Figure 2   Amniocentesis, 58
Figure 3   Immunofluorescent staining of antinuclear antibodies, 90
Figure 4   Catheter insertion for renal angiogram, 130
Figure 5   Arthroscopy, 139
Figure 6   Bilirubin metabolism and excretion, 158
Figure 7   Bone marrow aspiration, 186
Figure 8   Bronchoscopy, 208
Figure 9   Cardiac catheterization, 235
Figure 10   Chorionic villus sampling, 271
Figure 11   Hemostasis and fibrinolysis, 282
Figure 12   Colposcopy, 289
Figure 13   Cardiac enzymes after myocardial infarction, 322
Figure 14   Cystoscopic examination of the male bladder, 340
Figure 15   Ureteral catheterization through the cystoscope, 341
Figure 16   Disseminated intravascular coagulation, 364
Figure 17   Electrocardiography, 369
Figure 18   Endoscopic retrograde cholangiopancreatography, 397
Figure 19   Esophageal function studies, 408
Figure 20   Fetoscopy, 452
Figure 21   Glucose tolerance test, 493
Figure 22   Hematocrit, 512
Figure 23   Hysteroscopy, 551
Figure 24   Laparoscopy, 579
Figure 25   Liver biopsy, 595
Figure 26   Lumbar puncture, 608
Figure 27   Lung biopsy, 613
Figure 28   Lymphangiography, 625
Figure 29   Oximetry, 673
Figure 30   Papanicolaou (Pap) smear, 677
Figure 31   Paracentesis, 679
Figure 32   Pericardiocentesis, 699
Figure 33   Rectal ultrasonography, 753
Figure 34   Lung volumes and capacities, 776
Figure 35   Renal biopsy, 793
Figure 36   Renovascular hypertension, 801
Figure 37   Rectal culture of the female, 842
Figure 38   Urethral culture of the male, 843
Figure 39   Thoracentesis, 898
Figure 40   Transesophageal echocardiography, 934

Health care economics demands that laboratory and diagnostic testing be performed accurately and in the least amount of time possible. Tests should not have to be repeated because of problems with patient preparation, test procedure, or specimen collection technique. The following guidelines delineate the responsibilities for health care providers to ensure safety for test procedures and accuracy of test results. Guidelines are described for the following major types of tests: blood, urine, stool, x-ray, nuclear scanning, ultrasound, and endoscopy.

Blood tests

Overview

Blood studies are used to assess a multitude of body processes and disorders. Common studies include enzymes, serum lipids, electrolyte levels, red and white blood cell counts, clotting factors, hormone levels, and levels of breakdown products such as blood urea nitrogen.

Multiphasic screening machines can perform many blood tests quickly and simultaneously using a very small blood sample. The advantage of these machines is that results are available quickly and the cost is lower when compared with individually performing each test.

Appendix C provides a listing of disease and organ panels. For example, the basic metabolic panel and comprehensive metabolic panel have replaced the Chem-7 and Chem-12 panels. These changes are the result of recent federal guidelines that have standardized the nomenclature for chemistry panels.

Guidelines

- Observe universal precautions in collecting a blood specimen.
- Check whether fasting is required. Many studies, such as fasting blood sugar and cholesterol levels, require fasting for a designated time.
- If ordered, withhold medications until the blood is drawn. Indicate any drugs that the patient is taking.
- Record the time of day that the blood test is drawn. Some blood test results (such as those for cortisol) vary according to a diurnal pattern, and this must be considered when blood levels are interpreted.

- In general, two or three blood tests can be done per tube of blood collected (e.g., two or three chemistry tests from one red-top tube of blood).
- Note the patient's position for certain tests. For example, renin levels are affected by body position.
- Collect the blood in the proper color-coded test tube. Blood collection tubes have color-coded stoppers to indicate the presence or absence of different types of additives (preservatives and anticoagulants). A preservative prevents change in the specimen, and an anticoagulant inhibits clot formation or coagulation. Charts are available from the laboratory indicating the type of tube needed for each particular blood test. A representative chart is shown in Table 1, p. xv.
- Follow the recommended "order of draw" when collecting tubes. Draw specimens into nonadditive tubes (e.g., red-top) before drawing them into tubes with additives. Fill the tubes in the following order:
  1. Blood culture tubes (to maintain sterility)
  2. Nonadditive tubes (e.g., red-top)
  3. Coagulation tubes (e.g., blue-top)
  4. Heparin tubes (e.g., green-top)
  5. Ethylenediaminetetraacetic acid–K3 (EDTA-K3) tubes (e.g., lavender-top)
  6. Oxalate/fluoride tubes (e.g., gray-top)
- To obtain valid results, do not fasten the tourniquet for longer than 1 minute. Prolonged tourniquet application can cause stasis and hemoconcentration.
- Collect the blood specimen from the arm without an intravenous (IV) device, if possible. IV infusion can influence test results.
- Do not use the arm bearing a dialysis arteriovenous fistula for venipuncture unless the physician specifically authorizes it.
- Because of the risk of cellulitis, do not take specimens from the side on which a mastectomy or axillary lymph node dissection was performed.
- Follow the unit guidelines for drawing blood from an indwelling venous catheter, such as a triple-lumen catheter. Guidelines will specify the amount of blood to be drawn from the catheter and discarded before blood is collected for laboratory studies. The guidelines will also indicate the amount and type of solution needed to flush the catheter after drawing the blood to prevent it from being clogged by blood.
- Do not shake the blood specimen. Hemolysis may result from vigorous shaking and invalidate test results.

TABLE 1 Common blood collection tubes

Color of top	Additive	Purpose	Examples
Red	None	Allows blood sample to clot. This permits separation of serum when the serum needs to be tested.	Chemistry Bilirubin Blood urea nitrogen Calcium
Purple or lavender	Ethylenediamine-tetraacetic acid (EDTA)	Prevents blood from clotting	Hematology Complete blood cell count Platelet count
Gray	Sodium fluoride oxalate	Prevents glycolysis	Chemistry Glucose Lactose tolerance
Green	Heparin	Prevents blood from clotting when plasma needs to be tested	Chemistry Ammonia Carboxyhemoglobin
Blue	Sodium citrate	Prevents blood from clotting when plasma needs to be tested	Hematology Prothrombin time Partial thromboplastin time
Black	Sodium citrate	Binds calcium to prevent blood clotting	Westergren erythrocyte sedimentation rate (ESR)
Yellow	Citrate dextrose	Preserves red cells	Blood cultures
Gold serum separator tube (SST)	None	Collects serum	Chemistry

- Collect *blood cultures* before the initiation of antibiotic therapy. Blood cultures are often drawn when the patient manifests a fever. Often two or three cultures are taken at 30-minute intervals from different venipuncture sites.
- Skin punctures can be used for blood tests on capillary blood. Common puncture sites include the fingertips, earlobes, and heel surfaces. Fingertips are often used for small children, and the heel is the most commonly used site for infants.
- Ensure that the blood tubes are correctly labeled and delivered to the laboratory.
- After the specimen is drawn, apply pressure or a pressure dressing to the venipuncture site. Assess the site for bleeding.
- If the patient fasted before the blood test, reinstitute appropriate diet.

Urine tests

Overview

Urine tests are easy to obtain and provide valuable information about many body system functions, such as kidney function, glucose metabolism, and various hormone levels. The ability of the patient to produce specimens appropriately should be assessed to determine the need for assistance.

Guidelines

- Observe universal precautions in collecting a urine specimen.
- Use the first morning specimen for routine urinalysis because it is more concentrated. To collect a first morning specimen, have the patient void before going to bed and collect the first urine specimen immediately on rising.
- *Random* urine specimens can be collected at any time. They are usually obtained during daytime hours and without any prior patient preparation.
- If a *culture and sensitivity (C & S)* study is required or if the specimen is likely to be contaminated by vaginal discharge or bleeding, collect a *clean-catch* or *midstream* specimen. This requires meticulous cleansing of the urinary meatus with an iodine preparation to reduce contamination of the specimen by external organisms. Then the cleansing agent must be completely removed because it may contaminate the specimen. Obtain the *midstream* collection by:

1. Having the patient begin to urinate in a bedpan, urinal, or toilet and then stop urinating (This washes the urine out of the distal urethra.)
2. Correctly positioning a sterile urine container, into which the patient voids 3 to 4 ounces of urine
3. Capping the container
4. Allowing the patient to finish voiding

- One-time *composite* urine specimens are collected over a period that may range anywhere from 2 to 24 hours. To collect a timed specimen, instruct the patient to void and discard the first specimen. This is noted as the "start time" of the test. Instruct the patient to save all subsequent urine in a special container for the designated period. Remind the patient to void before defecating so that urine is not contaminated by feces. Also, instruct the patient not to put toilet paper in the collection container. A preservative is usually used in the collection container. At the end of the specified time period, have the patient void and then add this urine to the specimen container, thus completing the collection process.

- Collection containers for *24-hour urine specimens* should hold 3 to 4 L of urine and have tight-fitting lids. They should be labeled with the patient's name, the starting collection date and time, the ending collection date and time, the name of the test, the preservative, and storage requirements during collection.

- Many urine collections require preservatives to maintain their stability during the collection period. Some specimens are best preserved by being kept on ice or under refrigeration.

- *Urinary catheterization* may be needed for patients unable to void. This procedure is not preferred because of the risk of introducing organisms and because of patient discomfort.

- For patients with an *indwelling urinary catheter,* obtain a specimen by attaching a small-gauge (e.g., 25-gauge) needle to a syringe and aseptically inserting the needle into the catheter at a point distal to the sleeve leading to the balloon. Aspirate urine and then place it in a sterile urine container. The urine that accumulates in the plastic reservoir bag should never be used for a urine test.

- Urine specimens from infants and young children are usually collected in a disposable pouch called a *U bag.* This bag has

an adhesive backing around the opening to attach to the child. Once the bag is in place, check the child every 15 minutes to see if an adequate specimen has been collected. Remove the specimen as soon as possible after the collection, and then label it and transport it to the laboratory.
- Indicate on the laboratory slip any medications that may affect test results.

Stool tests

Overview

The examination of feces provides important information that aids in the differential diagnosis of various gastrointestinal disorders. Fecal studies may also be used for microbiologic studies, chemical determinations, and parasitic examinations.

Guidelines

- Observe universal precautions in collecting a stool specimen.
- Collect stool specimens in a clean container that has a fitted cover.
- Do not mix urine and toilet paper with the stool specimen. Both can contaminate the specimen and alter the results.
- Fecal analysis for occult blood, white blood cells, or qualitative fecal fat requires only a small amount of a randomly collected specimen.
- Quantitative tests for daily fecal excretion of a particular substance require a minimum of a 3-day fecal collection. This collection is necessary because the daily excretion of feces does not correlate well with the amount of food ingested by the patient in the same 24-hour period. Refrigerate specimens or keep them on ice during the collection period. Collect stool in a 1-gallon container.
- Some fecal collections require dietary restrictions before the collection (e.g., tests for occult blood).
- A small amount of fecal blood that is not visually apparent is termed *occult blood*. Chemical tests using commercially prepared slides are routinely used to detect fecal blood. Numerous commercial slide tests use guaiac as the indicator. These guaiac tests are routinely done on nursing units in the hospital.
- Consider various factors (such as other diagnostic tests and medications) in planning the stool collection. For example, if the patient is scheduled for x-ray studies using barium sulfate,

collect the stool specimen first. Various medications (e.g., tetracyclines and antidiarrheal preparations) affect the detection of intestinal parasites.

- Correctly label and deliver stool specimens to the laboratory within 30 minutes after collection. If you are unable to deliver the specimen within 30 minutes, it may be refrigerated for up to 2 hours.

X-ray studies

Overview

Because of the ability of x-rays to penetrate tissues, x-ray studies provide a valuable picture of body structures. X-ray studies can be as simple as a routine chest x-ray film or as complex as dye-enhanced cardiac catheterization. With the increasing concern about radiation exposure, it is important to realize that the patient may want to know if the proposed benefit outweighs the risks involved.

Guidelines

- Assess the patient for any similar or recent x-ray procedures.
- Evaluate the patient for allergies to iodine dye.
  1. Many types of contrast media are used in radiographic studies. For example, organic iodides and iodized oils are frequently used.
  2. Allergic reactions to iodinated dye may vary from mild flushing, itching, and urticaria to severe life-threatening anaphylaxis (evidenced by respiratory distress, drop in blood pressure, or shock). In the unusual event of anaphylaxis, the patient is treated with diphenhydramine (Benadryl), steroids, and epinephrine. Oxygen and endotracheal equipment should be on hand for immediate use.
  3. The patient should always be assessed for allergies to iodine dye before it is administered. Inform the radiologist if an allergy to iodinated contrast is suspected. The radiologist may prescribe a Benadryl and steroid preparation to be administered before testing. Usually hypoallergenic nonionic contrast will be used during the test.
  4. After the x-ray procedure, evaluate the patient for delayed reaction to dye (e.g., dyspnea, rashes, tachycardia, hives). This usually occurs within 2 to 6 hours after the test. Treat with antihistamines or steroids.
- Women in their childbearing years should have x-ray examinations during menses or 10 to 14 days after the onset of menses to avoid possible exposure to a fetus.

- Pregnant women should not have x-ray procedures, if possible, because of the risk of damage to the fetus.
- Note if other x-ray studies are being planned; schedule them in the appropriate sequence. For example, x-ray examinations that do not require contrast should precede examinations that do require contrast. X-ray studies using barium should be scheduled after ultrasonography studies.
- Note the necessary dietary restrictions. Studies such as a barium enema and intravenous pyelogram (IVP) are more accurate if the patient is kept NPO for several hours before the test.
- Determine if bowel preparations are necessary. For example, barium enemas and IVPs require bowel-cleansing regimens.
- Determine if signed consent forms are required. These are necessary for most invasive x-ray procedures.
- Remove metal objects such as necklaces and watches because they can hinder visualization of the x-ray field.
- Patient aftercare is determined by the type of x-ray procedure. For example, a patient having a simple chest x-ray study will not require postprocedure care. However, invasive x-ray procedures involving contrast dyes (such as cardiac catheterization) require extensive nursing measures to detect potential complications.

Nuclear scanning

Overview

With the administration of a radionuclide and subsequent detection of the measurement of radiation of a particular organ, functional abnormalities of various body areas such as the brain, heart, lung, and bones can be detected. Because the half-lives of the radioisotopes are short, only minimal radiation exposure occurs.

Guidelines

- Radiopharmaceuticals concentrate in target organs by various mechanisms. For example, some labeled compounds such as hippuran are cleared from the blood and excreted by the kidneys. Some phosphate compounds concentrate in the bone and infarcted tissue. Lung function can be studied by imaging the distribution of inhaled gases or aerosols.
- Note whether the patient has had any recent exposure to radionuclides. The previous study could interfere with the interpretation of the current study.

- Note the patient's age and current weight. This information is used to calculate the amount of radioactive substance to be administered.
- Nuclear scans are contraindicated in pregnant women and nursing mothers.
- Many scanning procedures do not require special preparation. However, a few have special requirements. For example, for bone scanning, the patient is encouraged to drink several glasses of water between the time of the injection of the isotope and the actual scanning. For some studies, blocking agents may need to be given to prevent other organs from taking up the isotope.
- For most nuclear scans, a small amount of an organ-specific radionuclide is given orally or injected intravenously. After the radioisotope concentrates in the desired area, the area is scanned. The scanning procedure usually takes place in the nuclear medicine department.
- Instruct the patient to lie still during the scanning.
- Usually encourage the patient to drink extra fluids to enhance excretion of the radionuclide after the test is finished.
- Although the amount of radionuclide excreted in the urine is very low, rubber gloves are sometimes recommended if the urine must be handled. Some hospitals may advise the patient to flush the toilet several times after voiding.

Ultrasound studies

Overview

In diagnostic ultrasonography, harmless high-frequency sound waves are emitted and penetrate the organ being studied. The sound waves bounce back to the sensor and are electronically converted into a picture of the organ. Ultrasonography is used to assess a wide variety of body areas, including the pelvis, abdomen, heart, and pregnant uterus.

Guidelines

- Most ultrasound procedures require little or no preparation. However, the patient having a pelvic sonogram needs a full bladder, and the patient having an ultrasound examination of the gallbladder must be kept NPO before the procedure.
- Ultrasound examinations are usually performed in an ultrasound room; however, they can be performed in the patient unit.

- For ultrasound, a greasy paste is applied to the skin overlying the desired organ. This paste is used to enhance sound transmission and reception because air impedes transmission of sound waves to the body.
- Because of the noninvasive nature of ultrasonography, no special nursing measures are needed after the study except for helping the patient remove the ultrasound paste.
- Ultrasound examinations have no radiation risk.
- Ultrasound examinations can be repeated as many times as necessary without being harmful to the patient. No cumulative effect has been seen.
- Barium has an adverse effect on the quality of abdominal studies. For this reason, schedule ultrasound of the abdomen before barium studies.
- Large amounts of gas in the bowel will not permit visualization of the bowel. This is because bowel gas is a reflector of sound.

Endoscopy procedures

Overview

With the help of a lighted, flexible instrument, internal structures of many areas of the body such as the stomach, colon, joints, bronchi, urinary system, and biliary tree can be directly viewed. The specific purpose and procedure should be reviewed with the patient.

Guidelines

- Preparation for an endoscopic procedure varies with the internal structure being examined. For example, examination of the stomach (gastroscopy) will require the passage of an instrument through the esophagus to the stomach. The patient is kept NPO for 8 to 12 hours before the test to prevent gagging, vomiting, and aspiration. For colonoscopy, an instrument is passed through the rectum and into the colon. Therefore the bowel must be cleansed and free of fecal material to afford proper visualization. Arthroscopic examination of the knee joint is usually done with the patient under general anesthesia, which necessitates routine preoperative care.
- Schedule endoscopic examinations before barium studies.
- Obtain a signed consent for endoscopic procedures.
- Endoscopic procedures are preferably performed in a specially equipped endoscopy room or in the operating room by a

physician. However, some kinds can safely be performed at the bedside.

- Air is instilled into the bowel during colon examinations to maintain patency of the bowel lumen and to afford better visualization. This sometimes causes gas pains.
- In addition to visualization of the desired area, special procedures can be performed. Biopsies can be obtained, and bleeding ulcers can be cauterized. Also, knee surgery can be performed during arthroscopy.
- Specific postprocedure interventions are determined by the type of endoscopic examination performed. All procedures have the potential complication of perforation and bleeding. Most procedures use some type of sedation; safety precautions should be observed until the effects of the sedatives have worn off.
- After colonoscopy and similar studies, the patient may complain of rectal discomfort. A warm tub bath may be soothing.
- Usually keep the patient NPO for 2 hours after endoscopic procedures of the upper gastrointestinal system. Be certain that swallow, gag, and cough reflexes are present before permitting fluids or liquids to be ingested orally.

abdominal ultrasound (Abdominal sonogram; Echogram; Ultrasound of the kidney, liver, pancreatobiliary system, gallbladder, pancreas, biliary tree)

Type of test Ultrasound

Normal findings Normal abdominal aorta, liver, gallbladder, bile ducts, pancreas, kidneys, ureters, and bladder

Test explanation and related physiology

Through the use of reflected sound waves, ultrasonography provides accurate visualization of the abdominal aorta, liver, gallbladder, pancreas, bile ducts, kidneys, ureters, and bladder. The technique of ultrasonography requires the emission of high-frequency sound waves from a transducer to penetrate the particular organ being studied. The sound waves are bounced back to the transducer and then electronically converted into a pictorial image (Figure 1). Real-time ultrasound provides an accurate picture of the organ being studied. Doppler ultrasound provides information concerning blood flow to those organs.

The *kidney* is ultrasonographically evaluated to diagnose and locate renal cysts, to differentiate renal cysts from solid renal tumors, to demonstrate renal and pelvic calculi, to document hydronephrosis, and to guide a percutaneously inserted needle for cyst aspiration or biopsy. Ultrasound of the urologic tract is also used to detect malformed or ectopic kidneys and perinephric abscesses. Renal transplantation surveillance is possible with ultrasound. One advantage of a kidney sonogram over intravenous pyelography (see p. 560) is that it can be performed on patients with impaired renal function because no intravenous contrast is required.

The prostate and the testes are discussed on pp. 752 and 826.

Another use of sonography is in the assessment of the *abdominal aorta* for aneurysmal dilation. Sonographic evidence of an aortic aneurysm greater than 5 cm or any size aneurysm that is documented to be significantly enlarging is an indication for abdominal aorta aneurysm resection. Ultrasound is also an ideal way to evaluate aneurysm patients, before and after surgery.

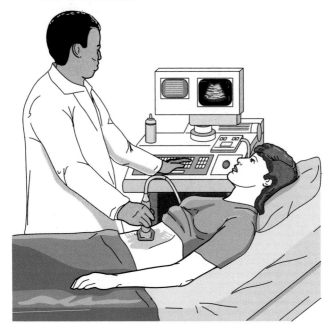

Figure 1 Ultrasound of the abdomen.

Ultrasound is used to detect cystic structures of the *liver* (e.g., benign cysts, hepatic abscesses, dilated hepatic ducts) and solid intrahepatic tumors (primary and metastatic). Hepatic ultrasound also can be performed intraoperatively by using a sterile probe. This technique allows for accurate location of small, nonpalpable hepatic tumors or abscesses. The *gallbladder* and *extrahepatic ducts* can be visualized and examined for evidence of gallstones, polyps, or dilation secondary to obstructive strictures or tumors. The *pancreas* is examined for evidence of tumor, pseudocysts, acute inflammation, chronic inflammation, or pancreatic abscess. Ultrasound of the pancreas is frequently performed serially to document and demonstrate resolution of acute pancreatic inflammatory processes.

Because this study requires no contrast material and has no associated radiation, it is especially useful in patients who are allergic to contrast and in those who are pregnant. Fasting may be preferred, but it is not mandatory. (See discussion of pelvic ultrasonography [p. 694] for sonographic evaluation of pelvic organs.)

Interfering factors

- Barium or gas will distort the sound waves and alter test results. Ultrasound tests should be performed before any x-ray testing with barium.
- The accuracy of ultrasonography is very dependent on the skills of the sonographer (the technician who performs the study).

Procedure and patient care

Before

PT Explain the procedure to the patient.

PT Tell the patient that fasting may or may not be required depending on the organ to be examined. No fasting is required for ultrasonography of the abdominal aorta, kidney, liver, spleen, or pancreas. Fasting, however, is preferred for ultrasound of the gallbladder and biliary tree.

During

- Note the following procedural steps:
  1. The patient is placed on the ultrasonography table in the prone or supine position, depending on the organ to be studied.
  2. A greasy conductive paste is applied to the patient's skin. This paste is used to enhance sound wave transmission and reception.
  3. A transducer is placed over the skin.
  4. Pictures are taken of the reflections from the organs being studied.
- The test is completed in approximately 20 minutes, usually by an ultrasound technologist, and interpreted by a radiologist.

PT Tell the patient that no discomfort is associated with the procedure.

After

- Remove the coupling agent (grease) from the patient's abdomen or back.
- Note that if a biopsy is done, refer to biopsy of the specific organ (e.g., liver or kidney biopsy).

Abnormal findings

Kidney

Renal cysts
Renal tumor
Renal calculi
Hydronephrosis
Ureteral obstruction
Perirenal abscess
Glomerulonephritis
Pyelonephritis
Perirenal hematoma

Gallbladder

Polyps
Tumor
Gallstone

Liver

Tumor
Abscess
Intrahepatic dilated bile ducts

Pancreas

Tumor
Cysts
Pseudocysts
Abscess
Inflammation

Bile ducts

Gallstone
Dilation
Stricture
Tumor

Abdominal aorta

Aneurysm

Abdominal cavity

Ascites
Abscess

acetylcholine receptor antibody (AChR Ab, Anti–acetylcholine receptor antibody)

Type of test Blood

Normal findings ≤0.03 nmol/L or negative

Test explanation and related physiology

This antibody may cause a block in neuromuscular transmission by interfering with the binding of *acetylcholine (ACh)* to AChR sites on the muscle membrane, thereby preventing muscle contraction. It is this phenomenon that characterizes myasthenia gravis (MG). Antibodies to AChR occur in more than 85% of patients with acquired MG. Lower levels are seen in patients with ocular MG only. The presence of this antibody is virtually diagnostic of MG, but a negative test does not exclude the disease. The measured titers do not correspond well with the severity of MG in different patients. In an individual patient, however, antibody levels are particularly useful in monitoring response to therapy. As the patient improves, antibody titers decrease.

There are three different AChR antibodies that test for MG. The AChR-*binding* antibody is most commonly used. The AChR-*modulating* antibody is more sensitive. A positive modulating antibody test may indicate subclinical MG, contraindicating the use of curare-like drugs during surgery. The AChR-*blocking* antibody is the least sensitive test (positive in only 61% of patients with MG), but can be quantified more accurately.

Interfering factors

- False-positive results may occur in patients with amyotrophic lateral sclerosis who have been treated with cobra venom.
- False-positive results may be seen in patients with penicillamine-induced, myasthenia-like symptoms.
- Drugs that may cause *increased* levels include muscle paralytic medicines (succinylcholine) and snake venom.
- Immunosuppressive drugs may suppress the formation of these antibodies in patients with subclinical MG.

Procedure and patient care

Before

PT Explain the procedure to the patient.
PT Tell the patient that no fasting is required.

During

- Collect a venous blood sample in a red-top tube.
- List on the laboratory slip all medications that the patient has taken in the last few days.

After

- Apply pressure or a pressure dressing to the venipuncture site.
- Assess the venipuncture site for bleeding.

Abnormal findings

▲   **Increased titer levels**

Myasthenia gravis
Ocular myasthenia gravis
Thymoma

notes

acid phosphatase (Prostatic acid phosphatase [PAP], Tartrate-resistant acid phosphatase [TRAP])

Type of test Blood

Normal findings

Adult/elderly: 0.13–0.63 units/L (Roy, Brower, Hayden; 37° C)
   or 2.2–10.5 units/L (SI units)
Child: 8.6–12.6 units/ml (30° C)
Newborn: 10.4–16.4 units/ml (30° C)

Test explanation and related physiology

Acid phosphatase is found in many tissues, including liver, red blood cells, bone marrow, and platelets. Highest levels are found in the prostate gland. Determination of the acid phosphatase level is primarily used to diagnose and stage prostatic carcinoma and to monitor the efficacy of treatment. Elevated levels are seen in patients with prostatic cancer that has metastasized beyond the capsule to other parts of the body, especially bone. If the tumor is successfully treated by surgery, acid phosphatase levels decrease in several days. If the tumor is treated by estrogen therapy, enzyme levels return to normal in several weeks. Rising levels of acid phosphatase may indicate a poor prognosis. The most clinically significant isoenzyme is the prostatic acid phosphatase (PAP). It is more accurate than total acid phosphatase in the prostatic cancer patient but less accurate than the prostate-specific antigen (PSA) (see p. 755).

Acid phosphatase is also found at high concentrations in seminal fluid; therefore, acid phosphatase tests may be performed on vaginal secretions to investigate alleged acts of rape.

The identification of *tartrate-resistant acid phosphatase (TRAP)* is very helpful in the diagnosis of hairy-cell leukemia (and occasionally other lymphoproliferative diseases). Five percent of patients with hairy-cell leukemia are not tartrate resistant.

Interfering factors

- Alkaline and acid phosphatase are very similar enzymes that differ in the pH at which they are identified. Any condition associated with very high levels of alkaline phosphatase may falsely indicate high acid phosphatase levels.

- Falsely high levels of acid phosphatase may occur in males after a digital examination or after instrumentation of the prostate (e.g., cystoscopy) because of prostatic stimulation.
- Drugs that may cause *elevated* levels include androgens (in females) and clofibrate (Atromid S).
- Drugs that may cause *decreased* levels include fluorides, phosphates, oxalates, and alcohol.

Procedure and patient care

Before

PT Explain the procedure to the patient.

PT Tell the patient that no food or drink restrictions are associated with this test.

- Note that some laboratories request they be notified before the blood sample is drawn so that immediate attention (<1 hr) can be given to the sample.

During

- Collect approximately 5 to 10 ml of blood in a red-top tube.
- Avoid hemolysis. Red blood cells contain acid phosphatase.
- Note on the laboratory slip if the patient has had a prostatic examination or instrumentation of the prostate within the last 24 hours.

After

- Apply pressure or a pressure dressing to the venipuncture site.
- Assess the venipuncture site for bleeding.
- Have the test performed without delay or freeze the specimen.
- Do *not* leave the specimen at room temperature for 1 hour or longer, because the enzyme is heat and pH sensitive and its activity will decrease.

Abnormal findings

▲ **Increased levels**

Prostatic carcinoma
Multiple myeloma
Paget's disease
Sickle cell crisis
Gaucher's disease
Renal impairment
Recent prostate
  manipulation

Benign prostatic hypertrophy
Prostatitis
Cancer of the breast and bone
Cirrhosis
Hyperparathyroidism
Thrombocytosis
Cancer metastasis to the bone

activated clotting time (ACT, Activated coagulation time)

Type of test Blood

Normal findings 70-120 sec

Therapeutic range for anticoagulation: 150-210 sec
(Normal ranges and anticoagulation ranges vary according to particular therapy.)

Possible critical values Depends upon use for the test and clinical situation

Test explanation and related physiology

The ACT is primarily used to measure the effect of heparin as an anticoagulant during cardiac angioplasty, hemodialysis, and cardiopulmonary bypass surgery (CPB). This test measures the time for whole blood to clot after the addition of particulate activators. It is similar to the activated partial thromboplastin time (APTT, p. 689) in that it measures the ability of the *intrinsic* pathway to begin clot formation by activating factor XII (see Figure 11, p. 282). By checking the blood clotting status with ACT, the response to heparin therapy can be monitored. Equally important is the use of the ACT in monitoring the dose of protamine sulfate required to reverse the effect of heparin in order to return the coagulation function to normal upon completion of surgical procedures and dialysis.

Both the APTT and the ACT can be used to monitor heparin therapy. However, the ACT has several advantages over the APTT. First, the ACT is more accurate than the APTT when high doses of heparin are used for anticoagulation. This makes it especially useful during clinical situations requiring high-dose heparin, such as during CPB when high-dose anticoagulation is necessary at levels 10 times those used for venous thrombosis. The APTT is not measurable at these high doses. The accepted goal for the ACT is 400 to 480 seconds during CPB.

Secondly, the ACT is both less expensive and more easily performed, even at the bedside. This allows for immediate accessibility and decreased turnaround time. The capability to perform the ACT at the "point of care" makes the ACT particularly useful for patients requiring angioplasty, hemodialysis, and CPB.

A nomogram adjusted to the patient's baseline ACT is often used as a guide to reach the desired level of anticoagulation during these procedures. This same nomogram is used in determining the dose of protamine to be administered to neutralize the heparin when a return to normal coagulation is desired upon completion of these procedures. The ACT is used in determining when it is safe to remove the vascular access upon completion of these procedures. The benefits of the *modified ACT* test are that it requires a smaller volume blood specimen; it can be automated; it can use standardized blood/reagent mixing; and it provides faster clotting time results than the conventional ACT. The modified ACT is being used even more frequently in vascular procedures that require high-dose heparin.

Interfering factors

- The ACT is affected by several biologic variables, including hypothermia, hemodilution, and platelet number and function.
- Factors affecting the pharmacokinetics of heparin (such as kidney or liver disease, and heparin resistance) can affect ACT measurements.
- Drugs such as aprotinin (a serine protease inhibitor used during CPB) can prolong the ACT when celite is used as the activator.

Procedure and patient care

Before

PT Explain the procedure to the patient.

During

- Less than 1 ml of blood is collected and placed in a machine at the bedside. When a clot is formed, the ACT value is displayed on the machine's panel.
- If the patient is receiving a continuous heparin drip, the blood sample is obtained from the arm without the intravenous catheter.

After

- Apply pressure to the venipuncture site. Remember that the bleeding time will be prolonged because of anticoagulation therapy.
- Assess the patient to detect possible bleeding. Check for blood in the urine and all other excretions, and assess the patient for bruises, petechiae, and low back pain.
- For clinical significance, the test results must be correlated with the time of heparin administration. A clinical flow sheet

is used to list the test results with the time and route of heparin administration.

Abnormal findings

▲ **Increased levels**

Heparin administration
Clotting factor deficiencies
Cirrhosis of the liver

▼ **Decreased levels**

Thrombosis

notes

adrenocorticotropic hormone (ACTH, Corticotropin)

Type of test   Blood

Normal findings

AM: <80 pg/ml or <18 pmol/L (SI units)
PM: <50 pg/ml or <11 pmol/L (SI units)

Test explanation and related physiology

The ACTH study is a test of anterior pituitary gland function that affords the greatest insight into the causes of either Cushing's syndrome (overproduction of cortisol) or Addison's disease (underproduction of cortisol). An elaborate feedback mechanism for cortisol exists to coordinate the function of the hypothalamus, pituitary gland, and adrenal glands. ACTH is an important part of this mechanism. Corticotropin-releasing hormone (CRH) is made in the hypothalamus. This stimulates ACTH production in the anterior pituitary gland. This, in turn, stimulates the adrenal cortex to produce cortisol. The rising levels of cortisol act as a negative feedback and curtail further production of CRH and ACTH.

In the patient with Cushing's syndrome, an elevated ACTH level can be caused by a pituitary or a nonpituitary (ectopic) ACTH-producing tumor, usually in the lung, pancreas, thymus, or ovary. ACTH levels over 200 pg/ml usually indicate ectopic ACTH production. If the ACTH level is below normal in a patient with Cushing's syndrome, an adrenal adenoma or carcinoma is probably the cause of the hyperfunction.

In patients with Addison's disease, an elevated ACTH level indicates primary adrenal gland failure, as in adrenal gland destruction caused by infarction, hemorrhage, or autoimmunity; surgical removal of the adrenal gland; congenital enzyme deficiency; or adrenal suppression after prolonged ingestion of exogenous steroids. If the ACTH level is below normal in a patient with adrenal insufficiency, hypopituitarism is most probably the cause of the hypofunction.

One must be aware that there is a diurnal variation of ACTH levels that corresponds to variation of cortisol levels. Levels in evening (8 PM to 10 PM) samples are usually one half to two thirds those of morning (4 AM to 8 AM) specimens. This diurnal variation is lost when disease (especially neoplasm) affects the pituitary or adrenal glands. Likewise, stress can blunt or eliminate this normal diurnal variation.

Interfering factors

- Stress (trauma, pyrogens, or hypoglycemia) and pregnancy can increase levels.
- Recently administered radioisotope scans can affect levels.
- ▼ Drugs that may cause *increased* levels include estrogens, ethanol, vasopressin, aminoglutethimide, amphetamines, insulin, metyrapone, and spironolactone.
- ▼ Corticosteroids may *decrease* ACTH levels.

Procedure and patient care

Before

- **PT** Explain the procedure to the patient. Allow plenty of time to answer questions so that the patient's stress is diminished as much as possible.
- Keep the patient NPO after midnight the day of the test.
- Evaluate the patient for stress factors that would invalidate the test results.
- Evaluate the patient for sleep pattern abnormalities. With a normal sleep pattern, the ACTH level is highest between 4 AM and 8 AM and lowest around 9 PM.

During

- Collect approximately 20 ml of heparinized venous blood in a green-top tube.
- Chill the blood tube to prevent enzymatic degradation of ACTH.

After

- Place the specimen in ice water and send it to the chemistry laboratory immediately. ACTH is a very unstable peptide in plasma and should be stored at −20° C to prevent artificially low values.
- Apply pressure or a pressure dressing to the venipuncture site.

Abnormal findings

▲   **Increased levels**

Addison's disease (primary
  adrenal insufficiency)
Cushing's disease (pituitary-
  dependent adrenal
  hyperplasia)
Ectopic ACTH syndrome
Stress
Adrenogenital syndrome
  (congenital adrenal
  hyperplasia)

▼   **Decreased levels**

Secondary adrenal
  insufficiency (pituitary
  insufficiency)
Cushing's syndrome
Hypopituitarism
Adrenal adenoma or
  carcinoma
Steroid administration

notes

adrenocorticotropic hormone stimulation test with cosyntropin (ACTH stimulation test, Cortisol stimulation test)

Type of test Blood

Normal findings

Rapid test: cortisol levels increase more than 7 mcg/dl above baseline
24-hour test: cortisol levels greater than 40 mcg/dl
3-day test: cortisol levels greater than 40 mcg/dl

Test explanation and related physiology

This test is performed on patients found to have an adrenal insufficiency. An increase in plasma cortisol levels after the infusion of an "ACTH-like" drug indicates that the adrenal gland is normal and capable of functioning if stimulated. In that case, the cause of the adrenal insufficiency would lie within the pituitary gland (hypopituitarism, which is called secondary adrenal insufficiency). If little or no rise in cortisol levels occurs after the administration of the ACTH-like drug, the adrenal gland is the source of the problem and cannot secrete cortisol. This is called primary adrenal insufficiency (Addison's disease), which may be caused by adrenal hemorrhage, infarction, autoimmunity, metastatic tumor, surgical removal of the adrenal glands, or congenital adrenal enzyme deficiency.

This test can also be used in the evaluation of patients with Cushing's syndrome. Patients with Cushing's syndrome caused by bilateral adrenal hyperplasia have an exaggerated cortisol elevation in response to the administration of the ACTH-like drug. Those experiencing Cushing's syndrome as a result of hyperfunctioning adrenal tumors (which are usually autonomous and relatively insensitive to ACTH) have little or no increase in cortisol levels over baseline values.

Cosyntropin (Cortrosyn) is a synthetic subunit of ACTH that has the same corticosteroid-stimulating effect as endogenous ACTH in healthy persons. During this test, cosyntropin is administered to the patient, and the ability of the adrenal gland to respond is measured by plasma cortisol levels.

The *rapid stimulation test* is only a screening test. A normal response excludes adrenal insufficiency. An abnormal response, however, requires a 1- to 3-day prolonged ACTH stimulation test to differentiate primary insufficiency from secondary insufficiency. It should be noted that the adrenal gland can also be stimulated by insulin-induced hypoglycemia as a stressing agent. When insulin is the stimulant, cortisol and glucose levels are measured.

Interfering factors

✓ Drugs that may cause artificially *increased* cortisol levels include corticosteroid, estrogens, and spironolactone.

Procedure and patient care

Before

PT Explain the procedure to the patient.

- Keep the patient NPO after midnight the day of the test.

During

Rapid test

- Obtain a baseline plasma cortisol level. This should be done within 30 minutes of cosyntropin (ACTH-like drug) administration.
- Administer an IV injection of cosyntropin over a 2-minute period as prescribed.
- Measure plasma cortisol levels 30 and 60 minutes after drug administration.

24-hour test

- Obtain a baseline plasma cortisol level.
- Start an IV infusion of synthetic cosyntropin in 1 L of normal saline.
- Administer the solution as prescribed for 24 hours.
- After 24 hours, obtain another plasma cortisol level.

3-day test

- Obtain a baseline plasma cortisol level.
- Administer the prescribed dose of cosyntropin IV over an 8-hour period on 2 to 3 consecutive days.
- The plasma cortisol is then measured at 12, 24, 36, 48, 60, and 72 hours after the start of the test.
- Collect plasma for cortisol levels in a red-top tube.

After

- Apply pressure to the venipuncture site.

Abnormal findings

In adrenal insufficiency

Increase above normal response (secondary adrenal insufficiency)

Hypopituitarism

Exogenous steroid ingestion

Endogenous steroid production from a nonendocrine tumor

Normal or below normal response (primary adrenal insufficiency)

Addison's disease

Adrenal infarction/hemorrhage

Metastatic tumor to the adrenal gland

Congenital enzyme adrenal insufficiency

Surgical removal of the adrenal gland

In Cushing's syndrome

Increase above normal response

Bilateral adrenal hyperplasia

Normal or below normal response

Adrenal adenoma

Adrenal carcinoma

ACTH-producing nonadrenal tumor

Chronic steroid use

notes

adrenocorticotropic hormone stimulation test with metyrapone (ACTH stimulation test with metyrapone)

Type of test Blood; urine (24-hour)

Normal findings

24-hour urine: baseline excretion of urinary 17-hydroxycorticosteroid (OCHS) more than doubled

Blood: 11-deoxycortisol increased to >7 mcg/dl and cortisol <10 mcg/dl

Test explanation and related physiology

Metyrapone is a potent blocker of an enzyme involved in cortisol production. Therefore cortisol production is reduced. When this drug is given, the resulting fall in cortisol production should stimulate pituitary secretion of ACTH by way of a negative feedback mechanism. Cortisol precursors (11-deoxycortisol and OCHS) can be detected in the urine or blood. This test is similar to the cosyntropin ACTH stimulation test (see p. 15).

In patients with adrenal hyperplasia caused by pituitary over-production of ACTH, the cortisol precursors are greatly increased, more than expected in normal patients. This is because the normal adrenal/pituitary response mechanism is still intact. No response to metyrapone occurs in patients with Cushing's syndrome resulting from adrenal adenoma or carcinoma because the tumors are autonomous and therefore insensitive to changes in ACTH secretion.

This test is also used to evaluate the pituitary reserve capacity to produce ACTH. It can document that adrenal insufficiency exists as a result of pituitary disease (secondary adrenal insufficiency) rather than primary adrenal pathology. This test should not be performed if primary adrenal insufficiency is likely. Severe, life-threatening adrenal crisis could be precipitated. A normal response to administration of ACTH should be demonstrated before the metyrapone is performed.

Contraindications

- Patients with possible adrenal insufficiency

Potential complications

- Addison's disease and addisonian crisis, because metyrapone inhibits cortisol production

Interfering factors

- Recent administration of radioisotopes will interfere with test results.
- Chlorpromazine (Thorazine) interferes with the response to metyrapone and should not be administered during the testing.

Procedure and patient care

Before

PT Explain the procedure to the patient.
- Obtain a baseline 24-hour urine specimen for 17-OCHS level (see p. 543) for the urine test.
- Obtain a baseline cortisol level (see p. 314) for the blood test.

During

Blood
- Administer 2 to 3 g of metyrapone at 11 PM the night before the blood specimen is to be collected. Collect a blood specimen in the morning.

Urine
- Obtain a 24-hour urine specimen for 17-OCHS level as a baseline. Then collect a 24-hour urine specimen for 17-OCHS level during and again 1 day after the oral administration of 500 to 750 mg of metyrapone, which is given every 4 hours for 24 hours.

After

- Assess the patient for impending signs of addisonian crisis (muscle weakness, mental and emotional changes, anorexia, nausea, vomiting, hypotension, hyperkalemia, vascular collapse).
- Note that addisonian crisis is a medical emergency that must be treated vigorously. Basically the immediate treatment includes replenishing steroids, reversing shock, and restoring blood circulation.

Abnormal findings

Increased cortisol precursors
Adrenal hyperplasia

No change in cortisol precursors
Adrenal tumor
Ectopic ACTH syndrome
Secondary adrenal insufficiency

notes

agglutinins, febrile/cold

Type of test Blood

Normal findings

Febrile (warm) agglutinins: no agglutination in titers ≤1:80
Cold agglutinins: no agglutination in titers ≤1:16

Test explanation and related physiology

Febrile agglutinin serologic studies are used to diagnose infectious diseases such as salmonellosis, rickettsial diseases, brucellosis, and tularemia. Neoplastic diseases such as leukemias and lymphomas are also associated with febrile agglutinins. Appropriate antibiotic treatment of the infectious agent is associated with a drop in the titer activity of febrile agglutinins.

Cold agglutinins occur in patients who are infected by other agents, most notably *Mycoplasma pneumoniae*. Other diseases include influenza, mononucleosis, rheumatoid arthritis, and lymphomas.

The febrile and cold agglutinins are antibodies that cause RBCs to aggregate at high or low temperatures, respectively. Agglutination occurring at titers greater than 1:16 for cold agglutinins and 1:80 for febrile agglutinins is considered abnormal and diagnostic of the infectious agent the agglutinins represent. High titers of either cold or warm agglutinins can interfere with blood typing, crossmatching, and transfusion.

Temperature regulation is important for the performance of these tests. Under no circumstances should the cold agglutinin specimen be refrigerated or the febrile agglutinin heated.

Interfering factors

✠ Some antibiotics (penicillin and cephalosporins) can interfere with the development of cold agglutinins.

Procedure and patient care

Before
PT Explain the procedure to the patient.
PT Tell the patient that no fasting is required.

During
- Collect approximately 7 ml of venous blood in a red-top tube (warmed or cooled; see previous discussion).

After
- Apply pressure to the venipuncture site.
- Transport the specimen immediately to the laboratory.

Abnormal findings

▲   **Increased febrile agglutinins**

Salmonellosis infection
Rickettsial disease
Brucellosis
Tularemia
Leukemia
Lymphoma

▲   **Increased cold agglutinins**
Mycoplasma pneumoniae infection
Viral illness
Infectious mononucleosis
Multiple myeloma
Scleroderma
Cirrhosis
Staphylococcemia
Thymic tumor
Influenza
Rheumatoid arthritis
Lymphoma

notes

A

AIDS serology (Acquired immunodeficiency serology, AIDS screen, Human immunodeficiency virus [HIV] antibody test, Western blot test antibody, Enzyme-linked immunosorbent assay [ELISA] for HIV antibody, p24 antigen capture assay, Detuned HIV antibody, Urine and saliva HIV antibody)

Type of test Blood

Normal findings No evidence of HIV antigen or antibodies

Test explanation and related physiology

Tests used to detect the antibody to HIV, which is the virus that causes AIDS, were first licensed for the screening of blood and plasma donors. The HIV virus is also known as human T-lymphotrophic virus, type III (HTLV-III), or the lymphadenopathy-associated virus (LAV). There are two types of HIV viruses (types 1 and 2). Type 1 is most prevalent in the United States and Western Europe. Type 2 is limited mostly to West African nations.

Those at high risk for AIDS include sexually active homosexual and bisexual men and women with multiple partners, IV drug abusers, persons receiving blood products tainted with HIV, and infants exposed to the virus during gestation and delivery.

Because of the medical and social significance of a positive test for HIV antibody, test results must be accurate and their interpretation correct. Therefore the U.S. Public Health Service has emphasized that an individual can be said to have serologic evidence of HIV infection only after an enzyme immunoassay (EIA) screening test is repeatedly reactive and another test, such as Western blot or immunofluorescence assay, validates the results. However, a positive EIA not confirmed by Western blot or immunofluorescence should not be considered negative. Repeat testing is required in 3 to 6 months. A person with a positive HIV test result does not have AIDS until the clinical criteria are fulfilled.

ELISA, which tests for antibodies to HIV in serum or plasma, is the most widely used and least expensive serologic test for AIDS. ELISA is used for clinical diagnosis, screening blood and blood products, and testing individuals who believe they may be infected with HIV. It is important to reiterate that ELISA detects antibodies to HIV. Because it does not detect viral antigens (see HIV viral load, p. 529), it cannot detect infection in its earliest stage (before antibodies are formed). There is a period (usually within 2 to 12 weeks, but possibly as long as 6 months) it takes for a person who has been infected with HIV to seroconvert (test positive for HIV antibodies). This time is called the window period.

The sensitivity (i.e., probability that the test results will be reactive if the specimen is a true positive) of the ELISA test is approximately 99% for blood from persons infected with HIV for 12 weeks or more. The probability of a false-negative test is remote, except during the first few weeks after infection before detectable antibodies appear.

The specificity (probability that test results will be nonreactive if the specimen is a true negative) of the ELISA test is approximately 99% when repeated. To increase the specificity of serologic tests further, a supplemental test (most often the Western blot) is done to validate repeatedly reactive ELISA results. Sensitivity of the blot test is comparable to or greater than a repeatedly reactive ELISA. The testing sequence of a repeatedly reactive ELISA and a positive Western blot test is highly predictive of HIV infection. A newer test, called a *detuned ELISA*, will become more widely available. The detuned test, which is used only after a Western blot, can determine whether the HIV infection is recent (within the past 6 months). This test may be useful for deciding upon early treatment options.

The diagnostic tests described in the preceding paragraphs detect HIV infection based on demonstration of *antibodies* to HIV. Recently it has become possible to diagnose HIV infection by the direct detection of HIV or one of its components. New tests are now available in the research laboratory and are of considerable help when the Western blot results are indeterminate. The simplest of these tests is the *p24 antigen capture assay*. This detects the viral protein p24 in the peripheral blood of HIV-infected individuals, where it exists either as a free antigen or complexed to anti-p24 antibodies.

The p24 antigen may be detectable as early as 2 to 6 weeks after infection. Throughout the course of HIV infection, an equilibrium exists between the p24 antigen and anti-p24 antibodies. During the first few weeks of infection, before the development of an immune response, there is a sharp increase in p24 antigen levels. These levels decline after the development of anti-p24 antibodies. Later in HIV disease, p24 antigen levels become detectable again.

The p24 antigen test is currently being used to assess the antiviral activity of experimental HIV therapies. The p24 antigen test also can be used to diagnose neonatal HIV infection, detect HIV before seroconversion, and determine the progression of AIDS.

The serologic identification of antibodies to HIV in blood is the most widely used method for diagnosing HIV infection. However, one barrier for individuals desiring HIV antibody testing has been the lack of alternatives to blood testing. Recently, the use of *oral fluids* for the detection of antibodies to HIV has become available as an alternative to serum testing. These new HIV-1 antibody tests use *oral mucosal transudate (OMT)*, a serum-derived fluid that enters saliva from the gingival crevice and across oral mucosal surfaces. These tests compare favorably to serum reliability because they are based on the same ELISA-Western blot algorithm. The OMT tests for HIV involve a simple, safe, and noninvasive method of specimen collection, thus providing an effective epidemiologic tool for HIV testing. OraSure, Orapette, and Omni-Sal are a few examples of these new oral testing kits. It is hoped that these portable, user-friendly diagnostic tests will facilitate identification of greater numbers of infected individuals, with the ultimate goals of early identification, early treatment, and prevention of disease transmission.

Another noninvasive alternative to blood testing is *urine testing* for HIV. In 1996, the U.S. Food and Drug Administration licensed the first screening EIA for the detection of urine HIV-1 antibodies, and in 1998 licensed a confirmation test for urine HIV-1 antibodies. Testing urine for HIV antibodies is valuable, especially when venipuncture is inconvenient, difficult, or unacceptable. Urine testing would certainly be safer, more convenient, and less costly than serum testing. Undoubtedly, this is another testing area ripe for additional research.

Home kits are now available that provide anonymous registration and pretest counseling via a toll-free call. Sample collection in the privacy of one's home, laboratory processing, and posttest counseling are components of this home-testing process. This test, which costs about $45 to $70, uses a fingerstick blood sample that is sent to a certified laboratory for testing. The methods used for these home tests are the same antibody methods (ELISA or Western blot) as mentioned above. In most cases, results are available in about 1 week.

Interfering factors

- False-positive results can occur in patients who have autoimmune disease, lymphoproliferative disease, leukemia, lymphoma, syphilis, or alcoholism.
- False-negative results can occur in the early incubation stage or end stage of AIDS.

Procedure and patient care

Before

PT Explain the procedure to the patient.
- Obtain an informed consent if required by the institution.
PT Tell the patient that no fasting or preparation is required.
- Maintain a nonjudgmental attitude toward the patient's sexual practices and allow the patient ample time to express his or her concerns regarding the results.

During

- Observe universal blood and body precautions. Wear gloves when handling blood products from all patients.
- Collect 7 ml of peripheral venous blood in a red-top tube. The blood is usually sent to an outside laboratory for testing.
- If the patient wishes to remain anonymous, use a number with the patient's name and record it accurately.
- Note that if the ELISA test is repeatedly reactive (i.e., test is positive twice consecutively), the Western blot test is performed on the same blood sample.
- If the Western blot test is equivocal, collect a second serum specimen 2 to 4 months later for testing.

After

- Apply pressure to the venipuncture site.
PT Inform the patient to observe the venipuncture site for infection. Patients with AIDS are immunocompromised and susceptible to infection.
- Follow the institution's policy regarding test result reporting. Do not give results over the telephone. Remember that positive results may have devastating consequences.
PT Explain to the patient that a positive Western blot test merely implies exposure to and presence of the AIDS virus within the body. It does not mean that the patient has clinical AIDS. Not all patients with positive antibodies will acquire the disease.
PT Encourage patients who test positive to identify their sexual contacts so that they can be informed and tested.

PT Inform the patient that subsequent sexual contact will put new partners at high risk for contracting AIDS.

PT Provide patient education regarding safe sexual practices.

🏠 Home care responsibilities

- Do not give the test results over the telephone.
- Positive results may have devastating consequences, including loss of job, insurance, relationships, and housing.
- Encourage patients who test positive to inform their sexual partners so they can be tested.
- Inform patients who test positive that subsequent sexual contact will put partners at high risk for contracting AIDS.

Abnormal findings

▲ **Increased levels**

AIDS

HIV infection

notes

alanine aminotransferase (ALT, Serum glutamic-pyruvic transaminase [SGPT])

Type of test Blood

Normal findings

Adult/child: 4-36 units/L at 37° C, or 4-36 units/L (SI units)
Elderly: may be slightly higher than adult
Infant: may be twice as high as adult

Test explanation and related physiology

ALT is found predominantly in the liver; lesser quantities are found in the kidneys, heart, and skeletal muscle. Injury or disease affecting the liver parenchyma will cause a release of this hepatocellular enzyme into the bloodstream, thus elevating serum ALT levels. Generally most ALT elevations are caused by liver disease. Therefore this enzyme is not only sensitive but also very specific in indicating hepatocellular disease. In hepatocellular disease other than viral hepatitis, the ALT/AST ratio *(DeRitis ratio)* is less than 1. In viral hepatitis, the ratio is greater than 1. This is helpful in the diagnosis of viral hepatitis.

Interfering factors

- Previous IM injections may cause elevated levels.
- Drugs that may cause *increased* ALT levels include acetaminophen, allopurinol, aminosalicylic acid (PAS), ampicillin, azathioprine, carbamazepine, cephalosporins, chlordiazepoxide, chlorpropamide, clofibrate, cloxacillin, codeine, dicumarol, indomethacin, isoniazid (INH), methotrexate, methyldopa, nafcillin, nalidixic acid, nitrofurantoin, oral contraceptives, oxacillin, phenothiazines, phenylbutazone, phenytoin, procainamide, propoxyphene, propranolol, quinidine, salicylates, tetracyclines, and verapamil.

Procedure and patient care

Before
PT Explain the procedure to the patient.
PT Tell the patient that no fasting is required.

During
- Collect approximately 7 to 10 ml of blood in a red-top tube and send it to the laboratory for analysis.

After

■ Apply pressure to the venipuncture site. Patients with liver dysfunction often have prolonged clotting times.

Abnormal findings

▲   **Increased levels**

Hepatitis
Hepatic necrosis
Hepatic ischemia
Cirrhosis
Cholestasis
Hepatic tumor
Hepatotoxic drugs
Obstructive jaundice
Severe burns
Trauma to striated muscle
Myositis
Pancreatitis
Myocardial infarction
Infectious mononucleosis
Shock

notes

aldolase

Type of test Blood

Normal findings
Adult: 3-8.2 Sibley-Lehninger units/dl or 22-59 mU/L at 37° C (SI units)
Child: approximately two times the adult values
Newborn: approximately four times the adult values

Test explanation and related physiology
Serum aldolase is very similar to the enzymes aspartate amino transferase AST (SGOT) (see p. 143) and CPK (see p. 322). Aldolase is an enzyme used in the glycolytic breakdown of glucose. As with AST and creatine phosphokinase, aldolase exists throughout the body in most tissues. This test is most useful for indicating muscular or hepatic cellular injury or disease. The serum aldolase level is very high in patients with muscular dystrophies, dermatomyositis, and polymyositis. Levels also are increased in patients with gangrenous processes, muscular trauma, and muscular infectious diseases (e.g., trichinosis). Elevated levels are also noted in chronic hepatitis, obstructive jaundice, and cirrhosis.

Neurologic diseases causing weakness can be differentiated from muscular causes of weakness with this test. Normal values are seen in patients with such neurologic diseases as poliomyelitis, myasthenia gravis, and multiple sclerosis. Elevated aldolase levels are seen in the primary muscular disorders.

Interfering factors
- Previous IM injections may cause elevated levels.
- ✗ Drugs that may cause *increased* aldolase levels include hepatotoxic agents.
- ✗ Drugs that may cause *decreased* aldolase levels include phenothiazines.

Procedure and patient care
Before
PT Explain the procedure to the patient.
- Note that a short period of fasting usually will provide more accurate results.

During

- Collect 7 to 10 ml of blood in a red-top tube.

After

- Apply pressure to the venipuncture site.

Abnormal findings

▲ **Increased levels**

Hepatocellular diseases
(e.g., hepatitis)

Muscular diseases
(e.g., muscular dystrophy,
dermatomyositis,
polymyositis)

Muscular trauma (e.g., severe
crush injuries)

Muscular infections (e.g.,
trichinosis)

Gangrenous processes (e.g.,
gangrene of the bowel)

Myocardial infarction

▼ **Decreased levels**

Late muscular
dystrophy

Hereditary fructose
intolerance

Muscle-wasting disease

notes

aldosterone

Type of test   Blood; urine (24-hour)

Normal findings

Blood

Supine: 3-10 ng/dl or 0.08-0.3 nmol/L (SI units)
Upright
   Female: 5-30 ng/dl or 0.14-0.8 nmol/L (SI units)
   Male: 6-22 ng/dl or 0.17-0.61 nmol/L (SI units)
Newborn: 5-60 ng/dl

1 week-1 year: 1-160 ng/dl	5-7 years: 5-50 ng/dl
1-3 years: 5-60 ng/dl	7-11 years: 5-70 ng/dl
3-5 years: 5-80 ng/dl	11-15 years: 5-50 ng/dl

Urine

2-26 mcg/24 hr or 6-72 nmol/24 hr (SI units)

Test explanation and related physiology

This test is used to diagnose hyperaldosteronism. Production of aldosterone, a hormone produced by the adrenal cortex, is regulated primarily by the renin-angiotensin system. Secondarily, aldosterone is stimulated by ACTH, low serum sodium levels, and high serum potassium levels. Aldosterone in turn stimulates the renal tubules to absorb sodium (water follows) and secrete potassium into the urine. In this way, aldosterone regulates serum sodium and potassium levels. Because water follows sodium transport, aldosterone also partially regulates water absorption (and plasma volume).

Increased aldosterone levels are associated with primary aldosteronism, in which a tumor (usually an adenoma) of the adrenal cortex (Conn's syndrome) or bilateral adrenal nodular hyperplasia causes increased production of aldosterone. Patients with primary aldosteronism characteristically have hypertension, weakness, polyuria, and hypokalemia.

Increased aldosterone levels also occur with secondary aldosteronism caused by nonadrenal conditions. These include the following:

1. Renal vascular stenosis or occlusion
2. Hyponatremia (from diuretic or laxative abuse) or low salt intake
3. Hypovolemia

4. Pregnancy or use of estrogens.
5. Malignant hypertension
6. Potassium loading
7. Edematous states such as congestive heart failure, cirrhosis, or nephrotic syndrome

The aldosterone assay can be done on a 24-hour urine specimen or a plasma blood sample. The advantage of the 24-hour urine sample is that short-term fluctuations are eliminated. Plasma values are more convenient to sample, but they are affected by the short-term fluctuations.

Primary aldosteronism can be diagnosed by demonstrating very little or no rise in serum renin levels during an *aldosterone stimulation test* (using salt restriction as the stimulant). This is because aldosterone is already maximally secreted by the pathologic adrenal gland. Failure to suppress aldosterone with saline infusion (1.5 to 2 L of NSS infused between 8 AM and 10 AM) *(aldosterone suppression test)* is further evidence of primary aldosteronism. Aldosterone can also be measured in blood obtained from adrenal venous sampling.

Interfering factors

- Strenuous exercise and stress can stimulate adrenocortical secretions and increase aldosterone levels.
- Excessive licorice ingestion can cause decreased levels because it produces an "aldosterone-like" effect.
- Values are influenced by posture, diet, diurnal variation, and pregnancy.
- Position can significantly affect aldosterone levels.
- Because the test is usually performed using radioimmunoassay, recently administered radioactive medications will affect test results.
- Drugs that may cause *increased* levels include diazoxide (Hyperstat), hydralazine (Apresoline), nitroprusside (Nipride), diuretics, laxatives, potassium, and spironolactone.
- Drugs that may cause *decreased* levels include fludrocortisone (Florinef), propranolol (Inderal), and angiotensin-converting inhibitor (e.g., captopril), as well as licorice.

Procedure and patient care

Before

PT Explain the procedure for the blood collection to the patient.
PT Note that the patient is asked to be in the upright position (at least sitting) for at least 2 hours before the blood is drawn.

PT Tell the patient that no fasting is necessary.

PT Explain the procedure for collecting a 24-hour urine sample if urinary aldosterone is ordered.

PT Give the patient verbal and written instructions regarding dietary and medication restrictions.

PT Instruct the patient to maintain a normal sodium diet (approximately 3 g/day) for at least 2 weeks before the blood or urine collection.

PT Have the patient ask the physician whether drugs that alter sodium, potassium, and fluid balance (e.g., diuretics, antihypertensives, steroids, oral contraceptives) should be withheld. Test results will be more accurate if these are suspended at least 2 weeks before either the blood or the urine test.

PT Inform the patient that renin inhibitors (e.g., propranolol) should not be taken 1 week before the test.

PT Tell the patient to avoid licorice for at least 2 weeks before the test because of its aldosterone-like effect.

During blood collection

- Collect approximately 5 to 10 ml of venous blood in a gold-top (serum separator) tube.
- Occasionally, for hospitalized patients, draw the sample with the patient in the supine position *before* he or she arises.
- Obtain the specimen in the morning.
- Note that sometimes a second specimen (upright sample) is collected 4 hours later, after the patient has been up and moving.
- Indicate on the laboratory slip if the patient was supine or standing during the venipuncture.
- Handle the blood specimen gently. Rough handling may cause hemolysis and alter the test results.
- Transport the specimen on ice to the laboratory.
- List on the laboratory slip any medications that can affect test results.

During urine collection

PT Instruct the patient to begin the 24-hour urine collection after urinating.

- Discard this specimen and note this time as the start of the 24-hour collection.
- Collect all the urine passed over the next 24 hours.

PT Instruct the patient to void before defecating so that the urine is not contaminated by feces.

PT Remind the patient not to put toilet paper in the collection container.

- Use a preservative with this 24-hour specimen.
- Keep the urine specimen on ice or refrigerated during the 24 hours.

PT Instruct the patient to collect the last specimen as close as possible to the end of the 24 hours. Add this urine to the container.

After blood collection

- Apply pressure to the venipuncture site.

After urine collection

- Transport the urine specimen promptly to the laboratory.

Abnormal findings

▲ **Increased levels**

Primary aldosteronism
Aldosterone-producing
   adrenal adenoma
   (Conn's disease)
Adrenal cortical nodular
   hyperplasia
Bartter's syndrome

Secondary aldosteronism
Hyponatremia
Hyperkalemia
Diuretic ingestion resulting
   in hypovolemia and
   hyponatremia
Laxative abuse
Stress
Malignant hypertension
Generalized edema
Renal arterial stenosis
Pregnancy
Oral contraceptives
Hypovolemia or
   hemorrhage
Cushing's syndrome

▼ **Decreased levels**

Aldosterone deficiency
Renin deficiency
Steroid therapy
Addison's disease
Patients on a
   high-sodium diet
Hypernatremia
Hypokalemia
Toxemia of pregnancy
Antihypertensive
   therapy

alkaline phosphatase (ALP)

Type of test Blood

Normal findings

Adult: 30-120 units/L or 0.5-2.0 μKat/L
Elderly: slightly higher than adults
Child/adolescent
  <2 years: 85-235 units/L
  2-8 years: 65-210 units/L
  9-15 years: 60-300 units/L
  16-21 years: 30-200 units/L

Test explanation and related physiology

Although ALP is found in many tissues, the highest concentrations are found in the liver, biliary tract epithelium, and bone. The intestinal mucosa and placenta also contain ALP. Detection of this enzyme is important for determining liver and bone disorders. Within the liver, ALP is present in Kupffer's cells. These cells line the biliary collecting system. This enzyme is excreted into the bile. Enzyme levels of ALP are greatly increased in both extrahepatic and intrahepatic obstructive biliary disease and cirrhosis. Other liver abnormalities, such as hepatic tumors, hepatotoxic drugs, and hepatitis, cause lesser elevations in ALP levels. Reports have indicated that the most sensitive test to indicate metastatic tumor to the liver is ALP.

Bone is the most frequent extrahepatic source of ALP; new bone growth is associated with elevated ALP levels, which explains why ALP levels are high in adolescents. Pathologic new bone growth occurs with osteoblastic metastatic (e.g., breast, prostate) tumors. Paget's disease, healing fractures, rheumatoid arthritis, hyperparathyroidism, and normal-growing bones are sources of elevated ALP levels as well.

Isoenzymes of ALP are sometimes used to distinguish between liver and bone diseases. The detection of isoenzymes can help differentiate the source of the pathology associated with the elevated total ALP. ALP_1 is from the liver. ALP_2 is from the bone.

Interfering factors

- Recent ingestion of a meal can increase ALP levels.
- Drugs that may cause *elevated* ALP levels include albumin made from placental tissue, allopurinol, antibiotics, azathioprine, colchicine, fluorides, indomethacin, isoniazid (INH),

methotrexate, methyldopa, nicotinic acid, phenothiazine, probenecid, tetracyclines, and verapamil.
▮ Drugs that may cause *decreased* levels include arsenicals, cyanides, fluorides, nitrofurantoin, oxalates, and zinc salts.

Procedure and patient care

Before
PT Explain the procedure to the patient.
PT Tell the patient that no fasting is usually required. Overnight fasting may be required for isoenzymes.

During
▪ Collect approximately 7 to 10 ml of blood in a red-top tube.

After
▪ Apply pressure to the venipuncture site. Patients with liver dysfunction often have prolonged clotting times.

Abnormal findings

▲ Increased levels	▼ Decreased levels
Cirrhosis	Hypothyroidism
Intrahepatic or extrahepatic biliary obstruction	Malnutrition
Primary or metastatic liver tumor	Milk-alkali syndrome
	Pernicious anemia
Normal pregnancy (third trimester, early postpartum)	Hypophosphatemia
Intestinal ischemia or infarction	Scurvy (vitamin C deficiency)
Metastatic tumor to the bone	Celiac disease
Healing fracture	Excess vitamin B ingestion
Hyperparathyroidism	
Paget's disease	
Rheumatoid arthritis	
Sarcoidosis	
Normal bones of growing children	

notes

allergy blood testing (IgE antibody test, Radioallergosorbent test [RAST])

Type of test Blood

Normal findings

Total IgE serum

Adult: 0-100 international units/ml

Child

    0-23 months: 0-13 international units/ml

    2-5 years: 0-56 international units/ml

    6-10 years: 0-85 international units/ml

Test explanation and related physiology

Measurement of serum immunoglobulin E (IgE) is an effective method by which to diagnose allergy and to specifically identify the allergen (the substance to which the person is allergic). Patients who have an allergy increase their serum IgE when exposed to the allergen. Various classes of allergens can initiate the allergic response. They include animal dander, foods, pollens, dusts, molds, insect venoms, drugs, and agents in the occupational environment.

Although skin testing (see p. 41) can also identify a specific allergen, measurement of serum levels of IgE is helpful when a skin test result is questionable, when the allergen is not available in a form for dermal injection, or when the allergen may incite an anaphylactic reaction if injected. IgE is particularly helpful in cases in which skin testing is difficult (e.g., in infants, or in patients with dermatographism or widespread dermatitis). However, it is important to note that an assay for IgE is expensive and the results are not available immediately. The decision concerning which method to use to diagnose an allergy and to identify the allergen depends on the elapsed time between exposure to an allergen and testing, class of allergen, age of patient, the possibility of anaphylaxis, and the affected target organ (skin, lungs, intestine, etc.)

IgE levels, like provocative skin testing, are used both to diagnose allergy and identify the allergen so that an immunotherapeutic regimen can be developed. In most patients, the treatment would include avoidance of the allergen and use of bronchodilators, antihistamines and, possibly, steroids. If aggressive antiallergy treatment is provided before testing, IgE levels may not rise despite the existence of an allergy.

Allergy to latex-containing products is increasingly common and certain industrial and most medical personnel are at risk. Latex allergy may develop in otherwise nonallergic patients because of overexposure. Furthermore, patients with latex exposure are at risk for allergic reaction if they undergo operative procedures or any procedure for which the health care personnel wear latex gloves. In these patients, a latex-specific IgE can be easily identified with the use of an enzyme-labeled immunometric assay. This test is 94% accurate.

There are many methods of measuring IgE. Among the most commonly used methods is the radioallergosorbent test (RAST). In this method, the serum of a patient suspected of having a specific allergy is mixed with a specific allergen. The antibody-allergen complex is then incubated with one or more radiolabeled monoclonal anti-IgE antibodies. The total amount of IgE can be measured.

Contraindications

- Patients with multiple allergies, because no information will be obtained regarding identification of the specific allergen

Interfering factors

- Concurrent diseases associated with elevated IgG levels will cause false-negative results.
- ✠ Drugs that may cause *increased* IgE levels include corticosteroids.

Procedure and patient care

Before

PT Explain the procedure to the patient.

PT Remind the patient that the suspected allergen will be mixed with the patient's blood specimen in the laboratory. The patient will not experience any allergic reaction by this method of testing.

- Determine if the patient has recently been treated with a corticosteroid for allergies.

During

- Collect 5 to 7 ml of venous blood in a serum tube (gold-top).

After

- Apply pressure to the venipuncture site.

Abnormal findings

Allergy-related diseases
Asthma
Dermatitis
Food allergy
Drug allergy
Occupational allergy
Allergic rhinitis
Angioedema

notes

allergy skin testing

Type of test Skin

Normal findings

<3 mm wheal diameter

<10 mm flare diameter

Test explanation and related physiology

When properly performed, skin testing is the most convenient and least expensive test for detecting allergic reactions. Since the early 1900s, skin testing has been a common practice for establishing a diagnosis by reexposure of the individual to a specific allergen. Skin testing provides useful confirmatory evidence when a diagnosis of allergy is suspected on clinical grounds. The simplicity, rapidity, low costs, sensitivity, and specificity explain the crucial position skin testing has in allergy testing.

In an allergic patient, an immediate wheal (swelling) and flare (redness) reaction follows injection of the specific allergen (that substance to which the person is allergic). This reaction is initiated by IgE and is mediated primarily by histamine secreted from mast cells. This usually occurs in about 5 minutes and peaks at 30 minutes. In some patients a "late phase reaction" occurs, which is highlighted by antibody and cellular infiltration into the area. This usually occurs within 1 to 2 hours.

There are two commonly accepted methods of injecting the allergen into the skin. The first method is called the *prick-puncture test*. In this method, the allergen is injected into the epidermis. Anaphylaxis reactions have not been reported with this method. The second method is called the *intradermal test*. Here the allergen is injected into the dermis (skin wheal). Large local reactions and anaphylaxis have been reported.

Patients with dermographism develop a skin wheal with any nonallergic skin irritation. In these patients, a false-positive reaction can occur with skin testing. To eliminate false positives, a "negative control" substance consisting of just the diluent without an allergen is injected at the same time as the other skin tests are performed. Likewise, patients who are immunosuppressed because of concurrent disease or medicines may have a blunted skin reaction even in the face of allergy. This would cause false-negative results. To avoid false negatives, a "positive control" substance consisting of a histamine analogue is injected into the forearm at the time of skin testing. This will cause a wheal and flare response even in the nonallergic patient, unless the patient is immunosuppressed.

For inhalant allergens, skin tests are extremely accurate. However, for food allergies, latex allergies, drug sensitivity, and occupational allergies, skin tests are less reliable. There is considerable variability in accuracy of skin testing because of poor injection techniques; however, when performed correctly, skin testing is a major tool in the diagnosis of allergy.

Contraindications

- Patients with a history of prior anaphylaxis

Potential complications

- Anaphylaxis

Interfering factors

- False-positive results may occur in patients with dermographism.
- False-positive results may occur if the patient has a reaction to the diluent used to preserve the extract.
- False-negative results may be caused by poor-quality allergen extracts, diseases that attenuate the immune response, or improper technique.
- Infants and the elderly may have decreased skin reactivity.
- ✗ Drugs that may *decrease* the immune response of skin testing include corticosteroids, theophylline, beta-blockers, ACE inhibitors, and nifedipine.

Procedure and patient care

Before
PT Explain the procedure to the patient.
- Observe skin testing precautions.
  1. Be sure that a physician is immediately available.
  2. Evaluate the patient for dermographism.
  3. Have medications and equipment available to handle anaphylaxis.
  4. Proceed with caution in patients with current allergic symptoms.
  5. Render great detail to the technique chosen for the skin test.
  6. Avoid bleeding due to injection.
  7. Avoid spreading of allergen solutions during the test.
  8. Record the skin reaction at the proper time.

- Obtain a history to evaluate the risk of anaphylaxis.
- Identify any immunosuppressive medications the patient may be taking.
- Evaluate the patient for dermographism by rubbing the skin with a pencil eraser and looking for a wheal at the site of irritation.
- Draw up 0.05 ml of 1:1000 aqueous epinephrine into a syringe before testing in the event of an exaggerated allergic reaction.
- A negative prick-puncture test should be performed prior to an intradermal test.

During

Prick-puncture method

- A drop of the allergen solution is placed onto the volar surface of the forearm or back.
- A 25-gauge needle is passed through the droplet and inserted into the epidermal space at an angle with the bevel facing up.
- The skin is lifted up and the fluid is allowed to seep in. Excess fluid is wiped off after about a minute.

Intradermal method

- With a 25-gauge needle, the allergen solution is injected into the dermis by creating a skin wheal. In this method, the bevel of the needle faces downward. A volume of between 0.01 and 0.05 ml is injected.
- In general, the allergen solution is diluted 100- to 1000-fold before injection.

After

- Evaluate the patient for exaggerated allergic response.
- In the event of a systemic reaction, a tourniquet should be placed above the testing site and epinephrine should be administered subcutaneously.
- With a pen, encircle the area of testing and mark the allergen used.
- Read the skin test at the appropriate time.
- Skin tests are read when the reaction is mature, after about 15 to 20 minutes. Both the largest and smallest diameter of the wheal are determined. The measurements (in millimeters) are averaged.
- The flare is measured in the same manner.
- The patient should be observed for 20 to 30 minutes prior to discharge.

Abnormal findings

Allergy-related diseases
Asthma
Dermatitis
Food allergy
Drug allergy
Occupational allergy
Allergic rhinitis
Angioedema

notes

alpha$_1$-antitrypsin (A1AT, AAT, alpha$_1$-antitrypsin phenotyping)

A

Type of test Blood

Normal findings 85-213 mg/dl or 0.85-2.13 g/L (SI units)

Test explanation and related physiology

Serum alpha$_1$-antitrypsin (α_1-antitrypsin) determinations should be obtained when an individual has a family history of emphysema, because a familial tendency to have a deficiency of this antienzyme exists. Deficient or absent serum levels of this enzyme are found in some patients with early onset of emphysema. These people usually develop severe, disabling emphysema. A similar deficiency is seen in children with cirrhosis and other liver diseases. AAT is also an acute-phase reactant that is elevated in the face of inflammation, infection, or malignancy. It is not specific as to the source of the inflammatory process.

Deficiencies of AAT can be genetic or acquired. Acquired deficiencies of AAT can occur in patients with protein deficiency syndromes (such as malnutrition, liver disease, nephrotic syndrome, and neonatal respiratory distress syndrome). People with AAT deficiency develop severe panacinar emphysema, although it is usually more severe in the lower third of the lungs in the third or fourth decade of life.

Routine serum protein electrophoresis (see p. 758) is a good screening test for AAT deficiency because AAT accounts for about 90% of the protein in the alpha$_1$-globulin region.

Inherited AAT deficiency is associated with symptoms earlier in life than acquired AAT deficiency. Inherited AAT is also commonly associated with liver and biliary disease. Individuals of the heterozygous state have diminished or low normal serum levels of alpha$_1$-antitrypsin. Approximately 5% to 14% of the adult population are in the heterozygous state and are considered to be at increased risk for the development of emphysema. Homozygous individuals have severe pulmonary and liver disease very early in life. AAT phenotyping is particularly helpful when blood AAT levels are suggestive but not definitive.

Interfering factors

- Serum levels of alpha$_1$-antitrypsin increase during pregnancy.
- Drugs that may cause *increased* levels include oral contraceptives.

Procedure and patient care

Before

PT Explain the procedure to the patient.

- Note that no fasting is usually required. Verify this with the laboratory performing the study.

During

- Collect approximately 5 to 10 ml of blood.

After

- Apply pressure to the venipuncture site.
- **PT** If the results show the patient is at risk for developing emphysema, begin patient teaching. Include such factors as avoidance of smoking, infection, and inhaled irritants; proper nutrition; adequate hydration; and education about the disease process of emphysema.

Abnormal findings

▲ **Increased levels**

Acute inflammatory disorders

Chronic inflammatory disorders

Stress

Infection

Thyroid infections

▼ **Decreased levels**

Early onset of emphysema (in adults)

Neonatal respiratory distress syndrome

Cirrhosis (in children)

Low serum proteins (e.g., nephrotic syndrome, malnutrition, end-stage cancer, protein-losing enteropathy)

notes

alpha-fetoprotein (AFP, α_1-Fetoprotein)

Type of test Blood

Normal findings

Adult: <40 ng/ml or <40 mcg/L (SI units)
Child (<1 year): <30 ng/ml
(Ranges are stratified by weeks of gestation and vary according to laboratory.)

Test explanation and related physiology

AFP is an oncofetal protein normally produced by the fetal liver and yolk sac. It is the dominant fetal serum protein in the first trimester of life and diminishes to very low levels by the age of 1 year. Increased serum levels of AFP are found in as many as 90% of patients with hepatomas. The higher the AFP level, the greater the tumor burden. A decrease in AFP would be seen if the patient were experiencing a response to antineoplastic therapy. AFP is not specific for hepatomas, although extremely high levels (above 500 ng/ml) are diagnostic for hepatoma. Other neoplastic conditions such as nonseminomatous germ cell tumors and teratomas of the testes, yolk sac and germ cell tumors of the ovaries, and, to a lesser extent, Hodgkin's disease, lymphoma, and renal cell carcinoma are also associated with elevated AFP levels. Noncancerous causes of elevated AFP levels occur in patients with cirrhosis or chronic active hepatitis.

AFP is also helpful in the diagnosis of fetal body wall defects. The most notable of these is neural tube defects (NTDs), which can vary from a small myelomeningocele to anencephaly. Although not widely used in United States, AFP can be used for widespread screening for NTDs.

Other examples of fetal body wall defects would include omphalocele and gastroschisis. Elevated serum AFP levels in pregnancy may also indicate multiple pregnancy, fetal distress, fetal congenital abnormalities, or intrauterine death. Low AFP levels after correction as to age of gestation, maternal weight, race, and presence of diabetes are found in mothers carrying offspring with trisomy 21 (Down syndrome).

Another test used to identify potential birth defects is the *maternal triple screen* test. It has become the standard of care to offer the maternal triple screen test to all pregnant women in their second trimester. This test includes serum AFP, human chorionic gonadotropin (see p. 740), and estriol (see p. 414). This test can indicate the chances that the child will be born with Down syndrome, neural tube defect, or anencephaly. Nearly 70% of women older than age 35 currently choose to be tested. Patients must understand that this test is for screening, and is not diagnostic. If the test results are abnormal, the test should be repeated. If the results are still abnormal and the age of the fetus is accurate, more specific tests such as amniocentesis (see p. 54), chorionic villus sampling (CVS) (see p. 269), or obstetrical ultrasound (see p. 694) should be performed. Now, a "*quadruple test*" is suggested to be more accurate. The fourth measurement is serum *inhibin A*, a protein that is associated with Down syndrome.

Interfering factors

- Recent administration of radioisotopes can affect values.

Procedure and patient care

Before

PT Explain the procedure to the patient.
PT Tell the patient that no food or fluid restriction is required.
- If AFP is to be performed on amniotic fluid, follow the Procedure and Patient Care for amniocentesis; see p. 57.

During

- Collect approximately 7 to 10 ml of blood in a red-top tube.

After

- Apply pressure to the venipuncture site.
- Include the gestational age on the laboratory slip.

Abnormal findings

▲ **Increased maternal serum AFP levels**

Neural tube defects
(e.g., anencephaly,
encephalocele,
spina bifida,
myelomeningocele)
Abdominal wall defects
(e.g., gastroschisis or
omphalocele)
Multiple pregnancy
Threatened abortion

▼ **Decreased maternal AFP**

Trisomy 21 (Down
syndrome)
Fetal wastage

Fetal distress or
congenital anomalies
Fetal death

▲ **Increased nonmaternal
AFP**

Primary hepatocellular
cancer (hepatoma)
Germ cell or yolk sac
cancer of the ovary
Embryonal cell or germ
cell tumor of the testes
Other cancers (e.g.,
stomach, colon, lung,
breast, and lymphoma)
Liver cell necrosis (e.g.,
cirrhosis or hepatitis)

notes

amino acid profiles (amino acid screen)

Type of test Blood; urine

Normal findings

Normal values vary for different amino acids.

Levels of amino acids are generally higher in infants and children, compared with adults.

Normal values vary widely, and only extremely abnormal results are diagnostic without genetic corroboratory evidence.

Test explanation and related physiology

Amino acids are the "building blocks" of proteins, hormones, nucleic acids, and pigments. They can act as neurotransmitters, enzymes, and coenzymes. Diet must provide eight essential amino acids to the body. The body can make the others. Amino acids must be transported across the gut and renal tubular lining cells. Their metabolism is essential to the production of other amino acids, proteins, carbohydrates, and lipids. Amino acid levels also may be affected by defects in renal tubule or gastrointestinal transport of amino acids.

When there is a defect in the metabolism or transport of any these amino acids, excesses of their precursors—or deficiencies of their "end product" amino acid—are evident in the blood, urine, or both. Most of these defects in amino acid metabolism are genetic and are, therefore, inherited. More than 90 diseases are associated with abnormal amino acid function. Sequelae of these diseases may be minimal or catastrophic (mental retardation, growth retardation, and seizures).

Clinical manifestations of these diseases may be precluded if diagnosis is early, and appropriate dietary replacement of missing amino acids are provided. Usually, urine testing (see phenylketonuria [PKU] testing, p. 702) for specific amino acids is used to screen for some of these errors in amino acid metabolism and transport. Once a presumptive diagnosis is made, amino acid levels can be determined by chromatographic methods on blood or amniotic fluid. The genetic defects for many of these diseases are becoming more defined, allowing for even earlier diagnosis to be made in utero. Common examples of amino acid diseases include PKU, cystinosis, and cystic fibrosis.

Interfering factors

- The circadian rhythm affects amino acid levels. Levels are usually lowest in the morning and highest by midday.
- Pregnancy is associated with reduced levels of some amino acids.
- ✗ Drugs that may *increase* amino acids include steroids and bismuth.
- ✗ Drugs that may *decrease* some amino acid levels include estrogens and oral contraceptives.

Procedure and patient care

Before

- Obtain a history of the patient's symptoms.
- Obtain a pedigree highlighting family members with amino acid disorders.
- **PT** A 12-hour fast is generally required before blood collection. Occasionally, a particular protein or carbohydrate load is ordered to stimulate production of a particular amino acid metabolite.

During

- Collect 5 ml of blood in a red-top tube.
- Usually a 24-hour random urine specimen is required. Screening is done on a spot urine using the first voided specimen in the morning.

After

- Generally genetic counseling is provided before testing. However, acute anxiety by the patient or parents often requires emotional support immediately after obtaining a specimen.

Abnormal findings

▲ **Increased blood levels**

Specific aminoacidopathies (e.g., PKU, maple syrup disease)
Specific aminoacidemias (e.g., glutaric aciduria)

▲ **Increased urine levels**

Specific aminoacidurias (e.g., cystinuria, homocystinuria)

▼ **Decreased blood levels**

Hartnup disease
Nephritis
Nephrotic syndromes

ammonia level

Type of test Blood

Normal findings

Adult: 10-80 mcg/dl or 6-47 µmol/L (SI units)
Child: 40-80 mcg/dl
Newborn: 90-150 mcg/dl

Test explanation and related physiology

Ammonia is used to support the diagnosis of severe liver diseases (fulminant hepatitis or cirrhosis). Ammonia levels are also used in the diagnosis and follow-up of hepatic encephalopathy.

Ammonia is a by-product of protein catabolism. Most of the ammonia is made by bacteria acting on proteins present in the gut. By way of the portal vein, ammonia goes to the liver, where it is normally converted into urea and then secreted by the kidneys. With severe hepatocellular dysfunction, ammonia cannot be catabolized. Further, when portal blood flow to the liver is altered (e.g., in portal hypertension), ammonia cannot reach the liver to be catabolized. Ammonia levels in the blood rise. Congenital enzymatic defects in the urea cycle also can cause a rise in ammonia levels. Finally, impaired renal function diminishes excretion of ammonia, and blood levels rise. High levels of ammonia are often associated with encephalopathy and coma. Arterial ammonia levels are more reliable than venous levels but are more difficult to obtain and not routinely used.

Interfering factors

- Hemolysis increases ammonia levels because the RBCs contain about three times the ammonia content of plasma.
- Muscular exertion can increase ammonia.
- Cigarette smoking can produce significant increases in ammonia levels.
- Ammonia levels may be falsely increased if the tourniquet is too tight for too long.
- Drugs that may cause *increased* ammonia levels include acetazolamide, alcohol, ammonium chloride, barbiturates, narcotics, parenteral nutrition, and diuretics (loop, thiazide).
- Drugs that may cause *decreased* levels include broad-spectrum antibiotics (e.g., neomycin), lactulose, levodopa, lactobacillus, and potassium salts.

Procedure and patient care

Before

PT Explain the procedure to the patient.
- Note that usually, no fasting is required.

During
- Collect approximately 5 to 7 ml of blood in a green-top tube. Note that some institutions require that the specimen be sent to the laboratory in an iced container.
- List on the laboratory slip any drugs that can affect test results.
- Avoid hemolysis and send the specimen promptly to the laboratory.

After
- Apply pressure to the venipuncture site. Many patients with liver disease have prolonged clotting times.

Abnormal findings

▲ **Increased levels**

Primary hepatocellular disease

Reye's syndrome

Asparagine intoxication

Portal hypertension

Severe heart failure with congestive hepatomegaly

Hemolytic disease of the newborn (erythroblastosis fetalis)

Gastrointestinal bleeding with mild liver disease

Gastrointestinal obstruction with mild liver disease

Hepatic encephalopathy and hepatic coma

Genetic metabolic disorder of the urea cycle

▼ **Decreased levels**

Essential or malignant hypertension

Hyperornithinemia

notes

amniocentesis (Amniotic fluid analysis)

Type of test Fluid analysis

Normal findings

Amniotic fluid volume (ml)	Weeks' gestation
450	15
750	25
1500	30-35
<1500	Full term

Amniotic fluid appearance: clear; pale to straw yellow
L/S ratio: ≥2:1
Bilirubin: <0.2 mg/dl
No chromosomal or genetic abnormalities
Phosphatidylglycerol (PG): positive for PG
Lamellar body count: >30,000
Alpha-fetoprotein: 2 mcg/ml

Test explanation and related physiology

Amniocentesis is performed on women to gather information about the fetus. The following can be evaluated by studying the amniotic fluid:

1. *Fetal maturity status*, especially pulmonary maturity (when early delivery is preferred). Fetal maturity is determined by analysis of the amniotic fluid in the following manner:

   a. *Lecithin/sphingomyelin (L/S) ratio.* The L/S ratio is a measure of fetal lung maturity, which is determined by measuring the phospholipids in amniotic fluid. Lecithin is the major constituent of surfactant, an important substance required for alveolar ventilation. If surfactant is insufficient, the alveoli collapse during expiration. This may result in respiratory distress syndrome (RDS), which is a major cause of death in immature babies. In immature fetal lungs, the sphingomyelin concentration in amniotic fluid is higher than the lecithin concentration. At 35 weeks of gestation, the concentration of lecithin rapidly increases, whereas sphingomyelin concentration decreases. An L/S ratio of 2:1 (3:1 in mothers with diabetes) or greater is a highly reliable indication that the fetal lungs and, therefore, the fetus are mature. In such a case, the infant would be unlikely to develop RDS after birth. As the L/S ratio decreases, the risk of RDS increases.

b. *Phosphatidylglycerol (PG)*. This is a minor component (about 10%) of lung surfactant phospholipids. However, since PG is almost entirely synthesized by mature lung alveolar cells, it is a good indicator of lung maturity. In healthy pregnant women, PG appears in amniotic fluid after 35 weeks of gestation, and levels gradually increase until term. The simultaneous determination of the L/S ratio and the presence of PG is an excellent method of assessing fetal maturity based on pulmonary surfactant.

c. *Lamellar body count.* This test to determine fetal maturity is also based on the presence of surfactant. These lamellar bodies represent the storage form of pulmonary surfactant. Lamellar body results are calculated in units of particle density per microliter of amniotic fluid. Some researchers have recommended cutoffs of 30,000/µl and 10,000/µl to predict low and high risk for RDS, respectively. If the count is greater than 30,000, there is 100% chance that the infant's lungs are mature enough to not experience RDS. If the lamellar body count is less than 10,000, the probability of RDS is high (67%). Values between 10,000 and 30,000/µl represent intermediate risk for RDS.

2. *Sex of the fetus.* Sons of mothers who are known to be carriers of X-linked recessive traits would have a 50:50 chance of inheritance.

3. *Genetic and chromosomal aberrations.* Genetic and chromosomal studies performed on cells aspirated within the amniotic fluid can indicate the gender of the fetus (important in sex-linked diseases such as hemophilia) or any of the described genetic and chromosomal aberrations (e.g., trisomy 21).

4. *Fetal status affected by Rh isoimmunization.* Mothers with Rh isoimmunization may have a series of amniocentesis procedures during the second half of pregnancy to assess the level of bilirubin pigment in the amniotic fluid. The quantity of bilirubin is used to assess the severity of hemolysis in Rh-sensitized pregnancy. Amniocentesis is usually initiated at 24 to 25 weeks when hemolysis is suspected.

5. *Hereditary metabolic disorders* such as cystic fibrosis.

6. *Anatomic abnormalities* such as neural tube closure defects (myelomeningocele, anencephaly, spina bifida). Increased levels of alpha-fetoprotein (AFP) in the amniotic fluid may indicate a neural crest abnormality (see p. 47).

Decreased AFP may be associated with increased risk of trisomy 21.

7. *Fetal distress*, detected by meconium staining of the amniotic fluid. This is caused by relaxation of the anal sphincter. In this case, the normally colorless and pale, straw-colored amniotic fluid may be tinged with green. Other color changes may also indicate fetal distress. For example, a yellow discoloration may indicate a blood incompatibility. A yellow-brown opaque appearance may indicate intrauterine death. A red color indicates blood contamination either from the mother or the fetus.

The timing of the amniocentesis varies according to the clinical circumstances. With advanced maternal age and if chromosomal or genetic aberrations are suspected, the test should be done early enough (at 14 to 16 weeks of gestation; at least 150 ml of fluid exists at this time) to allow a safe abortion. If information on fetal maturity is sought, performing the study during or after the 35th week of gestation is best.

Contraindications

- Patients with abruptio placentae
- Patients with placenta previa
- Patients with a history of premature labor (before 34 weeks of gestation, unless the patient is receiving antilabor medication)
- Patients with an incompetent cervix

Potential complications

- Miscarriage
- Fetal injury
- Leak of amniotic fluid
- Infection (amnionitis)
- Abortion
- Premature labor
- Maternal hemorrhage with possible maternal Rh isoimmunization
- Amniotic fluid embolism
- Abruptio placentae
- Inadvertent damage to the bladder or intestines

Interfering factors

- Fetal blood contamination can cause falsely elevated AFP levels.

A

- Hemolysis of the specimen can alter results.
- Contamination of the specimen with meconium or blood may give inaccurate L/S ratios.

Procedure and patient care

Before

PT Explain the procedure to the patient. Allay any fears and allow the patient to verbalize her concerns.

- Obtain an informed consent from the patient and her spouse.

PT Tell the patient that no food or fluid is restricted.

- Evaluate the mother's blood pressure and the fetal heart rate.
- Follow instructions regarding emptying the bladder, which depend on gestational age. Before 20 weeks of gestation, the bladder may be kept full to support the uterus. After 20 weeks, the bladder may be emptied to minimize the chance of puncture.
- Note that the placenta is localized before the study by ultrasound to permit selection of a site that will avoid placental puncture.

During

- Place the patient in the supine position.
- Note the following procedural steps:
  1. The skin overlying the chosen site is prepared and usually anesthetized locally.
  2. A long needle with a stylet is inserted through the midabdominal wall and directed at an angle toward the middle of the uterine cavity (Figure 2).
  3. The stylet is then removed, and a sterile plastic syringe attached.
  4. After 5 to 10 ml of amniotic fluid is withdrawn, the needle is removed.
  5. The specimen is placed in a light-resistant container to prevent breakdown of bilirubin.
  6. The site is covered with an adhesive bandage.
  7. If the amniotic fluid is bloody, the physician must determine whether the blood is maternal or fetal in origin. Kleinhauer-Boetke stain will stain fetal cells pink. Meconium in the fluid is usually associated with a compromised fetus.
  8. *Amniotic fluid volume* is calculated.

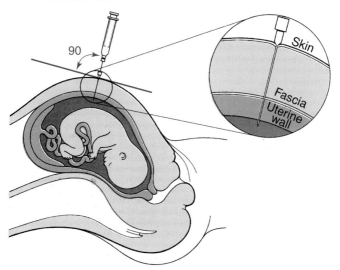

Figure 2 Amniocentesis. Ultrasound scanning is usually used to
determine the placental site and to locate a pocket of amniotic fluid.
The needle is then inserted. Three levels of resistance are felt as the
needle penetrates the skin, fascia, and uterine wall. When the needle is
placed within the uterine cavity, amniotic fluid is withdrawn.

- Note that this procedure takes approximately 20 to
  30 minutes.
- **PT** Tell the patient that the discomfort associated with amniocentesis is usually described as a mild uterine cramping that
  occurs when the needle contacts the uterus. Some women
  may complain of a "pulling" sensation as the amniotic fluid is
  withdrawn.
- Remember that many women are extremely anxious during
  this procedure.

After

- Place amniotic fluid in a sterile, siliconized glass container and
  transport it to a special chemistry laboratory for analysis.
  Sometimes the specimen may be sent by air mail to another
  commercial laboratory.

PT Inform the patient that the results of this study are usually not available for at least 2 weeks.

- For women who have Rh-negative blood, administer RhoGAM because of the risk of immunization from the fetal blood.

- Assess the fetal heart rate after the test to detect any ill effects related to the procedure. Compare this value with the preprocedure baseline value.

PT If the patient felt dizzy or nauseated during the procedure, instruct her to lie on her left side for several minutes before leaving the examining room.

- Observe the puncture site for bleeding or other drainage.

PT Instruct the patient to call her physician if she has any fluid loss, bleeding, temperature elevation, abdominal pain or cramping, fetal hyperactivity, or unusual fetal lethargy.

🏠 **Home care responsibilities**

- Instruct the patient to call her physician if she has any fluid loss, bleeding, temperature elevation, abdominal cramping, or unusual fetal movement.
- Inform the patient that the puncture site should be checked for bleeding and amniotic fluid loss.

Abnormal findings

Hemolytic disease of the newborn

Rh isoimmunization

Neural tube closure defects (e.g., myelomeningocele, anencephaly, spina bifida)

Abdominal wall closure defects (e.g., gastroschisis, omphalocele)

Sacrococcygeal teratoma

Meconium staining

Immature fetal lungs

Hereditary metabolic disorders (e.g., cystic fibrosis, Tay-Sachs disease, galactosemia)

Genetic or chromosomal aberrations (e.g., sickle cell anemia, thalassemia, Down syndrome)

Sex-linked disorders (e.g., hemophilia)

Polyhydramnios

Oligohydramnios

amylase

Type of test Blood; urine

Normal findings

Blood

60-120 Somogyi units/dl, or 30-220 units/L (SI units). Values may be slightly increased during normal pregnancy and in the elderly.

Urine (24-hour)

Up to 5000 Somogyi units/24 hr, or 6.5-48.1 units/hr (SI units)

Possible critical values Blood: More than three times the upper limit of normal (depending on the method)

Test explanation and related physiology

Serum amylase is an easily and rapidly performed test that is commonly used to diagnose and monitor the treatment of pancreatitis. Amylase is normally secreted from the pancreatic acinar cell into the pancreatic duct and then into the duodenum. Once in the intestine, it aids the catabolism of carbohydrates to their component simple sugars. Damage to acinar cells (as occurs in pancreatitis) or obstruction of the pancreatic duct flow (as a result of pancreatic carcinoma) causes an outpouring of this enzyme into the intrapancreatic lymph system and the free peritoneum. Blood vessels draining the free peritoneum and absorbing the lymph pick up the excess amylase. An abnormal rise in the serum level of amylase occurs within 12 hours of the onset of disease. Because amylase is rapidly cleared by the kidneys, serum levels return to normal 48 to 72 hours after the initial insult. Persistent pancreatitis, duct obstruction, or pancreatic duct leak (e.g., pseudocysts) will cause persistent elevated serum amylase levels.

Although serum amylase is a sensitive test for pancreatic disorders, it is not specific. Other nonpancreatic diseases can cause elevated amylase levels in the serum. For example, in a bowel perforation, intraluminal amylase leaks into the free peritoneum and is picked up by the peritoneal blood vessels. This results in an elevated serum amylase level. Also, a penetrating peptic ulcer into the pancreas will cause elevated amylase levels. Duodenal obstruction can be associated with less significant elevations in amylase. Because salivary glands contain amylase, elevations can be expected in patients with parotiditis (mumps). Amylase is also found in low levels in the ovaries and skeletal muscles. Ectopic pregnancy and severe diabetic ketoacidosis are also associated with hyperamylasemia.

Patients with chronic pancreatic disorders (e.g., chronic pancreatitis) that have previously resulted in pancreatic cell destruction often do not have high amylase levels associated with the above disorders, because less amylase is made within the pancreas.

Urine amylase levels rise after the blood levels. Several days after the onset of the disease process, serum amylase levels may be normal, but urine amylase levels are significantly elevated. Urine amylase is particularly useful in detecting pancreatitis late in the disease course.

As with serum amylase, urine amylase is sensitive but not specific for pancreatic disorders. A comparison of the renal clearance ratio of amylase to creatinine provides more specific diagnostic information than either the urine amylase level or the serum amylase level alone. When the *amylase/creatinine clearance* ratio is 5% or more, the diagnosis of pancreatitis can be made with certainty. With ratios less than 5% in a patient having elevated serum and urine amylase levels, nonpancreatic pathologic conditions should be suspected (e.g., perforated bowel, macroamylasemia).

Interfering factors

- IV dextrose solutions can cause a false-negative result.
- Serum lipemia falsely decreases amylase with the current laboratory methods.
- *Drugs that may cause *increased* serum amylase levels include* aminosalicylic acid, aspirin, azathioprine, corticosteroids, dexamethasone, ethyl alcohol, glucocorticoids, iodine-containing contrast media, loop diuretics (e.g., furosemide), methyldopa, narcotic analgesics, oral contraceptives, and prednisone.
- *Drugs that may cause *decreased* levels include* citrates, glucose, and oxalates.

Procedure and patient care

Before

PT Explain the procedure to the patient.
PT Tell the patient that no fasting is required.

During

Blood

- Collect 5 to 7 ml of venous blood in a red-top tube.
- Indicate on the laboratory slip any medications that may affect test results.

Urine

PT Instruct the patient to begin the 24-hour urine collection after urinating. Discard the initial specimen and start the 24-hour timing at that point.

- Collect all urine passed during the next 24 hours.
- A 2-hour spot urine can sometimes be sent instead of the 24-hour urine collection.

PT Show the patient where to store the urine specimen.

- Keep the specimen on ice or refrigerated during the collection period. No preservative is needed.
- Post the hours for urine collection in a prominent place to prevent accidental discarding of the specimen.

PT Instruct the patient to void before defecating so that urine is not contaminated by stool.

PT Remind the patient not to put toilet paper in the urine collection container.

PT Tell the patient to collect the last specimen as close as possible to the end of the collection period. Add this urine to the container.

- List on the laboratory slip any medications that may affect test results.

After

- Apply pressure to the venipuncture site.

Abnormal findings

▲   **Increased levels**

Acute pancreatitis
Penetrating peptic ulcer
Perforated peptic ulcer
Necrotic bowel
Perforated bowel
Acute cholecystitis
Parotiditis (mumps)
Ectopic pregnancy
Pulmonary infarction
Diabetic ketoacidosis
Chronic relapsing pancreatitis
Duodenal obstruction

A

amyloid beta protein precursor, soluble (sBPP)

Type of test Cerebrospinal fluid (CSF) analysis

Normal findings >450 units/L

Test explanation and related physiology

This test is performed on patients who become increasingly demented and confused and is used to diagnose Alzheimer's disease and other forms of senile dementia. Amyloid protein is a 42-amino-acid peptide that is broken off of a larger amyloid precursor protein (beta APP). These beta amyloid proteins have been shown to be neurotrophic and neuroprotective. For some unknown reason, beta amyloid is deposited on the brain in the form of plaques in patients with Alzheimer's. It has been discovered that these plaques contain damaged nerve cells in a compacted core of beta amyloid protein. As a result of this deposition, levels of beta amyloid are *decreased* in the cerebral spinal fluid of patients with Alzheimer's and other forms of dementia. Research has demonstrated the diagnostic potential of this biochemical marker for Alzheimer's. Further evidence of the importance of beta amyloid protein in Alzheimer's is found in patients with a genetic defect on chromosome 21. This gene normally encodes the synthesis of beta APP. In mutated forms of the gene, beta amyloid protein is low, and these patients experience familial Alzheimer's. This is a dominant genetic defect and is passed to 50% of the children.

Ongoing research has also focused on using CSF levels of *tau protein* as another biochemical marker for Alzheimer's. Neurofibrillary tangles, also noted in the brains of patients with Alzheimer's, are composed primarily of hyperphosphorylated tau. There is a consensus that CSF levels of tau are significantly *increased* in patients with Alzheimer's, as compared with healthy control subjects and patients with non-Alzheimer's neurologic disease.

Procedure and patient care

Before

PT Explain the procedure to the patient.

- Refer to the instructions for a lumbar puncture and CSF examination (see p. 602).

During
- Collect a CSF specimen as indicated in the lumbar puncture discussion.

After
- Follow the postprocedure guidelines after a lumbar puncture.

Abnormal findings

▼ **Decreased levels**
   Alzheimer's disease

notes

androstenediones (Androstenedione [AD], Dehydroepiandrosterone [DHEA], Dehydroepiandrosterone sulfate [DHEA S])

Type of test Blood

Normal findings

	Male	*Female*
AD	0.6-2.7 ng/ml	0.5-2.7 ng/ml
DHEA	1.0-9.5 ng/ml	0.4-3.7 ng/ml
DHEA S	280-640 mcg/dl	65-380 mcg/dl

Test explanation and related physiology

Androstenediones (ADs, DHEA, and its sulfuric ester, DHEA S) are precursors of testosterone and estrone and are made in the gonads and the adrenal gland. ACTH stimulates their adrenal secretion. The ADs are often elevated in cases of hirsutism and virilization. In the adult female, elevated levels of ADs can cause virilizing symptoms such as hirsutism, change in voice, and sterility. Children with congenital adrenal hyperplasia have enzyme defects in the synthesis of cortisol. ACTH secretion is stimulated by the lack of cortisol. As ACTH levels increase, production of ADs is stimulated, and levels increase. These hormones are converted into a relatively high level of testosterone by the peripheral tissues. In female children, pseudohermaphroditism results. In male children with similar congenital defects, precocious puberty will become obvious. This test is also used to assess delayed puberty.

Androstenedione and DHEA secretion is episodic and exhibits a diurnal variation similar to cortisol. DHEA S, on the other hand, does not show diurnal variation and is present in the serum at levels much higher than androstenedione or DHEA. Patients with polycystic ovary syndrome (Stein-Leventhal syndrome) have particularly elevated levels of androstenediones. DHEA S levels are particularly high in patients with adrenal carcinoma and to a lesser extent in patients with congenital adrenal hyperplasia and Cushing's disease. Patients with Cushing's syndrome caused by benign adrenal tumors, however, have normal androstenedione levels.

Interfering factors

- A radioactive scan performed 1 week before the test may invalidate the test results.
- ⚡ Drugs that may *increase* levels of androstenediones include corticotropin, clomiphene, and metyrapone.
- ⚡ Drugs that may *decrease* levels of androstenediones include steroids.

Procedure and patient care

Before

PT Explain the procedure to the patient.

PT Tell the female patient that the specimen should be collected 1 week before or after the menstrual period.

During

- Collect 6 ml of venous blood in a serum separator (gold) or red-top tube.
- Indicate the date of the last menstrual period (if applicable) on the laboratory form.

After

- Apply pressure to the venipuncture site.

Abnormal findings

▲ **Increased levels**

Adrenal tumor
Congenital adrenal
  hyperplasia
Ectopic ACTH-producing
  tumors
Cushing's syndrome
  (some cases)
Stein-Leventhal syndrome
Ovarian sex cord tumor

▼ **Decreased levels**

Gonadal failure
Primary or secondary
  adrenal insufficiency

notes

angiotensin-converting enzyme (ACE, Serum angiotensin-converting enzyme [SACE])

Type of test Blood

Normal findings <40 units/L or <670 nKat/L (SI units)

Test explanation and related physiology

ACE is used to detect and monitor the clinical course of sarcoidosis (a granulomatous disease that affects many organs, especially the lungs). Further, it is used to differentiate sarcoidosis from other granulomatous diseases. It is also used to differentiate between active and dormant sarcoid disease.

Elevated ACE levels are found in a high percentage of patients with sarcoidosis. This test is used primarily in patients with sarcoidosis to evaluate the severity of disease and the response to therapy. Levels are especially high with active pulmonary sarcoidosis and can be normal with inactive (dormant) sarcoidosis. Elevated ACE levels also occur in conditions other than sarcoidosis, including Gaucher's disease (a rare familial lysosomal disorder of fat metabolism), leprosy, alcoholic cirrhosis, active histoplasmosis, tuberculosis, Hodgkin's disease, myeloma, scleroderma, pulmonary embolism, and idiopathic pulmonary fibrosis.

Interfering factors

- Patients younger than 20 years of age normally have very high ACE levels.
- Hemolysis or hyperlipidemia may falsely decrease ACE levels.
- ☛ Drugs that may cause *decreased* ACE levels include ACE inhibitor antihypertensives and steroids.

Procedure and patient care

Before

PT Explain the procedure to the patient.

PT Tell the patient that no fasting is required.

During

- Collect approximately 5 ml of blood in a red-top tube.
- Note on the laboratory slip if the patient is taking steroids.

After

- Apply pressure to the venipuncture site.

Abnormal findings

▲   **Increased levels**

   Sarcoidosis
   Gaucher's disease
   Tuberculosis
   Leprosy
   Alcoholic cirrhosis
   Active histoplasmosis
   Hodgkin's disease
   Myeloma
   Idiopathic pulmonary fibrosis
   Diabetes mellitus
   Primary biliary cirrhosis
   Amyloidosis
   Hyperthyroidism
   Scleroderma
   Pulmonary embolism

notes

anion gap (AG, R factor)

Type of test Blood

Normal findings

16 ± 4 mEq/L (if potassium is used in the calculation)
12 ± 4 mEq/L (if potassium is not used in the calculation)
(Normal values of anion gap [AG] vary according to different
   normal values for electrolytes, depending on laboratory
   methods of measurement.)

Test explanation and related physiology

The AG is the difference between the cations and the anions in
the extracellular space that are routinely calculated in the laboratory (i.e., AG = [sodium + potassium] – [chloride + bicarbon-
ate]). In some laboratories, the potassium is not measured
because its level in acid/base abnormalities is so spurious. The
normal value is adjusted downward if potassium is eliminated
from the equation. The anion gap, although not real physiologically, is created by the small amounts of anions in the blood (such
as lactate, phosphates, sulfates, and proteins) that are not measured. Further, it is important to realize that the HCO_3 that is
measured is actually the venous CO_2, not the arterial HCO_3.

This calculation is most often helpful in identifying the cause of
metabolic acidosis. As acids such as lactic acid or ketoacids accumulate in the bloodstream, bicarbonate neutralizes them to maintain a normal pH within the blood. Mathematically, when
bicarbonate decreases, the AG increases. In general, most metabolic acidotic states (except Renal Tubular Acidosis) are associated
with an increased anion gap. The higher above normal the gap, the
more likely this will be the case. Most commonly, an increased AG
is more often the result of increased amounts of unmeasured
anions than of decreased amounts of unmeasured cations.

AG is also helpful in identifying the presence of a mixed acid base
situation. The arterial blood gasses do not always tell the story,
especially if there is a mixed metabolic acidosis and a concomitantly
occurring alkalosis. The AG increase will indicate the acidotic component. When combined with the ABGs and the electrolytes, these
complex clinical pictures can be more clearly elucidated. The AG
calculation is indicated when acid/base problems exist.

Proteins can have a significant effect on AG. For example, a
1 g/dl drop in serum protein is associated with a 2.5 mEq/L drop

in AG. Because the anion proteins are lost, the HCO_3 increases to maintain electrical neutrality. Except for hypoproteinemia, conditions that cause a reduced or negative anion gap are relatively rare compared with those associated with an elevated anion gap.

Interfering factors

☒ Drugs that *increase* AG are many. Examples include carbonic anhydrase inhibitors (e.g., acetazolamide), salicylate, ethanol, and methanol.

☒ Drugs that *decrease* AG are also many. Examples include lithium, acetazolamide, spironolactone, and sulindac.

Procedure and patient care

Before
PT Explain the procedure to the patient.
PT Tell the patient that neither food nor fluid is restricted.

During
- Collect 5 to 10 ml of venous blood in a red- or green-top tube.
- If the patient is receiving an IV infusion, obtain the blood from the opposite arm.
- List on the laboratory slip any drugs that may affect test results.

After
- The sodium, potassium, chloride, and bicarbonate levels are determined by an automated multichannel analyzer. The AG is then calculated as indicated in the test explanation section.
- Apply pressure to the venipuncture site.

Abnormal findings

▲ **Increased levels**
Lactic acidosis
Diabetic ketoacidosis
Alcoholic ketoacidosis
Starvation
Renal failure
Renal tubular acidosis
Increased gastrointestinal
   losses of bicarbonate
   (e.g., diarrhea or fistulae)
Hypoaldosteronism

▼ **Decreased levels**
Excess alkali ingestion
Multiple myeloma
Chronic vomiting or
   gastric suction
Hyperaldosteronism
Hypoproteinemia
Lithium toxicity
Bromide (cough syrup)
   toxicity

A

anticardiolipin antibodies (aCL antibodies, ACA)

Type of test Blood

Normal findings

Negative
> <23 GPL (IgG phospholipid units)
> <11 MPL (IgM phospholipid units)

Test explanation and related physiology

This test is positive in some patients with systemic lupus erythematosus (SLE). *Antiphospholipid antibodies* include *anticardiolipin antibodies* and the *"lupus anticoagulant."* Anticardiolipin antibodies (immunoglobulins G and M to cardiolipin) are found in approximately 40% of patients with SLE. SLE patients who are positive for anticardiolipin antibodies and the lupus anticoagulant are at higher risk for the development of the "antiphospholipid antibody syndrome." The clinical features include venous and arterial thrombosis, neuropsychiatric disorders, recurrent spontaneous abortion, and thrombocytopenia. Both antibodies may be found in drug-induced lupus, in nonautoimmune diseases (e.g., syphilis and acute infection), and in the normal elderly person.

Interfering factors

- Patients who have or had syphilis infections can have a false positive.
- Transient presence of these antibodies can occur in patients with infections, AIDS, inflammation, autoimmune diseases, or cancer.
- False-*positive* results have been seen in patients who take medications such as chlorpromazine, procainamide, dilantin, penicillin, hydralazine, and quinidine.

Procedure and patient care

Before
- **PT** Explain the procedure to the patient.
- **PT** Tell the patient that no fasting is required.

During
- Collect a venous blood sample according to the laboratory protocol.

After

- Apply pressure to the venipuncture site.

Abnormal findings

▲   **Increased levels**

Systemic lupus erythematosus
Thrombosis
Thrombocytopenia
Recurrent fetal loss
Syphilis
Acute infection
Elderly persons

notes

anticentromere antibody test (Centromere antibody)

Type of test Blood

Normal findings

Negative (if positive, serum will be titrated)

Weak positive: positive at the screening titer (1:40 for HEp-2 cells) (1:20 for kidney cells)

Moderately positive: one dilution above screening titer

Strong positive: two dilutions above screening titer

Test explanation and related physiology

A centromere is the region of the chromosome referred to as the "primary constriction" that divides the chromosome into "arms." During cell division, the centromere exists in the "pole" of the mitotic spindle.

Anticentromere antibodies are a form of *antinuclear antibodies*. They are found in a very high percentage of patients with CREST syndrome, a variant of scleroderma. CREST is characterized by calcinosis, Raynaud's phenomenon, esophageal dysfunction, sclerodactyly, and telangiectasia. Anticentromere antibodies, on the contrary, are present in only a small minority of patients with scleroderma, a disease that is difficult to differentiate from CREST. No correlation exists between antibody titer and severity of CREST disease.

Procedure and patient care

Before

PT Explain the procedure to the patient.

PT Tell the patient that no fasting is usually required.

During

- Collect one red-top tube of venous blood.

After

- Apply pressure to the venipuncture site.

Abnormal findings

Positive

CREST syndrome

antideoxyribonuclease-B titer (Anti-DNase-B [ADB], ADNase-B)

Type of test Blood

Normal findings

Adult: ≤85 Todd units/ml
Preschool: ≤60 Todd units/ml
School age: ≤170 Todd units/ml

Test explanation and related physiology

Like the antistreptolysin O titer (ASO titer) test (see p. 102), this immunologic test also detects antibodies directed against antigens produced by group A streptococci and is elevated in most patients with acute rheumatic fever (ARF) or poststreptococcal glomerulonephritis. This test is often run concurrently with the ASO titer; subsequent testing is usually performed to detect differences between the acute and convalescent blood samples. A rise in the titer of two or more dilution increments between acute and convalescent sera is significant and indicates that a streptococcal infection has occurred. The American Heart Association does not recommend performance of this test alone in the evaluation of patients with ARF. It may be more sensitive than the ASO titer, but its results are too variable. ASO titer is the recommended test, but when the two are done together, the results are better than either test alone.

Procedure and patient care

Before
PT Explain the procedure to the patient.
PT Inform the patient that no fasting is required.

During
■ Collect one red-top tube of venous blood.

After
■ Apply pressure to the venipuncture site.

Abnormal findings

▲ Increased levels

Acute rheumatic fever
Poststreptococcal glomerulonephritis

antidiuretic hormone (ADH, Vasopressin)

Type of test Blood

Normal findings

ADH: 1-5 pg/ml or <1.5 ng/L (SI units)

ADH suppression test (water load test):

    65% of water load excreted in 4 hours

    80% of water load excreted in 5 hours

    Urine osmolality (in second hour) ≤100 mmol/kg

    Urine to serum (U/S) osmolality ratio >100

    Urine specific gravity <1.003

Test explanation and related physiology

ADH, also known as *vasopressin*, is formed by the hypothalamus and stored in the posterior pituitary gland. It controls the amount of water resorbed by the kidney. ADH release is stimulated by an increase in serum osmolality or a decrease in intravascular blood volume. Physical stress, surgery, and even high levels of anxiety may also stimulate ADH release. With a release of ADH, more water is resorbed from the kidney. This increases the amount of free water within the bloodstream and causes a very concentrated urine. With low ADH levels, water is allowed to be excreted, thereby producing hemoconcentration and a more dilute urine.

Diabetes insipidus (DI) results when ADH secretion is inadequate or when the kidney is unresponsive to ADH stimulation. Inadequate ADH secretion is usually associated with central neurologic abnormalities (neurogenic DI) such as trauma, tumor, inflammation of the brain (hypothalamus), or surgical ablation of the pituitary gland. Patients with DI excrete large volumes of free water within a dilute urine. Their blood is hemoconcentrated, causing them to have a strong thirst.

Primary renal diseases may make the renal collecting system less sensitive to ADH stimulation (nephrogenic DI). Again, in this instance, a dilute urine created by excretion of high volumes of free water may occur. To differentiate neurogenic DI from nephrogenic DI, a *water deprivation ADH stimulation* test is performed. During this test, water intake is restricted, and urine osmolality is measured before and after vasopressin is administered. In neurogenic DI there is no rise in urine osmolality with water restriction, but there is a rise after vasopressin administration. In nephrogenic DI there is no rise in urine osmolality after water deprivation or vasopressin administration. The diagnosis indicated by this test can be corroborated by a serum ADH level. In neurogenic DI, ADH levels are low. In nephrogenic DI, ADH levels are high.

High serum ADH levels are also associated with the syndrome of inappropriate ADH secretion (SIADH). In response to the inappropriately high level of ADH secretion, water is resorbed by the kidneys greatly in excess of normal amounts. Thus the patient becomes very hemodiluted, and the urine concentrated. Blood levels of important serum ions diminish, causing severe neurologic, cardiac, and metabolic alterations. The most frequent cause of SIADH is the paraneoplastic syndrome, causing ectopic secretion of ADH. The most common tumors associated with SIADH include carcinoma of the lung and thymus; lymphomas; leukemia; and carcinomas of the pancreas, urologic tract, and intestine. SIADH is also associated with pulmonary diseases (e.g., tuberculosis, bacterial pneumonia), severe stress (e.g., surgery, trauma), CNS tumor, infection, or trauma. Patients with myxedema or Addison's disease also can experience SIADH.

The *water load test (ADH suppression test)* is used to differentiate the syndrome of inappropriate ADH (SIADH) from other causes of hyponatremia or edematous states. Usually this test is done concomitantly with measurements of urine and serum osmolality. Patients with SIADH will excrete none or very little of the "water load." Further, their urine osmolality will never be <100, and the urine/serum ratio is >100. Patients with other hyponatremia, edematous states, or chronic renal diseases will excrete up to 80% of the water load and will develop midrange osmolality results.

Interfering factors

- Patients with dehydration, hypovolemia, and stress may have increased ADH levels.
- Patients with overhydration, decreased serum osmolality, and hypervolemia may have decreased ADH levels.
- Use of a glass syringe or collection tube causes degradation of ADH.
- Drugs that *elevate* ADH levels include acetaminophen, barbiturates, cholinergic agents, estrogen, nicotine, oral hypoglycemic agents, some diuretics (e.g., thiazides), cyclophosphamide, narcotics, and tricyclic antidepressants.

✶ Drugs that *decrease* ADH levels include alcohol, beta-adrenergic agents, morphine antagonists, and phenytoin (Dilantin).

Procedure and patient care

Before

PT Explain the procedure to the patient.

PT Ensure that the patient is adequately hydrated. Tell the patient to fast for 12 hours.

- Evaluate the patient for high levels of physical or emotional stress.

During

- Collect approximately 7 ml of venous blood in a *plastic* red-top tube with the patient in the sitting or recumbent position.
- Record on the laboratory slip any drugs that may alter test results.

After

- Apply pressure to the venipuncture site.
- Note that the laboratory personnel usually freeze the serum and send it to a reference laboratory for testing.

Abnormal findings

▲ **Increased levels**

SIADH
Nephrogenic diabetes insipidus caused by primary renal diseases
Postoperative days 1 to 3
Severe physical stress (e.g., trauma, pain, prolonged mechanical ventilation)
Hypovolemia
Dehydration
Acute porphyria

▼ **Decreased levels**

Neurogenic (or central) diabetes insipidus
Surgical ablation of the pituitary gland
Hypervolemia
Decreased serum osmolality

notes

anti-DNA antibody test (Antideoxyribonucleic acid antibodies, Antibody to double-stranded DNA, Anti-double-stranded DNA, Anti-ds-DNA, DNA antibody, Native double-stranded DNA)

Type of test Blood

Normal findings

Negative: <70 international units/ml
Borderline: 70-200 international units/ml
Positive: >200 international units/ml

Test explanation and related physiology

The anti-ds-DNA test is useful for the diagnosis and follow-up of systemic lupus erythematosus (SLE). This antibody is found in approximately 65% to 80% of patients with active SLE and rarely in other diseases. High titers are characteristic of SLE. Low to intermediate levels of this antibody may be found in patients with other rheumatic diseases and in those with chronic hepatitis, infectious mononucleosis, and biliary cirrhosis. The anti-DNA titer decreases with successful therapy and increases with an exacerbation of SLE and especially with the onset of lupus glomerulonephritis. The test can return to near negative with dormant SLE.

The anti-DNA antibody is a subtype of the *antinuclear antibodies (ANAs)* (see p. 89). There are two types of anti-DNA antibodies. The first and most popular is the antibody against double-stranded DNA (anti-ds-DNA). The second type is the antibody against single-stranded DNA (anti-ss-DNA), which is less sensitive and specific for SLE but is positive in other autoimmune diseases. These antibody-antigen complexes that occur with autoimmune disease are not only diagnostic but are major contributors to the disease process. These complexes induce the complement system, which then may cause local or systemic tissue injury.

Interfering factors

- A radioactive scan performed within 1 week before the test may alter the test results.
- Drugs that may cause *increased* levels include hydralazine and procainamide.

Procedure and patient care

Before

PT Explain the procedure to the patient.

PT Tell the patient that no fasting is required.

During

- Collect one red-top tube of venous blood.

After

- Apply pressure to the venipuncture site.

Abnormal findings

▲   **Increased levels**

Systemic lupus erythematosus
Other autoimmune diseases
Chronic hepatitis
Infectious mononucleosis
Biliary cirrhosis

notes

anti-extractable nuclear antigens (Anti-ENA, Antibodies to extractable nuclear antigens, Anti-Jo-1 [antihistidyl transfer synthase], Antiribonucleoprotein [anti-RNP], Anti-Smith [anti-SM])

Type of test Blood

Normal findings Negative

Test explanation and related physiology

The anti-ENAs are used to assist in the diagnosis of systemic lupus erythematosus (SLE) and mixed connective tissue disease (MCTD) and to eliminate other rheumatoid diseases.

Anti-ENAs are a type of *antinuclear antibodies* to certain nuclear antigens that consist of RNA and protein. The ENA antigen is sometimes referred to as "saline-extracted antigen." The most common ENAs are Smith (SM) and ribonucleoprotein (RNP).

The *antinuclear Smith (anti-SM)* antibody is present in about 30% of patients with SLE and in about 8% of patients with MCTDs. However, it is not present in patients with most other rheumatoid-collagen diseases.

The *antinuclear ribonucleoprotein (anti-RNP)* is reported in nearly 100% of patients with MCTD and in about 25% of patients with SLE, discoid lupus, and progressive systemic sclerosis (scleroderma). In high titer, anti-RNP is suggestive of MCTD.

The *anti-Jo-1 (antihistidyl transfer synthase)* antibodies occur in patients with autoimmune interstitial pulmonary fibrosis and in a minority of patients with aggressive autoimmune myositis.

There are two other antibodies to ENAs. Anti-SS-A and anti-SS-B are described on p. 100 and are used mainly in the diagnostic evaluation of Sjögren's syndrome.

Procedure and patient care

Before

PT Explain the procedure to the patient.

PT Tell the patient that no fasting is required.

During

■ Collect a venous blood sample in a red-top tube.

After

■ Apply pressure to the venipuncture site.

- Check the venipuncture site for infection. Patients with autoimmune disease have a compromised immune system.

Abnormal findings

▲ **Increased anti-SM antibodies**

Systemic lupus erythematosus

▲ **Increased anti-RNP antibodies**

MCTD
SLE
Discoid lupus scleroderma

▲ **Increased anti-Jo-1 antibodies**

Pulmonary fibrosis
Autoimmune myositis

notes

antiglomerular basement membrane antibodies
(Anti-GBM antibody, AGBM, Glomerular basement antibody, Goodpasture's antibody)

Type of test
Blood; microscopic examination of tissue (lung or renal)

Normal findings
Tissue
Negative: no immunofluorescence noted on the renal or lung tissue basement membrane.
Blood: EIA (enzyme immunoassay)
Negative: <20 units EIA
Borderline: 20-100 units
Positive: >100 units

Test explanation and related physiology
This test is used to detect the presence of circulating glomerular basement membrane antibodies commonly present in autoimmune-induced nephritis (Goodpasture's syndrome).

Goodpasture's syndrome is an autoimmune disease characterized by the presence of antibodies circulating against antigens in the basement membrane of the renal glomerular and the pulmonary alveoli. These immune complexes activate the complement system and thereby cause tissue injury. Patients with this problem usually display a triad of glomerulonephritis (hematuria), pulmonary hemorrhage (hemoptysis), and antibodies to basement membrane antigens. About 60% to 75% of patients with immune-induced glomerular nephritis have these pulmonary complications.

Lung or renal biopsies are required to obtain tissue on which to demonstrate these antibodies with immunohistochemical techniques. Serum assays are a faster and more reliable method for diagnosing Goodpasture's syndrome, especially in patients in whom renal or lung biopsy may be difficult or contraindicated. Furthermore, serum levels can be used in monitoring response to therapy (plasmapheresis or immunosuppression).

Procedure and patient care

Before
PT Explain the procedure to the patient.
PT Tell the patient to fast for 8 hours before the test. Water is permitted.
PT If a lung biopsy (see p. 611) or renal biopsy (see p. 792) will be used to collect the specimen, explain these procedures to the patient.

During
▪ Collect one red-top tube of venous blood.

After
▪ Apply pressure to the venipuncture site.

Abnormal findings

Positive
Goodpasture's syndrome
Autoimmune glomerulonephritis
Lupus nephritis

notes

antimitochondrial antibody (AMA)

Type of test Blood

Normal findings No antimitochondrial antibodies (AMAs) at titers >1:5

Test explanation and related physiology

The AMA is used primarily to aid in the diagnosis of primary biliary cirrhosis. AMA is an anticytoplasmic antibody directed against a lipoprotein in the mitochondrial membrane. Normally the serum does not contain AMA at a titer greater than 1:5. AMA appears in 94% of patients with primary biliary cirrhosis. This disease may be an autoimmune disease that occurs predominantly in young or middle-aged women. It has a slow, progressive course marked by elevated liver enzymes, especially alkaline phosphatase and gamma-glutamyl transpeptidase (see pp. 36 and 463) and positive AMA. Liver biopsy (see p. 595) is usually required to confirm the diagnosis because AMA can be positive in patients with chronic active hepatitis, drug-induced cholestasis, autoimmune hepatitis (e.g., scleroderma, systemic lupus erythematosus), extrahepatic obstruction, or acute infectious hepatitis. There are subgroups of AMA. The M-2 subgroup is suspected to be very specific for primary biliary cirrhosis.

Procedure and patient care

Before
PT Explain the procedure to the patient.
PT Tell the patient that no fasting or special preparation is required.

During
- Collect 7 to 10 ml of venous blood in a red-top tube.

After
- Apply pressure to the venipuncture site. Patients with liver disease often have bleeding disorders.

Abnormal findings

▲   **Increased levels**

Primary biliary cirrhosis
Chronic active hepatitis
Systemic lupus erythematosus (SLE)
Syphilis
Drug-induced cholestasis
Autoimmune hepatitis (e.g., scleroderma, SLE)
Extrahepatic obstruction
Acute infectious hepatitis

notes

antimyocardial antibodies (AMA)

Type of test Blood

Normal findings Negative (if positive, serum will be titrated)

Test explanation and related physiology

This test is used to detect an autoimmune source of myocardial injury and disease. Antimyocardial antibodies may be detected in rheumatic heart disease, cardiomyopathy, postthoracotomy syndrome, and postmyocardial infarction syndromes. This test is used both in the detection of an autoimmune cause for these conditions and for monitoring their response to treatment. Antibodies against heart muscle are also found in 20% to 40% of postcardiac surgery patients and in a smaller number of postmyocardial infarction patients. These antibodies are usually associated with a pericarditis that follows the myocardial injury associated with cardiac surgery or myocardial infarction (Dressler's syndrome). AMA has also been detected with cardiomyopathy.

Procedure and patient care

Before

PT Explain the procedure to the patient.

PT Tell the patient that no fasting or special preparation is necessary.

During

- Collect a venous blood sample in a red-top tube.

After

- Apply pressure to the venipuncture site.

Abnormal findings

▲ **Increased levels**

Rheumatic heart disease
Cardiomyopathy
Postthoracotomy syndrome
Postmyocardial infarction
Rheumatic fever
Streptococcal infection

A

antineutrophil cytoplasmic antibody (ANCA)

Type of test Blood

Normal findings Negative

Test explanation and related physiology

This blood test is used to assist in the diagnosis of Wegener's granulomatosis (WG). It also is useful in following the course of the disease, monitoring the response to therapy, and providing early detection of relapse. WG is a regional systemic vasculitis in which the small arteries of the kidneys, lungs, and upper respiratory tract (nasopharynx) are damaged by a granulomatous inflammation. Diagnosis has been made by biopsy of clinically affected tissue. Recently serologic testing has begun to play a key role in the diagnosis of WG and other systemic vasculitis syndromes.

ANCAs are antibodies directed against cytoplasmic components of neutrophils. There are two types of antineutrophil cytoplasmic antibodies. The *C-ANCA* pattern is highly specific (95% to 99%) for WG. When the disease is limited to the respiratory tract, the C-ANCA is positive in only about 65% of patients. Nearly all patients with WG limited to the kidney do not have positive C-ANCA. When WG is inactive, the percentage of positives drops to about 30%.

The second type of ANCA is the *P-ANCA,* which produces a perinuclear pattern of staining in the neutrophil cytoplasm. P-ANCA pattern is found in 50% of patients with WG centered in the kidney. It also occurs in patients with non-WG glomerulonephritis. In patients with ulcerative colitis or sclerosing cholangitis, 75% will have positive P-ANCA.

Procedure and patient care

Before

PT Explain the procedure to the patient.
PT Tell the patient that no fasting is required.

During

- Collect venous blood in a tube as determined by the laboratory performing the test.

After

- Apply pressure to the venipuncture site.

Abnormal findings

▲ **Increased levels**

WG

Microscopic polyarteritis

Idiopathic crescentic glomerulonephritis

Ulcerative colitis

Primary sclerosing cholangitis

Autoimmune hepatitis

Churg-Strauss vasculitis

Active viral hepatitis

Crohn's disease

notes

antinuclear antibody (ANA)

Type of test Blood

Normal findings No ANA detected in a titer with a dilution >1:20

Test explanation and related physiology

ANA is a group of antinuclear antibodies used to diagnose systemic lupus erythematosus (SLE). Because almost all patients with SLE develop autoantibodies, a negative ANA test excludes the diagnosis. Positive results occur in approximately 95% of patients with this disease; however, many other rheumatic diseases are also associated with ANA.

There are several different patterns of fluorescence, seen through the UV microscope. When combined with the specific subtype of ANA, the pattern can increase specificity of the ANA subtypes for the various autoimmune diseases (Figure 3). As the diseases becomes less active because of therapy, the ANA titers can be expected to fall. As can be seen in Table 2, none of the ANA subtypes is exclusive for any one autoimmune disease.

TABLE 2 Autoimmune disease and positive ANAs

Autoimmune disease	Positive antibodies
SLE	ANA, SLE prep, ds-DNA, ss-DNA, anti-DNP, SS-A
Drug-induced SLE	ANA
Sjögren's syndrome	RF, ANA, SS-A, SS-B
Scleroderma	ANA, Scl-70, RNA, ds-DNA
Raynaud's disease	ACA, Scl-70
Mixed connective tissue disease	ANA, RNP, RF, ss-DNA
Rheumatoid arthritis	RF, ANA, RANA, RAP
Primary biliary cirrhosis	AMA
Thyroiditis	Antimicrosomal, antithyroglobulin
Chronic active hepatitis	ASMA

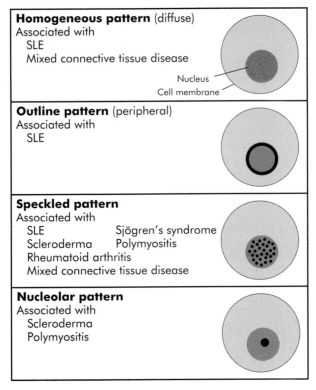

Figure 3 Patterns of immunofluorescent staining of antinuclear antibodies and the diseases with which they are associated.

Interfering factors

🖝 Drugs that may cause a *false-positive* ANA test include acetazolamide, aminosalicylic acid, chlorprothixene, chlorothiazides, griseofulvin, hydralazine, penicillin, phenylbutazone, phenytoin sodium, procainamide, streptomycin, sulfonamides, and tetracyclines.

🖝 Drugs that may cause a *false-negative* test include steroids.

Procedure and patient care

Before

PT Explain the procedure to the patient.

PT Tell the patient that no fasting or preparation is required.

During
- Collect 7 to 10 ml of venous blood in a red-top tube.
- Indicate on the laboratory slip any drugs that may affect the test results.

After
- Apply pressure to the venipuncture site.

Abnormal findings

▲   **Increased levels**

SLE
Rheumatoid arthritis
Chronic hepatitis
Periarteritis (polyarteritis) nodosa
Dermatomyositis
Scleroderma
Infectious mononucleosis
Raynaud's disease
Sjögren's syndrome
Other immune diseases
Leukemia
Myasthenia gravis
Cirrhosis

notes

anti-parietal cell antibody (APCA)

Type of test Blood

Normal findings Negative

Test explanation and related physiology

Parietal cells exist in the proximal stomach and produce hydrochloric acid and intrinsic factor. Intrinsic factor is necessary for the absorption of vitamin B_{12} (see p. 990). Anti-parietal cell antibodies are found in nearly 90% of patients with pernicious anemia. Nearly 60% of these patients also have antiintrinsic factor antibodies. It is thought that these antibodies contribute to the destruction of the gastric mucosa in these patients. APCA is also found in patients with atrophic gastritis, gastric ulcers, and gastric cancer.

APCA is present in other autoimmune-mediated diseases such as thyroiditis, myxedema, juvenile diabetes, Addison's disease, and iron-deficiency anemia. Nearly 10% to 15% of the normal population has APCA. As one ages, the incidence of having APCA increases (especially in relatives of patients with pernicious anemia).

APCA can cross-react with other antibodies, especially anticellular and antithyroid antibodies. Titer levels greater than 1:240 are considered positive.

Procedure and patient care

Before

PT Explain the procedure to the patient.

PT Tell the patient that no fasting or special preparation is necessary.

During

- Collect a venous blood sample in a red-top tube.

After

- Apply pressure or a pressure dressing to the venipuncture site.
- Check the venipuncture site for bleeding.

Abnormal findings

▲ **Increased levels**

Pernicious anemia
Atrophic gastritis
Hashimoto's thyroiditis
Myxedema
Juvenile diabetes
Addison's disease

notes

antiscleroderma antibody (Scl-70 antibody, Scleroderma antibody)

Type of test Blood

Normal findings Negative

Test explanation and related physiology

This antibody is diagnostic for scleroderma (progressive systemic sclerosis [PSS]) and is present in 45% of patients with that disease. Scl-70 antibody is an *antinuclear antibody* (see p. 89). PPS (scleroderma) is a multisystem disorder characterized by inflammation with subsequent fibrosis of the small blood vessels in skin and visceral organs, including the heart, lungs, kidneys, and gastrointestinal tract. A collagen-like substance is also deposited into the tissue of these organs. In general, the higher the titer of Scl-70 antibody, the more likely that PSS exists and the more active the disease is. As the disease becomes less active because of therapy, the Scl-70 antibody titers can be expected to fall.

The absence of this antibody does not exclude the diagnosis of scleroderma. The antibody is rather specific for PSS but is occasionally seen in other autoimmune diseases such as systemic lupus erythematosus, mixed connective tissue disease, Sjögren's syndrome, polymyositis, and rheumatoid arthritis.

Interfering factors

✱ Drugs that may cause *increased* levels include aminosalicylic acid, isoniazid, methyldopa, penicillin, propylthiouracil, streptomycin, and tetracycline.

Procedure and patient care

Before
PT Explain the procedure to the patient.
PT Tell the patient that no fasting is required.

During
■ Collect a venous sample of blood in a red-top tube.

After
■ Apply pressure to the venipuncture site.

Abnormal findings

Positive
Scleroderma
CREST syndrome

notes

anti-smooth muscle antibody (ASMA)

Type of test Blood

Normal findings No anti-smooth muscle antibodies (ASMAs) at titers >1:20

Test explanation and related physiology

The ASMA is used primarily to aid in the diagnosis of autoimmune chronic active hepatitis (CAH), which has also been referred to as "lupoid" CAH. ASMA is an *anticytoplasmic antibody* directed against actin, a cytoskeletal protein. Normally the serum does not contain ASMA at a titer greater than 1:20. ASMA is the most commonly recognized autoantibody in the setting of CAH. It appears in 70% to 80% of patients with CAH. Some types of CAH do not have positive ASMA antibodies. This disease may be an autoimmune disease that occurs predominantly in adult women. The clinical presentation of CAH is similar to viral hepatitis. That clinical picture, along with serologic and pathologic criteria, must exist for >6 months to be classified as CAH.

ASMA is not specific for CAH and can be positive in patients with viral infections, malignancy, multiple sclerosis, primary biliary cirrhosis, and *Mycoplasma* infections. Usually the titer of ASMA is low in these diseases. With CAH the titer is usually higher than 1:160. The titers are not helpful in predicting prognosis, nor do they indicate disease response to therapy.

Procedure and patient care

Before
PT Explain the procedure to the patient.
PT Tell the patient that no fasting or special preparation is required.

During
- Collect 7 to 10 ml of venous blood in a red-top tube.

After
- Apply pressure to the venipuncture site.
- Patients with liver disease can have bleeding disorders.

Abnormal findings

▲   **Increased levels**

CAH
Mononucleosis hepatitis
Primary biliary cirrhosis
Viral hepatitis
Multiple sclerosis
Malignancy
Intrinsic asthma

notes

antispermatozoal antibody (Sperm agglutination and inhibition, Sperm antibodies, Antisperm antibodies, Infertility screen)

Type of test Fluid analysis; blood

Normal findings Negative

Test explanation and related physiology

The antispermatozoal antibody test is an infertility screening test used to detect the presence of sperm antibodies. Antibodies directed toward sperm antigens can result in diminished fertility. This test is commonly used in the evaluation of an infertile couple. Antisperm antibodies may be found in the blood of men with blocked efferent ducts of the testes (a common cause of low sperm counts or poor sperm mobility) and in 30% to 70% of men who have had a vasectomy. Resorption of sperm from the blocked ducts results in the formation of autoantibodies to sperm as a result of sperm antigens interacting with the immune system. The IgA antisperm antibodies to the sperm tail are associated with poor motility and poor penetration of cervical mucus. IgG antisperm antibodies are associated with blockage of sperm-ovum fusion. High titers of IgG autoantibodies are often associated with postvasectomy degeneration of the testes, which explains why 50% of males remain infertile after successful repair of a previous vasectomy.

In men high serum titers of antispermatozoal antibody are considered strong evidence of infertility. Low titers are of unknown significance, as this is not an uncommon finding among normal fertile males. Serum antispermatozoal antibodies are found in nearly 20% of women. However, many of these women become pregnant. Therefore the significance of this antibody in women is uncertain.

Antispermatozoal antibodies can also be detected in the sperm of infertile males and in the cervical mucus of infertile females. It is often necessary to identify these antibodies in the serum and other body fluids in a thorough evaluation of infertility.

Procedure and patient care

Before

PT Explain the procedure to the patient.

Sperm specimen

PT Inform the man that a semen specimen should be collected after avoiding ejaculation for at least 3 days.

- Give the male patient the proper container for the sperm collection.

PT If the specimen is to be collected at home, be certain the patient is told that it must be taken to the laboratory for testing within 2 hours after collection.

During

- Collect a venous blood sample of approximately 7 to 10 ml from both the male and the female patient in red-top tubes.
- For a sperm specimen, collect the ejaculate in a plastic container.
- For a vaginal mucus specimen, collect 1 ml of cervical mucus and place in a plastic vial.

After

- Apply pressure to the venipuncture site.
- For a sperm, blood, or cervical specimen, place the specimen in a plastic vial, freeze, and send to a reference laboratory on dry ice.

PT Instruct the couple when and how to obtain the test results.

Abnormal findings

Infertility
Blocked efferent ducts in the testes
Vasectomy

notes

anti-SS-A (Ro), anti-SS-B (La), and anti-SS-C antibody (Anti-Ro, Anti-La, Sjögren's antibodies)

Type of test Blood

Normal findings Negative

Test explanation and related physiology

These three antinuclear antibodies are used to diagnose Sjögren's syndrome. Ro, La, and SS-C antibodies are a subtype of *antinuclear antibodies (ANA)* and react to nuclear antigens extracted from human B lymphocytes. Ro and La result in a speckled immunofluorescent pattern when seen in the UV microscope (see Figure 3, p. 90). Sjögren's syndrome is an immunogenic disease characterized by progressive destruction of the lacrimal and salivary exocrine glands leading to mucosal and conjunctival dryness. This disease can occur by itself (primary) or in association with other autoimmune diseases such as systemic lupus erythematosus (SLE), rheumatoid arthritis, and scleroderma. In the latter case, it is referred to as secondary Sjögren's syndrome.

Anti-SS-A antibodies may be found in approximately 60% to 70% of patients with primary Sjögren's syndrome. Anti-SS-B antibodies may be found in approximately half of patients with primary Sjögren's syndrome. When anti-SS-A and anti-SS-B antibodies are both positive, Sjögren's syndrome can be diagnosed. These antibodies are only occasionally found when secondary Sjögren's syndrome is associated with rheumatoid arthritis (RA). In fact anti-SS-B is found only in primary Sjögren's syndrome. However, anti-SS-C is positive in about 75% of patients with RA or patients with RA and secondary Sjögren's syndrome. Therefore these antibodies are also useful in differentiating primary from secondary Sjögren's syndrome.

Anti-SS-A can also be found in 25% of patients with SLE. This is particularly useful in "ANA (antinuclear antigen)-negative" cases of SLE, because these antibodies are present in the majority of such patients. Anti-SS-B is never found in SLE, however. In general, the higher the titer of anti-SS antibodies, the more likely that Sjögren's syndrome exists, and the more active is the disease. As Sjögren's syndrome becomes less active with therapy, the anti-SS antibody titers can be expected to fall.

Procedure and patient care

Before

PT Explain the procedure to the patient.
PT Tell the patient that no fasting is required.

During

- Collect a venous blood sample in a red-top tube.

After

- Apply pressure to the venipuncture site.

Abnormal findings

Positive

Sjögren's syndrome
Rheumatoid arthritis
ANA-negative SLE
Neonatal lupus

notes

antistreptolysin O titer (ASO titer)

Type of test Blood

Normal findings

Adult/elderly: ≤160 Todd units/ml
Newborn: similar to mother's value
6 months-2 years: ≤50 Todd units/ml
2-4 years: ≤160 Todd units/ml
5-12 years: 170-330 Todd units/ml

Test explanation and related physiology

This test is used primarily in determining that a previous *Streptococcus* infection has caused a poststreptococcal disease such as glomerulonephritis, rheumatic fever, bacterial endocarditis, or scarlet fever. Levels are highest in glomerulonephritis and rheumatic fever. The ASO titer is a serologic procedure demonstrating the reaction of the body to infection caused by group A beta hemolytic streptococci bacteria. The *Streptococcus* organism produces an enzyme called streptolysin O, which has the ability to destroy (lyse) red blood corpuscles. Because streptolysin O is antigenic, the body reacts by producing ASO, a neutralizing antibody. ASO appears in the serum 1 week to 1 month after the onset of a streptococcal infection. A high titer is not specific for a certain type of poststreptococcal disease (i.e., rheumatic fever versus glomerulonephritis), but merely indicates that a streptococcal infection is or has been present. When an ASO elevation is seen in a patient with glomerulonephritis or endocarditis, one can safely assume that the disease was caused by streptococcal infection. Serial rising titers of ASO over several weeks, followed by a slow fall in titers, is more supportive of the diagnosis of a previous streptococcal infection than is a single titer. The highest incidence of positive results is during the third week after the onset of acute symptoms of the poststreptococcal disease. By 6 months only about 30% of patients have abnormal titers.

Another immunologic test, *antideoxyribonuclease B (anti-DNase-B)* (see p. 74) also detects antigens produced by group A streptococci. The anti-DNase B level is elevated in most patients with acute rheumatic fever and poststreptococcal glomerulonephritis. When ASO and anti-DNase B are performed concurrently, 95% of previous streptococcal infections are detected.

Interfering factors

- Increased beta-lipoprotein levels inhibit streptolysin O and give a falsely high ASO titer.
- Drugs that may cause *decreased* ASO levels include antibiotics and adrenocorticosteroids.

Procedure and patient care

Before

PT Explain the procedure to the patient.
PT Tell the patient that no fasting is required.

During

- Collect approximately 5 to 10 ml of blood in a red-top tube.
- Avoid hemolysis of the blood specimen.
- Note on the laboratory slip any medications that may affect the test results.

After

- Apply pressure to the venipuncture site.
- Note that repeat ASO testing may be done to determine the highest level of increase.

Abnormal findings

▲ **Increased levels**

Streptococcal infection
Acute rheumatic fever
Acute glomerulonephritis
Bacterial endocarditis
Scarlet fever
Streptococcal pyoderma

notes

antithrombin III (AT-III, Functional antithrombin III assay, Heparin cofactor, Immunologic antithrombin III, Serine protease inhibitor)

Type of test Blood

Normal findings

Plasma: >50% of control value
Serum: 15% to 34% lower than plasma value
Immunologic: 17-30 mg/dl
Functional: 80% to 120%
(Values vary according to laboratory methods.)

Test explanation and related physiology

This test is used to evaluate patients suspected of having hypercoagulable states. It is also used to help identify the cause of "heparin resistance" in patients receiving heparin therapy. AT-III is an alpha$_2$ globulin produced in the liver. It inhibits the serum proteases involved in coagulation (II, X, IX, XI, XII). In normal homeostasis the coagulation system results from a balance between AT-III and thrombin. A deficiency of AT-III increases coagulation or the tendency toward thrombosis. A hereditary deficiency of AT-III is characterized by a predisposition toward thrombus formation. This is passed on as an autosomal-dominant abnormality. Individuals with hereditary AT-III deficiency typically develop thromboembolic events in their early twenties. These thrombotic events are usually venous. Acquired AT-III deficiency may be seen in patients with cirrhosis, liver failure, advanced carcinoma, nephrotic syndrome, disseminated intravascular coagulation, and acute thrombosis. AT-III is also decreased as much as 30% by pregnancy or with the use of exogenous estrogens. AT-III provides most of the anticoagulant effect of heparin. Heparin requires AT-III to express its effect. Patients who are deficient in AT-III may be heparin resistant and require unusually high doses to provide anticoagulation. In general, patients respond to heparin if more than 60% of normal AT-III levels exists.

Asymptomatic individuals with an antithrombin deficiency should receive prophylactic anticoagulation before any medical/surgical circumstances in which inactivity increases the risk of thrombosis. Increased levels of AT-III may occur in patients with acute hepatitis, obstructive jaundice, vitamin K deficiency, and kidney transplantation.

Interfering factors

▮ Drugs that may cause *increased* levels include anabolic steroids, androgens, oral contraceptives (containing progesterone), and sodium warfarin.
▮ Drugs that may cause *decreased* levels include fibrinolytics, heparin, L-asparaginase, and oral contraceptives (containing estrogen).

Procedure and patient care

Before

PT Explain the procedure to the patient.
PT Tell the patient that no fasting is required.

During

■ Collect a venous blood sample in a blue- or red-top tube.

After

■ Apply pressure to the venipuncture site.
■ Send the specimen to the laboratory immediately after collection.

Abnormal findings

▲ Increased levels

Kidney transplant
Acute hepatitis
Obstructive jaundice
Vitamin K deficiency

▼ Decreased levels

Disseminated intravascular coagulation
Hypercoagulation states (e.g., deep vein thrombosis)
Hepatic disorders (especially cirrhosis)
Nephrotic syndrome
Protein-wasting diseases (malignancy)
Hereditary familial deficiency of AT-III

notes

antithyroglobulin antibody (Thyroid autoantibody, Thyroid antithyroglobulin antibody, Thyroglobulin antibody)

Type of test Blood

Normal findings Titer <1:100

Test explanation and related physiology

This test is used primarily in the differential diagnosis of thyroid diseases such as Hashimoto's thyroiditis or chronic lymphocytic thyroiditis (in children). There are several antibodies to various thyroid gland components. Antithyroglobulin occurs when thyroglobulin, which normally exists in the blood (as a thyroid hormone carrier) and in the thyroid acts as an immune-stimulating antigen. Autoantibodies are developed and react against the thyroglobulin in the thyroid cells. This leads to thyroid inflammation and destruction.

Although many different thyroid diseases are associated with elevated antithyroglobulin levels, the most frequent is chronic thyroiditis (Hashimoto's thyroiditis in the adult and lymphocytic thyroiditis in children and young adults). The level must be extremely high to confirm the diagnosis of Hashimoto's thyroiditis. This antibody is present in only about 50% of patients with Hashimoto's thyroiditis. Both Hashimoto's and lymphocytic thyroiditis have been associated with other autoimmune (collagen vascular) diseases. The antithyroglobulin test is usually performed in conjunction with the antithyroid peroxidase antibody test (see p. 108). When this is done, the specificity and sensitivity are greatly increased.

A small percentage of the normal population have antithyroglobulin antibodies. Normally women tend to have higher levels than men.

Interfering factors

- Normal individuals, especially elderly women, may have antithyroglobulin antibodies.

Procedure and patient care

Before

PT Explain the procedure to the patient.

PT Tell the patient that no fasting is required.

During

- Collect approximately 3 to 5 ml of blood in a red-top tube.

After

- Apply pressure to the venipuncture site.

Abnormal findings

▲ **Increased levels**

Hashimoto's thyroiditis
Rheumatoid arthritis
Rheumatoid-collagen disease
Pernicious anemia
Thyrotoxicosis
Hypothyroidism
Thyroid carcinoma
Myxedema

notes

antithyroid peroxidase antibody (Anti-TPO, TPO-Ab, Antithyroid microsomal antibody, Antimicrosomal antibody, Microsomal antibody, Thyroid autoantibody, Thyroid antimicrosomal antibody)

Type of test Blood

Normal findings Titer <1:100

Test explanation and related physiology

This test is primarily used in the differential diagnosis of thyroid diseases such as Hashimoto's thyroiditis or chronic lymphocytic thyroiditis (in children). Thyroid microsomal antibodies are commonly found in patients with various thyroid diseases. They are found in 70% to 90% of patients with Hashimoto's thyroiditis. A microsomal antibody is an antibody for a section of microsome in the thyroid cell. The immune antibody–antigen complexes initiate inflammatory and cytotoxic effects on the thyroid follicle. There are several methods of measuring this antimicrosomal antibody. The most sensitive assay is for antithyroid peroxidase (anti-TPO) antibody. Anti-TPO is often performed in conjunction with the antithyroglobulin antibody test (see p. 106). When this is done, the specificity and sensitivity are greatly increased.

Anti-TPO is present in almost all patients with Hashimoto's thyroiditis, in more than 70% of those with Graves' disease, and, to a variable degree, in patients with nonthyroid autoimmune disease. Five percent to 10% of healthy people have elevated anti-TPO levels.

Procedure and patient care

Before

PT Explain the procedure to the patient.

PT Tell the patient that no fasting is required.

During

- Collect approximately 3 to 5 ml of venous blood in a red-top tube.

After

- Apply pressure to the venipuncture site.

Abnormal findings

A

▲ **Increased levels**

Chronic thyroiditis (Hashimoto's thyroiditis)
Rheumatoid arthritis
Rheumatoid-collagen disease
Pernicious anemia
Thyrotoxicosis
Hypothyroidism
Thyroid carcinoma
Myxedema

notes

apolipoproteins (Apolipoprotein A-I [Apo A-I], Apolipoprotein B [Apo B], Lipoprotein (a) [Lp (a)], Apolipoprotein E [Apo E])

Type of test Blood

Normal findings

Apo A-I

Adult/elderly
  Male: 75-160 mg/dl
  Female: 80-175 mg/dl
Child
  Newborn
    Male: 41-93 mg/dl
    Female: 38-106 mg/dl
  6 months-4 years
    Male: 67-167 mg/dl
    Female: 60-148 mg/dl
  5-17 years: 83-151 mg/dl

Apo B

Adult/elderly
  Male: 50-125 mg/dl
  Female: 45-120 mg/dl
Child
  Newborn: 11-31 mg/dl
  6 months-3 years: 23-75 mg/dl
  5-17 years:
    Male: 47-139 mg/dl
    Female: 41-132 mg/dl

Apo A-I/Apo B ratio

Male: 0.85-2.24
Female: 0.76-3.23

Lipoprotein (a)

Caucasian (5th-95th percentiles)
  Male: 2.2-49.4 mg/dl
  Female: 2.1-57.3 mg/dl
African-American (5th-95th percentiles)
  Male: 4.6-71.8 mg/dl
  Female: 4.4-75 mg/dl

Test explanation and related physiology

This test is used to evaluate the risks of atherogenic disease of the heart and peripheral arteries. These levels may be better indicators of atherogenic risks than lipoproteins such as HDL, LDL, and VLDL (see p. 592). The protein component of those lipoproteins, which plays an important role in lipid transport, is composed of several specific polypeptides called apolipoproteins. Apolipoproteins are also involved in binding lipoproteins to lipoprotein receptors at the cell surface, thus facilitating lipid uptake by cells.

Apolipoprotein A (apo A) is the major polypeptide component of HDL. Apo A has two major forms: apo A-I, which constitutes about 75% of the apo A in HDL, and apo A-II, which constitutes about 20% of the total HDL protein. In general, as HDL levels increase, apo A-I values increase. Because apo A-I reflects the HDL content of the serum and HDL levels are greater in females, apo A-I values are also higher in women than in men. Apo A-I has been proposed to be a better index of atherogenic risk than HDL assay.

Apolipoprotein B (apo B) is the major polypeptide component of LDL and makes up about 80% of that protein. Forty percent of the protein portion of very low-density lipoprotein (VLDL) is composed of apo B. Apo B has been shown to exist in two forms: apo B-100 and apo B-48. Apo B-100 is synthesized in the liver and found in lipoproteins of endogenous origin (VLDL and LDL). Apo B-100 is the principal transport mechanism for endogenous cholesterol. Apo B-100 has an affinity for the LDL receptor located on cell surfaces in peripheral tissues and is involved with cellular deposition of cholesterol. Because of this, some believe that apo B-100 may be a better indicator of atherosclerotic heart disease than LDL. The second apo B component is apo B-48, which is of intestinal origin and found mainly in chylomicrons. Apo B-48 serves to transport ingested lipids through the intestines and into the bloodstream.

Lipoprotein (a) [Lp(a)] (referred to as "lipoprotein little a") is another lipoprotein. The two polypeptide components of Lp(a) are apo (A) and an LDL-like protein containing apo B-100. Recent research has suggested that increased levels of Lp(a) may be an independent risk factor for atherosclerosis. It has been shown that apo (A) is a deformed relative of plasminogen, the precursor of the proteolytic enzyme plasmin, which is responsible for dissolving fibrin clots. This strong resemblance between an apolipoprotein and plasminogen may provide a link between lipids, the clotting mechanism, and atherogenesis. Microthrombi containing fibrin on the vessel wall become incorporated into the atherosclerotic plaque. It is suggested that, following endothelial damage, Lp(a) may insinuate itself into the arterial wall, inhibiting the cleavage of fibrin in microthrombi by competing with plasminogen for access for fibrin. Atherosclerotic damage of the arterial wall soon follows, leading to occlusive disease or aneurysm. Familial hypercholesterolemia, some forms of renal failure, nephrotic syndrome, and estrogen depletion in women over the age of 50 may also be associated with increased levels of Lp(a).

Decreased levels of apo A-I and increased levels of apo B-100 are associated with increased risk of coronary heart disease. Reports also indicate that a low ratio of apo A-I to apo B may be a good predictor of coronary heart disease. Individuals with increased concentrations of Lp(a) appear to have a significantly higher risk for coronary heart disease. Quantification of apolipoproteins is beginning to be performed as a routine clinical procedure.

These and other apolipoproteins are associated with the identification of other maladies. For example, *apolipoprotein E (apo E)* is involved in cholesterol transport and has three alleles: E-2, E-3, and E-4. The apo E-4 gene has been proposed as a risk factor for Alzheimer's disease (AD). The E-4 allele of apo E shows a strong association with AD in the general population. It is not clear how apo E functions as a risk factor modifying the age of onset of AD. Apo E is present in the neuritic amyloid plaques (see p. 63) and may also be involved in neurofibrillary tangle formation, because it binds to the tau protein. Ongoing research on apo E's functional role and its diagnostic usefulness is progressing rapidly.

Interfering factors

Apo A-I

- Physical exercise may increase apo A-I levels.
- Smoking may decrease levels.
- Diets high in carbohydrates or polyunsaturated fats may decrease apo A-I levels.
- ✗ Drugs that may *increase* apo A-I levels include carbamazepine, estrogens, ethanol, lovastatin, niacin, oral contraceptives, phenobarbital, pravastatin, and simvastatin.
- ✗ Drugs that may *decrease* apo A-I levels include androgens, beta-blockers, diuretics, and progestins.

Apo B

- Diets high in saturated fats and cholesterol may increase apo B levels.
- Drugs that may *increase* apo B levels include androgens, beta-blockers, diuretics, ethanol abuse, and progestins.
- Drugs that may *decrease* apo B levels include cholestyramine, estrogen (postmenopausal women), lovastatin, simvastatin, neomycin, niacin, and thyroxine.

Lipoprotein (a)

- Drugs that may *decrease* Lp(a) include estrogens, niacin, neomycin, and stanozolol.

Procedure and patient care

Before

PT Explain the procedure to the patient.

PT Instruct the patient to fast for 12 to 14 hours before testing. Only water is permitted.

PT Inform the patient that smoking is prohibited.

During

- Collect venous blood in a red-top tube.
- Indicate on the laboratory slip any drugs that may affect test results.

After

- Apply pressure to the venipuncture site.

Abnormal findings

▲ **Increased apo A-I**

Familial hyperalphalipoproteinemia
Pregnancy
Weight reduction

▼ **Decreased apo A-I**

Coronary artery disease
Ischemic coronary disease
Myocardial infarction
Familial hypoalphalipopro-teinemia
Fish eye disease
Uncontrolled diabetes mellitus
Tangier's disease
Nephrotic syndrome
Chronic renal failure
Cholestasis
Hemodialysis

▲ **Increased apo B**

Hyperlipoproteinemia
(types IIa, IIb, IV, V)
Nephrotic syndrome
Pregnancy
Hemodialysis
Biliary obstruction
Coronary artery disease
Diabetes
Hypothyroidism
Anorexia nervosa

▲ **Increased levels of Lp(a)**

Premature coronary artery
disease
Stenosis of cerebral arteries
Uncontrolled diabetes
mellitus
Severe hypothyroidism
Familial
hypercholesterolemia
Chronic renal failure
Estrogen depletion

▼ **Decreased apo B**

Tangier's disease
Hyperthyroidism
Malnutrition
Inflammatory joint
disease
Chronic pulmonary
disease
Weight reduction
Chronic anemia
Reye's syndrome

▼ **Decreased levels of Lp(a)**

Alcoholism
Malnutrition
Chronic liver
hepatocellular disease

notes

Apt test (Downey test, Qualitative fetal hemoglobin stool test, Stool for swallowed blood)

Type of test Stool

Normal findings

No newborn blood present
Maternal blood may be present

Test explanation and related physiology

Blood in the stool of a newborn must be rapidly evaluated. Whereas an adult can lose hundreds of milliliters of blood, that volume may represent the entire blood volume of a newborn child. Furthermore, some serious diseases present as rectal bleeding in the newborn. Much more commonly, however, newborns may simply be defecating maternal blood that was swallowed during birth or breast-feeding.

The Apt test is performed on the stool specimen to differentiate maternal from fetal blood in the stool. Fetal hemoglobin is resistant to denaturization; adult hemoglobin (hemoglobin A) is not. When sodium hydroxide is added to the blood, maternal blood will dissolve, leaving only a brown hematin stain. Newborn blood (containing hydroxide-resistant hemoglobin) will not dissolve, and red blood will remain in the specimen. This test can be performed on stool, a stool-stained diaper, amniotic fluid, or vomitus.

Procedure and patient care

Before
PT Explain the procedure to the newborn's parents.
- It is always important to assess vital signs of a newborn who develops possible intestinal bleeding.

During
- Obtain an adequate stool or vomitus specimen. Only a small amount is required.
- In the laboratory, 1% NaOH is added to the specimen. Vomitus is diluted and centrifuged first. Maternal blood turns brown; newborn blood stays red or pink.

After
- If maternal blood is present, reassure the parents and examine the mother for nipple erosion and/or cracking.

- If newborn blood is present, obtain intravenous access and begin close observation and support during further diagnostic procedures.

Abnormal findings

Active gastrointestinal bleeding
Necrotizing enterocolitis

notes

arterial blood gases (ABGs, blood gases) A

Type of test Blood

Normal findings

pH
Adult/child: 7.35-7.45
Newborn: 7.32-7.49
2 months-2 years: 7.34-7.46
pH (venous): 7.31-7.41

Pco_2
Adult/child: 35-45 mm Hg
Child <2 years: 26-41 mm Hg
Pco_2 (venous): 40-50 mm Hg

HCO_3
Adult/child: 21-28 mEq/L
Newborn/infant: 16-24 mEq/L

Po_2
Adult/child: 80-100 mm Hg
Newborn: 60-70 mm Hg
Po_2 (venous): 40-50 mm Hg

O_2 saturation
Adult/child: 95%-100%
Elderly: 95%
Newborn: 40%-90%

O_2 content
Arterial: 15-22 vol %
Venous: 11-16 vol %

Base excess: 0 ± 2 mEq/L

Possible critical values

pH: <7.25, >7.55
Pco_2: <20, >60
HCO_3: <15, >40
Po_2: <40
O_2 saturation: 75% or lower
Base excess: ± 3 mEq/L

Test explanation and related physiology

Measurement of ABGs provides valuable information in assessing and managing a patient's respiratory (ventilation) and metabolic (renal) acid/base and electrolyte homeostasis. It is also used to assess adequacy of oxygenation. ABGs are used to monitor patients on ventilators, monitor critically ill nonventilator patients, establish preoperative baseline parameters, and enlighten electrolyte therapy.

pH

The pH is inversely proportional to the actual hydrogen ion concentration. Therefore, as the hydrogen ion concentration decreases, the pH increases, and vice versa. The pH is a measure of alkalinity (pH >7.4) and acidity (pH <7.35). In respiratory or metabolic alkalosis, the pH is elevated; in respiratory or metabolic acidosis, the pH is decreased (Table 3).

P_{CO_2}

The P_{CO_2} is a measure of the partial pressure of CO_2 in the blood. P_{CO_2} is a measurement of ventilation capability. The faster and more deeply one breathes, the more CO_2 is blown off, and P_{CO_2} levels drop. Therefore P_{CO_2} is referred to as the *respiratory* component in acid-base determination because this value is controlled primarily by the lungs. As the CO_2 level increases, the pH decreases. The CO_2 level and the pH are inversely proportional. The P_{CO_2} in the blood and cerebrospinal fluid is a major stimulant to the breathing center in the brain. As P_{CO_2} levels rise, breathing is stimulated. If P_{CO_2} levels rise too high, breathing cannot keep up with the demand to blow off or ventilate. As P_{CO_2} levels rise further, the brain is depressed, and ventilation decreases further, causing coma.

The P_{CO_2} level is elevated in primary respiratory acidosis and decreased in primary respiratory alkalosis (see Table 3). Because the lungs compensate for primary metabolic acid-base derangements, P_{CO_2} levels are affected by metabolic disturbances as well. In metabolic acidosis the lungs attempt to compensate by "blowing off" CO_2 to raise pH. In metabolic alkalosis the lungs attempt to compensate by retaining CO_2 to lower pH (Table 4).

Bicarbonate (HCO_3) or CO_2 content

Most of the CO_2 content in the blood is HCO_3. The bicarbonate ion is a measure of the *metabolic (renal/kidney)* component of the acid-base equilibrium. It is regulated by the kidneys. This ion can be measured directly by the bicarbonate value or

TABLE 3 Normal values for arterial blood gases and abnormal values in uncompensated acid-base disturbances

Acid-base disturbances	pH	P_{CO_2} (mm Hg)	HCO_3 (mEq/L)	Common causes
None (normal values)	7.35-7.45	35-45	22-26	
Respiratory acidosis	↓	↑	Normal	Respiratory depression (drugs, central nervous system trauma) Pulmonary disease (pneumonia, chronic obstructive pulmonary disease, respiratory underventilation)
Respiratory alkalosis	↑	↓	Normal	Hyperventilation (emotions, pain, respirator overventilation)
Metabolic acidosis	↓	Normal	↓	Diabetes, shock, renal failure, intestinal fistula
Metabolic alkalosis	↑	Normal	↑	Sodium bicarbonate overdose, prolonged vomiting, nasogastric drainage

TABLE 4 Acid-base disturbances and compensatory mechanisms

Acid-base disturbance	Mode of compensation
Respiratory acidosis	Kidneys will retain increased amounts of HCO_3 to increase pH.
Respiratory alkalosis	Kidneys will excrete increased amounts of HCO_3 to lower pH.
Metabolic acidosis	Lungs "blow off" CO_2 to raise pH.
Metabolic alkalosis	Lungs retain CO_2 to lower pH.

indirectly by the CO_2 content (see p. 226). As the HCO_3 level increases, the pH also increases; therefore the relationship of bicarbonate to pH is directly proportional. HCO_3 is elevated in metabolic alkalosis and decreased in metabolic acidosis (see Table 3). The kidneys also are used to compensate for primary respiratory acid-base derangements. For example, in respiratory acidosis the kidneys attempt to compensate by resorbing increased amounts of HCO_3. In respiratory alkalosis the kidneys excrete HCO_3 in increased amounts in an attempt to lower pH through compensation. (See Table 4.)

Po_2

This is an indirect measure of the oxygen content of arterial blood. Po_2 is a measure of the tension (pressure) of oxygen dissolved in the plasma. This pressure determines the force of O_2 to diffuse across the pulmonary alveoli membrane. The Po_2 level is decreased in:

1. Patients who are unable to oxygenate the arterial blood because of O_2 diffusion difficulties (e.g., pneumonia, shock lung, and congestive failure)
2. Patients who have premature mixing of venous blood with arterial blood (e.g., in congenital heart disease)
3. Patients who have underventilated and overperfused pulmonary alveoli (Pickwickian syndrome [i.e., obese patients who cannot breathe properly when in the supine position], or patients with significant atelectasis)

O_2 saturation

Oxygen saturation is an indication of the percentage of hemoglobin saturated with O_2. When 92% to 100% of the hemoglobin carries O_2, the tissues are adequately provided with O_2, assuming normal O_2 dissociation. As the Po_2 level decreases, the percentage of hemoglobin saturation also decreases. When the Po_2 level drops below 60 mm Hg, small decreases in the Po_2 level cause large decreases in the percentage of hemoglobin saturated with O_2. At O_2 saturation levels of 70% or lower, the tissues are unable to extract enough O_2 to carry out their vital functions.

O_2 saturation is calculated by the blood gas machine using the following formula:

$$\text{Percentage of } O_2 \text{ saturation} = 100 \times \frac{\text{Volume of } O_2 \text{ content Hgb}}{\text{Volume of } O_2 \text{ Hgb capacity}}$$

Pulse oximetry is a noninvasive method of determining O_2 saturation (p. 672). This can be done easily and continuously. The machine measures O_2 saturation. It actually measures all forms of oxygen-saturated hemoglobin, including carboxyhemoglobin (which rises during smoke inhalation or with the use of some inhalants). Therefore, in cases of carbon monoxide poisoning in which carboxyhemoglobin is high, oximetry will indicate an inaccurately high O_2 saturation. During oximetry monitoring a small cliplike sensor is applied to the tip of the finger or earlobe. The oximeter transmits light from one side and records the amount of light on the other side, thus determining O_2 saturation.

O_2 content

This is a calculated number that represents the amount of O_2 in the blood. The formula for calculation is:

$$O_2 \text{ content} = O_2 \text{ saturation} \times \text{Hgb} \times 1.34 + Po_2 \times 0.003$$

Nearly all O_2 in the blood is bound to hemoglobin. O_2 content decreases with the same diseases that diminish Po_2.

Base excess/deficit

This number is calculated by the blood gas machine using the pH, Pco_2, and the hematocrit. It represents the amount of buffering anions in the blood. HCO_3 is the largest of these. Others include hemoglobin, proteins, and phosphates. Base excess is a way to take all these anions into account when determining acid/base treatment based on the *metabolic* component. Negative base excess (deficit) indicates a metabolic acidosis (e.g., lactic acidosis). A positive base excess indicates metabolic alkalosis or compensation to prolonged respiratory acidosis.

Contraindications

- Patients with negative Allen test indicating that there is no ulnar artery
- Patients with AV fistula proximal to the site of proposed access
- Patients with severe coagulopathy

Potential complications

- Occlusion of the artery used for access
- Penetration of other important structures anatomically juxtaposed to the artery (e.g., nerve)

Interfering factors

- O_2 saturation can be falsely increased with the inhalation of carbon monoxide.
- Respiration can be inhibited by the use of sedative hypnotics or narcotics.

Procedure and patient care

Before

PT Explain the procedure to the patient.

PT Tell the patient that the arterial puncture is associated with more discomfort than a venous puncture.

- Notify the laboratory before drawing ABGs so that the necessary equipment can be calibrated before the blood sample arrives.
- Perform the Allen test to assess collateral circulation.
- To perform the Allen test, make the patient's hand blanch by obliterating both the radial and the ulnar pulses, and then release the pressure over the ulnar artery only. If flow through the ulnar artery is good, flushing will be seen immediately. The Allen test is then positive, and the radial artery can be used for puncture.
- If the Allen test is negative (no flushing), repeat it on the other arm.
- If both arms give a negative result, choose another artery for puncture.
- Note that the Allen test ensures collateral circulation to the hand if thrombosis of the radial artery should follow the puncture.

During

- Note that arterial blood can be obtained from any area of the body where strong pulses are palpable, usually from the radial, brachial, or femoral artery.
- Cleanse the arterial site.
- Consider applying 0.5 ml of lidocaine in the skin overlying the proposed access site.
- Attach a 20-gauge needle to a syringe containing approximately 0.2 ml of heparin.
- After drawing 3 to 5 ml of blood, remove the needle and apply pressure to the arterial site for 3 to 5 minutes.
- Expel any air bubbles in the syringe.
- Cap the syringe and gently rotate to mix the blood and heparin.
- Indicate on the laboratory slip if the patient is receiving oxygen therapy or is attached to a ventilator.
- Note that an arterial puncture is performed by laboratory technicians, respiratory-inhalation therapists, nurses, or physicians in approximately 10 minutes.

After

- Place the arterial blood on ice and immediately take it to the chemistry laboratory for analysis.
- Apply pressure or a pressure dressing to the arterial puncture site for 3 to 5 minutes to avoid hematoma formation.
- Assess the puncture site for bleeding. Remember that an artery rather than a vein has been stuck.
- If the patient has an abnormal clotting time or is taking anticoagulants, apply pressure for a longer period (approximately 15 minutes).

Abnormal findings

▲ **Increased pH
   (alkalosis)**

Metabolic alkalosis
Hypokalemia
Hypochloremia
Chronic and high volume
   gastric suction
Chronic vomiting
Aldosteronism
Mercurial diuretics

Respiratory alkalosis
Chronic heart failure
Cystic fibrosis
Carbon monoxide poisoning
Pulmonary emboli
Shock
Acute severe pulmonary
   diseases
Anxiety neuroses
Pain
Pregnancy

▼ **Decreased pH
   (acidosis)**

Metabolic acidosis
Ketoacidosis
Lactic acidosis
Severe diarrhea
Renal failure

Respiratory acidosis
Respiratory failure

▲ **Increased P_{CO_2}**

Chronic obstructive
   pulmonary disease
   (COPD) (bronchitis,
   emphysema)
Oversedation
Head trauma
Overoxygenation in a
   patient with COPD
Pickwickian syndrome

▼ **Decreased P_{CO_2}**

Hypoxemia
Pulmonary emboli
Anxiety
Pain
Pregnancy

▲ **Increased P_{O_2}, increased O_2 content**

Polycythemia
Increased inspired O_2
Hyperventilation

▼ **Decreased P_{O_2}, decreased O_2 content**

Anemias
Mucus plug
Bronchospasm
Atelectasis
Pneumothorax
Pulmonary edema
Adult respiratory
  distress syndrome
Restrictive lung disease
Atrial or ventricular
  cardiac septal defects
Emboli
Inadequate O_2 in
  inspired air
  (suffocation)
Severe hypoventilation
  (e.g., oversedation,
  neurologic
  somnolence)

▲ **Increased HCO_3**

Chronic vomiting
Chronic high volume
  gastric suction
Aldosteronism
Use of mercurial diuretics
COPD

▼ **Decreased HCO_3**

Chronic and severe
  diarrhea
Chronic use of loop
  diuretics
Starvation
Diabetic ketoacidosis
Acute renal failure

notes

arteriography (Angiography)

Type of test   X-ray with contrast dye

Normal findings   Normal arterial vasculature

Test explanation and related physiology

With the injection of radiopaque contrast material into arteries, blood vessels can be visualized to determine arterial anatomy, vascular disease, or neoplasms. With a catheter usually placed through the femoral artery and into the desired artery, radiopaque contrast is rapidly injected while x-ray films are obtained. Blood flow dynamics, abnormal blood vessels, vascular anomalies, normal and abnormal vascular anatomy, and tumors are easily seen. With the use of *digital subtraction angiography (DSA)*, bony structures can be obliterated from the picture.

DSA is a sophisticated type of computerized fluoroscopy that, when used with arterial angiography, can better visualize the arteries of the body, especially the carotid and cerebral arteries. It is especially useful when adjacent bone inhibits visualization of the blood vessel to be evaluated. For DSA an image (mask) is made of the area of clinical interest and stored in the computer program. After intraarterial injection of contrast material, subsequent images are made. The computer then subtracts the preinjection "mask" image from the postinjection image. This removes all the undesired images (e.g., bone) and leaves an arterial image of high contrast and quality.

Although nearly all major blood vessels can be visualized through the technique of arteriography, the kidneys, adrenal glands, brain, and abdominal aorta (with lower extremities) are most usually visualized. Coronary arteriography is described under cardiac catheterization (see p. 232).

Renal angiography permits evaluation of blood flow dynamics, demonstration of abnormal blood vessels, and differentiation of a vascular renal cyst from hypervascular renal cancers. Arteriosclerotic narrowing (stenosis) of the renal artery is best demonstrated with this study. The angiographic location of the stenotic area is helpful for the vascular surgeon considering repair. Complete transection of the renal artery by blunt or penetrating trauma can also be seen as total vascular obstruction. Highly vascular renal cancers can produce a "blush" of contrast material during angiography.

The adrenal gland and its arterial system can also be visualized by *adrenal arteriography*. Both benign and malignant tumors of the adrenal gland can be detected easily by this technique. Bilateral adrenal hyperplasia can also be identified.

Cerebral angiography provides radiographic visualization of the cerebral vascular system with the injection of radiopaque dye into the carotid or vertebral arteries. Abnormalities of the cerebral circulation such as aneurysms, occlusions, stenosis, or arteriovenous (AV) malformations can be identified by using this procedure. A vascular tumor is seen as a mass containing small, abnormal blood vessels. A nonvascular tumor, abscess, or hematoma appears as a mass distorting the normal vascular contour.

Lower extremity arteriography allows for accurate identification and location of occlusions within the abdominal aorta and lower extremity arteries. After the catheter is placed in the aorta or more selectively into the femoral artery, radiopaque dye is injected. X-ray films are taken in timed sequence to allow radiographic visualization of the arterial system of the lower extremities. Total or near-total occlusion of the flow of dye is seen in arteriosclerotic vascular occlusive disease. Emboli are seen as total occlusions of the artery. Arterial traumas such as lacerations or intimal tears (laceration of the arterial inner lining) likewise appear as total or near-total obstruction of the flow of dye. Aneurysmal dilation of the arteries or its branches also can be seen. Unusual arterial disorders such as Buerger's disease and fibromuscular dysplasia have the classic arterial "beading," which is pathognomonic.

Arterial vascular balloon dilation can be performed if a short segment arterial stenosis is identified. In these instances the wire is placed through the angiocatheter into the area of narrowing. A balloon catheter is inserted over the wire. The dilating balloon is inflated, and the arteriosclerotic plaque is gently and persistently dilated.

Contraindications

- Patients with allergies to shellfish or iodinated dye
- Patients who are uncooperative or agitated
- Patients who are pregnant, unless the benefits outweigh the risks
- Patients with renal disorders, because iodinated contrast is nephrotoxic
- Patients with a bleeding propensity
- Patients with unstable cardiac disorders
- Patients who are dehydrated, because they are especially susceptible to dye-induced renal failure

Potential complications

- Allergic reaction to iodinated dye
- Hemorrhage from the arterial puncture site used for arterial access
- Arterial embolism from dislodgment of an arteriosclerotic plaque
- Soft tissue infection around the puncture site
- Renal failure, especially in elderly patients who are chronically dehydrated or have a mild degree of renal failure
- Dissection of the intimal lining of the artery causing complete or partial arterial occlusion
- Pseudoaneurysm development as a result of failure of the puncture site to seal
- With adrenal angiography, fatal hypertensive crisis may occur in patients with pheochromocytoma. Propranolol (Inderal), a beta-adrenergic blocker, and phenoxybenzamine (Dibenzyline), an alpha-adrenergic blocker, are given for several days before the study to avoid precipitation of a malignant hypertensive episode
- In adrenal angiography, hemorrhage of the adrenal gland, which may lead to adrenal insufficiency
- Hypoglycemia or acidosis may occur in patients who are taking metformin (Glucophage) and receive iodine dye.

Procedure and patient care

Before

PT Explain the procedure to the patient. Allay any fears and allow the patient to verbalize concerns.
- Ensure that written and informed consent for this procedure is in the patient's chart.
PT Inform the patient that a warm flush may be felt when the dye is injected.
- Assess the possibility of allergies to iodinated dye.
- Determine if the patient has been taking anticoagulants.
- Keep the patient NPO for 2 to 8 hours before testing.
- Mark the site of the patient's peripheral pulses with a pen before arterial catheterization. This will permit assessment of the peripheral pulses after the procedure.
- If the patient does not have peripheral pulses before arteriography, document that fact so that arterial occlusion will not be suspected on the postangiogram assessment.

- Administer preprocedure medications as ordered.
- If the patient is suspected of having pheochromocytoma, administer propranolol and phenoxybenzamine as ordered to prevent a potentially fatal hypertensive episode.
- Ensure that the appropriate coagulation studies have been performed and are normal.
- For cerebral angiograms, perform a baseline neurologic assessment to compare subsequent assessments. This is to potentially diagnose any strokes that may be precipitated by cerebral arteriography.
- Remove all valuables and dental prostheses.
- **PT** Instruct the patient to void before the study because the iodinated dye can act as an osmotic diuretic.
- **PT** Inform the patient that bladder distention may cause some discomfort during the study.

During

- Note the following preprocedure steps:
  1. The patient may be sedated before being taken to the angiography room, which is usually within the radiology department.
  2. The patient is placed on the x-ray table in the supine position.
  3. If the femoral artery is to be used, the groin is shaved, prepared, and draped in a sterile manner.
  4. The femoral artery is cannulated, and a wire is threaded up that artery and into or near the opening of the desired artery to be examined (Figure 4).
  5. A catheter is then placed over the wire. The wire and catheter are both placed under fluoroscopic visualization. Because the catheter and wire have a curled tip at the end, both can be manipulated directly into the artery to be studied. The wire is removed.
  6. Through the catheter, iodinated contrast material is injected by the use of an automated injector at a preset, controlled rate. This occurs over several seconds.
  7. Serial x-ray films are taken in timed sequence to show the arterial injection, and subsequent x-ray films are taken to show the venous phase of the injection.
- Note that this procedure is usually performed by an angiographer (radiologist) in approximately 1 to 2 hours.

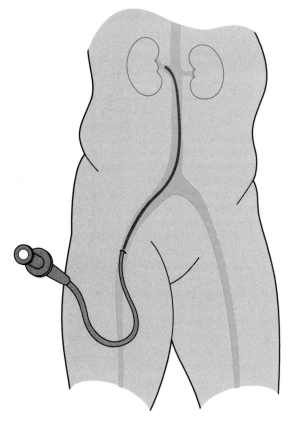

Figure 4 Catheter insertion for renal angiogram. The angiocatheter with attached syringe is inserted into the femoral artery and advanced into the renal artery.

PT During the dye injection, remind the patient that an intense, burning flush may be felt throughout the body but lasts only a few seconds.
PT Tell the patient that the most significant discomfort is the groin puncture necessary for arterial access.
PT Remind the patient of the discomfort of lying on a hard x-ray table for a long period.
- During adrenal angiography, monitor blood pressure for evidence of malignant hypertensive storm.

After

- X-ray studies are completed, the catheter is removed, and a pressure dressing is applied to the puncture site.
- Monitor the patient's vital signs for indications of hemorrhage.
- Assess the peripheral arterial pulse in the extremity used for vascular access and compare it with the preprocedure baseline values.
- Perform a neurologic assessment for any signs of catheter-induced embolic stroke syndrome if cerebral arteriography is performed.
- Observe the arterial puncture site frequently for signs of bleeding or hematoma.
- Maintain pressure at the puncture site with a 1- to 2-1b sandbag or an IV bag.
- Keep the patient on bed rest for about 8 hours after the procedure to allow for complete sealing of the arterial puncture site.
- Assess the patient's extremities for signs of loss of blood supply (e.g., loss of pulses, numbness, pallor, tingling, pain, loss of sensory/motor function).
- Note and compare the color and temperature of the extremity with that of the uninvolved extremity.
- Administer mild analgesics for minor discomfort at the arterial puncture site.
- Notify the physician if the patient has severe, continuous pain.
- **PT** Instruct the patient to drink fluids to prevent dehydration caused by the diuretic action of the dye.
- Evaluate the patient for delayed allergic reaction to the dye.

🏠 Home care responsibilities

- Check the arterial puncture site for bleeding and hematoma.
- Monitor the vital signs for evidence of bleeding (increased pulse and decreased BP).
- Instruct the patient to report any signs of numbness, tingling, pain, or loss of function in the involved extremity.
- Encourage the patient to drink fluids to prevent dehydration.

Abnormal findings

Adrenal angiography

Pheochromocytoma
Adrenal adenoma
Adrenal carcinoma
Bilateral adrenal hyperplasia

Arteriography of the lower extremity

Arteriosclerotic occlusion
Embolus occlusion
Primary arterial diseases (e.g., fibromuscular dysplasia,
  Buerger's disease)
Aneurysm
Aberrant arterial anatomy
Tumor neovascularity
Neoplastic arterial compression

Brain arteriography

Vascular aneurysm
Vascular occlusion or stenosis
Vascular AV malformations
Tumor
Abscess
Hematoma
Cerebral vascular thrombosis

Kidney arteriography

Anatomic aberrant blood vessels
Renal cyst
Renal solid tumor
Atherosclerotic narrowing of the renal artery
Renal vascular causes of hypertension

notes

arthrocentesis with synovial fluid analysis (Synovial fluid analysis, Joint aspiration)

Type of test Fluid analysis

Normal findings

Synovial fluid: clear and straw colored with few white blood cells (WBCs), no crystals, and a good mucin clot

Chemical test values (e.g., glucose determination): approximating those found in the bloodstream

Test explanation and related physiology

Arthrocentesis is performed to establish the diagnosis of joint infection, arthritis, crystal-induced arthritis (gout and pseudo-gout), synovitis, or neoplasms involving the joint. This procedure is also used to identify the cause of joint inflammation or effusion, to monitor chronic arthritic diseases, and to inject antiinflammatory medications (usually corticosteroids) into a joint space.

Arthrocentesis is performed by inserting a sterile needle into the joint space of the involved joint to obtain synovial fluid for analysis. Synovial fluid is a liquid found in small amounts within the joints. Aspiration (withdrawal of the fluid) may be performed on any major joint such as the knee, shoulder, hip, elbow, wrist, or ankle.

The fluid sample is examined microscopically and chemically. A culture of the fluid is usually performed. Normal joint fluid is clear, straw colored, and quite viscous due to the hyaluronic acid, which acts as a lubricant. Viscosity is reduced in patients with inflammatory arthritis. Viscosity can be roughly estimated by forcing some synovial fluid from a syringe. Fluid of high viscosity forms a "string" several inches long; fluid of low viscosity drips similar to water.

The synovial fluid glucose value is usually within 10 mg/dl of the serum glucose value. For proper interpretation, the synovial fluid glucose and serum glucose samples should be drawn simultaneously after the patient has fasted for 6 hours. The synovial fluid glucose level falls with increasing severity of inflammation. Although lowest in septic arthritis (the synovial fluid glucose value may be less than 50% of the serum glucose value), a low synovial glucose level also may be seen in patients with rheumatoid arthritis. The synovial fluid is also tested for protein, uric acid, and lactate levels. Increased uric acid levels would indicate gout. Increased protein and lactate levels indicate bacterial infection.

Cell counts are also performed on the synovial fluid. Normally the joint fluid contains less than 200 WBCs/mm³ and 2000 red blood cells (RBCs)/μl. An increased WBC count with a high percentage of neutrophils (over 75%) supports the diagnosis of acute bacterial infectious arthritis. Leukocytes can also occur in other conditions such as acute gouty arthritis and rheumatoid arthritis. The differential white cell count, however, will indicate monocytosis or lymphocytosis with these later-mentioned diseases.

Bacterial and fungal cultures are usually requested and performed when infection is suspected. Gonococci are a cause of joint infection. Smears for acid-fast stains for tubercle bacilli are also performed on the synovial fluid.

The synovial fluid is also analyzed for complement levels (see p. 292). Complement levels are decreased in patients with systemic lupus erythematosus, rheumatoid arthritis, or other immunologic arthritis. These decreased joint complement levels are caused by consumption of the complement induced by the antigen-antibody immune complexes within the joint cavity.

Synovial fluid is also examined under polarized light for the presence of crystals, which permits differential diagnosis between gout and pseudogout (the calcium pyrophosphate dihydrate crystals of pseudogout are birefringent [blue on red background] when examined with a polarized light microscope). Cholesterol crystals occur in rheumatoid arthritis.

Contraindications

- Patients with skin or wound infections in the area of the needle puncture, because of the risk of sepsis

Potential complications

- Joint infection
- Hemorrhage in the joint area

Procedure and patient care

Before

PT Explain the procedure to the patient.
PT Obtain an informed consent if this is the institution's policy.
- Keep the patient NPO after midnight on the day of the test. This is done to prevent alterations of the chemical determinations (e.g., glucose) that may be performed with the study. However, this study may be done more conveniently in a physician's office without the patient fasting.

During

- Have the patient lie on his or her back with the joint fully extended.
- Note the following procedural steps:
  1. The skin is locally anesthetized to minimize pain.
  2. The area is aseptically cleansed, and a needle is inserted through the skin and into the joint space.
  3. Fluid is obtained for analysis. The joint area sometimes may be wrapped with an elastic bandage to compress free fluid within a certain area, thereby ensuring maximal collection of fluid.
  4. If a corticosteroid is to be administered, a syringe containing the steroid preparation is attached to the needle, and the drug is injected.
  5. The needle is removed, and a pressure dressing may be applied to the site.
  6. Sometimes a peripheral venous blood sample is taken to compare chemical tests on the blood with chemical studies on the synovial fluid.
- Note that a physician performs this procedure in an office or at the patient's bedside in approximately 10 minutes.
- PT Tell the patient that the only discomfort associated with this test is the injection of the local anesthetic.
- Be aware that joint-space pain may worsen after fluid aspiration, especially in patients with acute arthritis.

After

- Assess the joint for any pain, fever, or swelling, which may indicate infection.
- Apply ice to decrease pain and swelling.
- Keep a pressure dressing on the joint to avoid recollection of joint fluid or development of a hematoma.
- PT Tell the patient to avoid strenuous use of the joint for the next several days.

🏠 **Home care responsibilities**

- Teach the patient to walk on crutches.
- Educate the patient to observe for signs of bleeding into the joint (significant swelling, increasing pain, or joint weakness).
- Teach the patient to observe for signs of infection of the joint (fever, swelling, redness about the joint, and increasing pain).
- Educate the patient to observe for signs of phlebitis. This is not uncommon in a person immobilized by joint pain. The involved leg may get swollen, painful, and edematous.
- Instruct the patient not to drive until approved by the physician.
- Ice should be applied at home to minimize the normal swelling that may occur around the involved joint.

Abnormal findings

Infection
Degenerative arthritis (osteoarthritis)
Synovitis
Neoplasm
Joint effusion
Septic arthritis
Systemic lupus erythematosus
Rheumatoid arthritis
Gout
Pseudogout

notes

arthrography (Arthrogram)

Type of test X-ray with contrast dye

Normal findings Normal bursae, menisci, ligaments, and articular cartilage of the joint

Test explanation and related physiology

Arthrography affords radiographic visualization of a joint after the injection of a radiopaque substance, air, or both into the joint cavity to outline the soft tissue structures not normally seen on routine x-ray films. Bones, meniscus, cartilage, and ligaments are clearly visualized with this procedure. Joint derangement and synovial cysts are also diagnosed with arthrography.

Arthrography is usually performed on the knee and shoulder joints; however, it can also be done on other joints such as the ankles, hips, wrists, or temporomandibular joint. This procedure is usually performed on patients with persistent, unexplained joint pain, swelling, or dysfunction.

Contraindications

- Patients who are pregnant, unless the benefits outweigh the risks
- Patients with active arthritis
- Patients with joint infection

Potential complications

- Infection at the puncture site
- Allergic reaction to the iodinated dye
  This rarely occurs because the dye is not administered intravenously.

Procedure and patient care

Before

PT Explain the procedure to the patient.
- Obtain an informed consent if required by the institution.
PT Tell the patient that neither fasting nor sedation is required.

During

- Place the patient in the supine position on the examining table.
- Note the following procedural steps:
  1. The skin overlying the joint is aseptically cleansed and anesthetized.
  2. A needle is inserted into the joint space.

3. Fluid is aspirated to minimize dilution of the contrast material, which could diminish the quality of the x-ray films.
4. With the needle still in place, the aspirating syringe is removed and a syringe containing dye is inserted.
5. The contrast agent is injected.
6. The needle is removed, and the joint is manipulated to help distribute the contrast material. The patient may be asked to walk several steps or to pass the joint through range-of-motion exercises.
7. X-ray films are taken with the joint held in various positions.

- Note that the physician performs this procedure in approximately 30 minutes.
- **PT** Tell the patient that pressure or a tingling sensation may be felt as the contrast medium is injected and that some discomfort in the joint may occur.

After

- Assess the joint for swelling after the test. Apply ice if necessary.
- Administer a mild analgesic (e.g., aspirin, acetaminophen) if the patient has mild discomfort.
- Report any increase in pain or swelling to the physician.
- **PT** Inform the patient that crepitant noises (crackling tissue-paper sounds) in the joint may be heard after the test. These symptoms are normal and usually disappear in 1 to 2 days. The sounds are caused by the air injected into the joint during the procedure.

Abnormal findings

Joint derangement
Cysts
Arthritis
Fractured knee meniscus
Muscle tendon tears
Cartilaginous diseases (e.g., chondromalacia)
Ligamentous injury
Synovial tumor
Synovitis

arthroscopy

Type of test Endoscopy

Normal findings Normal ligaments, menisci, and articular surfaces of the joint

Test explanation and related physiology

Arthroscopy is an endoscopic procedure that allows examination of a joint interior with a specially designed endoscope. Arthroscopy is a highly accurate test because it allows direct visualization of an anatomic site (Figure 5). Although this technique can visualize many joints of the body, it is most often used to evaluate the knee for meniscus cartilage or ligament injury. It is also used in the differential diagnosis of acute and chronic disorders of the knee (e.g., arthritic inflammation vs. injury).

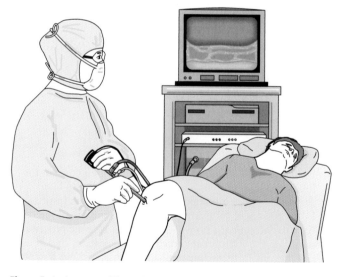

Figure 5 Arthroscopy. The arthroscope is placed within the joint space of the knee. Video arthroscopy requires a water source to distend the joint space, a light source to see the contents of the joint, and a television monitor to project the image. Other trocars are used for access of the joint space for other operative instruments.

Physicians can now perform corrective surgery on the knee through the endoscope. Meniscus removal, spur removal, ligamentous repair, and biopsy are but a few of the procedures that are done through the arthroscope. Arthroscopy provides a safe, convenient alternative to open surgery (arthrotomy) because surgery is done through small trocars that are placed into the joint. Surgical maneuvers are carried out under direct vision of the camera, which is attached to the arthroscope. Because a large incision is avoided, recovery is faster and more comfortable.

Arthroscopy is also used to monitor the progression of disease and the effectiveness of therapy. Visual findings may be recorded by attaching a video camera to the arthroscope. Joints that can be evaluated by the arthroscope include the tarsal, ankle, knee, hip, carpal, wrist, shoulder, and temporomandibular joints.

Contraindications

- Patients with ankylosis
- Patients with local skin or wound infections
- Patients who have recently had an arthrogram

Potential complications

- Infection
- Hemarthrosis
- Swelling
- Thrombophlebitis
- Joint injury
- Synovial rupture

Procedure and patient care

Before

PT Explain the procedure to the patient.
- Ensure that the physician has obtained written consent for this procedure.
- Follow the routine preoperative procedure of the institution.
- Keep the patient NPO after midnight on the day of the test.
PT Instruct the patient who will use crutches after the procedure regarding the appropriate crutch gait. The patient should use crutches after arthroscopy until able to walk without limping.
- Shave the hair in the area 6 inches above and below the joint before the test (as ordered).

During

- Place the patient on his or her back on an operating room table.

- Note the following procedural steps:
  1. Local or general anesthesia is used.
  2. The leg is carefully scrubbed, elevated, and wrapped with an elastic bandage from the toes to the lower thigh to drain as much blood from the leg as possible.
  3. A tourniquet is placed on the patient's leg. If the tourniquet is not used, a fluid solution may be instilled into the patient's knee immediately before insertion of the arthroscope to distend the knee and help reduce bleeding.
  4. The foot of the table is lowered so that the patient's knee is at a 45-degree angle.
  5. A small incision is made in the skin around the knee.
  6. The arthroscope (a lighted instrument) is inserted into the joint space to visualize the inside of the knee joint. In the past the surgeon looked directly into the scope. More recently, a video camera is attached to the scope, and the image is projected on a TV monitor.
  7. Although the entire joint can be viewed from one puncture site, additional punctures for better visualization are often necessary.
  8. After the area is examined, biopsy or appropriate surgery can be performed.
  9. Before removing the arthroscope, the joint is irrigated. Pressure is then applied to the knee to remove the irrigating solution.
  10. After a few stitches are placed into the skin, a pressure dressing is applied over the incision site.
- Note that this procedure is performed in the operating room by an orthopedic surgeon in approximately 15 to 30 minutes.
- **PT** Tell the patient receiving local anesthesia that there may be transient discomfort from the injection of the local anesthetic and the pressure of the tourniquet on the leg.
- **PT** Inform the patient that a thumping sensation may be felt as the arthroscope is inserted into the joint and that the joint may be painful for several days.

After
- Assess the patient's neurologic and circulatory status.
- Assess vital signs and observe the patient for signs of infection, including fever, swelling, increased pain, and redness or drainage at the incision site.

PT Instruct the patient to elevate the knee when sitting and to avoid overbending the knee so that swelling is minimized.

PT Inform the patient that he or she can usually walk with the assistance of crutches; however, this depends on the extent of the procedure and the physician's protocol.

PT Tell the patient to minimize use of the joint for several days.

- Examine the incision site for bleeding.
- Apply ice to reduce pain and swelling.

PT Inform the patient that the sutures will be removed in approximately 7 to 10 days.

🏠 Home care responsibilities

- Teach the patient to walk on crutches.
- Educate the patient to observe for signs of bleeding into the joint (significant swelling, increasing pain, or joint weakness).
- Teach the patient to observe for signs of infection of the joint (fever, swelling, redness about the joint, and increasing pain).
- Educate the patient to observe for signs of phlebitis. This is not uncommon in a person immobilized by joint pain. The involved leg may become swollen, painful, and edematous.
- Instruct the patient not to drive until approved by the physician.
- Ice should be applied at home to minimize the normal swelling that may occur around the involved joint.

Abnormal findings

Torn cartilage	Synovitis
Torn ligament	Osteoarthritis
Patellar disease	Rheumatoid arthritis
Patellar fracture	Degenerative arthritis
Chondromalacia	Meniscal disease
Osteochondritis dissecans	Osteochondromatosis
Cyst (e.g., Baker's)	Trapped synovium

aspartate aminotransferase (AST; formerly called Serum glutamic-oxaloacetic transaminase [SGOT])

Type of test Blood

Normal findings

Adult: 0-35 units/L, or 0-0.58 µKat/L (SI units); females tend
   to have slightly lower values than males
Elderly: values slightly higher than adult
Child: values similar to adult
Newborn/infant: 15-60 units/L

Test explanation and related physiology

   This test is used in the evaluation of suspected coronary occlusive heart disease or suspected hepatocellular diseases. When disease or injury affects the cells of these tissues, the cells lyse. The AST is released and picked up by the blood, and the serum level rises. The amount of AST elevation is directly related to the number of cells affected by the disease or injury. Further, the elevation depends on the time after the injury that the blood is drawn. AST is cleared from the blood in a few days. Serum AST levels become elevated 8 hours after cell injury, peak at 24 to 36 hours, and return to normal in 3 to 7 days. If the cellular injury is chronic, levels will be persistently elevated.

   AST was formerly known as *SGOT*. The AST/SGOT enzyme was once tested in the cardiac enzyme series for evaluation of myocardial infarction (MI). The AST has been replaced by newer cardiac markers.

   Because AST also exists within the liver cells, diseases that affect the hepatocyte cause elevated levels of this enzyme. In acute hepatitis AST levels can rise 20 times the normal value. In acute extrahepatic obstruction (e.g., gallstone), AST levels quickly rise to 10 times the normal and swiftly fall. In cirrhotic patients the level of AST depends on the amount of active inflammation.

   Serum AST levels are often compared with alanine aminotransferase (ALT, see p. 28) levels. The AST/ALT ratio is usually greater than 1.0 in patients with alcoholic cirrhosis, liver congestion, and metastatic tumor of the liver. Ratios less than 1.0 may be seen in patients with acute hepatitis, viral hepatitis, or infectious mononucleosis. The ratio is less accurate if AST levels exceed 10 times normal.

Patients with acute pancreatitis, acute renal diseases, musculoskeletal diseases, or trauma may have a transient rise in serum AST. Patients with red blood cell abnormalities such as acute hemolytic anemia and severe burns also can have elevations of this enzyme.

Interfering factors

- Exercise may cause increased levels.
- Pyridoxine deficiency (beriberi or pregnancy), severe long-standing liver disease, uremia, or diabetic ketoacidosis may cause decreased levels.
- Drugs that may cause *increased* levels include antihypertensives, cholinergic agents, coumarin-type anticoagulants, digitalis preparations, erythromycin, isoniazid, methyldopa, oral contraceptives, opiates, salicylates, hepatotoxic medications, and verapamil.

Procedure and patient care

Before

- **PT** Explain the procedure to the patient.
- If possible, avoid giving the patient any IM injection because increased enzyme levels may result.
- If possible, hold drugs that could interfere with test results for 12 hours before the test.

During

- Collect a venous sample of blood in a red-top tube.
- Rotate the venipuncture site.
- Avoid hemolysis.
- Indicate on the laboratory slip any drugs that may cause false-positive results.
- Record the time and date of any IM injection given.
- Record the exact time and date when the blood test is performed. This aids in the interpretation of the temporal pattern of enzyme elevations.

After

- Apply pressure to the venipuncture site.

Abnormal findings

▲ Increased levels

Heart diseases
Myocardial infarction
Cardiac operations
Cardiac catheterization and
  angioplasty
Liver diseases
Hepatitis
Hepatic cirrhosis
Drug-induced liver injury
Hepatic metastasis
Hepatic necrosis (initial
  stages only)
Hepatic surgery
Infectious mononucleosis
  with hepatitis
Hepatic infiltrative process
  (e.g., tumor)
Skeletal muscle diseases
Skeletal muscle trauma
Recent noncardiac surgery
Multiple traumas
Severe, deep burns
Progressive muscular
  dystrophy
Recent convulsions
Heat stroke
Primary muscle diseases
  (e.g., myopathy, myositis)
Other diseases
Acute hemolytic anemia
Acute pancreatitis

▼ Decreased values

Acute renal disease
Beriberi
Diabetic ketoacidosis
Pregnancy
Chronic renal dialysis

notes

barium enema (BE, Lower GI series)

Type of test X-ray with contrast dye

Normal findings

Normal filling, contour, patency, and positioning of barium in the colon
Normal filling of the appendix and terminal ileum

Test explanation and related physiology

The BE study consists of a series of x-ray films visualizing the colon. It is used to demonstrate the presence and location of polyps, tumors, and diverticula. Anatomic abnormalities (e.g., malrotation) also can be detected. Therapeutically the BE may be used to reduce nonstrangulated ileocolic intussusception in children. Bleeding from diverticula can cease with barium enema.

The BE is occasionally used to assess filling of the appendix. When the clinical picture suggests possible appendicitis, failure of the appendix to fill with barium may support the diagnosis. Although the colon is the main organ evaluated by a BE, reflux of barium into the terminal ileum also allows adequate visualization of the distal part of the small intestine. Diseases that affect the terminal ileum, especially Crohn's disease (regional enteritis), can be identified. Inflammatory bowel disease involving the colon can be detected with BE. Fistulas involving the colon can be demonstrated by BE.

In many instances, air is insufflated into the colon after the instillation of barium. This provides an air contrast to the barium. With air contrast, the colonic mucosa can be much more accurately visualized. This is called an *air-contrast barium enema*. It is used especially when small polyps are suspected. The accuracy of the regular BE in detecting small colonic tumors is approximately 60%; however, the accuracy of an air-contrast BE in detecting small colonic tumors exceeds 85%.

Contraindications

- Patients suspected of a perforation of the colon
  In these patients, diatrizoate (Gastrografin), a water-soluble contrast medium, is used.
- Patients who are unable to cooperate
  This test requires the patient to hold the barium in the rectum and colon. This is especially difficult for elderly patients.

- Patients with megacolon
  Barium may worsen the disease.

Potential complications

B

- Colonic perforation, especially when the colon is weakened by inflammation, tumor, or infection
- Barium fecal impaction

Interfering factors

- Barium within the abdomen from previous barium tests
- Significant residual stool within the colon
  This precludes adequate visualization of the entire bowel wall. Stool may be confused for polyps.
- Spasm of the colon
  Spasm can mimic the radiographic signs of a cancer. The use of IV glucagon minimizes spasm.

Procedure and patient care

Before

PT Explain the procedure to the patient. Encourage the patient to verbalize questions and fears.

- Assist the patient with the bowel preparation, which varies among institutions. In elderly patients this preparation can be exhausting and may even cause severe dehydration. A typical preparation for most adults would include the following actions.

Day before examination

- Give the patient clear liquids for lunch and supper (no dairy products).

PT Instruct the patient to drink one glass of water or clear fluid every hour for 8 to 10 hours.

- Administer a cathartic (10 ounces of magnesium citrate) or X-Prep (extract of senna fruit) at 2 PM. In children lesser volumes may be used.
- Administer three 5-mg bisacodyl (Dulcolax) tablets at 7 PM.
- A pediatric Fleet enema the night before testing and repeated 3 hours before testing may be adequate prep for an infant.
- Keep the patient NPO after midnight the day of the test.

Day of examination

- Keep the patient NPO.
- Administer a bisacodyl suppository at 6 AM and/or a cleansing enema.

- Note that pediatric patients will have individualized bowel preparations.
- Note that special preparations will be ordered for patients with an ileostomy or colostomy.
- Determine whether the bowel is adequately cleansed. When the fecal return is similar to clear water, preparation is adequate; if large, solid fecal waste is still being evacuated, preparation is inadequate. Notify the radiologist, who may want to extend the bowel preparation.

PT Suggest that the patient take reading material to the x-ray department to occupy the time while expelling the barium.

During

- Note the following procedural steps:
    1. The test begins with placement of a balloon rectal catheter.
    2. The balloon on the catheter is inflated tightly against the anal sphincter to hold the barium within the colon.
    3. The patient is asked to roll in the lateral, supine, and prone positions.
    4. The barium is dripped into the rectum by gravity. The colon of the young child is not able to tolerate the volume and pressure of instillation of barium that an adult can. Both volume and pressure should be reduced.
    5. The barium flow is monitored fluoroscopically.
    6. The colon is thoroughly examined as the barium flow progresses through the large colon and into the terminal ileum.
    7. The barium is drained out.
    8. If an air-contrast BE has been ordered, air is insufflated into the large bowel.
    9. The patient is asked to expel the barium, and a postevacuation x-ray film is taken.
    10. The standard procedure for administering the barium through a colostomy is to instill the contrast medium through an irrigation cone placed in the stoma. When the x-ray series is completed, the barium is allowed to be expelled from the stoma. A gentle stream of clean water for irrigation is helpful in expelling residual barium.
- Note that this test is usually performed in the radiology department by a radiologist in approximately 45 minutes.

PT Inform the patient that abdominal bloating and rectal pressure will occur during instillation of barium.

After

- Ensure that the patient defecates as much barium as possible.
- **PT** Suggest the use of soothing ointments on the anal area to minimize any anorectal pain that may result from the aggressive test preparation.
- **PT** Encourage ingestion of fluids to avoid dehydration caused by the cathartics.
- **PT** Encourage rest after the procedure. The cleansing regimen and BE procedure may be exhausting.
- **PT** Be aware of dehydration and electrolyte abnormalities. Instruct parents to hydrate the child well with electrolyte-containing fluids after the BE.

🏠 Home care responsibilities

- Inform the patient that bowel movements will be white. When all the barium has been expelled, the stool will return to normal color.
- Note that laxatives may be ordered to facilitate evacuation of barium.

Abnormal findings

Malignant tumor

Polyps

Diverticula

Inflammatory bowel diseases (e.g., ulcerative colitis, Crohn's disease)

Colonic stenosis secondary to ischemia, infection, or previous surgery

Perforated colon

Colonic fistula

Appendicitis

Extrinsic compression of the colon from extracolonic tumors (e.g., ovarian)

Extrinsic compression of the colon from an abscess

Malrotation of the gut

Colon volvulus

Intussusception

Hernia

barium swallow

Type of test　X-ray with contrast dye

Normal findings　Normal size, contour, filling, patency, and positioning of the esophagus

Test explanation and related physiology

This barium contrast study provides a more thorough examination of the esophagus than most upper GI series (see p. 949). As in most barium contrast studies, defects in normal filling and narrowing of the barium column indicate tumor, strictures, or extrinsic compression from extraesophageal tumors or an abnormally enlarged heart and great vessels. Varices also can be seen as serpiginous, linear-filling defects. Anatomic abnormalities such as hiatal hernia, Schatzki's rings, and diverticula (Zenker's or epiphrenic) can be seen as well.

In patients with esophageal reflux, the radiologist may identify reflux of the barium from the stomach back into the esophagus. Muscular abnormalities such as achalasia, as well as diffuse esophageal spasm, can be detected easily by a barium swallow. If perforations or rupture of the esophagus are suspected, it is best not to use barium; rather, water-soluble x-ray contrast should be used. If swallowing function is to be evaluated and there is a concern for the potential of aspiration during the test, barium should be used instead of Gastrografin, which can cause a chemical pneumonitis.

Contraindications

- Patients with evidence of bowel obstruction
  Barium may create a stonelike impaction.
- Patients with a perforated viscus
  If barium were to leak, the degree and duration of infection would be much worse. Usually, when perforation is suspected, diatrizoate (Gastrografin), a water-soluble contrast medium, is used.
- Patients whose vital signs are unstable
- Patients who are unable to cooperate for the test

Potential complications

- Barium-induced fecal impaction

Interfering factors

- Food within the esophagus prevents adequate visualization.

B

Procedure and patient care

Before

PT Explain the procedure to the patient.

PT Instruct the patient not to take anything by mouth for at least 8 hours before testing. Usually the patient is kept NPO after midnight on the day of the test.

- Assess the patient's ability to swallow. If the patient tends to aspirate, inform the radiologist.
- Accompany the hospitalized patient to the x-ray department if vital signs are not stable and the test still needs to be performed.

During

- Note the following procedural steps:
  1. The fasting patient is asked to swallow the contrast medium. Usually this is barium sulfate in a milkshake-like substance; however, if a perforated viscus is possible, Gastrografin is used.
  2. As the patient drinks the contrast through a straw, the x-ray table is tilted to the near-erect position.
  3. The patient is asked to roll into various positions so that the entire esophagus can be adequately visualized.
  4. With fluoroscopy, the radiologist follows the barium column through the entire esophagus.
- Note that this procedure is usually performed in the radiology department by a radiologist in approximately 15 to 20 minutes.

PT Tell the patient that no discomfort is associated with this test.

After

PT Inform the patient of the need to evacuate all the barium. Cathartics are recommended. Initially stools are white but should return to normal color with complete evacuation.

🏠 Home care responsibilities

- Inform the patient that initially stools will be white. When all the barium has been expelled, the stool will return to normal color.
- Note that laxatives may be ordered to facilitate evacuation of barium.

Abnormal findings

Total or partial esophageal obstruction
Cancer
Scarred strictures
Lower esophageal rings
Peptic esophageal ulcers
Varices
Peptic or corrosive esophagitis
Achalasia
Esophageal motility disorders (e.g., presbyesophagus, diffuse esophageal spasm)
Diverticula
Chalasia
Extrinsic compression from extraesophageal tumors, cardiomegaly, or aortic aneurysm

notes

Bence Jones protein

B

Type of test Urine

Normal findings No Bence Jones protein present

Test explanation and related physiology

The detection of Bence Jones protein in the urine most commonly indicates multiple myeloma (especially when the urine levels are high). The test is used to detect and monitor the treatment and clinical course of multiple myeloma and other similar diseases.

Bence Jones proteins are light chain portions of immunoglobulins found in 75% of the patients with multiple myeloma. These proteins are made most notably by the plasma cells in these patients. They also may be associated with tumor metastases to the bone, chronic lymphocytic leukemias, lymphoma, macroglobulinemia, and amyloidosis.

Normally there is no protein in the urine because the glomerular spaces do not allow filtration of large molecules such as proteins. Bence Jones proteins, however, are very small and are easily filtrated by the kidney and excreted into the urine. Because the Bence Jones protein is rapidly cleared from the blood by the kidney, it is very difficult to detect in the blood; therefore, only urine is used for this study. Normally urine should contain no Bence Jones proteins.

Routine urine testing for proteins using reagent strips often does not reflect the type or amount of proteins in the urine. In fact, the strip may show a completely negative result, despite large amounts of Bence Jones globulins in the urine. Proteins in the urine are best identified by *protein electrophoresis* of the urine. With this method, the proteins are separated based on size and electrical charge in an electric field when the urine specimen is applied to a gel plate. Once the various proteins are separated, antisera to specific proteins can be added to the gel and specific precipitin arcs can be identified *(immunoelectrophoresis)*. When these arcs are compared to controls, even unusual pathologic proteins can be identified. Greater specificity is gained by applying *immunofixation* techniques to the electrophoresis. See p. 758 (protein electrophoresis).

Interfering factors

- Dilute urine may yield a false-negative result.

Procedure and patient care

Before

PT   Explain the procedure to the patient.

PT   Instruct the patient not to contaminate the urine specimen with toilet paper or stool.

During

PT   Instruct the patient to collect an early morning specimen of at least 50 ml of uncontaminated urine in a container. It may be helpful to know the amount of these proteins excreted over 24 hours. If so, a 24-hour collection is ordered.

After

- Immediately transport the specimen to the laboratory. If it cannot be taken to the laboratory immediately, refrigerate it, because heat-coagulable proteins can decompose, causing a false-positive test.

Abnormal findings

▲   **Increased levels**

     Multiple myeloma (plasmacytoma)

     Various metastatic tumors

     Chronic lymphocytic leukemia

     Amyloidosis

     Lymphoma

     Waldenstrom's macroglobulinemia

notes

beta-$_2$ microglobulin (B$_2$M)

Type of test Blood; urine; fluid analysis

Normal findings
Blood: 1.1-2.4 mg/L
Urine: 0-160 mcg/L
CSF: 0-2.4 mg/L

Test explanation and related physiology

Beta-$_2$ microglobulin (*B$_2$M*) is a protein found on the surface of all cells. It is an HLA major histocompatibility antigen that exists in increased numbers on white blood cells and particularly on lymphatic cells. Production of this protein increases as these cells are produced or destroyed. Therefore, *B$_2$M* is increased in patients with malignancies (especially lymphoma, leukemia, or multiple myeloma) and in patients with chronic severe inflammatory diseases. It is an accurate measurement of tumor disease activity, stage of disease, and prognosis and, as such, is an important tumor marker.

Blood levels are increased in HIV patients and are a measure of the disease activity. Cytomegalovirus infection is also associated with increased blood levels.

B$_2$M is excreted in the glomeruli and is partially reabsorbed back into the blood by the renal tubule. In a patient with renal disease, when blood and urine *B$_2$M* levels are obtained simultaneously, one can differentiate glomerular from tubular disease. In glomerular disease, blood levels are high and urine levels are low. In tubular disease, the blood levels are low and urine levels are high. Blood levels increase early in kidney transplant rejection.

In patients with aminoglycoside toxicity, *B$_2$M* becomes elevated even before creatinine. Increased urine levels are found in patients with kidney disease caused by high exposure to heavy metals, such as cadmium or mercury. Periodic testing is performed on these patients to detect kidney disease at its earliest stage.

Interfering factors
- Results could be affected by recent nuclear imaging because *B$_2$M* testing is performed by radioimmunoassay.
- *B$_2$M* is unstable in acid urine.

Procedure and patient care

Before
PT Explain the procedure to the patient to minimize anxiety.

During
Blood
- Collect approximately 5 ml of venous blood in a red-top tube.

Urine
PT Instruct the patient to begin the 24-hour collection after voiding. Discard the first volded specimen.
- Collect all urine passed by the patient during the next 24 hours.
- Note that it is not necessary to measure each urine specimen.
PT Remind the patient to void before defecating so that the urine is not contaminated by feces.
PT Tell the patient not to put toilet paper in the collection container.
PT Encourage the patient to drink fluids during the 24 hours unless this is contraindicated for medical purposes.
PT Instruct the patient to collect the last specimen as close as possible to the end of the 24-hour period. Add this to the collection.

After
- Apply pressure to the venipuncture site.

Abnormal findings

▲ **Increased urine levels**

Renal tubule disease
Drug-induced renal toxicity
Heavy metal-induced renal disease
Lymphomas, leukemia, myeloma
AIDS

▲ **Increased serum levels**

Lymphomas, leukemia, myeloma
Glomerular renal disease
Renal transplant rejection
Viral infections
Chronic inflammatory processes

bilirubin

B

Type of test Blood

Normal findings

Adult/elderly/child

Total bilirubin: 0.3-1.0 mg/dl or 5.1-17 μmol/L (SI units)

Indirect bilirubin: 0.2-0.8 mg/dl or 3.4-12.0 μmol/L (SI units)

Direct bilirubin: 0.1-0.3 mg/dl or 1.7-5.1 μmol/L (SI units)

Newborn total bilirubin: 1.0-12.0 mg/dl or 17.1-205 μmol/L (SI units)

Test explanation and related physiology

Bile, which is formed in the liver, has many constituents, including bile salts, phospholipids, cholesterol, bicarbonate, water, and bilirubin. Bilirubin metabolism begins with the breakdown of red blood cells (RBCs) in the reticuloendothelial system (Figure 6). Hemoglobin is released from RBCs and broken down to heme and globin molecules. Heme is then catabolized to form biliverdin, which is transformed to bilirubin. This form of bilirubin is called *unconjugated (indirect) bilirubin*. In the liver, indirect bilirubin is conjugated with a glucuronide, resulting in *conjugated (direct) bilirubin*. The conjugated bilirubin is then excreted from the liver cells and into the intrahepatic canaliculi, which eventually lead to the hepatic ducts, the common bile duct, and the bowel.

Jaundice is the discoloration of body tissues caused by abnormally high blood levels of bilirubin. This yellow discoloration is recognized when the total serum bilirubin exceeds 2.5 mg/dl.

Physiologic jaundice of the newborn occurs if the newborn's liver is immature and does not have enough conjugating enzymes. This results in a high circulating blood level of unconjugated bilirubin, which can pass through the blood-brain barrier and deposit in the brain cells of the newborn. This can cause encephalopathy *(kernicterus)*.

Once the jaundice is recognized either clinically or chemically, it is important (for therapy) to differentiate whether it is predominantly caused by unconjugated or conjugated bilirubin. This in turn will help differentiate the etiology of the defect. In general, jaundice caused by hepatocellular dysfunction (e.g., hepatitis) results in elevated levels of unconjugated bilirubin. Jaundice resulting from extrahepatic obstruction of the bile

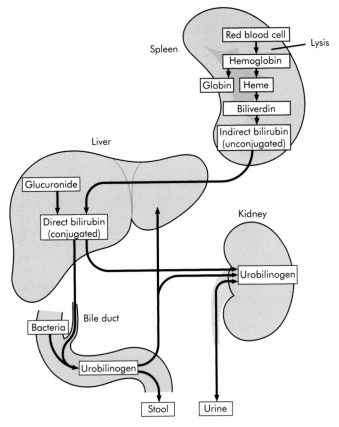

Figure 6 Bilirubin metabolism and excretion. The spleen, liver, kidney, and gastrointestinal tract contribute to this process.

ducts (e.g., gallstones or tumor blocking the bile ducts) results in elevated conjugated bilirubin levels; this type of jaundice usually can be resolved surgically or endoscopically.

The total serum bilirubin level is the sum of the conjugated (direct) and unconjugated (indirect) bilirubin. These are separated out when "fractionation or differentiation" of the total bilirubin to its direct and indirect parts is requested from the laboratory. Normally the unconjugated bilirubin makes up 70% to 85% of the total bilirubin. In patients with jaundice, when more than 50% of the bilirubin is conjugated, it is considered a conjugated hyperbilirubinemia from gallstones, tumor, inflammation, scarring, or obstruction of the extrahepatic ducts. Unconjugated hyperbilirubinemia exists when less than 15% to 20% of the total bilirubin is conjugated. Diseases that typically cause this form of jaundice include accelerated erythrocyte (RBC) hemolysis or hepatitis.

Delta bilirubin is a form of bilirubin that is covalently bound to albumin. It has a longer half-life than the other bilirubins; therefore, it remains elevated during the convalescent phases of hepatic disorders when the conjugated bilirubin would have already returned to normal. It can be derived by the following calculation: delta bilirubin equals total bilirubin minus the sum of the conjugated and unconjugated bilirubin.

Interfering factors

- Blood hemolysis and lipemia can produce erroneous results.
- Drugs that may cause *increased* levels of total bilirubin include allopurinol, anabolic steroids, antibiotics, antimalarials, ascorbic acid, azathioprine, chlorpropamide (Diabinese), cholinergics, codeine, dextran, diuretics, epinephrine, meperidine, methotrexate, methyldopa, monoamine oxidase inhibitors, morphine, nicotinic acid (large doses), oral contraceptives, phenothiazines, quinidine, rifampin, salicylates, steroids, sulfonamides, theophylline, and vitamin A.
- Drugs that may cause *decreased* levels of total bilirubin include barbiturates, caffeine, penicillin, and salicylates (high-dose).

Procedure and patient care

Before

PT Explain the procedure to the patient.
- Note that fasting requirements vary among different laboratories. Some require keeping the patient NPO after midnight the day of the test except for water.

During

- Collect 5 to 7 ml of venous blood in a red-top tube.
- Use a heel puncture for blood collection in infants.
- Prevent hemolysis of blood during phlebotomy.
- Do *not* shake the tube; inaccurate test results may occur.
- Protect the blood sample from bright light. Prolonged exposure (longer than 1 hr) to sunlight or artificial light can reduce bilirubin content.

- List on the laboratory slip any drugs that may affect test results.

After

- Apply pressure to the venipuncture site. Patients who are jaundiced may have prolonged clotting times.

Abnormal findings

▲ **Increased levels of conjugated (direct) bilirubin**

Gallstones
Extrahepatic duct obstruction (tumor, inflammation, gallstone, scarring, or surgical trauma)
Extensive liver metastasis
Cholestasis from drugs
Dubin-Johnson syndrome
Rotor's syndrome

▲ **Increased levels of unconjugated (indirect) bilirubin**

Erythroblastosis fetalis
Hemolytic jaundice
Large-volume blood transfusion
Resolution of a large hematoma
Hepatitis
Sepsis
Neonatal hyperbilirubinemia
Hemolytic anemia
Crigler-Najjar syndrome
Gilbert's syndrome
Pernicious anemia
Cirrhosis
Transfusion reaction
Sickle cell anemia

notes

bioterrorism infectious agents testing

Type of test Various (e.g., blood, urine, stool, tissue culture, sputum, lymph node biopsy, skin)

Normal findings Negative for evidence of infectious agent

Test explanation and related physiology

Infectious agents used in bioterrorism are many and it would be difficult to discuss each possible agent. In this test, we comment on those agents to which humans are most likely to be exposed, either in war or a civilian terrorist attack. Refer to Table 5 for specific information on each agent. All documented cases must be reported to the Department of Public Health.

Botulism infection

The botulinum toxin produced by *Clostridia botulinum* causes this disease. The GI tract usually absorbs this organism after eating undercooked meat or sauces exposed to room temperature for prolonged periods. The organism also can be inhaled by handling these items or by open wound contamination of soil that contains *C. botulinum*.

Blurred vision, dysphagia, and muscle weakness progressing to flaccid paralysis are symptoms of the disease. Symptoms begin 6 to 12 hours after ingestion of the contaminated food or approximately 1 week after wound contamination.

The test used to diagnose this disease involves the identification of the toxin in the blood, stool, or vomitus of the affected individual. The food itself can also be tested. The toxin can be identified by the biologic Mouse Neutralization test. *C. botulinum* can also be cultured in an anaerobic environment from the stool or from contaminated food.

Treatment involves the use of botulinum antitoxin that can be obtained from the Centers for Disease Control and Prevention (CDC). However, this antitoxin presents a risk of "serum sickness" in nearly one fourth of the patients who receive it.

Anthrax

Anthrax is caused by *Bacillus anthracis*, which is a spore-forming gram-positive rod. Gastrointestinal anthrax is contracted by eating undercooked meat. Pulmonary anthrax results from inhalation of spores or tissues from infected animals. Once inhaled, it is always fatal without treatment. Cutaneous anthrax

TABLE 5 Bioterrorism infectious agents testing

Infection/Infectious agent	Site of entry	Sources	Specimen	Tests
Botulism/ *Clostridium botulinum*	GI mucosal surfaces, lung, wound contamination	Undercooked meats, soil, dust	Blood, stool, vomitus, food	Botulinum toxin, mouse bioassay
Anthrax, *Bacillus anthracis*	Lung, GI	Undercooked meats, inhalation of spores from animal products, skin	Sputum, blood, stool, skin vesicle, food, spores	Culture, Gram's stain
Yellow fever/ Hantavirus, Ebola virus, multiple other viruses	Skin bite	Rodent or mosquito bites	Blood, sputum, tissue	Culture, serology for viral antigens
Plague infections/ *Yersinia pestis*	Skin bite	Infected fleas	Blood, sputum, lymph node aspirate	Culture of organism

Brucellosis/ *Brucella abortus, canis,* etc.	GI, lung, wound	Infected meats and milk products	Blood, sputum, food	Culture of organism
Smallpox/ *Variola virus*	Lungs	Respiratory droplets, direct contact, contaminated clothing	Vesicle	Viral culture or viral identification with electron microscopy
Tularemia/ *Francisella tularensis*	Skin, GI tract, lungs	Ingestion of contaminated plants or water	Blood, sputum, stool	Culture of organism

occurs after contact with contaminated meat, wool, hides, or leather from infected animals.

The three forms of the disease are cutaneous, GI, and pulmonary. Symptoms include fever, malaise, fatigue progressing to cutaneous lesions, or pulmonary failure. Symptoms occur about 2 to 6 days after exposure.

Culturing the organism in sheep blood agar makes the diagnosis. Appropriate specimens for culture would be stool, blood, sputum, or the cutaneous vesicle. Treatment for this disease is early institution of antibiotics and supportive care.

Hemorrhagic fever (yellow fever)

This disease complex has many causative viruses, including arenavirus, bunyavirus (including hantavirus), filovirus (including Ebola), and flavivirus. Symptoms include fever, thrombocytopenia, shock, multiorgan failure, lung edema, and jaundice. Symptoms develop 4 to 21 days after a mosquito or rodent bite (depending on the disease). This disease is contagious, and patients with suspicious symptoms should be quarantined.

The diagnosis is determined by clinical evaluation. However, viral cultures with polymerase chain reaction identification, serology, and immunohistochemistry of tissue specimens are possible. There is no specific treatment other than aggressive medical therapy and support of organ failure.

Plague

This disease is caused by *Yersinia pestis* and has three forms: bubonic (enlarged lymph nodes), septicemic (blood-borne), and pneumonic (aerosol). Pneumonic is, by far, the deadliest form of the infection. Symptoms may include fever, chills, weakness, enlarged lymph nodes, or pneumonia and respiratory failure.

The diagnosis is made by culture of the blood, sputum, or lymph node aspirate. This disease complex can be treated with antibiotics when started early in the course of the disease. The risk for bioterrorism is attack or spread by aerosol transmission.

Smallpox

Smallpox is a serious, contagious, and sometimes fatal infectious disease caused by the variola virus (a DNA virus). There is no specific treatment for smallpox disease, and the only prevention is vaccination. There are two clinical forms of smallpox. Variola major is the severe and most common form of smallpox, with a more extensive rash and higher fever. Variola minor is a less common presentation of smallpox and a much less severe disease. The disease was eradicated after a successful worldwide vaccination program. It is very easily spread and is, therefore, considered a potential bioterrorism weapon.

   The first symptoms of smallpox include fever, malaise, head and body aches, and sometimes vomiting. Next a rash occurs in the mouth and then on the skin. This rash proceeds to become pustular. As the pustules dry up and scab, the patient is no longer contagious.

   Viral culture, serology, immunohistochemistry, or electron microscopy can make the diagnosis. The best specimen is the vesicular rash. There is no treatment for the disease, but vaccination is available and is offered to all those at risk for bioterrorism.

Tularemia

   This disease is caused by a bacterium called *Francisella tularensis*. It is contracted by drinking contaminated water or eating vegetation contaminated by infected animals. When it enters through the skin, tularemia can be recognized by the presence of a lesion and swollen glands. Ingestion of the organism may produce a throat infection, intestinal pain, diarrhea, and vomiting. Symptoms generally appear from 2 to 10 days—but usually 3 days—after exposure.

   Inhalation of the organism may produce a fever alone or fever combined with a pneumonia-like illness. Diagnosis is made by culture of the blood, sputum, or stool. The specimen must be cultured in cysteine heart agar.

Brucellosis

   This disease is caused by *Brucella abortis, suis, melitensis*, or *canis*. It is contracted by ingestion of contaminated milk products, direct puncture of the skin (in butchers and farmers), or by inhalation. The illness is characterized by acute or insidious onset of fever, night sweats, undue fatigue, anorexia, weight loss, headache, and arthralgia. *Brucella* can be cultured from a blood, sputum, or food specimen. Serology testing is also possible. Diagnosis is confirmed by a fourfold or greater rise in *Brucella* agglutination titer between acute- and convalescent-phase serum specimens obtained 2 weeks or more apart and studied at the same laboratory. Demonstration by immunofluorescence of a *Brucella* organism in a clinical specimen is another method of diagnosis.

Procedure and patient care

Before

- Maintain strict adherence to all procedures to avoid violations in isolation or contamination.

- Biohazard precautions are to be taken with each specimen.
- Laboratory personnel must strictly adhere to all universal standard precautions.

During

- If an enema is used to obtain a botulinum stool specimen, use sterile water. Saline can negate results.
- Send enough blood for adequate testing. Usually two red-top tubes are adequate. It is best to send it on ice.
- If food is sent for testing, it should be sent in its original containers.
- For anthrax or smallpox testing of a cutaneous lesion, soak one or two culture swabs with fluid from a previously unopened lesion.

After

- Identify all potential sources of contamination.
- Isolate individuals who are suspected of having a contagious disease.

Abnormal findings

See Table 5.

notes

bladder cancer markers (Bladder tumor antigen [BTA], Nuclear matrix protein 22 [NMP22])

Type of test Urine

Normal findings

BTA <14 units/ml
NMP22 <10 units/ml

Test explanation and related physiology

The recurrence rate for bladder cancers that have been resected by transurethral cystoscopy is high. Surveillance testing requires frequent urine testing for cytology and frequent cystoscopic evaluations. The use of bladder tumor markers may provide improved accuracy in diagnosing recurrent bladder cancer by an easier and cheaper method. BTA is a factor H-related protein that is produced by bladder tumor cells. NMP22 is a nuclear matrix protein that is deposited into the urine during apoptosis (nuclear disruption) of bladder cancer cells.

Normally, none or very little levels of these proteins are found in the urine. Elevated levels are associated with bladder cancer. It has been suggested that BTA and NMP22 be used in surveillance testing of patients after curative resection of bladder cancer. When normal, cystoscopy rarely yields positive results. When significantly elevated, bladder tumor recurrence is strongly suspected. Furthermore, when NMP22 is performed 10 days after bladder cancer extirpative surgery, it is extremely accurate in identifying patients who are at great risk for recurrence. NMP22 may also be a good screening test for those patients at increased risk for developing bladder cancer. BTA, however, is not a good screening test, because increased BTA levels can also be elevated in other circumstances such as recent urologic surgery, urinary tract infection, or calculi. Cancers involving the ureters and renal pelvis may also be associated with increased BTA and NMP22.

Interfering factors

- These proteins are very unstable. If the urine is not immediately stabilized, false negatives may occur.

Procedure and patient care

Before

PT Explain the procedure to the patient.
PT Tell the patient that no fasting is required.

During

- A single voided specimen should be collected before noon.
- The specimen should be transported to the lab immediately to avoid deterioration of the protein.
- If a time delay is required, the specimen should be refrigerated.

After

PT Explain any other surveillance testing that may be required for bladder cancer follow-up.

Abnormal findings

Bladder cancer

notes

bleeding time (Ivy bleeding time)

Type of test Blood

Normal findings 1-9 minutes (Ivy method)
(Results vary among laboratories.)

Possible critical values >15 minutes

Test explanation and related physiology

The bleeding time test is used to evaluate the vascular and platelet factors associated with hemostasis. It is frequently performed on preoperative patients to ensure adequate hemostasis. When vascular injury occurs, the first hemostatic response is a spastic contraction of the lacerated microvessels. Next, platelets adhere to the wall of the vessel at the area of laceration in an attempt to plug the hole. Failure of either process results in a prolonged bleeding time. If platelets are present in inadequate quantities (usually less than 50,000), if the platelet function is inadequate (as in patients with uremia or with recent ingestion of aspirin), or if vessel constriction is inadequate (such as exists in the elderly or with increased capillary fragility), the bleeding time is prolonged.

For this study, a small, standard superficial incision is made in the forearm, and the time required for the bleeding to stop is recorded. This is called the *bleeding time*. Normal values vary according to the method used; the method most often used today is the *Ivy bleeding time test*.

Because vessel constriction and platelet adherence are not affected by coagulation (intrinsic and extrinsic system), defects in coagulation do not affect the bleeding time. Therefore, this test only evaluates platelet function and quantity and vascular constriction capability. It is not an accurate test of platelet numbers. This can better be quantified by a direct platelet count (see p. 714).

Contraindications

- Patients with low platelet counts
- Patients who are unable to cooperate
- Patients who cannot have a blood pressure cuff placed on the arm (e.g., those with cellulitis)
- Patients with a history of keloid formation
- Patients with senile skin changes

- Patients who have had a mastectomy or axillary lymph node dissection
  Avoid the arm on the affected side.

Potential complications

- Skin infection
- Excessive bleeding from test site

Interfering factors

- Aggressively wiping the site of laceration can prolong the test results.
- Extremes in body temperatures can alter results. High body temperatures can prolong results; low temperatures can falsely shorten results.
- Drugs that may cause *increased* bleeding times include anticoagulants, dextran, indomethacin, salicylates, streptokinase, allopurinol, some antibiotics, halothane, nonsteroidal antiinflammatory drugs, urokinase, and warfarin.

Procedure and patient care

Before

- PT Explain the procedure to the patient.
- Obtain a consent form if required by the institution.
- PT Tell the patient that no fasting is required.
- Obtain a drug history to detect if the patient has recently had aspirin, anticoagulants, or any other medications that may affect test results.
- PT Inform the patient that minor discomfort may occur with this test because of the skin laceration.

During

- Note the following procedural steps:
  1. The skin of the inner part of the forearm is cleansed with alcohol or povidone-iodine (Betadine).
  2. A blood pressure cuff is applied on the arm above the elbow, inflated to 40 mm Hg, and maintained at this pressure during the study.
  3. A small laceration is then made 1 mm deep into the skin, and the time is recorded.
  4. Bleeding ensues, and the blood is wiped clean at 30-second intervals.
  5. When no new bleeding occurs, the time is again noted.
  6. The interval from the beginning to the end of bleeding is calculated. This is the bleeding time.

7. The blood pressure cuff is then removed, and an adhesive dressing is applied to the patient's arm.

8. If bleeding persists more than 10 minutes, the test is stopped, and a pressure dressing is applied.

B

- Indicate on the laboratory slip any medications that may affect test results.
- Note that this test is usually performed by a laboratory technician in less than 10 minutes.

PT Inform the patient that minor discomfort may occur with this test because of the skin laceration.

After

- Apply pressure or pressure dressing to the puncture site.
- Assess the puncture site for bleeding.
- Abnormal results should be repeated.

Abnormal findings

▲ **Prolonged times or increased values**

Bone marrow failure
Primary or metastatic tumor infiltration of bone marrow
Disseminated intravascular coagulation
Thrombocytopenia
Hypersplenism
von Willebrand's disease
Collagen vascular disease
Cushing's syndrome
Henoch-Schönlein syndrome
Severe liver disease
Clotting factor deficiency
Capillary fragility
Leukemia
Uremia
Bernard-Soulier syndrome
Connective tissue disorder
Hereditary telangiectasia
Glanzmann's thrombasthenia

blood culture and sensitivity

Type of test Blood

Normal findings Negative

Test explanation and related physiology

Blood cultures are obtained to detect the presence of bacteria in the blood. Bacteremia (the presence of bacteria in the blood) can be intermittent and transient, except in endocarditis or suppurative thrombophlebitis. An episode of bacteremia is usually accompanied by chills and fever; thus the blood culture should be drawn when the patient manifests these signs to increase the chances of growing out bacteria on the cultures. It is important that at least two culture specimens be obtained from two different sites. If one produces bacteria and the other does not, it is safe to assume that the bacteria in the first culture may be a contaminant and not the infecting agent. When both cultures grow the infecting agent, bacteremia exists and is caused by the organism that is growing out in the culture. If the patient is receiving antibiotics during the time that the cultures are drawn, the laboratory should be notified. Resin can be added to the culture medium to negate the antibiotic effect in inhibiting growth of the offending bacteria in the culture. If cultures are to be performed while the patient is on antibiotics, the blood culture specimen should be taken shortly before the next dose of the antibiotic is administered. All cultures preferably should be performed before antibiotic therapy is initiated.

Culture specimens drawn through an IV catheter are frequently contaminated, and tests using them should not be performed unless catheter sepsis is suspected. In these situations, blood culture specimens drawn through the catheter help identify the causative agent more accurately than a culture specimen from the catheter tip.

Most organisms require approximately 24 hours to grow in the laboratory, and a preliminary report can be given at that time. Often, 48 to 72 hours are required for growth and identification of the organism. Anaerobic organisms may take longer to grow.

Interfering factors

- Contamination of the blood specimen, especially by skin bacteria, may occur.

Procedure and patient care

Before

PT Explain the procedure to the patient.
PT Tell the patient that no fasting is required.

During

- Carefully prepare the proposed venipuncture site with povidone-iodine (Betadine). Allow the skin to dry.
- Clean the tops of the Vacutainer tubes or culture bottles with povidone-iodine and allow them to dry. Some laboratories suggest cleaning with 70% alcohol after cleaning with povidone-iodine and air drying.
- Collect approximately 10 to 15 ml of venous blood by venipuncture from each site in a 20-ml syringe.
- Discard the needle on the syringe and replace with a second sterile needle before injecting the blood sample into the culture bottle.
- Inoculate the anaerobic bottle first if both anaerobic and aerobic cultures are needed.
- Mix gently after inoculation.
- Label the specimen with the patient's name, date, time, and tentative diagnosis.
- Indicate on the laboratory slip any medications that may affect test results.

After

- Transport the culture bottles immediately to the laboratory (or at least within 30 minutes).
- Notify the physician of any positive results so that appropriate antibiotic therapy can be initiated.

Abnormal findings

Bacteremia

notes

blood smear (Peripheral blood smear, Red blood cell morphology, RBC smear)

Type of test Blood

Normal findings

Normal quantity of red and white blood cells (RBCs, WBCs)
  and platelets
Normal size, shape, and color of RBCs
Normal WBC differential count

Test explanation and related physiology

Examination of the peripheral blood smear can provide a significant amount of information concerning drugs and diseases that affect RBCs and WBCs. Furthermore, other congenital and acquired diseases can be diagnosed. When special stains are applied to the blood smear, leukemia, infection, infestation, and other diseases can be identified.

When adequately prepared and examined microscopically by an experienced technologist and pathologist, a smear of peripheral blood is the most informative of all hematologic tests. All three hematologic cell lines—erythrocytes (RBCs), platelets, and leukocytes (WBCs)—can be examined. In the peripheral blood, five different types of leukocytes can routinely be identified: neutrophils, eosinophils, basophils, lymphocytes, and monocytes. The first three are also referred to as granulocytes. Please see the discussion in "bone marrow biopsy/aspiration" (p. 183) for more information concerning the various elements of blood.

Microscopic examination of the RBCs can reveal variations in RBC size (anisocytosis), shape (poikilocytosis), color, or intracellular content. Classification of RBCs according to these variables is most helpful in identifying the causes of anemia and the presence of other diseases.

RBC size abnormalities
  Microcytes (small RBCs)
      Iron deficiency
      Hereditary spherocytosis
      Thalassemia
  Macrocytes (larger size)
      Vitamin B_{12} or folic acid deficiency
      Reticulocytosis secondary to increased erythropoiesis
        (RBC production)

Occasional liver disorder
Postsplenectomy anemia
RBC shape abnormalities
Spherocytes (small and round)
Hereditary spherocytosis
Acquired immunohemolytic anemia
Elliptocytes (crescent or sickle shaped)
Hereditary elliptocytosis
Sickle cell anemia
Leptocytes, or "target cells" (thin cells and with less hemoglobin)
Hemoglobinopathies
Thalassemia
Spicule cell
Uremia
Liver disease
Bleeding ulcer
RBC color abnormalities
Hypochromic (pale)
Iron deficiency
Thalassemia
Cardiac disease
Hyperchromasia (more colored)
Concentrated hemoglobin, usually caused by dehydration
RBC intracellular structure
Nucleated (normoblasts) (Usually RBCs do not have a
nucleus, but immature RBCs do. Immature nucleated cells
indicate increased RBC synthesis.)
Anemia
Chronic hypoxemia
"Normal" for an infant
Marrow-occupying neoplasm or fibrotic tissue
Basophilic stippling (refers to bodies enclosed or
included in the cytoplasm of the RBCs)
Lead poisoning
Howell-Jolly bodies (small, round remnants of nuclear
material remaining within the RBC)
After a surgical splenectomy
Hemolytic anemia
Megaloblastic anemia
Heinz bodies (small, irregular particles of hemoglobin)
Drug-induced RBC injury
Hemoglobinopathies
Hemolytic anemia

The WBCs are examined for total quantity, differential count, and degree of maturity. An increased number of immature WBCs may indicate leukemia or infection. A decreased WBC count indicates failure of marrow to produce WBCs, resulting from drugs, chronic disease, neoplasia, or fibrosis.

Finally, an experienced cell examiner also can estimate platelet number (see p. 714) on a peripheral blood smear.

Procedure and patient care

Before

PT Explain the procedure to the patient.
PT Tell the patient that no fasting is required.

During

- Collect a drop of blood from a finger stick or heel stick and place it on a slide.
- If necessary, perform a venipuncture and collect the blood in a lavender-top tube.
- Note that a blood smear is first studied with an automated calculator programmed to recognize abnormal blood cell shapes and other variations. A more accurate smear is performed by a technologist. Low counts may be "hand counted" to ensure accuracy. The most accurate smear requires review by a pathologist.

After

- Apply pressure to the venipuncture site.

Abnormal findings

See listing under Test Explanation and Related Physiology (pp. 174-175).

notes

blood typing

B

Type of test Blood

Normal findings Compatibility

Test explanation and related physiology

With blood typing, ABO and Rh antigens can be detected in the blood of prospective blood donors and potential blood recipients. This test is also used to determine the blood type of expectant mothers and newborns. A description of the ABO system, Rh factors, and blood crossmatching is reviewed here.

ABO system

Human blood is grouped according to the presence or absence of A or B antigens. The surface membranes of group A red blood cells (RBCs) contain A antigens; group B RBCs contain B antigens on their surface; group AB RBCs have both A and B antigens; and group O RBCs have neither A nor B antigens. In general, a person's serum does not contain antibodies to match the surface antigen on their RBCs. That is, persons with group A antigens (type A blood) will not have anti-A antibodies. However, they may have anti-B antibodies. Vice versa is true for persons with group B antigens. Group O blood may have both anti-A and anti-B antibodies (see Table 6). Blood transfusions are actually transplantations of tissue (blood) from one person to another. It is important that the recipient not have antibodies to the donor's RBCs. If this were to occur, there could be a hypersensitivity reaction, which can vary from mild fever to anaphylaxis with severe intravascular hemolysis. If donor ABO antibodies are present against the recipient antigens, usually only minimal reactions occur.

TABLE 6 Blood typing

Blood type	Antigen	Antibody
Group A	A	B
Group B	B	A
Group AB (universal receiver)	A, B	None
Group O (universal donor)	None	A, B

Persons with group O blood are considered "universal donors" because they do not have antigens on their RBCs. People with group AB blood are considered "universal recipients" because they have no antibodies to react to the transfused blood. Group O blood is usually transfused in emergent situations in which rapid, life-threatening blood loss occurs and immediate transfusion is required. The chance of a transfusion reaction is least when type O is used. Women of childbearing potential should receive group O negative blood, and men generally receive group O positive blood when emergency transfusion prior to type-specific or crossmatched blood is required.

Rh factors

The presence or absence of Rh antigens on the RBC's surface determines the classification of Rh positive or Rh negative. After ABO compatibility, Rh factor is the next most important antigen affecting the success of a blood transfusion. The major Rh factor is $Rh_o(D)$. There are several minor Rh factors. If $Rh_o(D)$ is absent, the minor Rh antigens are tested. If negative, the patient is considered "Rh negative" (Rh^-).

Procedure and patient care

Before
PT Explain the procedure to the patient.
PT Tell the patient that no fasting is required.

During
- Collect approximately 7 to 14 ml of venous blood in a red-top tube. (This may vary among laboratories.)
- Avoid hemolysis.
- Appropriately label the blood tube before sending it to the laboratory.

After
- Assess the venipuncture site for bleeding.

Abnormal findings

See Test Explanation and Related Physiology.

notes

bone densitometry (Bone mineral content [BMC], Bone absorptiometry, Bone mineral density [BMD])

B

Type of test X-ray

Normal findings

Normal: <1 standard deviation below normal (>–1)

Osteopenia: 1-2.5 standard deviations below normal (–1 to –2.5)

Osteoporosis: >2.5 standard deviations below normal (<–2.5)

Test explanation and related physiology

Bone densitometry is used to determine bone mineral content and density to diagnose osteoporosis as early as possible. Osteoporosis and osteopenia are terms used for bone that becomes weakened and fractures easily. This most commonly occurs in postmenopausal women. However, other diseases are associated with osteoporosis, such as malnourishment or osteopenic endocrinopathies (e.g., hyperparathyroidism) in patients.

The earlier that osteoporosis is recognized, the more effective the treatment and the milder the clinical course. If the diagnosis of osteoporosis is delayed until fractures occur or even until plain film x-rays identify "thin" bones, the success of treatment is less likely. Because therapy can be expensive and is not without risks, the diagnosis of osteoporosis must be made on the basis of accurate data. Bone densitometry can provide early and accurate measurements of bone strength based on bone density.

Several groups of bones are routinely evaluated because they accurately represent the entire skeleton. The lumbar spine is the best representative of cancellous bone. The radius is the most easily studied cortical bone. The proximal hip (neck of the femur) is the best representative of mixed (cancellous and cortical) bone. However, specific bone sites can be evaluated if they are particularly symptomatic.

Dual energy densitometry (absorptiometry) is most commonly used. There are two types of dual photon energy and, therefore, two different methods of performing dual energy densitometry. *Dual-photon absorptiometry (DPA)* and *dual-energy x-ray absorptiometry (DEXA)* are most commonly used. Because DPA and DEXA use two photons, more energy is produced so that bones (spine and hip [femoral neck]) surrounded by a lot of soft tissue can be more easily penetrated. The source of the photon is placed on one side of the bone to be studied. The gamma detector is placed on the other side. Increased bone density is associated with increased bone photon absorption and, therefore, less photon recognition at the site of the gamma detector.

Several other methods are available to measure BMD. *Quantitative computed tomography (QCT)* uses CT technology to measure central bones, especially the spine. *Single x-ray absorptiometry* uses a single x-ray beam to measure the density of a peripheral bone (finger, wrist, or heel). *Ultrasound absorption* (quantitative ultrasound) can be used to measure peripheral bones (heel [calcaneus], patella, or mid-tibia). Which method will ultimately be used for diagnosis and which will be used in mass screening remains to be seen. All methods seem to have an accuracy rate in excess of 85%.

The diagnosis of osteoporosis can be made when vertebral bone density is more than 10% below that expected according to a chart based on sex, age, height, weight, and race. Usually bone density is reported in terms of standard deviation (SD) removed from mean values. T scores compare the patient's results to a group of young healthy adults. Z scores compare the patient's results to a group of age-matched controls. The World Health Organization has defined osteopenia as a bone density value of greater than 1 SD below peak bone mass levels of young women, and osteoporosis as a value of greater than 2.5 SD below that same measurement scale. Positive T scores indicate bone stronger than normal. Negative T scores indicate bone weaker than normal.

This test is also used to monitor patients who are undergoing treatment for osteoporosis.

Interfering factors

- Barium may falsely increase the density of the lumbar spine. Bone density measurements should not be performed for about 10 days after barium studies.
- Calcified abdominal aortic aneurysm may falsely increase bone density of the spine.
- Internal fixation devices of the hip or radius will falsely increase bone density of those bones.
- Overlying metal jewelry or other objects may falsely increase bone density of the bones.
- Previous fractures of the bone to be studied can falsely increase bone density of the bone.

- Metallic clips placed in the plane of the vertebrae of patients who have had previous abdominal surgery can falsely increase bone density of the bone.
- Prior bone scans can falsely decrease bone density because the photons generated from the bone (as a result of the previously administered bone scan radionuclide) will be detected by the scintillator detector.

Procedure and patient care

Before

PT Explain the procedure to the patient.

PT Tell the patient that no fasting or sedation is required.

- The machine is usually calibrated by the x-ray or nuclear medicine technician before the patient's arrival.

PT Instruct the patient to remove all metallic objects (e.g., belt buckles, zippers, coins, keys) that might be in the scanning path.

During

- Note the following procedural steps:
  1. The patient lies supine on an imaging table with his or her legs supported and placed on a padded box to flatten the pelvis and lumbar spine.
  2. Under the table, a photon generator is slowly successively passed under the lumbar spine.
  3. A scintillator (gamma or x-ray) detector/camera is passed over the patient in a manner parallel to the generator. An image of the lumbar spine and hip bone is obtained by the scintillator camera and projected onto a computer monitor.
  4. Next, the appropriate foot is applied to a brace that internally rotates the nondominant hip, and the procedure is repeated over the hip. A similar procedure is performed for radius evaluation.
  5. When the radius is examined, the nondominant arm is preferred, unless there is a history of fracture to that bone.
- Note that the data are interpreted by a radiologist or a physician trained in nuclear medicine.
- Note that bone density studies take about 30 to 45 minutes to perform and are free of any discomfort. Only minimal radiation is used for this procedure.
- Note that there are numerous types of bone densitometry machines. Peripheral units that quickly scan the finger, heel,

or forearm are often used to find patients at risk for osteoporosis. Abnormal results are followed up with the more comprehensive table procedure described.

After

- On the computer screen, a small window of the lumbar spine, femoral neck, or distal radius is drawn. The computer calculates the amount of photons not absorbed by the bone. This is called the bone mineral content (BMC). Bone mineral density (BMD) is computed as follows:

$$\text{BMD} = \frac{\text{BMC}}{\text{Surface area of the bone}} \quad (\text{gm} \cdot \text{cm}^2)$$

Abnormal findings

Osteopenia
Osteoporosis

notes

bone marrow biopsy (Bone marrow examination, Bone marrow aspiration)

B

Type of test Microscopic examination of tissue

Normal findings

Cell type	Range (%)
Myeloblasts	<5
Promyelocytes	1-8
Myelocytes	
Neutrophilic	5-15
Eosinophilic	0.5-3
Basophilic	<1
Metamyelocytes	
Neutrophilic	15-25
Eosinophilic	<1
Basophilic	<1
Mature myelocytes	
Neutrophilic	10-30
Eosinophilic	<5
Basophilic	<5
Mononuclear	
Monocytes	<5
Lymphocytes	3-20
Plasma cells	<1
Megakaryocytes	<5
M/E ratio	<4
Normoblasts	25-50

Normal iron content is demonstrated by staining with Prussian blue

Test explanation and related physiology

Bone marrow examination is an important part of the evaluation of patients with hematologic diseases. Indications for bone marrow examination include the following:

1. To confirm the diagnosis of megaloblastic anemias
2. To diagnose leukemia or myeloma
3. To determine if the marrow is the cause of reduced blood cells in the peripheral bloodstream
4. To document deficient iron stores

5. To document bone marrow infiltrative diseases (neoplasm or fibrosis)
6. Identification of tumor, as staging lymphomas

The bone marrow is located in the central fatty core of cancellous bone (sternum, rib, and pelvis) and the long bones (femur, tibia, and humerus). There, blood-forming cells produce the blood cells and release them into the circulatory system.

By examining a bone marrow specimen, a hematologist can fully evaluate hematopoiesis. Examination of the bone marrow reveals the number, size, and shape of the red and white blood cells (RBCs, WBCs) and megakaryocytes (platelet precursors) as these cells evolve through their various stages of development in the bone marrow. Microscopic examination includes estimation of cellularity, determination of the presence of fibrotic tissue or neoplasms (both primary and metastatic), and estimation of iron storage.

To estimate cellularity, the specimen is examined, and the relative quantity of each cell type determined. Leukemias or leukemoid drug reactions are suspected when increased numbers of leukocyte precursors are present. Physiologic marrow leukemoid compensation for infection also will be recognized by the presence of an increased number of leukocyte precursors. Decreased numbers of marrow leukocyte precursors occur in patients with myelofibrosis, metastatic neoplasia, or agranulocytosis; in elderly patients; and after radiation therapy or chemotherapy.

Increased numbers of marrow RBC precursors occur with polycythemia vera or as physiologic compensation to hypoxemia or hemorrhagic or hemolytic anemias. Decreased numbers of marrow RBC precursors occur with erythroid hypoplasia after chemotherapy, radiation therapy, administration of other toxic drugs, iron deficiency, or marrow replacement by fibrotic tissue or neoplasms.

Increased numbers of platelet precursors (megakaryocytes) are seen in the marrow of patients who are compensating after an episode of acute hemorrhage. They are also seen in some forms of chronic myeloid leukemia. This increase also may be compensatory in patients with secondary hypersplenism associated with portal hypertension or other conditions. In these patients the spleen prematurely extracts platelets from the circulatory system. Platelet counts decrease, and the marrow compensates by increasing production. Decreased numbers of megakaryocytes occur in patients who have had radiation therapy, chemotherapy, or other drug therapy, and in patients with neoplastic or fibrotic marrow infiltrative diseases. Patients with aplastic anemia also have decreased numbers of megakaryocytes.

Increased numbers of lymphocyte precursors occur in chronic, viral, or mycoplasma infections (e.g., mononucleosis), lympho-cytic leukemia, and lymphoma. Plasma cells (plasmocytes) are increased in number in patients with multiple myelomas, Hodgkin's disease, hypersensitivity states, rheumatic fever, and other chronic inflammatory diseases.

Estimation of cellularity also can be expressed as a ratio of myeloid (WBC) to erythroid (RBC) cells (M/E ratio). The nor-mal M/E ratio is approximately 3:1. The M/E ratio is greater than normal in those diseases mentioned previously in which increased leukocyte precursors are present or erythroid precur-sors are decreased. The M/E ratio is below normal when either leukocyte precursors are decreased or erythroid precursors are increased. A more detailed listing of diseases affecting the M/E ratio can be found in most hematology textbooks.

Drug-induced or idiopathic myelofibrosis can be detected by examination of the bone marrow. Using special stains, one can estimate iron stores with a marrow biopsy. Although fibrosis or neoplasia occasionally can be detected in aspiration studies, biopsy is the best method. Leukemias, multiple myelomas, and polycythemia vera can be detected easily in biopsy specimens. Similarly, lymphomas and other metastatic tumors (e.g., cancers of the breast, kidney, and lung) can be seen. Bone marrow biopsy is an important part of staging for lymphomas and Hodgkin's disease.

Contraindications

- Patients with acute coagulation disorders because of the risk of excessive bleeding
- Patients who cannot cooperate and remain still during the procedure

Potential complications

- Hemorrhage, especially if the patient has a coagulopathy
- Infection, especially if the patient is leukopenic
- Sternal fracture as a result of too aggressive application of pressure to the sternum at the time of biopsy
- Inadvertent puncture of the heart or great vessels when the test is performed on the sternum

Procedure and patient care

Before
PT Explain the procedure to the patient.
- Obtain a written and informed consent for this procedure.
- Encourage the patient to verbalize fears, because many patients are anxious concerning this study.
- Assess the coagulation studies. Report any evidence of coagulopathy to the physician.
- Obtain an order for sedatives if the patient appears extremely apprehensive.

PT Remind the patient to remain very still throughout the procedure.

During
- Note the following procedural steps for *bone marrow aspiration*, which is performed on the sternum, iliac crest, anterior or posterior iliac spines, and proximal tibia (in children):
  1. The procedure is usually performed at the patient's bedside using local anesthesia.
  2. A preferred site is the posterior iliac crest, with the patient placed prone or on the side (Figure 7).
  3. The area overlying the bone is prepared and draped in a sterile manner.
  4. The overlying skin and soft tissue, along with the periosteum, is infiltrated with lidocaine.

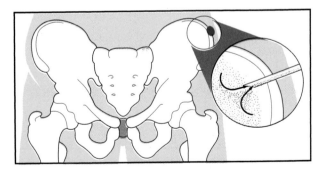

Figure 7 Bone marrow aspiration. Samples of the bone marrow are taken from along the posterior superior iliac crest.

5. A large-bore needle containing a stylus is slowly advanced through the soft tissue and into the outer table of the bone.
6. Once inside the marrow, the stylus is removed, and a syringe is attached.
7. One half to 2 ml of bone marrow is aspirated, smeared on slides, and allowed to dry.
8. The slides are sprayed with a preservative and taken to the pathology laboratory.

- Note the following procedural steps for *bone marrow biopsy*:
  1. The skin and soft tissues overlying the bone are incised.
  2. A core biopsy instrument is "screwed" into the bone.
  3. The biopsy specimen is obtained and sent to the pathology laboratory for analysis.
- Note that aspiration is performed by a trained nurse or physician. Bone marrow biopsy is usually performed by a physician. The duration of these studies is approximately 20 minutes.
- PT Inform the patient that he or she may have some apprehension when pressure is applied to puncture the outer table of the bone during biopsy specimen removal or aspiration.
- PT Tell the patient that he or she probably will feel pain during lidocaine infiltration and pressure when the syringe plunger is withdrawn for aspiration.

After

- Apply pressure to the puncture site to arrest minimal bleeding. Apply an adhesive bandage.
- Observe the puncture site for bleeding. Ice packs may be used to help control bleeding.
- Assess for tenderness and erythema, which may indicate infection. Report this to the physician.
- Evaluate the patient for signs of shock (increased pulse rate, decreased blood pressure) and pain.
- Normally place the patient on bed rest for 30 to 60 minutes after the test.
- Note that some patients complain of tenderness at the puncture site for several days after this study. Mild analgesics may be ordered.

🏠 Home care responsibilities

- Instruct the patient to observe the puncture site for bleeding.
- Inform the patient that tenderness and erythema may indicate infection. This should be reported to the physician.
- Mild analgesics may be needed for several days after this procedure for complaints of tenderness at the puncture site.

Abnormal findings

Neoplasm
Viral infection
Bacterial infection
Fungal infection
Myelofibrosis
Agranulocytosis
Polycythemia vera
Multiple myelomas
Hodgkin's disease
Hypersensitivity states
Acute hemorrhagic marrow hyperplasia
Anemia
Lymphoma
Chronic inflammatory disease
Leukemia
Rheumatic fever
AIDS

notes

bone scan

Type of test Nuclear scan

Normal findings No evidence of abnormality

Test explanation and related physiology

The bone scan permits examination of the skeleton by a scanning camera after IV injection of a radionuclide material, usually technetium (Tc)-99m. After injection of the Tc, the radiopharmaceutical is taken up by the bone. Gamma rays are emitted from the Tc through the body and detected by a scintillator. The scintillator emits light with each photon it receives from the gamma ray. When these light patterns are arranged in a spatial order, a realistic image of the bones is apparent.

The degree of radionuclide uptake is related to the metabolism of the bone. Normally a uniform concentration should be seen throughout the bones of the body. An increased uptake of isotope is abnormal and may represent tumor, arthritis, fracture, degenerative bone and joint changes, osteomyelitis, bone necrosis, osteodystrophy, and Paget's disease. These areas of concentrated radionuclide uptake are often called *hot spots* and are detectable months before an ordinary x-ray film can reveal the pathology. Hot spots occur because new bone growth is usually stimulated around areas of pathology. If pathology exists and there is no new bone formation around the lesion, the scan will not pick up the abnormality.

The major reason a bone scan is performed is to detect metastatic cancer to the bone. All malignancies capable of metastasis may reach the bone, especially those of the prostate, breast, lung, kidney, urinary bladder, and thyroid gland. Bone scans may be serially repeated to monitor tumor response to antineoplastic therapy.

Bone scans also provide valuable information in the evaluation of patients with trauma or unexplained pain. Bone scanning is much more sensitive than routine x-ray films in detecting small and difficult-to-find fractures, especially in the spine, ribs, face, and small bones of the extremities. Bone scans are used to determine the age of a fracture as well. If a fracture line is seen on a plain x-ray film and the uptake around that fracture is not increased on a bone scan, the injury is said to be an "old" fracture, exceeding several months in age.

Although the bone scan is extremely sensitive, unfortunately it is not very specific. Fractures, infections, tumors, and arthritic changes all appear similar in this scan. Bone scans are helpful in identifying infection (osteomyelitis) when plain films fail to identify the classic findings of infection.

Contraindications

- Patients who are pregnant, unless the benefits outweigh the risk of fetal damage
- Patients who are lactating, because of the risk of contaminating the infant

Procedure and patient care

Before

PT Explain the procedure to the patient.

PT Assure patients they will not be exposed to large amounts of radioactivity, because only tracer doses of the isotope are used.

PT Tell the patient that no fasting or sedation is required.

During

- Note the following procedural steps:
  1. The patient receives an IV injection of an isotope, usually sodium pertechnetate (technetium-99m) in a peripheral vein.
  2. The patient is encouraged to drink several glasses of water between the time of radioisotope injection and the scanning. This facilitates renal clearance of the circulating tracer not picked up by the bone. The waiting period before scanning is approximately 1 to 3 hours.
  3. The patient is instructed to urinate.
  4. The patient is positioned in the supine position on the scanning table in the nuclear medicine department.
  5. A radionuclide detector is placed over the patient's body and records the radiation emitted by the skeleton.
  6. This information is translated into a two-dimensional view of the skeleton, which is then visualized on Polaroid or x-ray film.
  7. The patient is repositioned in the prone and lateral positions during the test.
- Note that this scan is performed by a nuclear medicine technician in 30 to 60 minutes. It is interpreted by a physician trained in nuclear medicine imaging.

PT Tell the patient that the injection of the radioisotope causes slight discomfort.
PT Inform patients in significant pain that lying on the hard scanning table can be uncomfortable.

B

After
- Because only tracer doses of radioisotope are used, remember that no precautions need to be taken to prevent radioactive exposure to other personnel or family present.
PT Assure the patient that the radioactive substance is usually excreted from the body within 6 to 24 hours.

🏠 Home care responsibilities

- Instruct the patient to observe the injection site for redness or swelling.
- Encourage the patient to drink fluids to aid in the excretion of the radioactive substance.

Abnormal findings

Primary or metastatic tumor of the bone
Fracture
Degenerative arthritis
Rheumatoid arthritis
Osteomyelitis
Bone necrosis
Renal osteodystrophy
Paget's disease
Osteomyelitis

notes

bone turnover biochemical markers (N-telopeptide [NTx], Osteocalcin [bone G1a protein, BGP, osteocalc], Pyridinium [PYD] crosslinks)

Type of test Blood; urine

Normal findings

	NTx urine (nm BCE*/ mm creatinine)	NTx serum (nm BCE*)	Osteocalc serum (ng/ml)	PYD urine (nm/mm)
Female	26-124	6.2-19	0.7-6.4	15.3-33.6
Male	21-83	5.4-24.2	1.1-6.4	10.3-33.6

*BCE = bone collagen equivalents

Test explanation and related physiology

With the increased use of bone density scans (see p. 179), osteoporosis can now be diagnosed and treated more easily. This has prompted an interest in biochemical markers of bone metabolism. Bone is continuously being turned over—bone resorption by osteoclasts and bone formation by osteoblasts. Osteoporosis is a common disease of postmenopausal women and is associated with increased bone resorption and decreased bone formation. The result is thin and weak bones that are prone to fracture. The same process is now becoming increasingly recognized in elderly men, as well. Early diagnosis allows therapeutic intervention to prevent bone fracture.

Bone mineral density studies (p. 179) are valuable tools in the identification of osteoporosis; however, they cannot recognize small changes in bone metabolism. Although bone density studies can be used to monitor the effectiveness of therapy, it takes years to detect measurable changes in bone density. Biochemical markers, however, can identify significant improvement in a few months after instituting successful therapy. Furthermore, the cost of bone density studies limits the feasibility of performing this test as frequently as may be required to monitor treatment.

Because the levels of bone turnover biochemical markers vary according to the time of day and bone volume, these studies are not helpful in screening for detection of osteoporosis. Their use is in determining the effect of treatment as these markers are compared to pretreatment levels. Levels will decline with the use of antiresorption drugs (such as estrogen, alendronate, calcitonin, and raloxifene).

N-telopeptide (NTx) is the protein used in type 1 collagen that makes up nearly 90% of the bone matrix. The N terminals of these proteins are crosslinked to provide tensile strength to the bone. When bone is broken down, NTx is released into the bloodstream and excreted in the urine.

Osteocalcin, or *bone Gla protein (BGP),* is a noncollagenous protein in the bone and is made by osteoblasts. It enters the circulation during bone resorption as well as bone formation and is a good indicator of bone metabolism. Serum levels of BGP correlate with bone formation and destruction (turnover). Increased levels are associated with increased bone mineral density loss. BGP is a vitamin K–dependent protein. A reduced vitamin K intake is associated with reduced BGP levels. This probably explains the pathophysiology of vitamin K–dependent deficiency osteoporosis.

Pyridinium (PYD) crosslinks are formed during maturation of the type 1 collagen during bone formation. During bone resorption, these pyridinium crosslinks are released into the circulation.

These bone turnover biochemical markers cannot indicate the risk of bone fracture nearly as well as a bone density measurement scan. These markers can be used to monitor the activity and treatment of Paget's disease, hyperparathyroidism, and bone metastasis.

Biochemical markers are normally high in children because of increased bone resorption associated with growth and remodeling of the ends of the long bones. The levels reach a peak at about age 14, and then gradually decline to adult values. Because estrogen is a strong inhibitor of osteoclastic (bone resorption) activity, loss of bone density begins soon after menopause begins. Marker levels therefore rise after menopause. Most urinary assays are correlated with creatinine excretion for normalization.

Interfering factors

- Measurements of these urinary markers can differ by as much as 30% in one person even on the same day. Collecting double-voided specimens in the morning can minimize variability.
- Bodybuilding treatments, such as testosterone, can cause reduced levels of NTx.

Procedure and patient care

Before

PT Explain the procedure to the patient.
- It is important to obtain baseline levels before instituting therapy.
- Note that some labs require a 24-hour urine collection.

During

Urine
- Preferably, obtain a double-voided specimen.
- Collect the urine specimen 30 to 40 minutes before the time the specimen is needed.
- Discard this first specimen.
- Give the patient a glass of water to drink.
- At the requested time, obtain a second specimen.

Blood
- Collect 7 ml of venous blood in a red-top tube for NTx and/or a lavender- or green-top tube for osteocalcin.

After
- Send the specimen to the laboratory for testing.

Abnormal findings

▲ Increased levels

Osteoporosis
Paget's disease
Advanced bone tumors
  (primary or metastatic)
Acromegaly
Hyperparathyroidism
Hyperthyroidism

▼ Decreased levels

Hypoparathyroidism
Hypothyroidism
Cortisol therapy

notes

bone x-ray

Type of test X-ray

Normal findings No evidence of fracture, tumor, infection, or congenital abnormalities

Test explanation and related physiology

X-ray films of the long bones are usually taken when the patient has complaints about a particular body area. Fractures or tumors are readily detected by x-ray studies. In patients who have a severe or chronic infection overlying a bone, an x-ray film may detect the infection involving that bone (osteomyelitis). X-ray studies of the long bones also can detect joint destruction and bone spurring as a result of persistent arthritis. Growth patterns can be followed by serial x-ray studies of a long bone, usually the wrists and hands. Healing of a fracture can be documented and followed. X-ray films of the joints reveal the presence of joint effusions and soft tissue swelling as well. Calcifications in the soft tissue indicate chronic inflammatory changes of the nearby bursa or tendons. Soft tissue swelling also can be seen on these bone x-rays. Because the cartilage and tendons are not directly visualized, cartilage fractures, sprains, or ligamentous injuries cannot be seen.

At least two x-rays at 90-degree angles are required so that the bone region being studied can be visualized from two different angles (usually anterior to posterior and lateral). Some bone studies (e.g., skull, spine, hip) require oblique views to visualize all the parts that need to be seen.

Interfering factors

- Jewelry or clothing can obstruct radiographic visualization of part of the bone to be evaluated.
- Prior barium studies can diminish the full radiographic visualization of some of the bones surrounding the abdomen (e.g., spine and pelvis).

Procedure and patient care

Before

PT Explain the procedure to the patient.
- Handle carefully any injured parts of the patient's body.
PT Instruct the patient that he or she will need to keep the extremity still while the x-ray film is being taken. This can

sometimes be difficult, especially when the patient has severe pain associated with a recent injury.

- Shield the patient's testes, ovaries, or pregnant abdomen to avoid exposure from scattered radiation.

PT Tell the patient that no fasting or sedation is required.

During

- Note that in the x-ray department, the patient is asked to place the involved extremity in several positions. An x-ray film is taken of each position.
- Note that this test is routinely performed by a radiologic technologist within several minutes.

PT Tell the patient that no discomfort is associated with this test, except possibly from moving an injured extremity.

After

- Administer an analgesic for relief of pain if indicated.

Abnormal findings

Fractures
Congenital bone disorders (e.g., achondroplasia, dysplasia, dysostosis)
Tumors (osteogenic sarcoma, Paget's disease, myeloma, or metastatic)
Infection/osteomyelitis
Osteoporosis/osteopenia
Joint destruction (arthritis)
Bone spurring
Abnormal growth pattern
Joint effusion
Foreign bodies

notes

breast cancer tumor analysis (Breast cancer predictors, DNA ploidy status, S-phase fraction, Cathepsin D, HER 2 [c erbB2, neu] protein, p53 protein, Ki67 protein)

Type of test   Microscopic examination

Normal findings

DNA ploidy
   Aneuploid is unfavorable
   Diploid is favorable
S-phase fraction
   >5.5% is unfavorable
   <5.5% is favorable
Cathepsin D
   >10% is unfavorable
   <10% is favorable
HER 2 protein
   Moderate or strong staining in 10% of the cancer cells is
      unfavorable.
   Partial staining in ≤10% of the cancer cells is favorable.
p53 protein
   >10% is unfavorable
   <10% is favorable
Ki67 protein
   >20% is unfavorable
   10%-20% is borderline
   <20% is favorable

Test explanation and related physiology

Nearly 30% of the patients whose tumor has been completely removed and who have no evidence of lymph node metastasis will also develop recurrence. It would be helpful to predict the patients who are destined for recurrence so that they can be selected for systemic therapy, whereas patients who will not have a recurrence can be spared the morbidity of a treatment that is not needed. Conventional predictors such as tumor size, grade, histologic type, and hormone receptors have not proven to be reliable. As a result, there has been a marked increase in the efforts to identify newer markers that more accurately reflect cellular function and growth.

DNA ploidy status and S-phase fraction

Measurement of the rapidity with which the cells in a breast cancer grow includes ploidy status and S-phase analysis. Normally, cells are diploid (one set of paired chromosomes) and have a small number of cells in the S phase of cell division. During the mitotic phase of cell division, the amount of DNA doubles (two sets of paired chromosomes) in preparation for cell division. Because the more aggressive cancer cells divide more rapidly, many cells are in various stages of the mitotic phase. These cells may have a variable number of chromosome sets (aneuploid).

It has been noted that the more aggressive cancer cells are more often in S phase (a time of intracellular protein synthesis in preparation for division). This is usually reported as S-phase fraction (SPF), that is, the number of cells in S phase divided by the total number of cancer cells in the particular specimen.

Cathepsin D

This protein catabolic enzyme was found to be absent in resting breast tissue but significantly elevated in malignant tissue. It was thought that this protein on the cellular membrane contributed, in some way, to the malignant potential of the tumor. The exact cutoff point between favorable prognosis and unfavorable prognosis has yet to be standardized.

HER 2 (c erbB2, neu) protein

The HER 2 gene encodes the synthesis of a protein called tyrosine kinase and HER 2 protein. These proteins are epidermal growth factors that exist on the membrane of cells. It has been found that more aggressive breast cancers are associated with an overamplification of the HER 2 gene resulting in increased levels of the HER 2 protein. As a result, elevated levels of this protein found in breast cancer cells are associated with an unfavorable prognosis.

HER 2 testing is also helpful in making treatment decisions. Some oncologists feel that HER 2–positive tumors, despite their estrogen and progesterone receptor status, will not respond to hormone manipulation. Further, it was found that non-adriamycin-containing chemotherapy may not be as effective in HER 2–positive patients. Finally, it has been found that the HER 2 gene can act as a target for an antineoplastic drug called trastuzumab (Herceptin). By affecting this epidermal growth regulator, trastuzumab may be able to control some breast cancers that have not responded to other treatments.

B

p53 protein

The p53 gene is a tumor suppressor gene that is overexpressed in more aggressive breast cancer cells. Mutation of the gene causes overexpression and a buildup of mutant proteins on the surface of the cancer cells.

Ki67 protein

The Ki67 gene encodes the synthesis for Ki67 protein that is associated with a more aggressive breast cancer.

Interfering factors

- Delay in tissue fixation may cause deterioration of marker proteins and produce lower values.
- Preoperative use of some chemotherapy agents may cause decreased levels of some marker proteins.

Procedure and patient care

Before

PT Indicate to the patient that an examination for these tumor predictor markers may be performed on their breast cancer tissue.
- Provide psychologic and emotional support to the breast cancer patient.

During

- The surgeon obtains tumor tissue.
- This tissue should be placed on ice or in formalin.
- Part of the tissue is used for routine histology. A portion of the paraffin block is sent to a reference laboratory.

After

PT Explain to the patient that results are usually available in 1 week.

Abnormal findings

Unfavorable

notes

breast ductal lavage

Type of test Fluid analysis

Normal findings No atypical cells in the effluent

Possible critical values

Cancer cells in the effluent

Test explanation and related physiology

The theory behind ductal lavage is that by washing out exfoliated cells from a few breast ducts, the risk of breast cancer developing in the near future can be assessed. If atypical cells are obtained, the risk of breast cancer developing in the next decade may be as high as 4 to 10 times normal. Once that risk is identified, the patient may choose to attempt to alter that risk by using chemopreventative medications, such as tamoxifen.

Initially, it was hoped that ductal lavage would be able to identify ductal carcinoma of the breast at its earliest stages. The results of several large studies did not support that fact. Its use has now been limited to women who have been found to be at a statistically higher personal risk for breast cancer by *Gail or Claus breast cancer risk models.* These statistical models are based on age at menarche, age at first pregnancy, prior breast surgery, family history, and history of atypical changes in previous breast biopsies. Many women found to be at increased risk would like more data before they decide to take a medication designed to reduce those risks. If these women were found to have atypical cells in the lavage, most would choose to take the medication. If no atypical cells were found, they may choose close observation only.

There are still no data to confirm that the findings do accurately reflect a true risk for breast cancer. Furthermore, there are no data to indicate what a negative lavage means.

Contraindications

- Patients with prior breast cancer surgery because their risks are already known to be high

Potential complications

- Infection

Procedure and patient care

Before

PT Explain the procedure to the patient. Often these women have already received extensive counseling regarding their risk of breast cancer.

■ Be sure the breast exam and mammogram are normal.

■ Apply a topical anesthetic to the nipple area about ½ hour before the test.

During

■ Note the following procedural steps:

1. A suction apparatus is applied to the nipple area. Ducts that reveal fluid with the suction are then chosen for cannulation.

2. A tiny catheter is gently placed into the nipple duct and the duct is lavaged with 1 to 3 ml of saline.

3. The effluent is collected in a small tube and sent for cytology.

4. The procedure is then repeated for the other ducts that produced fluid with nipple suction.

■ This procedure is performed by a surgeon in the office. There is minimal to moderate discomfort associated with the nipple suction, duct cannulation, and lavage.

After

PT Inform the patient of the possibility of mild breast discomfort.

■ Arrange for follow-up to discuss test results.

■ Provide counseling if results indicate atypical or malignant cells.

Abnormal findings

Atypical cells
Ductal cancer cells

notes

breast scintigraphy (Breast scan, Sestamibi breast scan, Scintimammography)

Type of test Nuclear

Normal findings Negative: minimal, symmetric bilateral and uniform breast uptake equal to soft tissue uptake

Test explanation and related physiology

Nuclear scans of the breast using sestamibi are used to identify breast cancer in patients whose dense breast tissue precludes accurate evaluation by conventional mammography. This test has been used as an adjunct in patients with an indeterminate mammogram and in women with lumpy breasts. This scan may miss as many as 10% to 15% of cancers, however. Furthermore, the false-positive rate is about 15%. Areas of benign cellular hyperplasia also trap the radiotracer. Because cellular hyperplasia is a common finding in the breast just before menses, imaging at this time in the menstrual cycle should be avoided.

Breast nuclear scans will not replace the role of mammography in breast imaging. Nor will it ever be an effective screening tool for the early detection of breast cancer among large populations. However, its role as a second-line imaging modality is growing.

This scan may be helpful in staging breast cancer patients. The radiotracer often goes directly to axillary lymph nodes that contain metastatic breast cancer.

Contraindications

- Patients who are pregnant, unless the benefits outweigh the risk of fetal injury
- Patients who are lactating, because of the risk of contaminating maternal milk

Procedure and patient care

Before

PT Explain the procedure to the patient.

PT Assure patients that they will not be exposed to large amounts of radioactivity because only tracer doses of the isotope are used.

PT Tell the patient that no fasting or sedation is required.

During

- Note the following procedural steps:
  1. The patient may be positioned in the supine, prone, or sitting position.
  2. 20 mCi of Tc-99m sestamibi is injected intravenously into the arm contralateral to the suspicious breast.
  3. Imaging begins 10 minutes after injection. A scintillator camera is placed over the breast and records the radiation emitted.
  4. This information is translated into a two-dimensional view of the skeleton, which is then visualized on film.
  5. These images are compared to surrounding soft tissue readings.

After

PT Because only tracer doses of radioisotope are used, no precautions need to be taken to prevent radioactive exposure to other personnel or family present.

PT Assure the patient that the radioactive substance is usually excreted from the body within 6 to 24 hours.

PT Encourage the patient to drink fluids to aid in the excretion of the radioactive substance.

- Observe the injection site for redness or swelling.

Abnormal findings

Breast cancer
Hyperplasia of the breast tissue

notes

breast sonogram (Ultrasound mammography)

Type of test Ultrasound

Normal findings No evidence of cyst or tumor

Test explanation and related physiology

Ultrasound examination of the breast is most commonly used to determine if a mammographic abnormality or a palpable lump is a cyst (fluid-filled) or solid tumor (benign or malignant). In diagnostic real-time ultrasound, harmless high-frequency sound waves are emitted and penetrate the breast. The sound waves are bounced back to the sensor and arranged in a pictorial image by electronic conversion. Ultrasound of the breast is a useful test for differentiating cystic and solid breast lesions. It can be used to monitor a cyst to determine if it enlarges or disappears. Ultrasound is especially useful in patients with an abnormal mass on a mammogram to determine if the abnormality is cystic or solid.

Ultrasound of the breast is also useful in the examination of symptomatic women for whom the radiation of mammography is potentially harmful. These include:

1. Pregnant women
   Radiation may be harmful to the fetus.
2. Women under the age of 25
   These women may experience a greater oncologic risk from the radiation of mammography.
3. Women who have silicone prosthesis–augmented breasts
   The prosthesis can be penetrated by the ultrasound beam. Ordinarily these prostheses would obscure residual tissue on physical examination and x-ray mammography.
4. Women who refuse to have x-ray mammography because of unreasonable fear of diagnostic radiation.

Diagnostic accuracy is improved when breast ultrasound is combined with x-ray mammography (see p. 637). Ultrasound can be used to locate a nonpalpable breast abnormality for biopsy or aspiration.

Procedure and patient care

Before

PT Explain the procedure to the patient.

PT Assure the patient that no discomfort is associated with this study.

PT Inform the patient that no fasting or sedation is required before the tests. Instruct the patient not to apply any lotions or powders to the breasts on the examination day.

During

- Note the following procedural steps:
  1. The patient lies in the prone position on the examining table, which contains a tank that holds heated and chlorinated water.
  2. One breast at a time is immersed in the water.
  3. The transducer that produces the ultrasound waves and detects their echoes is positioned at the bottom of the water tank.
  4. Alternatively the patient is placed in the supine position, and the transducer is directly applied to the breast using contact gel to improve sound transmission.
- Note that this test is performed by an ultrasound technician in approximately 15 minutes.
- Although there is no discomfort associated with this procedure, women with back problems or limited flexibility may have difficulty maintaining the position for this procedure.

After

- After the test is completed, the breasts are dried and the conductive paste is removed.

Abnormal findings

Cyst
Hematoma
Cancer
Fibroadenoma
Fibrocystic disease
Abscess

bronchoscopy

Type of test Endoscopy

Normal findings Normal larynx, trachea, bronchi, and alveoli

Test explanation and related physiology

Bronchoscopy permits endoscopic visualization of the larynx, trachea, and bronchi by either a flexible fiberoptic bronchoscope or a rigid bronchoscope. There are many diagnostic and therapeutic uses for bronchoscopy. *Diagnostic* uses of bronchoscopy include:

1. Direct visualization of the tracheobronchial tree for abnormalities (e.g., tumors, inflammation, strictures)
2. Biopsy of tissue from observed lesions
3. Aspiration of "deep" sputum for culture and sensitivity and for cytology determinations
4. Direct visualization of the larynx for identification of vocal cord paralysis, if present

Therapeutic uses of bronchoscopy include:

1. Aspiration of retained secretions in patients with airway obstruction or postoperative atelectasis
2. Control of bleeding within the bronchus
3. Removal of foreign bodies that have been aspirated
4. Brachytherapy, which is endobronchial radiation therapy using an iridium wire placed via the bronchoscope
5. Palliative laser obliteration of bronchial neoplastic obstruction

The *flexible fiberoptic bronchoscope* has accessory lumens through which cable-activated instruments can be used for removing biopsy specimens of pathologic lesions. Also, the collection of bronchial washings (obtained by flushing the airways with saline solution), pulmonary toilet, and the instillation of anesthetic agents can be carried out through these extra lumens. Double-sheathed, plugged-protected brushes also can be passed through this accessory lumen. Specimens for cytology and bacteriology can be obtained with these brushes. This allows more accurate determination of pulmonary infectious agents. Needles can be placed through the scope to obtain biopsies from tissue immediately adjacent to the bronchi. Laser therapy to burn out endotracheal lesions can now be performed through the bronchoscope.

Contraindications

- Patients with hypercapnia and severe shortness of breath who cannot tolerate interruption of high-flow oxygen
  However, bronchoscopy can be performed through a special oxygen mask or an endotracheal tube so that the patient can receive oxygen if required.
- Severe tracheal stenosis may make it difficult to pass the scope.

Potential complications

- Fever
- Hypoxemia
- Laryngospasm
- Bronchospasm
- Pneumothorax
- Aspiration
- Hemorrhage (after biopsy)

Procedure and patient care

Before

- PT Explain the procedure to the patient. Allay any fears and allow the patient to verbalize any concerns.
- Obtain informed consent for this procedure.
- Keep the patient NPO for 4 to 8 hours before the test to reduce the risk of aspiration.
- PT Instruct the patient to perform good mouth care to minimize the risk of introducing bacteria into the lungs during the procedure.
- Remove and safely store the patient's dentures, glasses, or contact lenses before administering the preprocedure medications.
- Administer the preprocedure medications as ordered.
- PT Reassure the patient that he or she will be able to breathe during this procedure.
- PT Instruct the patient not to swallow the local anesthetic sprayed into the throat. Provide a basin for expectoration of the lidocaine.

During

- Note the following procedural steps for *fiberoptic bronchoscopy*:
  1. This test is performed by a pulmonary specialist or a surgeon at the bedside or in an appropriately equipped room.

2. The patient's nasopharynx and oropharynx are anesthetized topically with lidocaine spray before insertion of the bronchoscope.

3. The patient is placed in a sitting or supine position, and the tube is inserted through the nose or mouth and into the pharynx (Figure 8).

4. After the tube passes into the larynx and through the glottis, more lidocaine is sprayed into the trachea to prevent the cough reflex.

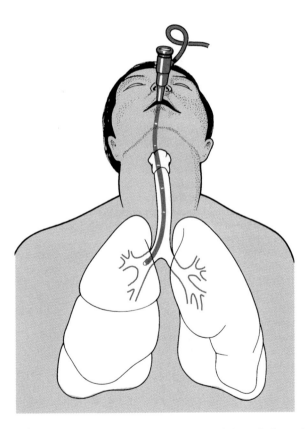

Figure 8 Bronchoscopy. A bronchoscope is inserted through the trachea and into the bronchus.

B

5. The tube is passed farther, well into the trachea, bronchi, and first- and second-generation bronchioles, for systematic examination of the bronchial tree.
6. Biopsy specimens and washings are taken if pathology is suspected.
7. If bronchoscopy is performed for pulmonary toilet (removal of mucus), each bronchus is aspirated until clear.

- Note that this procedure is performed by a physician in approximately 30 to 45 minutes.

PT Tell the patient that because of sedation, no discomfort is usually felt.

After

PT Instruct the patient not to eat or drink anything until the tracheobronchial anesthesia has worn off and the gag reflex has returned, usually in approximately 2 hours.

- Observe the patient's sputum for hemorrhage if biopsy specimens were removed. A small amount of blood streaking may be expected and is normal for several hours. Large amounts of bleeding can cause a chemical pneumonitis.

- Observe the patient closely for evidence of impaired respiration or laryngospasm. The vocal cords may go into spasms after intubation. Emergency resuscitation equipment should be readily available.

PT Inform the patient that postbronchoscopy fever often develops within the first 24 hours.

- If a tumor is suspected, collect a postbronchoscopy sputum sample for a cytology determination.

PT Inform the patient that warm saline gargles and lozenges may be helpful if a sore throat develops.

🏠 Home care responsibilities

- Suggest that the patient gargle with saline or soothing mouthwash to minimize a sore throat.
- Fever is not uncommon after bronchoscopy. High, persistent fever should be reported immediately.
- Bronchospasm or laryngospasm should be reported immediately to emergency personnel.
- Inform the patient that biopsy or culture reports will be available in 2 to 7 days.

Abnormal findings

Inflammation
Strictures
Tuberculosis
Cancer
Hemorrhage
Foreign body
Abscess
Infection

notes

CA 15-3 and CA 27.29 tumor markers (Cancer antigen 15-3)

Type of test Blood

Normal findings

CA 15-3: <22 units/ml or <22 kU/L (SI units)
CA 27.29: <38 units/ml or <38 kU/L (SI units)

Test explanation and related physiology

The CA 15-3 and CA 27.29 antigens are tumor-associated serum markers available for staging breast cancer and monitoring its treatment. CA 15-3 or CA 27.29 levels are high in less than 50% of patients who have a localized breast cancer or a small tumor burden. Of patients with metastatic breast cancer, however, 80% do have elevated CA 15-3 levels, and 65% have elevated CA 27.29 levels; therefore, the usefulness of these antigen tests as a screening technique in early breast cancers (the most common cancer of women) is quite limited. These tumor markers are not used for screening patients for breast cancer. Benign breast disease and nonbreast malignancies (such as lung, pancreas, ovary, and prostate) also can cause elevation of these antigen levels.

The use of these antigens should be limited to monitoring the treatment of advanced disease. CA 15-3 was the first breast tumor marker available.

Interfering factors

- Some of the other benign and malignant diseases associated with elevations of these antigens include cancer of the lung, ovary, pancreas, prostate, and colon; fibrocystic disease of the breast; cirrhosis; and hepatitis.

Procedure and patient care

Before

PT Explain the procedure to the patient.
PT Tell the patient that no fasting is required.

During

- Collect 7 to 10 ml of venous blood in a red-top tube.
- Have the blood sample sent to a central diagnostic laboratory. The results are available to the local hospital in 7 to 10 days.

After
- Apply pressure to the venipuncture site.

Abnormal findings

▲ **Increased levels**

Metastatic breast cancer

notes

CA 19-9 tumor marker (Cancer antigen 19-9)

Type of test Blood

Normal findings <37 units/ml or <37 kU/L (SI units)

Test explanation and related physiology

CA 19-9 antigen is a tumor marker used in diagnosis, evaluation of a patient's response to treatment, and surveillance of patients with pancreatic or hepatobiliary cancer. CA 19-9 is a carbohydrate antigen that exists on the surface of cancer cells. In the diagnosis of pancreatic carcinoma, the presence of a pancreatic mass or biliary obstruction and greatly elevated CA 19-9 levels would support pancreatic cancer as the diagnosis over benign pancreatitis. Likewise, patients whose symptoms are ascites, jaundice, and elevated CA 19-9 levels would be suspected of having hepatobiliary cancer. But CA 19-9 levels may not be elevated in all patients with pancreatic carcinoma. Approximately 70% of patients with pancreatic carcinoma and 65% of patients with hepatobiliary cancer have elevated levels.

CA 19-9 levels are used in the posttreatment surveillance of those who have had pancreatic or hepatobiliary cancers. In the few patients with pancreatic or biliary cancer who have a positive response to surgery, chemotherapy, or radiation therapy, a decline in serum levels of CA 19-9 will confirm this response. A rapid rise in CA 19-9 levels may be associated with a recurrent or progressive tumor growth. Mildly elevated levels may exist in patients with gastric cancer, colorectal cancer, or hepatoma, and even in 6% to 7% of patients with nongastrointestinal malignancies. Patients who have pancreatitis, gallstones, cirrhosis, inflammatory bowel disease, or cystic fibrosis also can have minimally elevated levels of CA 19-9.

Because of its lack of sensitivity and specificity, CA 19-9 is not effective in screening for pancreaticobiliary tumors in the general population.

Procedure and patient care

Before

PT Explain the procedure to the patient.

PT Tell the patient that no fasting is required.

During
- Collect 7 to 10 ml of blood in a red-top tube.
- Have the blood sent to a central diagnostic laboratory for CA 19-9 determinations. The results are available to the local hospital in 7 to 10 days.

After
- Apply pressure to the venipuncture site.

Abnormal findings

▲   **Increased levels**

Pancreatic carcinoma
Hepatobiliary carcinoma
Pancreatitis
Cholecystitis
Cirrhosis
Gastric cancer
Colorectal cancer
Gallstones
Cystic fibrosis
Lung cancer

notes

CA-125 tumor marker (Cancer antigen-125)

C

Type of test Blood

Normal findings 0-35 units/ml or <35 kU/L (SI units)

Test explanation and related physiology

CA-125 is an extremely accurate marker for nonmucinous epithelial tumors of the ovary. It is elevated in more than 80% of women with ovarian cancer. This tumor marker has a high degree of sensitivity and specificity for ovarian cancer and has been of great benefit to clinicians.

The CA-125 serum tumor marker is also used to determine a patient's response to therapy. Serial comparative testing will show a progressive decline in CA-125 levels for patients responding to treatment. Also, CA-125 tumor markers can predict whether a second-look (repeat) diagnostic laparotomy will be positive. A second-look laparotomy will detect a residual tumor in 97% of patients whose CA-125 level is greater than 35 units/ml, whereas only 56% of patients with ovarian cancer whose CA-125 level is less than 35 units/ml will have a positive second-look laparotomy. A precipitous fall in CA-125 after two courses of chemotherapy is an accurate predictor of a complete response to chemotherapy and is used as a good prognostic sign.

Finally, CA-125 determinations can be used in posttreatment surveillance of patients with ovarian cancer. In a patient who has had a complete response as a result of radiation therapy, chemotherapy, or surgery, a delayed rise in the CA-125 level is an early predictor of a recurrent tumor in 93% of patients. Abnormal levels can antedate the appearance of obvious recurrent ovarian cancer by 2 to 7 months.

CA-125 is not an effective screening test for the asymptomatic general public because of its lack of specificity. It is used in a "high-risk" population of women who have a strong family history of ovarian cancer. Elevated levels in the general population indicate that either benign or malignant disease is present in 95% of patients.

Other tumors and benign processes can cause elevated CA-125 levels as well. Diseases that affect the peritoneum such as cirrhosis, pancreatitis, peritonitis, endometriosis, and pelvic inflammatory disease can create elevated levels of CA-125. Other malignancies occurring in the female genital tract, pancreas, colon, lung, and breast can also be associated with elevated levels of this protein. Of the normal population, 1% to 2% have CA-125 levels in excess of 35 units/ml.

Interfering factors

- The first trimester of pregnancy and normal menstruation may be associated with mild elevations of CA-125 levels.
- Patients with benign peritoneal diseases (e.g., cirrhosis, endometriosis) have mildly increased levels.

Procedure and patient care

Before
PT Explain the procedure to the patient.
PT Tell the patient that no fasting or sedation is required.

During
- Collect 7 to 10 ml of blood in a red-top tube.
- Have the blood sent to a central diagnostic laboratory for determination of CA-125 level. The results are available to the local hospital in 3 to 7 days.

After
- Apply pressure to the venipuncture site.

Abnormal findings

▲   Increased levels

Malignant disorders
Cancer of the ovary
Cancer of the pancreas
Cancer of the nonovarian female genital tract
Cancer of the breast
Cancer of the colon
Cancer of the lung
Lymphoma
Peritoneal carcinomatosis
Benign disorders
Cirrhosis
Peritonitis
Pregnancy
Endometriosis
Pancreatitis
Pelvic inflammatory disease

---

calcitonin (Human calcitonin [HCT], Thyrocalcitonin)

Type of test   Blood

Normal findings

Basal (plasma)
    Males: ≤19 pg/ml or ≤19 ng/L (SI units)
    Females: ≤14 pg/ml or ≤14 ng/L (SI units)
Calcium infusion (2.4 mg/kg)
    Males: ≤190 pg/ml or ≤190 ng/L
    Females: ≤130 pg/ml or ≤130 ng/L
Pentagastrin injection (0.5 mcg/kg)
    Males: ≤110 pg/ml or ≤110 ng/L
    Females: ≤30 pg/ml or ≤30 ng/L

Test explanation and related physiology

Calcitonin is a hormone secreted by the parafollicular or C cells of the thyroid gland. Its secretion is stimulated by elevated serum calcium levels. The purpose of calcitonin is to contribute to calcium homeostasis. It decreases serum calcium levels by inhibiting bone resorption and increasing calcium excretion by the kidneys.

This test is usually used in the evaluation of patients with or suspected to have medullary carcinoma of the thyroid. Seventy-five percent of these patients have hypersecretion of calcitonin despite normal serum calcium levels. Calcitonin is also useful in monitoring response to therapy and predicting recurrences of medullary thyroid cancer, and as a screening test for those with a family history of medullary cancer who are therefore at high risk (20%) for medullary cancer. This is a cancer of the thyroid with a familial tendency; if it is found late, it has a poor prognosis. Routine screening for elevated calcitonin levels can detect medullary cancer early and improve chances for cure. C-cell hyperplasia, a benign calcitonin-producing disease that also has a familial tendency, is also associated with elevated calcitonin levels.

Equivocal elevations in calcitonin levels should be followed with further provocative testing using pentagastrin or calcium to stimulate calcitonin secretion. *Pentagastrin stimulation* involves an IV infusion over 5 to 10 seconds, with blood samples drawn before the injection and at 90 seconds, 2 minutes, and 5 minutes after the infusion. The *calcium infusion test* can be performed in a variety of ways but is most commonly administered over a 1-minute interval with baseline and 5- and 10-minute postinfusion blood levels. With medullary cancer of the thyroid, the provocative tests can cause the calcitonin to rise significantly.

Elevated levels of calcitonin also may be seen in people with cancer of the lung, breast, and pancreas. This is probably a form of paraneoplastic syndrome in which there is an ectopic production of calcitonin by the nonthyroid cancer cells.

Interfering factors

- Levels are often elevated in normal pregnant females and newborns.
- ✘ Drugs that may cause *increased* levels include calcium, cholecystokinin, epinephrine, glucagon, pentagastrin, and oral contraceptives.

Procedure and patient care

Before
PT Explain the procedure to the patient.
PT Tell the patient that an overnight fast is required. Water is permitted.

During
- Collect a venous sample of blood in a heparinized green-top or chilled red-top tube according to the laboratory's protocol.
- The specimen should be placed on ice immediately. The blood is frozen and sent to a reference laboratory.

After
- Apply pressure to the venipuncture site.
PT Tell the patient that results may not be available for several days.

Abnormal findings

▲ **Increased levels**

Medullary carcinoma of the thyroid
C cell hyperplasia
Oat cell carcinoma of the lung
Breast carcinoma
Pancreatic cancer
Primary hyperparathyroidism
Secondary hyperparathyroidism because of chronic renal
   failure
Pernicious anemia
Zollinger-Ellison syndrome
Alcoholic cirrhosis
Thyroiditis

notes

calcium (Total/ionized calcium, Ca, Serum calcium)

Type of test Blood; urine

Normal findings

Age	mg/dl	mmol/L
Total calcium		
<10 days	7.6-10.4	1.9-2.6
Umbilical	9-11.5	2.25-2.88
10 days-2 years	9-10.6	2.3-2.65
Child	8.8-10.8	2.2-2.7
Adult*	9-10.5	2.25-2.75
Ionized calcium		
Newborn	4.20-5.58	1.05-1.37
2 months-18 years	4.80-5.52	1.20-1.38
Adult	4.5-5.6	1.05-1.3

*In elderly individuals, values tend to decrease.

Possible critical values

<6 mg/dl (may lead to tetany)
>14 mg/dl (may lead to coma and cardiac arrest)

Test explanation and related physiology

The serum calcium test is used to evaluate parathyroid function and calcium metabolism by directly measuring the total amount of calcium in the blood. Determination of serum calcium is used to monitor patients with renal failure, renal transplantation, hyperparathyroidism, and various malignancies. It is also used to monitor calcium levels during and after large-volume blood transfusions.

About half the total calcium in the blood exists in its free (ionized) form, and about half exists in its protein-bound form (mostly with albumin). The serum calcium level is a measure of both. As a result, when the serum albumin level is low (as in malnourished patients), the serum calcium level will also be low, and vice versa. As a rule of thumb, the total serum calcium level decreases by approximately 0.8 mg for every 1-g decrease in the serum albumin level. Serum albumin should be measured with serum calcium. An advantage of measuring only the ionized form is that it is unaffected by changes in serum albumin levels.

When the serum calcium level is elevated on at least three separate determinations, the patient is said to have hypercalcemia. The most common cause of hypercalcemia is hyperparathyroidism. Parathormone (see p. 684) causes elevated calcium levels by increasing gastrointestinal absorption, decreasing urinary excretion, and increasing bone resorption. Malignancy, the second most common cause of hypercalcemia, can cause elevated calcium levels in two main ways. First, tumor metastasis (myeloma, lung, breast, renal cell) to the bone can destroy the bone, causing resorption and pushing calcium into the blood. Second, the cancer (lung, breast, renal cell) can produce a parathyroid hormonelike substance that drives the serum calcium up (ectopic PTH). Excess vitamin D ingestion can increase serum calcium by increasing renal and gastrointestinal absorption. Granulomatous infections such as sarcoidosis or tuberculosis are associated with hypercalcemia.

Hypocalcemia occurs in patients with hypoalbuminemia. The most common causes of hypoalbuminemia are malnutrition (especially in alcoholics) and large-volume IV infusions. Large blood transfusions are associated with low serum calcium levels because the citrate additives used in banked blood for anticoagulation bind the free calcium in the recipient's bloodstream. Intestinal malabsorption, renal failure, rhabdomyolysis, alkalosis, and acute pancreatitis (caused by saponification of fat) are also known to be associated with low serum calcium levels. Hypomagnesemia can be associated with refractory hypocalcemia.

Urinary calcium can be measured and is used most commonly to identify and support the diagnosis of hypercalcemia. Excretion of calcium in the urine is increased in all patients with hypercalcemia. Urinary calcium levels are decreased in patients with hypocalcemia. Urinary calcium measurement is not commonly used today because the development of assays for parathyroid hormone has replaced the need for urine calcium measurements to make the diagnosis of hyperparathyroidism. The test is still helpful in determining the cause of recurrent nephrolithiasis.

Interfering factors

- Vitamin D intoxication may cause increased serum calcium levels.
- Excessive ingestion of milk may cause increased levels.
- Serum pH can affect calcium values. A decrease in pH causes increased calcium levels.

- Prolonged tourniquet time will lower pH and falsely increase calcium levels.
- There is normally a small diurnal variation in calcium, with peak levels occurring around 9 PM.
- Hypoalbuminemia is artifactually associated with decreased levels of total calcium.
- ☤ Drugs that may cause *increased* serum levels include calcium salts, hydralazine, lithium, thiazide diuretics, parathyroid hormone (PTH), thyroid hormone, alkaline antacids, Ca salts, ergocalciferol, androgens, and vitamin D.
- ☤ Drugs that may cause *decreased* serum levels include acetazolamide, anticonvulsants, asparaginase, aspirin, calcitonin, cisplatin, corticosteroids, heparin, laxatives, loop diuretics, magnesium salts, diuretics, estrogens, albuterol, and oral contraceptives.

Procedure and patient care

Before
PT Explain the procedure to the patient.
PT Tell the patient that no fasting is required; however, the serum calcium may be part of a multichemical analysis in which fasting is required for the other studies.

During
- Collect approximately 7 ml of venous blood in a red-top tube. Avoid prolonged tourniquet use.
- List on the laboratory slip any medications that may affect test results.

After
- Apply pressure to the venipuncture site.

Abnormal findings

▲ **Increased levels (hypercalcemia)**

Hyperparathyroidism
Nonparathyroid PTH-producing tumor (e.g., lung or renal carcinoma)
Metastatic tumor to the bone
Paget's disease of bone
Prolonged immobilization
Milk-alkali syndrome
Vitamin D intoxication
Lymphoma
Granulomatous infections (e.g., sarcoidosis and tuberculosis)
Addison's disease
Acromegaly
Hyperthyroidism

▼ **Decreased levels (hypocalcemia)**

Hypoparathyroidism
Renal failure
Hyperphosphatemia secondary to renal failure
Rickets
Vitamin D deficiency
Osteomalacia
Malabsorption
Pancreatitis
Fat embolism
Alkalosis

notes

caloric study (Oculovestibular reflex study)

Type of test Electrodiagnostic

Normal findings Nystagmus with irrigation

Test explanation and related physiology

Caloric studies are used to evaluate the vestibular portion of the eighth cranial nerve (CN VIII) by irrigating the external auditory canal with hot or cold water. Normally stimulation with cold water causes rotary nystagmus (involuntary rapid eye movement) away from the ear being irrigated; hot water induces nystagmus toward the side of the ear being irrigated. If the labyrinth is diseased or CN VIII is not functioning (e.g., from tumor compression), no nystagmus is induced. This study aids in the differential diagnosis of abnormalities that may occur in the vestibular system, brainstem, or cerebellum.

Contraindications

- Patients with a perforated eardrum
  Cold air may be substituted for the fluid.
- Patients with an acute disease of the labyrinth (e.g., Ménière's syndrome)
  The test can be performed when the acute attack subsides.

Interfering factors

✘ Drugs such as sedatives and antivertigo agents can alter test results.

Procedure and patient care

Before
PT Explain the procedure to the patient.
- Hold solid foods before the test to reduce the incidence of vomiting.

During
- Although the exact procedures for caloric studies vary, note the following steps in a typical test:
  1. Before the test, the patient is examined for the presence of nystagmus, postural deviation (Romberg's sign), and past-pointing. This examination provides the baseline values for comparison during the test.

2. The ear canal should be examined and cleaned by a physician before testing to ensure that the water will freely flow to the middle ear area.

3. The ear on the suspected side is irrigated first because the patient's response may be minimal.

4. After an emesis basin is placed under the ear, the irrigation solution is directed into the external auditory canal until the patient complains of nausea and dizziness or nystagmus is seen. Usually this occurs in 20 to 30 seconds.

5. If after 3 minutes no symptoms occur, the irrigation is stopped.

6. The patient is tested again for nystagmus, past-pointing, and Romberg's sign.

7. After approximately 5 minutes, the procedure is repeated on the other side.

- Note that this procedure is usually performed by a physician or technician in approximately 15 minutes.

PT Tell the patient that he or she will probably experience nausea and dizziness during the test.

After

- Usually place the patient on bed rest for approximately 30 to 60 minutes until nausea or vomiting subsides.
- Ensure patient safety related to dizziness.

Abnormal findings

Brainstem inflammation, infarction, or tumor
Cerebellar inflammation, infarction, or tumor
Vestibular or cochlear inflammation or tumor
Acoustic neuroma
Eighth nerve neuritis/neuropathy

notes

carbon dioxide content (CO_2 content, CO_2 combining power)

Type of test Blood

Normal findings

Adult/elderly: 23-30 mEq/L or 23-30 mmol/L (SI units)
Child: 20-28 mEq/L
Infant: 20-28 mEq/L
Newborn: 13-22 mEq/L

Possible critical values <6 mEq/L

Test explanation and related physiology

The CO_2 content is a measure of CO_2 in the blood. In the peripheral venous blood, this is used to assist in evaluating the pH status of the patient and to assist in evaluation of electrolytes. The serum CO_2 test is usually included with other assessments of electrolytes. It is usually done with a multiphasic testing machine which also measures sodium, potassium, chloride, BUN, and creatinine. It is important not to get this test confused with P_{CO_2}. This CO_2 content measures the H_2CO_3, dissolved CO_2, and bicarbonate ion (HCO_3) that exists in the serum. Because the amounts of H_2CO_3 and dissolved CO_2 in the blood are so small, CO_2 content is an indirect measure of HCO_3 anion. HCO_3 anion is second in importance to the chloride ion in electrical neutrality (negative charge) of extracellular and intracellular fluid; its major role is in acid-base balance.

Levels of HCO_3 are regulated by the kidneys. Increases cause alkalosis, and decreases cause acidosis. See further discussion of this test as it is performed on arterial blood (p. 117). When CO_2 content is measured in the laboratory with other serum electrolytes, air affects the specimen, and the CO_2 partial pressure can be altered. Therefore, venous blood specimens are not very accurate for true CO_2 content or HCO_3. This test is used mostly as a rough guide to the patient's acid-base balance.

Interfering factors

- Underfilling the tube with blood allows CO_2 to escape from the serum specimen and may significantly reduce HCO_3 values.

¶ Drugs that may cause *increased* serum CO_2 and HCO_3 levels include aldosterone, barbiturates, bicarbonates, ethacrynic acid, hydrocortisone, loop diuretics, mercurial diuretics, and steroids.

¶ Drugs that may cause *decreased* levels include methicillin, nitrofurantoin (Furadantin), paraldehyde, phenformin hydrochloride, tetracycline, thiazide diuretics, and triamterene.

Procedure and patient care

Before

PT Explain the procedure to the patient.

PT Tell the patient that no fasting is required.

During

- Collect approximately 7 to 10 ml of venous blood in a red- or green-top tube.

After

- Apply pressure to the venipuncture site.

Abnormal findings

▲ **Increased levels**

Severe diarrhea
Starvation
Severe vomiting
Aldosteronism
Emphysema
Metabolic alkalosis
Gastric suction

▼ **Decreased levels**

Renal failure
Salicylate toxicity
Diabetic ketoacidosis
Metabolic acidosis
Shock
Starvation

notes

carboxyhemoglobin (COHb, Carbon monoxide)

Type of test Blood

Normal findings

Saturation of hemoglobin

Nonsmoker: <3%

Smoker: ≤12%

Newborn: ≥12%

Possible critical values

20% to 30%: Dizziness, headache, disturbances in judgment

30% to 40%: Tachycardia, hyperpnea, hypotension, confusion

50% to 60%: Coma

>60%: Death

Test explanation and related physiology

This test is used to detect carbon monoxide poisoning. It measures the amount of serum COHb, which is formed by the combination of carbon monoxide (CO) and hemoglobin (Hb). CO combines with Hb 200 times more readily than oxygen (O_2) can combine with Hb (oxyhemoglobin). The result is fewer Hb bonds available to combine with O_2. Further, when CO occupies the O_2 binding sites, the hemoglobin molecule is changed to bind the remaining O_2 more tightly. This greater affinity of CO for Hb and change in O_2 binding strength does not allow the O_2 to pass readily from the RBCs to the tissue. Less O_2 is therefore available for tissue cell respiration. This results in hypoxemia.

CO poisoning is documented by Hb analysis for COHb. A specimen should be drawn as soon as possible after exposure, because CO is rapidly cleared from the Hb by breathing normal air. O_2 saturation studies and oximetry are inaccurate in CO-exposed patients because they measure all forms of oxygen-saturated hemoglobin, including carboxyhemoglobin. In these circumstances the patient's oximetry will be good, yet the patient is hypoxemic.

This test can also be used to evaluate patients with complaints of headache, irritability, nausea, vomiting, and vertigo, who unknowingly may have been exposed to CO. Its greatest use, however, is in patients exposed to smoke inhalation, exhaust fumes, and fires. Other sources of CO include tobacco smoke, petroleum and natural-gas fuel fumes, automobile exhaust, unvented natural-gas heaters, and defective gas stoves. The treatment of CO toxicity is administration of high concentrations of O_2 to displace the carboxyhemoglobin.

C

Procedure and patient care

Before

PT Explain the procedure to the patient or family.

- Obtain the patient's history related to any possible source of CO inhalation.
- Assess the patient for signs and symptoms of mild CO toxicity (e.g., headache, weakness, dizziness, malaise, dyspnea) and moderate to severe CO toxicity (e.g., severe headache, bright red mucous membranes, cherry red blood). Maintain patient safety precautions if confusion is present.

During

- Collect approximately 5 to 10 ml of venous blood in a lavender- or green-top tube.

After

- Apply pressure to the venipuncture site.
- Treat the patient as indicated by the physician. Usually the patient receives high concentrations of O_2.
- PT Encourage respirations to allow the patient to clear CO from the Hb.

Abnormal findings

Carbon monoxide poisoning

notes

carcinoembryonic antigen (CEA)

Type of test Blood

Normal findings <5 ng/ml or <5 mcg/L (SI units)

Test explanation and related physiology

The CEA is a protein that normally occurs in fetal gut tissue. By the time of birth, detectable serum levels disappear. In the early 1960s CEA was found to exist in the bloodstream of adults who had colorectal tumors. Thus the antigen was thought to be a specific indicator of the presence of colorectal cancer. Subsequently, however, this protein has been found in patients who have a variety of carcinomas (e.g., breast, pancreatic, gastric, hepatobiliary), sarcomas, and even many benign diseases (e.g., ulcerative colitis, diverticulitis, cirrhosis). Chronic smokers also have elevated CEA levels.

Because the CEA level can be elevated in both benign and malignant diseases, it is not considered to be a specific test for colorectal cancer. As a result, CEA is not a reliable screening test for the detection of colorectal cancer in the general population. Its use is limited to determining the prognosis and monitoring the response of tumor to antineoplastic therapy in a patient with cancer. This is especially helpful in patients with breast and gastrointestinal cancers. The CEA level on the initial test is an indicator of tumor burden and prognosis. Smaller and early-staged tumors are likely to have minimal CEA elevations, if not normal CEA levels. A drastic reduction of normal CEA levels is expected with complete eradication of tumor. Therefore this test is used to determine the adequacy of treatment.

This test also is used in the surveillance of patients with cancer. A steadily rising CEA level is occasionally the first sign of tumor recurrence. This makes CEA testing very valuable in the follow-up of patients who have had potentially curative therapy. It is important to note that many patients with advanced breast or gastrointestinal tumors may not have elevated CEA levels.

CEA can also be detected in body fluids other than blood. Its presence in those body fluids indicates metastasis. This antigen is commonly measured in peritoneal fluid or chest effusions. An elevated CEA in these fluids indicates metastasis to the peritoneum or pleurae, respectively. Likewise, elevated CEA levels in the CSF would indicate central nervous system metastasis.

Interfering factors

- Smokers tend to have higher CEA levels than nonsmokers.
- Benign diseases (e.g., cholecystitis, colitis, diverticulitis) are associated with elevated CEA levels.
- Liver diseases (e.g., hepatitis, cirrhosis) are associated with elevated CEA levels.

Procedure and patient care

Before

PT Explain the procedure to the patient.

PT Tell the patient that no fasting is required.

During

- Collect a peripheral blood specimen. The collecting tube varies according to the commercial laboratory. (The two most frequently used laboratories for this test are Abbott Laboratories and Roche Labs.)
- Indicate on the laboratory slip if the patient smokes or has diseases that can affect test results.

After

- Apply pressure to the venipuncture site.

Abnormal findings

▲   Increased levels

Cancer (gastrointestinal, breast, lung, pancreatic, hepatobiliary)

Inflammation (colitis, cholecystitis, pancreatitis, diverticulitis)

Cirrhosis

Peptic ulcer

notes

cardiac catheterization (Coronary angiography, Angiocardiography, Ventriculography)

Type of test X-ray with contrast dye

Normal findings Normal heart-muscle motion, normal coronary arteries, normal great vessels, and normal intracardiac pressures and volumes

Test explanation and related physiology

Cardiac catheterization is used to visualize the heart chambers, arteries, and great vessels. It is used most often to evaluate patients with chest pain. Patients with a positive stress test are also studied to locate the region of coronary occlusion. This test is also used to determine the effects of valvular heart disease. Right heart catheterization is performed to calculate cardiac output. This is the most accurate method to determine cardiac output. Right heart catheterization is also used to identify pulmonary emboli (see pulmonary angiography, p. 771).

For cardiac catheterization, a catheter is passed into the heart through a peripheral vein or artery, depending on whether catheterization of the right or left side of the heart is being performed. Pressures are recorded through the catheter, and radiographic dyes are injected. With the assistance of a computer, cardiac output and other measures of cardiac functions can be determined. Cardiac catheterization is indicated for the following reasons:

1. To identify, locate, and quantitate the severity of atherosclerotic, occlusive coronary artery disease
2. To evaluate the severity of acquired and congenital cardiac valvular or septal defects
3. To determine the presence and degree of congenital cardiac abnormalities such as transposition of great vessels, patent ductus arteriosus, and anomalous venous return to the heart
4. To evaluate the success of previous cardiac surgery or balloon angioplasty
5. To evaluate cardiac muscle function
6. To identify and quantify ventricular aneurysms
7. To identify and locate acquired disease of the great vessels such as atherosclerotic occlusion or aneurysms within the aortic arch

8. To evaluate patients with acute myocardial infarction and facilitate infusion of thrombolytic agents into the occluded coronary arteries
9. To insert a catheter to monitor right-sided heart pressures such as pulmonary artery and pulmonary wedge pressures (Table 7 provides pressures and volumes used in cardiac monitoring.)
10. To perform dilation of stenotic coronary arteries (angioplasty), place coronary artery stents, or perform laser atherectomy

Cardiac catheterization is performed under sterile conditions. In right-sided heart catheterization, usually the subclavian, brachial, or femoral vein is used for vascular access. In left-sided heart catheterization, usually the right femoral artery is cannulated; alternatively, however, the brachial artery may be chosen (Figure 9). As the catheter is placed into the great vessels of the heart chamber, pressures are monitored and recorded. Blood samples for analysis of O_2 content are also obtained. The catheter is advanced with appropriate guidance into the desired position. After pressures are obtained, angiographic visualization of the heart chambers, valves, and coronary arteries is achieved with the injection of radiographic dye.

Transluminal coronary angioplasty is a therapeutic procedure that can be performed during coronary angiography in medical centers where open heart surgery is available. During this procedure a specific, specially designed balloon catheter is introduced into the coronary arteries and placed across the stenotic area of the coronary artery. This area can then be dilated by controlled inflation of the balloon. The coronary arteriogram is then repeated to document the effects of the forceful dilation of the stenotic area. Coronary arterial stents can be placed at the site of previous stenosis after angioplasty and maintain patency for longer periods of time. Likewise, laser atherectomy of coronary arterial plaques can be performed to more permanently open hard, atheromatous plaques.

Contraindications

- Patients who are unable to cooperate during the test
- Patients who would refuse intervention if an amenable lesion were found
- Patients with an iodine dye allergy who have not received preventive medication for allergy

TABLE 7 Pressures and volumes used in cardiac monitoring

Pressures	Description	Normal values
Routine blood pressure	Routine brachial artery pressure	90-140/60-90 mm Hg
Systolic left ventricular pressure	Peak pressure in the left ventricle during systole	90-140 mm Hg
End-diastolic left ventricular pressure	Pressure in the left ventricle at the end of diastole	4-12 mm Hg
Central venous pressure	Pressure in the superior vena cava	2-14 cm H_2O
Pulmonary wedge pressure	Pressure in the pulmonary venules, an indirect measurement of left atrial pressure and left ventricular end-diastolic pressure	Left atrial: 6-15 mm Hg
Pulmonary artery pressure	Pressure in the pulmonary artery	15-28/5-16 mm Hg
Aortic artery pressure	Same as routine blood pressure	
End-diastolic volume (EDV)	Amount of blood present in the left ventricle at the end of diastole	50-90 ml/m^2
End-systolic volume (ESV)	Amount of blood present in the left ventricle at the end of systole	25 ml/m^2
Stroke volume (SV)	Amount of blood ejected from the heart in one contraction (SV = EDV – ESV)	45 ± 12 ml/m^2
Ejection fraction (EF)	Proportion (fraction) of EDV ejected from the left ventricle during systole (EF = SV/EDV)	0.67 ± 0.07
Cardiac output (CO)	Amount of blood ejected by the heart in 1 minute	3-6 L/min
Cardiac index (CI)	Amount of blood ejected by the heart in 1 minute per square meter of body surface area (CI = CO/body surface area)	2.8-4.2 L/min/m^2 for a patient with 1.5 m^2 of body surface area

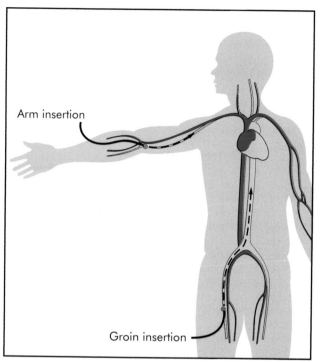

Arm insertion

Groin insertion

Figure 9 Cardiac catheterization. Brachial (arm) or femoral (groin) arterial insertion for cardiac catheterization.

- Patients who are pregnant, because of radiation exposure to the fetus
- Patients with renal disorders, because iodinated contrast is nephrotoxic
- Patients with a bleeding propensity

Potential complications

- Cardiac arrhythmias (dysrhythmias)
- Perforation of the heart myocardium
- Catheter-induced embolic stroke (cerebrovascular accident) or myocardial infarction
- Complications associated with the catheter insertion site such as arterial thrombosis, embolism, or pseudoaneurysm

- Infection at the catheter insertion site
- Pneumothorax following subclavian vein catheterization of the right side of the heart
- Hypoglycemia or acidosis in patients who are taking Glucophage and receive iodine dye

Procedure and patient care

Before

PT Explain the procedure to the patient.
- Obtain written permission from the fully informed patient.
- Allay the patient's fears and anxieties regarding this test. Although this test creates tremendous fear in a patient, it is performed often, and complications are rare.

PT Instruct the patient to abstain from oral intake for at least 4 to 8 hours before the test.
- Prepare the catheter insertion site by shaving and scrubbing the skin.
- Mark the patient's peripheral pulses with a pen before catheterization. This will facilitate postcatheterization assessment of the pulses at the affected and nonaffected extremities.
- Provide appropriate precatheterization sedation as ordered by the physician.

PT Instruct the patient to void before going to the catheterization laboratory.
- Remove all valuables and dental prostheses before transporting the patient to the catheterization laboratory.
- Obtain IV access for delivery of IV fluids and cardiac drugs if necessary.

During

- Take the patient to the cardiac catheterization laboratory.
- Note the following procedural steps:
  1. The chosen catheter insertion site is prepared and draped in a sterile manner.
  2. The desired vessel is punctured with a needle.
  3. A wire is placed through the needle and into the catheter.
  4. The angiographic catheter is threaded on top of the wire.
  5. Once the catheter is in the desired location, the appropriate cardiac pressures and volumes are measured.
  6. Cardiac ventriculography is performed with controlled injection of contrast.

7. Each coronary artery is catheterized. Cardiac angiography is then carried out with a controlled injection of contrast material.
8. During the injection, x-ray films are rapidly made.
9. The patient's vital signs must be monitored constantly during this procedure.
10. If *angioplasty* is performed, the cardiologist appropriately places the catheter and balloon at the stenotic area. Note the following procedural steps:
    a. As the ECG tracing is observed, the balloon is inflated, and the stenotic areas are forcefully dilated.
    b. If signs of myocardial ischemia develop, the balloon is immediately deflated.
    c. Usually inflation of the balloon is continued only for a few seconds.
11. After obtaining all the required information, the catheter is removed.

- Note that this test is usually performed by a cardiologist in approximately 1 hour.
- **PT** Tell the patient that during the injection he or she may experience a severe hot flush. This is uncomfortable but lasts only 10 to 15 seconds.
- Note that some patients have a tendency to cough as the catheter is placed into the pulmonary artery.
- Verbally support the patient as the x-ray films are taken, because the loud noises may be frightening.

After

- Monitor the patient's vital signs.
- Apply pressure to the site of vascular access.
- Keep the patient on bed rest for 4 to 8 hours to allow for complete sealing of the arterial puncture.
- Keep the affected extremity extended and immobilized with sandbags to decrease bleeding.
- Assess the puncture site for signs of bleeding, hematoma, or absence of pulse.
- Assess the patient's pulses of both extremities. Compare with preprocedure baseline values.
- **PT** Encourage the patient to drink fluids to maintain adequate hydration. Dehydration may be caused by the diuretic action of the dye. Monitor urinary output.
- See p. xix for appropriate interventions concerning care of patients with iodine allergy.

PT Instruct the patient that the test will be reviewed by the cardiologist and the results will be available in 1 or 2 days.

🏠 Home care responsibilities

- Instruct the patient in proper positioning of the extremity to decrease bleeding.
- Check for signs of bleeding (decreased BP and increased pulse).
- Assess the puncture site for bleeding and hematoma.
- Instruct the patient to report any signs of numbness, tingling, pain, or loss of function in the involved extremity.

Abnormal findings

Anatomic variation of the cardiac chambers and great vessels
Coronary artery occlusive disease
Ventricular aneurysm
Ventricular mural thrombi
Intracardiac tumor
Aortic root arteriosclerotic or aneurysmal disease
Anomalies in pulmonary venous return
Acquired or congenital septal defects and valvular abnormalities
Pulmonary emboli
Pulmonary hypertension

notes

cardiac exercise stress testing (Stress testing; Exercise testing; Electrocardiograph [ECG] stress testing, exercise testing; Nuclear stress testing; Echo stress testing)

C

Type of test Electrodiagnostic; nuclear

Normal findings Patient able to obtain and maintain maximal heart rate of 85% for predicted age and gender with no cardiac symptoms or ECG change. No cardiac muscle wall dysfunction present.

Test explanation and related physiology

Stress testing is used in the following situations:
1. To evaluate chest pain in a patient suspected of having coronary disease (Occasionally a person may have significant coronary stenosis that is not apparent during normal physical activity. If, however, the pain can be reproduced with exercise, one may infer that coronary occlusion is present.)
2. To determine the limits of safe exercise during a cardiac rehabilitation program or to assist patients with cardiac disease in maintaining good physical fitness
3. To detect labile or exercise-related hypertension
4. To detect intermittent claudication in patients with suspected vascular occlusive disease in the extremities. (In this situation, the patient may experience leg muscle cramping while performing the exercise.)
5. To evaluate the effectiveness of treatment in patients who take antianginal or antiarrhythmic medications
6. To evaluate the effectiveness of cardiac intervention (such as bypass grafting or angioplasty)

Stress testing is a noninvasive study that provides information about the patient's cardiac function. In stress testing the heart is stressed in some way and then evaluated during the stress. Changes indicating ischemia suggest coronary occlusive disease. By far the most commonly used method of stress is *exercise stress testing* (bike or treadmill). *Chemical stress testing* methods are becoming more commonly used because of their safety and increased accuracy. A third method, less commonly used, is *pacer stress testing*.

During *exercise stress testing*, the ECG, heart rate, and blood pressure are monitored while the patient engages in some type of physical activity (stress). Two methods of stress testing include pedaling a stationary bike and walking on a treadmill. With the stationary bicycle, the pedaling tension is slowly increased to increase the heart rate. With the treadmill test, the speed and grade of incline are increased. The treadmill test is the most frequently used, because it is the most easily standardized and reproducible. The various grades of exercise are determined by the cardiologist in attendance based on estimation of cardiac function capabilities.

The usual goal of exercise stress testing is to increase the heart rate to just below maximal levels or to the "target heart rate." Usually this target heart rate is 80% to 90% of the maximal heart rate. The test is usually discontinued if the patient reaches that target heart rate or develops any symptoms or ECG changes. The maximal heart rate is determined by a chart that takes into account the patient's age (about 230 minus the patient's age) and gender. The normal maximal heart rate for adults varies from 150 to 200 beats/min; patients taking calcium channel blockers and sympathetic blockers have a lower-than-expected maximal heart rate.

Exercise stress testing is based on the principle that occluded arteries will be unable to meet the heart's increased demand for blood during the testing. This may become obvious with symptoms (e.g., chest pain, fatigue, dyspnea, tachycardia, cardiac arrhythmias [dysrhythmias], fall in blood pressure) or ECG changes (e.g., ST-segment variance >1 mm, increasing premature ventricular contractions, or other rhythm disturbances). An advantage of stress testing is that these symptoms can be stimulated and identified in a safe environment. Besides the electrodiagnostic method of cardiac evaluation, the stressed heart can also be evaluated by nuclear scanning or echocardiography. Findings of ischemia are discussed in following paragraphs.

When exercise testing is not advisable or the patient is unable to exercise to a level adequate to stress the heart (patients with an orthopedic, arthritic, neurologic, or pulmonary limitation), *chemical stress testing* is recommended. Chemical stress testing is becoming increasingly used because of its accuracy and ease of performance. Although chemical stress testing is less physiologic than exercise testing, it is safer and more controllable. *Dipyridamole (Persantine)* is a coronary vasodilator. If one coronary artery is significantly occluded, the coronary blood flow is diverted to the opened vessels.

Adenosine works similarly to dipyridamole. *Dobutamine* is another chemical that can stress the heart. Dobutamine stimulates the heart muscle function. This entails administration of progressively greater amounts of dobutamine over 3-minute intervals. The normal heart muscle increases (augments) its contractility (wall motion). Ischemic muscle has no augmentation. In fact, in time the ischemic area becomes hypokinetic. Infarcted tissue is akinetic. In chemical stress testing, the stressed heart is evaluated by nuclear scanning or echocardiography.

Pacing is another method of stress testing. In patients with permanent pacemakers, the rate of capture can be increased to a rate that would be considered a cardiac stress. The heart is then evaluated electrodiagnostically or with nuclear scanning or echocardiography.

The methods of evaluation of the heart are electrophysiologic parameters (such as ECG, blood pressure, and heart rate), cardiac nuclear scanning, and echocardiography. These other tests are discussed separately (see pp. 244 and 365). Echocardiography is fast becoming the method of choice for urgent and elective cardiac evaluation with or without stress testing.

Contraindications

- Patients with unstable angina
- Patients with severe aortic valvular heart disease
- Patients who cannot participate in an exercise program because of their impaired lung or motor function
- Patients who have recently had a myocardial infarction
  In this case, however, limited stress testing can be done.
- Patients with severe congestive heart failure
- Patients who have severe claudication and cannot walk adequately to stress their hearts

Potential complications

- Fatal cardiac arrhythmias
- Severe angina
- Myocardial infarction
- Fainting

Interfering factors

- Heavy meals before testing can divert blood to the gastrointestinal tract.
- Nicotine from smoking can cause coronary artery spasm.

- Medical problems such as left ventricular hypertrophy, hypertension, valvular heart disease (especially of the aortic valve), left bundle-branch block, severe anemia, hypoxemia, and chronic pulmonary disease can affect results.
- Drugs that can affect test results include beta-blockers (e.g., propranolol [Inderal]), calcium channel blockers, digoxin, and nitroglycerin.

Procedure and patient care

Before

PT Explain the procedure to the patient.

PT Instruct the patient to abstain from eating, drinking, and smoking for 4 hours.

PT Inform the patient about the risks of the test and obtain informed consent.

PT Instruct the patient to bring comfortable clothing and shoes in which to exercise. Slippers are not acceptable.

PT Inform the patient if any medications should be discontinued before testing.

- Obtain a pretest ECG.
- Record the patient's vital signs for baseline values.
- Apply and secure appropriate ECG electrodes.

During

- Note that a physician usually is present during stress testing.
- After the patient begins to exercise, adjust the treadmill machine settings to apply increasing levels of stress at specific intervals. It is helpful to encourage and support the patient at each level of increased stress.

PT Encourage patients to verbalize any symptoms.

- Note that during the test the ECG tracing and vital signs are monitored continuously.
- Terminate the test if the patient complains of chest pain, exhaustion, dyspnea, fatigue, or dizziness.
- Note that testing usually takes approximately 45 minutes.

PT Inform the patient that the physician in attendance usually interprets the results and will explain them to the patient.

After

- Place the patient in the supine position to rest after the test.
- Monitor the ECG tracing and record vital signs at poststress intervals, until recordings and values return to pretest levels.
- Remove electrodes and paste.

Abnormal findings

Coronary artery occlusive disease
Exercise-related hypertension
Intermittent claudication
Abnormal cardiac rhythms: stress induced

notes

cardiac nuclear scanning (Myocardial scan, Cardiac scan, Nuclear cardiac scanning, Heart scan, Thallium scan, MUGA scan, Isonitrile scan, Sestamibi cardiac scan, Cardiac flow studies)

Type of test Nuclear scan

Normal findings Normal myocardial ejection fraction and coronary perfusion

Test explanation and related physiology

Cardiac nuclear scanning is used to detect myocardial ischemia, infarction, wall dysfunction, and decreased ejection fraction. It is commonly used as the imaging method part of cardiac stress testing (see discussion in cardiac stress testing). Specific indications for cardiac nuclear scanning include:

1. Screening of adults for past and recent infarction
2. Evaluation of patients with chest pain and uninterpretable or equivocal ECG changes caused by drugs, bundle-branch block, or left ventricular hypertrophy
3. Evaluation of myocardial perfusion before and after coronary artery bypass surgery
4. Quantification and surveillance of myocardial infarction
5. Evaluation of medical and surgical therapy for coronary artery perfusion
6. Evaluation of ventricular function in patients with myocardial disease
7. Evaluation of patients receiving cardiotoxic drugs (e.g., adriamycin chemotherapy)

Cardiac radionuclear scanning is a noninvasive and safe method of recognizing alterations of left ventricular muscle function and coronary artery blood distribution. Many different radionuclear materials can be used, most often technetium-99m pertechnetate, thallium-201, or technetium-99m pyrophosphate. When these compounds are injected intravenously and a radiation detector is placed over the heart, an image of the heart can be recorded and photographed.

In evaluating the patency of the coronary arteries, the characteristic abnormality varies according to the type of radiocompound used. When thallium is used, all normal myocardial cells take up the substance and appear on the photoscan. Ischemic or infarcted cells do not take up the substance and appear as "cold spots," devoid of nuclear material and surrounded by normal cells. Technetium sestamibi (isonitrile) presents a similar picture.

It is an even better cardiac imaging agent. Higher quality images can be obtained on the first pass, providing information similar to angiocardiography. Perfusion images, ventricular function, and gated-pool ejection fractions can all be obtained with a single injection. This is often called a *myocardial perfusion scan*. Furthermore, with the use of isonitrile, an ischemic area will be visible several hours after an ischemic event.

Technetium pyrophosphate is a radionuclide that binds with calcium. When ischemia or early infarction has occurred, intracellular calcium leaks out of the cardiac muscle cells. The calcium in the area of injury is very high. The technetium pyrophosphate binds to that calcium and creates an area of increased radionuclide uptake (hot spot). This is often called a *myocardial infarction scan*. If these patients have chest pain and the pyrophosphate scan is positive, muscle injury has occurred. This type of scan is especially helpful if the patient has had chest pain 5 to 10 days before seeing a doctor. Because the pyrophosphate scan stays positive for a long time, the delayed diagnosis of a myocardial infarction can be made.

Using these radionuclides, cardiac nuclear scanning is performed to indicate myocardium ischemia or infarction. Cardiac scanning also can be used to assess myocardial ischemia during stress testing (see p. 239). In some cases, no evidence of diminished blood supply to the myocardium is evident during the resting state. When stress testing is performed, however, evidence of myocardial ischemia can become quite obvious and is easily detected by nuclear stress testing. In this form of nuclear cardiac scanning, the radionuclide is injected intravenously at the point of maximal cardiac stress. The radionuclide accumulates in the myocardium in direct proportion to the regional myocardial blood flow. The normal myocardium will have much greater radionuclide activity than the ischemic myocardium. When this stress scan is compared to a resting cardiac nuclear scan, exercise-induced ischemia can be seen. This test is beneficial in detecting coronary occlusive disease, and is successful in assessing postoperative patency of a coronary bypass graft.

For an evaluation of myocardial function, technetium pertechnetate or technetium-labeled albumin is used to measure the part of blood ejected from the ventricle during one cardiac cycle *(ejection fraction)*. Normally, more than 65% of the blood is ejected from the ventricle during systole. Values less than this indicate decreased contractility of the heart caused by ischemia, infarction, or cardiomyopathy. Computers can be synchronized with the electrocardiogram (ECG) during scanning. The amount of blood ejected during systole also can be calculated based on the size of the heart at end-systole and end-diastole. This form of determination of ventricular function is called *gated pool imaging* or the *gated pool ejection fraction. Multigated acquisition (MUGA) scan* is another name for this test, based on the name of the computer machinery originally required for this determination.

This computer-assisted gated (synchronized) cardiac scan can also allow the myocardial wall to be photographed while in motion. This allows visualization of the myocardium during several cardiac cycles, and contractility of the myocardium can be determined. This imaging technique is called *nuclear ventriculography* and can provide the same information as radiographic ventriculography, which is performed during cardiac catheterization (see p. 232); however, the nuclear scans are noninvasive and much safer. Ischemic areas are seen to be hypokinetic on scan. Infarcted areas are akinetic on scan. This is also evident after stress during a cardiac stress test.

Cardiac flow studies can be performed by the rapid injection of the radionuclide into a vein (jugular or antecubital), and by then obtaining images immediately after the "first pass" of the radionuclide through the heart and great vessels. This provides excellent information about the direction of blood flow to and from the heart ventricles. It is particularly helpful in the evaluation of children suspected of having congenital heart disorders. Ventricular septal defects cause shunting of blood from the left ventricle to the right ventricle. Transposition of great vessels is easily demonstrated. Valvular regurgitation is also obvious. This test also allows the physician to quantify the amount of blood flow affected by those disorders.

Single-photon emission (the radionuclear materials discussed in previous paragraphs emit single photons) computed tomography (SPECT) has been used to visualize the heart from many different angles. These images are then reconstructed using techniques similar to CT scanning, and three-dimensional images of the physiologic cardiac processes are obtained. Areas of myocardial ischemia can be seen with far greater resolution and more accurately quantified.

Contraindications

- Patients who are uncooperative
- Patients who are pregnant, unless the benefits outweigh the risk of fetal exposure to radionuclide material

Interfering factors

- Myocardial trauma
- Recent nuclear scans (e.g., thyroid or bone scan)
- Cardiac flow studies can be altered by excessive changes in chest pressures (e.g., as with excessive crying in the pediatric patient).
- Drugs such as long-acting nitrates

Procedure and patient care

Before

PT Explain the procedure to the patient.

PT Instruct the patient that a short fasting period may be required.

During

- Take the patient to the nuclear medicine department.
- Note the following procedural steps:
  1. An IV injection of radionuclide material is performed.
  2. Depending on the radionuclide used, scanning is performed 15 minutes to 4 hours later.
  3. A gamma ray detector is placed over the precordium.
  4. The patient is placed in a supine position, then in the lateral position, and then in both the right and left oblique positions.
  5. The gamma-ray scanner records the image of the heart, and a photograph is immediately developed.
  6. For a *thallium exercise stress test*, radioactive thallium is injected during exercise when the patient reaches a maximum heart rate. The patient then lies on a table, and scanning is done. A repeat scan may be done 3 to 4 hours later.
  7. If an *isonitrile stress test* is needed, the patient is injected and scanned 30 to 60 minutes later for the resting phase. Four hours later, cardiac stress testing is done. After a second injection, scanning is repeated. Milk and a muffin are usually given after each isonitrile injection to facilitate clearing of the radionuclide from the hepatobiliary system.

PT Tell the patient that the only discomfort associated with this test is the venipuncture required for injection of the radioisotope.

- Note that myocardial scans are usually performed in less than 30 minutes by a nuclear medicine technician.

After

- Because only tracer doses of radioisotopes are used, note that no precautions need to be taken against radioactive exposure to personnel or family.
- **PT** Encourage the patient to drink fluids to aid in the excretion of the radioactive substance.
- Apply pressure or a pressure dressing to the venipuncture site.
- If stress testing was performed, evaluate the patient's vital signs at frequent intervals (as indicated).

Abnormal findings

Coronary artery occlusive disease

Decreased myocardial function associated with ischemia, myocarditis, cardiomyopathy, or congestive heart failure

notes

carotid artery duplex scanning (Carotid ultrasound)

Type of test Ultrasound

C

Normal findings Carotid artery free of plaques and stenosis

Test explanation and related physiology

Carotid duplex scanning is a noninvasive, ultrasound test used on the extracranial carotid artery to detect occlusive disease directly. It is recommended for patients with headaches and with neurologic symptoms, such as transient ischemic attacks (TIA), hemiparesis, paresthesia, and acute speech or visual deficits.

This scan is called "duplex" because it combines the benefits of two methods of ultrasonography—Doppler and B-mode. With the use of the transducer, a B-mode ultrasound grayscale image of the carotid vessel is obtained. A pulsed Doppler probe within the transducer is used to evaluate blood flow velocity and direction in the artery and to measure the amplitude and waveform of the carotid arterial pulse. A computer combines that information and provides a two-dimensional image of the carotid artery along with an image of blood flow. With this technique, one is able to directly visualize areas of stenotic or occluded arteries and arterial flow disruption. The degree of occlusion is measured in percentage of the entire lumen that is occluded.

Color Doppler ultrasound (CDU) can be added to duplex scanning. CDU assigns color for direction of blood flow within the vessel, and the intensity of that color is dependent on the mean computed velocity of blood traveling in the vessel. This allows visualization of stenotic areas by seeing slowing or reversal of direction of blood flow at a particular area of the artery. Reversal of blood flow is sometimes associated with contralateral arterial occlusion, which can be easily demonstrated using this technique.

Procedure and patient care

Before
- **PT** Explain the procedure to the patient.
- **PT** Tell the patient that no special preparation is required.
- **PT** Assure the patient that the study is painless.

During
- Place the patient in the supine position with the head supported to prevent lateral motion.

- Note the following procedural steps:
  1. A water-soluble gel is used to couple the sound from the transducer to the skin surface.
  2. Images of the carotid artery and pulse waveform are obtained.
- Note that this test is performed by an ultrasound technologist in the ultrasound or radiology department in approximately 15 to 30 minutes.
- **PT** Tell the patient that no discomfort is associated with this test.

After

- Remove the water-soluble gel from the patient.

Abnormal findings

Carotid artery occlusive disease

notes

cervical biopsy (Punch biopsy, Endocervical biopsy, LEEP cervical biopsy, Cone biopsy, Conization)

C

Type of test Microscopic examination

Normal findings Normal squamous cells

Possible critical values

Cancer cells

Test explanation and related physiology

When a PAP smear reveals an "epithelial cell abnormality" or when a pelvic exam reveals a possible abnormality in the cervix, a biopsy of that structure is performed. There are several different methods of biopsy, all of which obtain an increasing amount of tissue. Cervical biopsy procedures include:

- A *simple cervical biopsy*, sometimes called a *punch biopsy*, removes a small piece of tissue from the surface of the cervix. This is often performed during colposcopy, see page 289.
- An *endocervical biopsy (endocervical curettage)* removes tissue from high in the cervical canal by scraping with a sharp instrument.
- *Loop electrosurgical excision procedure (LEEP)* uses a thin, low-voltage electrified wire loop to cut out abnormal tissue on the cervix and high in the endocervical canal (sometimes called a *large loop excision of the transformation zone [LLETZ]*).
- A *cone biopsy (conization)* is a more extensive form of a cervical biopsy. It is called a cone biopsy because a cone-shaped wedge of tissue is removed from the cervix. Both normal and abnormal cervical tissues are removed. This can be performed by LEEP, surgical knife (scalpel), or a carbon dioxide laser.

After colposcopy and a cervical biopsy, LEEP may be used to treat abnormal, precancerous cells found on biopsy. It can also be used to assess the extent of and sometimes to treat noninvasive cervical cancers.

Contraindications

- Patients with active menstrual bleeding
- Pregnant patients

Potential complications

- After the surgery, a small number of women (less than 10%) may have significant bleeding that requires vaginal packing or a blood transfusion.
- Infection of the cervix or uterus may occur. (This is rare.)
- Narrowing of the cervix (cervical stenosis) that can cause infertility. (This is rare.)

Procedure and patient care

Before
PT Explain the procedure to the patient.
- Obtain informed consent if required by the institution.

During
- Note the following procedural steps:
  1. The patient is placed in the lithotomy position and a vaginal speculum is used to expose the vagina and cervix.
  2. The cervix is cleansed with a 3% acetic acid solution or iodine to remove excess mucus and cellular debris and to accentuate the difference between normal and abnormal epithelial tissues.
  3. Medication is injected to numb the cervix *(cervical block)*.
  4. With the instrument chosen by the doctor, a punch biopsy, endocervical biopsy, LEEP, or cone biopsy is performed.
- Note that the physician performs the procedure in approximately 5 to 10 minutes.
- While cone biopsy is done in the operating room, the other procedures can be performed in the doctor's office.
- PT Tell the patient that some women complain of pressure pains from the vaginal speculum and that discomfort may be felt if biopsy specimens are obtained.
- Most women can return to normal activities immediately after a simple cervical biopsy or an endocervical biopsy.
- Most women will be able to return to normal activities within 2 to 4 days after LEEP or cone biopsies. This can vary, depending on the amount of tissue removed during the procedure.

After
PT Inform the patient that it is normal to experience the following:
  Vaginal bleeding if biopsy specimens were taken. Suggest that she wear a sanitary pad.

Mild cramping for several hours after the procedure.
Brownish-black vaginal discharge during the first week.
Vaginal discharge or spotting for about 1 to 3 weeks.

PT Instruct the patient that sanitary napkins should be used instead of tampons for 1 to 3 weeks.

PT Tell the patient to avoid sexual intercourse for 3 to 4 weeks.

PT Inform the patient not to douche for 3 to 4 weeks.

PT Inform the patient when and how to obtain the results of this study.

PT Instruct the patient to call the doctor for any of the following symptoms:

Fever
Spotting or bleeding that lasts longer than 1 week
Bleeding that is heavier than a normal menstrual period and contains blood clots
Increasing pelvic pain
Bad-smelling, yellowish vaginal discharge, which may indicate an infection

Abnormal findings

Cervical chronic infection
Cervical intraepithelial neoplasia
Cervical carcinoma in situ
Invasive cervical carcinoma
Endocervical adenocarcinoma

notes

---

chest x-ray (CXR, Chest radiography)

Type of test X-ray

Normal findings Normal lungs and surrounding structures

Test explanation and related physiology

The chest x-ray film is important in a complete evaluation of the pulmonary and cardiac systems. This procedure is often part of the general admission screening workup in adult patients. Much information can be provided by the chest x-ray film. One can identify or follow (by repeated chest x-ray films) the following:

1. Tumors of the lung (primary and metastatic), heart (myxoma), chest wall (soft-tissue sarcomas), and bony thorax (osteogenic sarcoma)
2. Inflammation of the lung (pneumonia), pleura (pleuritis), and pericardium (pericarditis)
3. Fluid accumulation in the pleura (pleural effusion), pericardium (pericardial effusion), and lung (pulmonary edema)
4. Air accumulation in the lung (chronic obstructive pulmonary disease) and pleura (pneumothorax)
5. Fractures of the bones of the thorax or vertebrae
6. Diaphragmatic hernia
7. Heart size, which may vary depending on cardiac function
8. Calcification, which may indicate large-vessel deterioration or old lung granulomas
9. Location of centrally placed intravenous access devices

Most chest x-ray films are taken with the patient standing. The sitting or supine position also can be used, but x-ray films taken with the patient in the supine position will not demonstrate fluid levels. A *posteroanterior (PA)* view, with the x-rays passing through the back of the body (posterior) to the front of the body (anterior), is taken first. Then a *lateral* view, with the x-rays passing through the patient's side, is taken.

Oblique views may be taken with the patient turned at different angles as the x-rays pass through the body. *Lordotic* views provide visualization of the apices (rounded upper portions) of the lungs and are usually used for detection of tuberculosis. *Decubitus* films are taken with the patient in the recumbent lateral position to localize fluid, which becomes dependent within the pleural space (pleural effusion).

Chest x-ray studies are best performed in the radiology department. Studies using a portable x-ray machine may be done at the bedside and are often performed on critically ill patients who cannot leave the nursing unit.

Contraindications

- Patients who are pregnant, unless the benefits outweigh the risks

Interfering factors

- Conditions (e.g., severe pain) that prevent the patient from taking and holding a deep breath
- Scarring from previous lung surgery, which makes interpretation difficult
- Obesity, which requires more x-ray to penetrate the body to provide a readable picture

Procedure and patient care

Before

PT Explain the procedure to the patient.

PT Tell the patient that no fasting is required.

PT Instruct the patient to remove clothing to the waist and to put on an x-ray gown.

PT Inform the patient to remove all metal objects (e.g., necklaces, pins) so that they do not block visualization of part of the chest.

PT Tell the patient that he or she will be asked to take a deep breath and hold it while the x-ray films are taken.

PT Instruct men to ensure that their testicles are covered and women to have their ovaries covered, using a lead shield to prevent radiation-induced abnormalities.

During

PT After the patient is correctly positioned, tell him or her to take a deep breath and hold it until the x-ray films are taken.

- Note that x-ray films are taken by a radiologic technologist in several minutes.

PT Inform the patient that no discomfort is associated with chest radiography.

After

- Note that no special care is required following the procedure.

Abnormal findings

Lung

Lung tumor (primary or
  metastatic)
Pneumonia
Pulmonary edema
Pleural effusion
Chronic obstructive
  pulmonary disease
Pneumothorax
Atelectasis
Tuberculosis
Lung abscess
Congenital lung diseases
  (hypoplasia)
Pleuritis
Foreign bodies (chest,
  bronchus, or esophagus)

Heart

Cardiac enlargement
Pericarditis
Pericardial effusion

Chest wall

Soft tissue sarcoma
Osteogenic sarcoma
Fracture (ribs or thoracic spine)
Thoracic spine scoliosis
Metastatic tumor to the
  bony thorax

Diaphragm

Diaphragmatic/hiatal hernia

Mediastinum

Aortic calcinosis
Enlarged lymph nodes
Dilated aorta
Thymoma
Lymphoma
Substernal thyroid
Widened mediastinum

notes

Chlamydia

Type of test Microscopic examination or blood test

Normal findings

Negative culture
Antibodies: Immunoglobulin test ≤1:640

Test explanation and related physiology

There are many *Chlamydia* species that cause various diseases within the human body. *Chlamydia psittaci* causes respiratory tract infections and occurs as a result of close contact with infected birds. *C. pneumoniae*, another species, causes pneumonia. *C. trachomatis* infection is probably the most frequently occurring sexually transmitted disease in developed countries. Infections of the genitalia are most common, followed by those of the conjunctiva, pharynx, urethra, and rectum. Lymphogranuloma venereum was the first form of venereal disease recognized as a *C. trachomatis* infection. The second serotype of *C. trachomatis* causes the eye disease trachoma, which is the most common form of preventable blindness. A third serotype produces genital and urethral infections different from lymphogranuloma. This later type is transmitted by direct contact of an infant with the mother's cervix during vaginal delivery, or by direct contact of genitalia during sexual activity. *Chlamydia* may be associated with cases of pelvic inflammatory disease, particularly in adolescents. Most women colonized with *Chlamydia* are asymptomatic.

Chlamydia infection is thought to be the most prevalent sexually transmitted disease in the United States. Strategies to control its spread include screening all at-risk groups, particularly sexually active adolescents and those with other sexually transmitted disease, for disease.

The *Chlamydia* organism can be detected in many different ways. It seems to be most accurately demonstrated by tissue culture. Although these cultures require a special cell culture line, which takes several days, they are used as the gold standard against which other methods of detection of *Chlamydia* are measured. It is now possible to detect the antigen by direct fluorescent antibody slide staining and the enzyme-linked immunosorbent assay (ELISA) technique. The sensitivity and specificity of these newer techniques are lower than culture techniques, however.

Interfering factors

- Women presently having routine menses
- Patients undergoing antibiotic therapy

Procedure and patient care

Before

PT Explain the procedure to the patient.
- Note that many different methods are used to perform chlamydial tests.

During

- Collect venous blood in a red-top tube.
- Acute and convalescent serum should be drawn 2 to 3 weeks apart.
- A conjunctival smear is obtained by swabbing the eye lesion with a cotton-tipped applicator or scraping with a sterile ophthalmic spatula and smearing on a clean glass slide.
- Sputum cultures (see p. 872) are used to check for *C. psittaci* respiratory infections.
- Note the following procedural steps for *cervical culture:*
  1. The female patient should refrain from douching and bathing in a tub before the cervical culture is performed.
  2. The patient is placed in the lithotomy position.
  3. A nonlubricated vaginal speculum is inserted to expose the cervix.
  4. The mucus is removed from the squamocolumnar junction of the cervix.
  5. A sterile, cotton-tipped swab is inserted into the endocervical canal and moved from side to side for 30 seconds to obtain the culture.
- Note the following procedural steps for *urethral culture:*
  1. The urethral specimen should be obtained from the man before voiding.
  2. A culture is taken by inserting a sterile thin swab gently into the urethra for about 3 to 4 cm.
- Note that these tests are performed by a physician or nurse in several minutes.
PT Tell the patient that minimal discomfort is associated with these procedures.

After

- Treat patients who have positive smears with antibiotics.
- PT Tell affected patients to have their sexual partners examined.

Abnormal findings

Chlamydia infection

notes

chloride, blood (Cl)

Type of test Blood

Normal findings

Adult/elderly: 98-106 mEq/L or 98-106 mmol/L (SI units)
Child: 90-110 mEq/L
Newborn: 96-106 mEq/L
Premature infant: 95-110 mEq/L

Possible critical values

<80 or >115 mEq/L

Test explanation and related physiology

This test is performed as a part of *multiphasic testing* in what is usually called "electrolytes." By itself, not much information is obtained. However, with interpretation of the other electrolytes, chloride can give an indication of acid-base balance and hydrational status.

Chloride is the major extracellular anion. Its main purpose is to maintain electrical neutrality, mostly as a salt with sodium. It follows sodium (cation) losses and accompanies sodium excesses to maintain electrical neutrality. For example, when aldosterone encourages sodium resorption, chloride follows to maintain electrical neutrality. Because water moves with sodium and chloride, chloride also affects water balance. Finally, chloride also serves as a buffer to assist in acid-base balance. As carbon dioxide (and H cation) increases, bicarbonate must move from the intracellular space to the extracellular space. To maintain electrical neutrality, chloride will shift back into the cell.

Hypochloremia and hyperchloremia rarely occur alone and are usually part of parallel shifts in sodium or bicarbonate levels (see p. 118). Signs and symptoms of hypochloremia include hyperexcitability of the nervous system and muscles, shallow breathing, hypotension, and tetany. Signs and symptoms of hyperchloremia include lethargy, weakness, and deep breathing.

Interfering factors

- Excessive infusions of saline can result in increased chloride levels.
- ✍ Drugs that may cause *increased* serum chloride levels include acetazolamide, ammonium chloride, androgens, chlorothiazide, cortisone preparations, estrogens,

guanethidine, hydrochlorothiazide, methyldopa, and nonsteroidal antiinflammatory drugs.

✗ Drugs that may cause *decreased* levels include aldosterone, bicarbonates, corticosteroids, cortisone, hydrocortisone, loop diuretics, thiazide diuretics, and triamterene.

C

Procedure and patient care

Before

PT Explain the procedure to the patient.
PT Tell the patient that no fasting is required.

During

■ Collect 5 to 10 ml of venous blood in a red- or green-top tube.

After

■ Apply pressure or a pressure dressing to the venipuncture site.

Abnormal findings

▲ **Increased levels (hyperchloremia)**

Dehydration
Renal tubular acidosis
Excessive infusion of normal saline
Cushing's syndrome
Eclampsia
Multiple myeloma
Kidney dysfunction
Metabolic acidosis
Hyperventilation
Anemia
Respiratory alkalosis
Hyperparathyroidism

▼ **Decreased levels (hypochloremia)**

Overhydration
Congestive heart failure
Syndrome of inappropriate antidiuretic hormone
Vomiting
Chronic gastric suction
Chronic respiratory acidosis
Salt-losing nephritis
Addison's disease
Burns
Metabolic alkalosis
Diuretic therapy
Hypokalemia
Aldosteronism
Respiratory acidosis

notes

cholesterol

Type of test Blood

Normal findings

Adult/elderly: <200 mg/dl or <5.20 mmol/L (SI units)

Child: 120-200 mg/dl

Infant: 70-175 mg/dl

Newborn: 53-135 mg/dl

(Values vary with age and testing center.)

Test explanation and related physiology

Cholesterol is the main lipid associated with arteriosclerotic vascular disease. However, cholesterol is required for the production of steroids, sex hormones, bile acids, and cellular membranes. Most of the cholesterol we eat comes from foods of animal origin. The liver metabolizes the cholesterol to its free form, and cholesterol is transported in the bloodstream by lipoproteins. Nearly 75% of the cholesterol is bound to low-density lipoproteins (LDLs) (see p. 592), and 25% is bound to high-density lipoproteins (HDLs) (see p. 592). Therefore, cholesterol is the main component of LDLs and only a minimal component of HDLs and very low-density lipoproteins. It is the LDL that is most directly associated with increased risk of coronary heart disease (CHD).

The purpose of cholesterol testing is to identify patients at risk for arteriosclerotic heart disease. Cholesterol testing is usually done as a part of *lipid profile* testing, which also evaluates lipoproteins (see p. 592) and triglycerides (see p. 937), because by itself cholesterol is not a totally accurate predictor of heart disease. There is considerable overlap in what are considered "normal" and "high-risk" levels. "Normal" levels have been derived from a group of patients who have no obvious evidence of CHD. However, these findings may not be accurate because these patients may have preclinical CHD and may not truly reflect a "no-risk" population.

Because of these significant variabilities, elevated results should be corroborated by repeating the study. The two results should be averaged to obtain an accurate cholesterol for risk assessment.

Because the liver is required to make cholesterol, low serum cholesterol levels are indicative of severe liver diseases. Further, because our main source of cholesterol is our diet, malnutrition is also associated with low cholesterol levels. Certain illnesses can affect cholesterol levels. For example, patients with an acute myocardial infarction may have as much as a 50% reduction in cholesterol level for as many as 6 to 8 weeks.

C

In 1984 the National Institutes of Health developed a consensus in regard to total cholesterol levels and risk of CHD (Table 8). The cholesterol-to-HDL ratio has been used to assess the risk of CHD (Table 9). Familial hyperlipidemias and hyperlipoproteinemias are often associated with high cholesterol.

Interfering factors

- Pregnancy is usually associated with elevated cholesterol levels.
- Oophorectomy increases levels.
- Recumbent position is associated with decreased levels.

TABLE 8 Total cholesterol as an indicator of risk of CHD (mg/100 ml [SI units: mmol/L])*

Age	Low risk	Moderate risk	High risk
2-19	<170 [4.4]	171-185	>185 [4.8]
20-29	<200 [5.5]	201-220	>220 [5.7]
30-39	<220 [5.7]	221-240	>240 [6.2]
>40	<240 [6.2]	241-260	>260 [6.8]

*When cholesterol testing is combined with lipoproteins, risk of CHD can be more accurately calculated.

TABLE 9 Cholesterol to HDL ratio as an indicator of risk of CHD

	Ratio	
Risk	Male	Female
1/2 Average	3.4	3.3
Average	5.0	4.4
2× Average	10.0	7.0
3× Average	24.0	11.0

✔ Drugs that may cause *increased* levels include adrenocorticotropic hormone, anabolic steroids, beta-adrenergic blocking agents, corticosteroids, epinephrine, oral contraceptives, phenytoin (Dilantin), sulfonamides, thiazide diuretics, cyclosporine, and vitamin D.

✔ Drugs that may cause *decreased* levels include allopurinol, androgens, bile salt-binding agents, captopril, chlorpropamide, clofibrate, colchicine, colestipol, erythromycin, isoniazid, liothyronine (Cytomel), lovastatin (Mevacor), monoamine oxidase inhibitors, neomycin (oral), niacin, and nitrates.

Procedure and patient care

Before

PT Instruct the patient to fast 12 to 14 hours after eating a low-fat diet before testing. Only water is permitted.

PT Indicate to the patient that dietary intake at least 2 weeks before testing will affect results.

PT Tell the patient that no alcohol should be taken 24 hours before the test.

During

■ Collect 5 to 10 ml of blood in a red-top tube.

■ Indicate on the laboratory slip any drugs that may affect cholesterol levels.

■ Finger stick method is often used in mass screening.

After

■ Apply pressure to the venipuncture site.

PT Instruct patients with high levels regarding a low-cholesterol diet, exercise, and appropriate body weight.

Abnormal findings

▲ **Increased levels**

Hypercholesterolemia
Hyperlipidemia
Hypothyroidism
Uncontrolled diabetes
  mellitus
Nephrotic syndrome
Pregnancy
High-cholesterol diet
Xanthomatosis
Hypertension
Myocardial infarction
Atherosclerosis
Biliary cirrhosis
Stress
Nephrosis

▼ **Decreased levels**

Malabsorption
Malnutrition
Hyperthyroidism
Cholesterol-lowering
  medication
Pernicious anemia
Hemolytic anemia
Sepsis
Stress
Liver disease
Acute myocardial
  infarction

notes

---

cholinesterase (CHS, Pseudocholinesterase, Cholinesterase RBC, Red cell cholinesterase, Acetylcholinesterase)

Type of test   Blood

Normal findings

Serum cholinesterase 8-18 units/ml or 8-18 units/L (SI units)
RBC cholinesterase 5-10 units/ml or 5-10 units/L (SI units)
Dibucaine inhibition 79%-84%
(Values vary with laboratory test methods.)

Test explanation and related physiology

This test is done to identify patients with pseudocholinesterase deficiency before anesthesia or to identify patients who may have been exposed to phosphate poisoning. Cholinesterases hydrolyze acetylcholine and other choline esters and thereby regulate nerve impulse transmission at the nerve synapse and neuromuscular junction. There are two types of cholinesterases: acetylcholinesterase, also known as "true cholinesterase," and pseudocholinesterase. True cholinesterase exists primarily in the red blood cell and nerve tissue. It is not in the serum. Pseudocholinesterase, on the other hand, exists in the serum. Deficiencies in either of these enzymes can be acquired or congenital.

Because succinylcholine (the most commonly used muscle relaxant during anesthesia induction) is inactivated by pseudocholinesterase, people with an inherited pseudocholinesterase enzyme deficiency exhibit increased prolonged effects of succinylcholine. Patients with a genetic variant of pseudocholinesterase may have a nonfunctioning form of pseudocholinesterase and will also experience prolonged effects of succyinlcholine administration. Prolonged muscle paralysis and apnea will occur after anesthesia in these patients. This situation can be avoided by measuring serum cholinesterase (pseudocholinesterase) in all patients with a family history of prolonged apnea after surgery. Because patients with a nonfunctioning variant of pseudocholinesterase will have normal total quantitative pseudocholinesterase levels, yet still have prolonged paralytic effects of succynlcholine, a second test (dibucaine inhibition) usually is also performed. Dibucaine is a known local anesthetic that inhibits the function of normal pseudocholinesterase. The dibucaine number is the percent of pseudocholinesterase activity that is inhibited when dibucaine is added to the patient's serum sample. If total pseudocholinesterase is normal and dibucaine numbers are low, the presence of a nonfunctioning pseudocholinesterase variant is suspected and the patient will be at risk for succinylcholine-induced prolonged paralysis.

A common form of acquired cholinesterase deficiency, either true or pseudocholinesterase, is caused by overexposure to pesticides or organophosphates. Persons with jobs associated with chronic exposure to these chemicals are often monitored by the frequent testing of RBC cholinesterase levels. Other potential causes of reduced cholinesterase levels include chronic liver diseases, malnutrition, and hypoalbuminemia. An increased cholinesterase level, when found in the amniotic fluid, represents strong evidence for a *neural tube defect.*

Interfering factors

- Pregnancy decreases test values.
- ⚕ Drugs that may cause *decreased* values include atropine, caffeine, codeine, estrogens, morphine sulfate, neostigmine, oral contraceptives, phenothiazines, theophylline, quinidine, and vitamin K.

Procedure and patient care

Before

- PT Explain the procedure to the patient.
- PT Tell the patient that no fasting is required.
- If the test is done to identify the presurgical patient who may be at risk for cholinesterase deficiency, be sure the test is completed several days before the planned surgery.
- It may be recommended to withhold medications that could alter test results for 12 to 24 hours before the test.

During

- Collect a venous blood sample in a red-top tube.
- On the laboratory requisition slip, include a listing of all medications taken by the patient.

After

- Apply pressure or a pressure dressing to the venipuncture site.

Abnormal findings

▲ **Increased serum levels**

Hyperlipidemia
Nephrosis
Diabetes

▲ **Increased RBC levels**

Reticulocytosis
Sickle cell disease

▼ **Decreased serum levels**

Poisoning from organic
  phosphate insecticides
Hepatocellular disease
Persons with congenital
  pseudocholinesterase
  enzyme deficiency
Malnutrition

▼ **Decreased RBC levels**

Congenital
  cholinesterase
  deficiency
Poisoning from organic
  phosphate insecticides

notes

chorionic villus sampling (CVS, Chorionic villus biopsy [CVB])

C

Type of test   Cell analysis

Normal findings   No genetic or biochemical disorders

Test explanation and related physiology

CVS is performed on women whose unborn child may be at risk for life-threatening or significant life-altering genetic defects. This would include women who:

- Are older than age 35 to 40 years at the time of pregnancy
- Have had frequent spontaneous abortions
- Have had previous pregnancies with fetuses or infants with chromosomal or genetic defects (e.g., Down syndrome)
- Have a genetic defect in themselves (e.g., hemoglobinopathies)

The CVS test can be performed between 8 and 12 weeks of gestation for the early detection of genetic and biochemical disorders. Because CVS detects congenital defects early, first-trimester therapeutic abortions can be performed if indicated and desired.

For this study, a sample of chorionic villi from the chorion frondosum, which is the trophoblastic origin of the placenta, is obtained for analysis. These villi are present from 8 to 12 weeks on and reflect fetal chromosome, enzyme, and deoxyribonucleic acid content, thus permitting a much earlier diagnosis of prenatal problems than amniocentesis (see p. 54), which cannot be done before 14 to 16 weeks. Further, the cells derived by chorionic villus sampling are more easily grown in tissue culture for karyotyping (determination of chromosomal/genetic abnormalities). The cells obtained at amniocentesis take a longer time to grow in culture, further adding to the delay in obtaining answers. Although amniocentesis is a safer procedure, the information obtained is available much later in the pregnancy. At this late point, therapeutic abortion for severe genetic defects is more difficult.

Potential complications

- Accidental abortion
- Infection
- Bleeding
- Fetal limb deformities

Procedure and patient care

Before

PT Explain the procedure to the patient.

■ Be certain that the physician has obtained a signed consent for the procedure.

PT Tell the patient that no food or fluid restrictions are necessary.

PT Encourage the patient to drink at least 1 to 2 glasses of fluid before testing.

PT Instruct the patient not to urinate for several hours before testing. A full bladder is an excellent reference point for pelvic ultrasound.

■ Assess the vital signs of the mother and the fetal heart rate of the fetus before testing. These are baseline studies that should be repeated during and on completion of the test.

During

■ Note the following procedural steps:

1. The patient is placed in the lithotomy position.
2. A cannula is inserted into the cervix and uterine cavity (Figure 10).
3. Under ultrasound guidance the cannula is rotated to the site of the developing placenta.
4. A syringe is attached, and suction is applied to obtain several samples of villi.
5. As many as three or more samples may be obtained to get sufficient tissue for accurate sampling.
6. If ultrasound indicates that the trophoblastic tissue is remote from the cervix, a transabdominal approach similar to that described for amniocentesis (p. 54) may be used.

■ Note that this procedure is performed by an obstetrician in approximately 30 minutes.

PT Inform the patient that discomfort associated with this test is similar to that of a Pap smear.

After

■ Note that some Rh-negative patients may receive RhoGAM. RhoGAM is given because of the risk of Rh incompatibility from the fetal blood, which could threaten the fetus.

■ Monitor the vital signs and check the patient for signs of bleeding.

■ Schedule the patient for an ultrasound in 2 to 4 days to affirm the continued viability of the fetus.

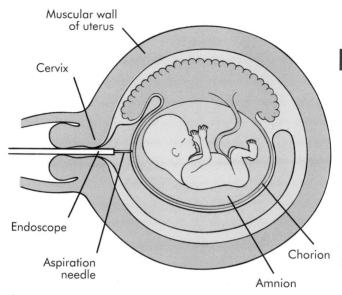

Figure 10 Chorionic villus sampling. Diagram of an 8-week pregnancy showing endoscopic aspiration of extraplacental villi.

- Assess the vaginal area for discharge and drainage; note the color and amount.
- **PT** Assess and educate the patient for signs of spontaneous abortion (e.g., cramps, bleeding).
- **PT** Inform the patient how she can obtain the results from her physician. Make sure she understands that the results are usually not available for several weeks. (Results may be available much sooner at major medical centers that perform this test.)
- **PT** Inform the patient about genetic counseling services if needed.

🏠 Home care responsibilities

- Instruct the patient to immediately report signs of spontaneous abortion (e.g., cramps and bleeding).
- Educate the mother to identify and report signs of endometrial infection (vaginal discharge, fever, crampy abdominal pain).

Abnormal findings
Genetic and biochemical disorders

notes

chromosome karyotype (Blood chromosome analysis, Chromosome studies, Cytogenetics, Karyotype)

C

Type of test Blood

Normal findings

Female: 44 autosomes + 2 X chromosomes; karyotype: 46,XX
Male: 44 autosomes + 1 X, 1 Y chromosome; karyotype: 46,XY

Test explanation and related physiology

This test is used to study an individual's chromosome makeup to determine chromosomal defects associated with disease or the risk of developing disease. The term *karyotyping* refers to the arrangement and pairing of cell chromosomes in order from the largest to the smallest to analyze their number and structure. Variations in either can produce numerous developmental abnormalities and diseases. A normal karyotype of chromosomes consists of a pattern of 22 pairs of autosomal chromosomes and a pair of sex chromosomes: XY for the male and XX for the female. Chromosomal karyotype abnormalities can be congenital or acquired. These karyotype abnormalities can occur because of duplication, deletion, translocation, reciprocation, or genetic rearrangement.

Chromosome karyotyping is useful in evaluating congenital anomalies, mental retardation, growth retardation, delayed puberty, infertility, hypogonadism, primary amenorrhea, ambiguous genitalia, chronic myelogenous leukemia, neoplasm, recurrent miscarriage, prenatal diagnosis of serious congenital diseases (especially in situations of advanced maternal age), Turner's syndrome, Klinefelter's syndrome, Down syndrome, and other suspected genetic disorders. The products of conception also can be studied to determine the cause of stillbirth or miscarriage.

Procedure and patient care

Before

PT Explain the procedure to the patient.
- Determine how the specimen will be collected. Obtain preparation guidelines from the laboratory if indicated.
- Many patients are fearful of the test results and require considerable emotional support.
- In some states, informed consent is required.

During

- Specimens for chromosome analysis can be obtained from numerous sources. Leukocytes from a peripheral venipuncture are most easily and most often used for this study.
- Bone marrow biopsies and surgical specimens also can be used sometimes as sources for analysis.
- During pregnancy, specimens can be collected by amniocentesis (see p. 54) and chorionic villus sampling (see p. 269).
- Fetal tissue or products of conception can be studied to determine the reason for loss of a pregnancy.
- Smears and stains of buccal mucosal cells are less costly but not as accurate as other tissue for karyotyping.

After

- Aftercare depends on how the specimen was collected.
- **PT** Inform the patient that test results are generally not available for several months.
- If an abnormality is identified, often the entire family line must be tested. This can be exhaustive and expensive.
- If the test results show an abnormality, encourage the patient to verbalize his or her feelings. Provide emotional support.

Abnormal findings

Congenital anomalies
Mental retardation
Growth retardation
Delayed puberty
Infertility
Hypogonadism
Primary amenorrhea
Ambiguous genitalia
Chronic myelogenous leukemia
Neoplasm
Recurrent miscarriage
Down syndrome
Tay-Sachs disease
Sickle cell anemia
Turner's syndrome
Klinefelter's syndrome

clostridial toxin assay (*Clostridium difficile*, Antibiotic-associated colitis assay; Pseudomembranous colitis toxic assay)

C

Type of test Stool

Normal findings Negative (no *Clostridium* toxin identified)

Test explanation and related physiology

Clostridium difficile bacterial infection of the intestine may occur in patients who are immunocompromised or taking broad-spectrum antibiotics (e.g., clindamycin, ampicillin, and cephalosporins). The infection results from depression of the normal flora of the bowel through the administration of antibiotics. This increases the number of *C. difficile* bacteria within the intestines. The overgrowth of *C. difficile* causes diarrhea, which is usually watery and voluminous. Abdominal cramps, fever, and leukocytosis are noted in most patients. Occasionally a patient has abdominal bloating and fever without diarrhea. Symptoms usually begin 4 to 10 days after the initiation of antibiotic therapy.

The clostridial bacterium releases a toxin that causes necrosis of the colonic epithelium. The detection of this toxin in the stool is therefore diagnostic of clostridial enterocolitis (pseudomembranous colitis). *C. difficile* can also be diagnosed by obtaining colonic-rectal tissue for this toxin. Finally, stool cultures (p. 876) for *C. difficile* can be performed. The patient must wait longer for stool culture results to be available than for results of the toxin assay.

Procedure and patient care

Before

PT Explain the method of stool collection to the patient. Be matter-of-fact to avoid embarrassment to the patient.

PT Instruct the patient not to mix urine and toilet paper with the stool specimen.

■ Handle the specimen carefully, as though it were capable of causing infection. If the nurse is assisting with the specimen collection, gloves should be worn.

During

PT Instruct the patient to defecate into a clean container. A rectal swab cannot be used because it collects inadequate amounts of stool.

- Note that a stool specimen also can be collected by proctoscopy.
- Place the specimen in a closed container and transport it to the laboratory to prevent deterioration of the toxin.
- If the specimen cannot be processed immediately, refrigerate it.

After

- Maintain enteric isolation precautions on all patients until appropriate therapy is completed.

Abnormal findings

Antibiotic-related (pseudomembranous) *C. difficile* colitis

notes

clot retraction test (Whole-blood clot retraction test)

Type of test Blood

Normal findings

50% to 100% clot retraction in 1 to 2 hours
Complete retraction within 24 hours

Test explanation and related physiology

The clot retraction test is used to evaluate bleeding disorders. Clot retraction is prolonged in thrombocytopenia (i.e., decreased platelet count), and Glanzmann's thrombasthenia (abnormal platelet function). Blood is collected in a tube free of anticoagulants. The time required to form a clot and for the edges of the clot to retract from the sides of the glass tube is the clot retraction time. The clot should be separate from the clear serum. It should maintain its shape (a mold of the glass tube) after being removed from the tube. If the platelet count is reduced or the function of the platelets is inadequate, the clot may only be weakly formed and may have very little if any retraction from the tube side walls. On removal, the clot is shapeless and dissipates. Clot retraction is rarely used today because of availability of accurate platelet counts and more accurate methods of determining platelet dysfunction.

If fibrinolysins are present, no clot retraction will occur. This test is only reliable if the hematocrit and fibrinogen (factor I) concentrations are within normal limits.

If the hematocrit is high (polycythemia or hemoconcentration), clot retraction time is reduced. If fibrinogen is reduced, clot retraction time is prolonged. Poor whole-blood clot retraction also occurs in patients with thrombasthenia (abnormal platelets) and Waldenström's macroglobulinemia.

Contraindications

- Patients with low platelet counts
- Patients with hypofibrinogenemia
- Patients taking aspirin

Interfering factors

- Uremia
- Drugs that may alter test results include aspirin and nonsteroidal antiinflammatory agents.

Procedure and patient care

Before

PT Explain the procedure to the patient.

PT Tell the patient that no fasting is required.

During

- Avoid excessive probing during venipuncture if a coagulation disorder is suspected.
- Collect approximately 5 to 7 ml of venous blood in a red-top tube.
- Avoid hemolysis.
- Indicate on the laboratory slip if the patient is taking aspirin or a nonsteroidal antiinflammatory agent.

After

- Transport the specimen to the laboratory within 1 hour of collection.
- Apply pressure or a pressure dressing to the venipuncture site.

Abnormal findings

▲ **Increased clot retraction**
Severe anemia
Hypofibrinogenemia

▼ **Decreased or poor clot retraction**
Thrombocytopenia
von Willebrand's disease
Thrombasthenia (abnormal platelets)
Waldenström's macroglobulinemia

notes

coagulating factors concentration (Factor assay, Coagulating factors, Blood-clotting factors)

Type of test Blood

Normal findings

Factor	Normal value (% of "normal")
II	80-120
V	50-150
VII	65-140
VIII	55-145
IX	60-140
X	45-155
XI	65-135
XII	50-150

Test explanation and related physiology

These tests measure the quantity of each specific factor thought to be responsible for suspected defects in hemostasis. Testing is available to measure the quantity of the factors listed above. When these factors exist in concentrations below their "minimal hemostatic level," clotting is impaired. These minimal hemostatic levels vary according to the factor involved.

Deficiencies of these factors may be a result of inherited genetic defects, acquired diseases, or drug therapy. Common medical conditions associated with decreased factor concentrations are listed in Table 10. It is important to identify the exact factor or factors involved in the coagulating defect so that appropriate blood component replacement can be administered.

The hemostasis and coagulation system is a homeostatic balance between factors encouraging clotting and those encouraging clot dissolution (Figure 11). See Table 11 for a list of factor names and routine coagulation test abnormalities associated with factor deficiency.

Fibrinogen (factor I, p. 454), like many of the coagulation proteins, is considered an acute reactant protein and is elevated in many severe illnesses. It is also considered a risk factor for coronary heart disease and stroke.

Prothrombin is a vitamin K–dependent clotting factor. Its production in the liver requires vitamin K. This vitamin is fat soluble and is dependent on bile for absorption. Bile duct

Text continued on p. 284.

TABLE 10 Conditions that may result in coagulation factor excess or deficiency

Factor	Increased (excess)	Decreased (deficiency)
I (Fibrinogen)	Acute inflammatory reactions	Liver disease (hepatitis or cirrhosis)
	Trauma	DIC
	Coronary heart disease	Fibrinolysis
	Cigarette smoking	Congenital deficiency
II (Prothrombin)	ND	Vitamin K deficiency
		Liver disease
		Congenital deficiency
		Warfarin ingestion
V (Proaccelerin)	ND	Liver disease
		DIC
		Fibrinolysis
VII (Proconvertin [stable factor])	ND	Congenital deficiency
		Vitamin K deficiency
		Liver disease
		Warfarin ingestion
VIII (Antihemophilic factor)	Acute inflammatory reactions	Hemophilia A
	Trauma/stress	Congenital deficiency
	Pregnancy	DIC
		Autoimmune disease
von Willebrand factor	ND	von Willebrand's disease
		Congenital deficiency
		Autoimmune disease

Continued

TABLE 10 Conditions that may result in coagulation factor excess or deficiency—cont'd

Factor	Increased (excess)	Decreased (deficiency)
IX (Christmas factor)	ND	Congenital deficiency Hemophilia B Liver disease Nephrotic syndrome Warfarin ingestion DIC Vitamin K deficiency
X (Stuart factor)	ND	Congenital deficiency Liver disease Warfarin ingestion Vitamin K deficiency
XII (Hageman factor)	ND	Congenital deficiency Vitamin K deficiency Liver disease Warfarin ingestion DIC

ND, there is no common disease state known to be associated with an excess of this factor; *DIC,* disseminated intravascular coagulation.

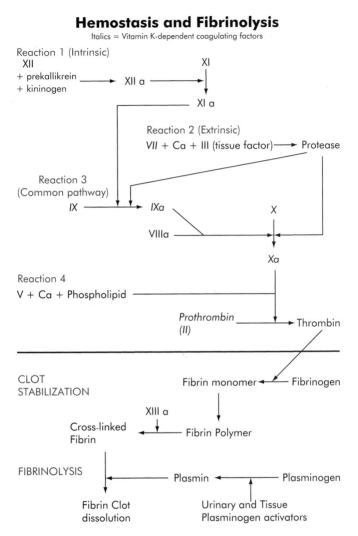

Figure 11 Secondary hemostasis (fibrin clot formation) and fibrinolysis (fibrin clot dissolution). Primary hemostasis involves platelet plugging of the injured blood vessel. Secondary hemostasis, as described here, takes place most rapidly on the platelet surface after attachment to the fractured endothelium. Four different reactions result in the formation of fibrin. As seen beneath the dark line in the figure, the fibrin clot supports the platelet clump so that the clot does not get swept away by the tremendous "shear forces" of the fast-moving blood cells. Fibrinolysis follows formation of the fibrin clot in order to prevent complete occlusion of the injured blood vessel.

TABLE 11 List of minimum concentration of coagulation factors required for fibrin production

Factor	Name	Quantitation minimum hemostatic level (mg/dl)	Abnormal coagulation tests associated with deficiency	Blood components to provide specific factor
I	Fibrinogen	60-100		C, FFP, FWB
II	Prothrombin	10-15	PT	P, WB, FFP FWB
III	Tissue factor or thromboplastin	QNA	PT	
IV	Calcium	see calcium, p. 220		
V	Proaccelerin	5-10	PT, APTT	FFP, FWB
VII	Stable factor	5-20	PT	P, WB, FFP, FWB
VIII	Antihemophilic factor	30	APTT	C, FFP, VIII CONC
IX	Christmas factor	30	APTT	FFP, FWB
X	Stuart factor	8-10	PT, APTT	P, WB, FFP, FWB
XI	Plasma thromboplastin antecedent	25	APTT	P, WB, FFP, FWB
XII	Hageman factor	yes	APTT	
XIII	Fibrin stabilizing factor	no	APTT, WBC	

APTT, activated partial thromboplastin time; *PT*, prothrombin time; *WBC*, whole blood clotting; *C*, cryoprecipitate; *FFP*, fresh frozen plasma; *FWB*, fresh whole blood (less than 24 hours old); *P*, unfrozen banked plasma; *WB*, banked whole blood; *VII CONC*, factor VIII concentrate.

Text continued from p. 279.

obstruction or malabsorption causes a vitamin K deficiency and results in reduced quantity of prothrombin and other vitamin K–dependent factors (VII, IX, X). It usually takes about 3 weeks before body stores of vitamin K are exhausted.

Factor VIII is actually a complex molecule with two components. The first component is related to hemophilia A and is involved in the hemostatic mechanism as described in previous paragraphs. The second component is the von Willebrand factor and is related to von Willebrand's disease. This second component is involved in platelet adhesion and aggregation. Patients with factor XII deficiency have been observed to have an increased risk of myocardial infarction and venous thrombosis.

Interfering factors

- Many of these proteins are heat sensitive, and their levels are decreased the longer the specimen is kept at room temperatures.
- Pregnancy or the use of contraceptive medication can increase levels of several of these factors, especially VIII and IX. A mild deficiency can be masked.
- Many of these protein coagulation factors are "acute reactant" proteins. Acute illness, stress, exercise, or inflammation can raise levels.

Procedure and patient care

Before
PT Explain the procedure to the patient.
PT Tell the patient that no fasting is required.

During
- Collect approximately 7 to 10 ml of venous blood in a blue-top tube.

After
- Apply pressure to the venipuncture site.
- Deliver the blood specimen to the laboratory as soon as possible.

Abnormal findings

Table 10 on p. 280 lists conditions that may result in a coagulation factor excess or deficiency.

colonoscopy

Type of test Endoscopy

Normal findings Normal colon

Test explanation and related physiology

With fiberoptic colonoscopy, the entire colon from anus to cecum can be examined in most patients. As with sigmoidoscopy, benign and malignant neoplasms, polyps, mucosal inflammation, ulceration, and sites of active hemorrhage can be visualized. Diseases such as cancer, polyps, ulcers, and arteriovenous (AV) malformations also can be visualized. Cancers, polyps, and inflammatory bowel diseases can be biopsied through the colonoscope with cable-activated instruments; and sites of active bleeding can be coagulated with the use of laser, electrocoagulation, and injection of sclerosing agents.

This test is recommended for patients who have obvious or occult blood in the stool, lower gastrointestinal bleeding, a change in bowel habits, or who are at high risk for colon cancer. The latter group includes patients with a strong personal or family history of colon cancer, polyps, or ulcerative colitis. It is recommended for patients who have abdominal pain and is used as a surveillance tool for patients who have had colorectal cancer, inflammatory bowel disease, or polyposis.

Contraindications

- Patients whose medical condition is not stable
  This test requires sedation, which may induce hypotension in the medically unstable patient.
- Patients who are bleeding profusely from the rectum
  The viewing lens will become covered with blood clots, preventing visualization of the lower intestinal tract.
- Patients with a suspected perforation of the colon
- Patients with toxic megacolon
  These patients may worsen with the test preparation.
- Patients with a recent colon anastomosis (within the last 14 to 21 days)
  The anastomosis may break down with significant insufflation of CO_2.

Potential complications

- Bowel perforation
- Persistent bleeding from a biopsy site
- Oversedation, resulting in respiratory depression

Interfering factors

- Poor bowel preparation may result in the stool immediately obstructing the lens and precluding adequate visualization of the colon.
- Active bleeding obstructs the lens system and precludes adequate visualization of the colon.

Procedure and patient care

Before

PT Explain the procedure to the patient.

PT Fully inform the patient about the risks of the procedure and obtain an informed consent.

PT Instruct the patient as to the appropriate bowel preparation. One type is the *2-day bowel preparation*, which uses clear liquids for 2 days, along with a strong cathartic such as magnesium citrate and bisacodyl (Dulcolax). On the day of examination, an enema is given. A *1-day preparation* using a glycol (CoLyte) bowel preparation has become more widely used. After the patient ingests a gallon of CoLyte, enemas are not usually needed. The 1 gallon should be consumed within 4 hours if possible. Lemonade powder may be added to the glycol cathartic.

- Avoid an oral bowel preparation in patients with upper gastrointestinal obstruction, suspected acute diverticulitis, or recent bowel resectional surgery.
- Assure patients that they will be appropriately draped to avoid unnecessary embarrassment.
- Administer appropriate preendoscopy sedation, usually meperidine (Demerol) and midazolam hydrochloride (Versed).

During

- Note the following procedural steps:
  1. IV access is obtained.
  2. After a rectal examination indicates adequate bowel preparation, the patient is sedated.
  3. The patient is placed in the lateral decubitus position, and the colonoscope is placed into the rectum.

4. Under direct visualization, the colonoscope is directed to the cecum. Often a significant amount of manipulation is required to obtain this position.

5. As in all endoscopy, air is insufflated to distend the bowel for better visualization.

6. Complete examination of the large bowel is carried out.

7. Polypectomy, biopsy, and other endoscopic surgery is performed after appropriate visualization.

8. When the laser or coagulator is used, the air is removed, and carbon dioxide is used as an insufflating agent to avoid explosion.

▪ Note that this test is performed by a physician trained in gastrointestinal endoscopy in approximately 30 to 60 minutes.

PT Tell the patient that minimal discomfort is associated with the test.

After

PT Explain to patients that air has been insufflated into the bowel. They may experience flatulence or gas pains.

▪ Examine the abdomen for evidence of colon perforation (abdominal distention and tenderness).

▪ Assess the patient's vital signs. Watch for a decrease in blood pressure and an increase in pulse as an indication of hemorrhage.

▪ Inspect the stool for gross blood.

▪ Notify the physician if the patient develops increased pain or significant gastrointestinal bleeding.

▪ Allow the patient to eat when fully alert if no evidence of bowel perforation exists.

PT Encourage the patient to drink a lot of fluids when intake is allowed. This will make up for the dehydration associated with the bowel preparation.

🏠 Home care responsibilities

- Observe for increasing abdominal pain, which may indicate bowel perforation.
- Inform the patient that frequent, bloody bowel movements may indicate poor hemostasis if biopsy or polypectomy was performed.
- Observe for abdominal bloating and inability to pass flatus, which may indicate colon obstruction if a neoplasm was identified.
- Assess for weakness and dizziness, which may indicate orthostasis and hypovolemia due to dehydration.
- Evaluate for fever and chills, which may indicate a bowel perforation.

Abnormal findings

Colon cancer
Colon polyps
Inflammatory bowel disease (e.g., ulcerative or Crohn's colitis)
AV malformations
Hemorrhoids
Ischemic or postinflammatory strictures
Diverticulosis

notes

colposcopy

Type of test Endoscopy

Normal findings Normal vagina and cervix

Test explanation and related physiology

Colposcopy provides an in situ macroscopic examination of the vagina and cervix with a colposcope, which is a macroscope with a light source and a magnifying lens (Figure 12). With this procedure, tiny areas of dysplasia, carcinoma in situ, and invasive cancer that would be missed by the naked eye can be visualized, and biopsy specimens can be obtained. The study is performed on patients with abnormal vaginal epithelial patterns, cervical lesions, or suspicious Pap smear results and on those exposed to

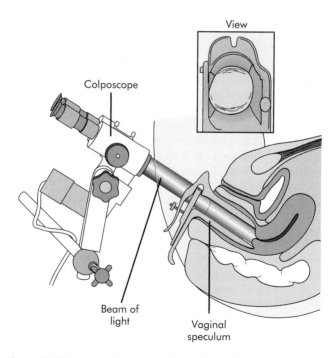

Figure 12 Colposcopy. A colposcope is used to evaluate clients with an abnormal Pap smear and a grossly normal cervix.

diethylstilbestrol in utero. It may be a sufficient substitute to cone biopsy (removal and examination of a cone of tissue from the cervix) in evaluating the cause of abnormal cervical cytologic findings.

It is important to realize that colposcopy is useful only in identifying a suspicious lesion. Definitive diagnosis requires biopsy of the tissue. One of the major advantages of this procedure is that of directing the biopsy to the area most likely to be truly representative of the lesion. A biopsy performed without colposcopy may not necessarily be representative of the lesion's true pathologic condition, resulting in a significant risk of missing a serious lesion.

The patient will need to have diagnostic conization if:

1. Colposcopy and endocervical curettage do not explain the problem or match the cytologic findings of the Pap smear within one grade.
2. The entire transformation zone is not seen.
3. The lesion extends up the cervical canal beyond the vision of the colposcope.

The need for up to 90% of cone biopsies is eliminated by an experienced colposcopist. Endocervical curettage may routinely accompany colposcopy to detect unknown lesions in the endocervical canal.

Contraindications

- Patients with heavy menstrual flow

Interfering factors

- Failure to cleanse the cervix of foreign materials (e.g., creams, medications) may impair visualization.

Procedure and patient care

Before

PT Explain the procedure to the patient.

- Obtain informed consent if required by the institution.

During

- Note the following procedural steps:
  1. The patient is placed in the lithotomy position, and a vaginal speculum is used to expose the vagina and cervix.
  2. After the cervix is sampled for cytologic findings, it is cleansed with a 3% acetic acid solution to remove excess mucus and cellular debris. The acetic acid also accentuates the difference between normal and abnormal epithelial tissues.

3. The colposcope is focused on the cervix, which is then carefully examined.

4. Usually the entire lesion can be outlined, and the most atypical areas selected for biopsy specimen removal.

- Note that colposcopy is performed by a physician in approximately 5 to 10 minutes.

PT Tell the patient that some women complain of pressure pains from the vaginal speculum and that momentary discomfort may be felt if biopsy specimens are obtained.

After

PT Inform the patient that she may have vaginal bleeding if biopsy specimens were taken. Suggest that she wear a sanitary pad.

PT Instruct the patient to abstain from intercourse and not to insert anything (except a tampon) into the vagina until healing of a biopsy is confirmed.

PT Inform the patient when and how to obtain the results of this study.

Abnormal findings

Dysplasia
Carcinoma in situ
Invasive cancer
Cervical lesions

notes

complement assay (C3 and C4 complement)

Type of test Blood

Normal findings

Total complement: 75-160 units/ml or 75-160 kU/L (SI units)
C3: 55-120 mg/dl or 0.55-1.20 g/L (SI units)
C4: 20-50 mg/dl or 0.20-0.50 g/L (SI units)

Test explanation and related physiology

Measurements of complement are used primarily to diagnose angioedema and to monitor the activity of disease in patients with systemic lupus erythematosus nephritis, membranoproliferative nephritis, or poststreptococcal nephritis.

Serum complement is a group of globulin proteins that act as enzymes. These enzymes facilitate the immunologic and inflammatory response. The total complement, sometimes labeled CH 50, is made up of nine major components: C1 through C9. Besides these major components, there are some subcomponent and "inhibitor" components involved in the system. Once activated, complement acts to increase vascular permeability, allowing antibodies and white blood cells (WBCs) to be delivered to the area of the immune/antigen complex. Complement also acts to increase chemotaxis (attracting WBCs to the area), phagocytosis, and immune adherence of the antibody to antigen. These processes are vitally important in the normal inflammatory response.

Reduced complement levels can be congenital, as in hereditary angioedema. Hereditary angioedema is a congenital lack of a C1 "inhibitor" (often called C1 esterase). The complement system is overly activated, and the complement components are "consumed" or used up. Serum levels fall.

In the chronic presence of antibody/antigen complexes, the complement system is overly activated, and the complement components are "consumed" or used up. Serum levels fall. Diseases associated with these immune complexes include serum sickness, lupus erythematosus, infectious endocarditis, renal transplant rejection, vasculitis, and some forms of glomerulonephritis. As these diseases are successfully treated, complement levels can be expected to return to normal.

Complement components are increased after the onset of various acute or chronic inflammatory diseases or acute tissue damage. This is very similar to an "acute reaction" protein.

Interfering factors

- C3 is very unstable at room temperatures.

Procedure and patient care

Before

PT Explain the procedure to the patient.

PT Tell the patient that no fasting or special preparations are required.

During

- Collect 7 to 10 ml of venous blood in a red-top tube.

After

- Apply pressure to the venipuncture site.

Abnormal findings

▲ **Increased levels**

Rheumatic fever (acute)
Myocardial infarction (acute)
Ulcerative colitis
Cancer

▼ **Decreased levels**

Cirrhosis
Autoimmune disease (e.g., systemic lupus erythematosus)
Serum sickness (immune complex disease)
Glomerulonephritis
Lupus nephritis
Renal transplant rejection (acute)
Protein malnutrition
Anemia
Malnutrition
Hepatitis
Rheumatoid arthritis
Sjögren's syndrome
Severe sepsis

notes

complete blood count and differential count
(CBC and diff)

The CBC and differential count are a series of tests of the peripheral blood that provide a tremendous amount of information about the hematologic system and many other organ systems. They are inexpensively, easily, and rapidly performed as a screening test. The CBC and differential count include automated measurement of the following studies, which are discussed separately:

Red blood cell count (RBC, see p. 782)
Hemoglobin (Hgb, see p. 514)
Hematocrit (Hct, see p. 511)
Red blood cell indices (RBC indices, see p. 785)
    Mean corpuscular volume (MCV)
    Mean corpuscular hemoglobin (MCH)
    Mean corpuscular hemoglobin concentration (MCHC)
    Red blood cell distribution width (RDW)
White blood cell count (WBC) and differential count
    (see p. 994)
    Neutrophils (polynucleated cells or "polys," segmented
        cells or "segs," band cells, stab cells)
    Lymphocytes
    Monocytes
    Eosinophils
    Basophils
Blood smear (see p. 174)
Platelet count (see p. 714)
Platelet volume, mean (MPV), (see p. 717)

notes

computed tomography of the abdomen (CAT scan of the abdomen, CT scan of the abdomen, Helical/spiral CT scan of the abdomen, CT angiography, CT arteriography, CT colonoscopy, Virtual colonoscopy)

C

Type of test X-ray with contrast dye

Normal findings No evidence of abnormality

Test explanation and related physiology

The CT scan of the abdomen is a noninvasive, yet very accurate, x-ray procedure used to diagnose pathologic conditions such as tumors, cysts, abscesses, inflammation, perforation, bleeding, obstruction, aneurysms, and calculi of the abdominal and retroperitoneal organs. The CT scan image results from passing x-rays through the abdominal organs at many angles. The variation in density of each tissue allows for a variable penetration of the x-rays. Each density is given a numeric value called a *density coefficient,* which is digitally computed into shades of gray. This is then displayed on a television screen as thousands of dots in various shades of gray. The final display appears as an actual photograph of the anatomic area sectioned by x-rays. The image can be enhanced by repeating the CT scan after IV administration of iodine containing-contrast dye. These images can be recorded on Polaroid or x-ray film.

Liver tumors, abscesses, trauma, cysts, and anatomic abnormalities can be seen; and pancreatic tumors, pseudocysts, inflammation, calcification, bleeding, and trauma can be detected. The kidneys and urinary outflow tract are well visualized.

Renal tumors and cysts, ureteral obstruction, calculi, and congenital renal and ureteral abnormalities are easily seen with the use of IV contrast injection. Extravasation of urine secondary to trauma or obstruction can also be demonstrated easily. Adrenal tumors and hyperplasia are best diagnosed with this technique. Some radiology literature indicates that the histology of the tumor can be suggested based on the density coefficients shown on the scan.

Although the bowel can be better visualized by an upper GI series, small bowel follow-through, or barium enema, large tumors and perforations of the bowel can be identified with the CT scan, especially when oral contrast is ingested. The spleen can be well visualized for hematoma, laceration, fracture, tumor infiltration, and splenic vein thrombosis with CT scanning. The retroperitoneal lymph nodes can be evaluated. These are usually present, but all nodes with a diameter greater than 2 cm are considered abnormal. The abdominal aorta and its major branches can be evaluated for aneurysmal dilation and intramural thrombi, and the pelvic structures (including the uterus, ovaries, tubes, prostate, and rectum) and musculature can be evaluated for tumors, abscesses, infection, or hypertrophy. Ascites and hemoperitoneum can easily be demonstrated with the CT scan.

With the development of new and faster scanners, dynamic scanning can be performed during arterial injection of dye to the organ being studied. Dynamic scanning can indicate blood flow and degree of vascularity of an organ or part of an organ in the abdomen. This is called *dynamic CT scanning*. (See CT portogram, p. 307, as an example.)

Helical (also called spiral, or volume-averaging) *CT scanning* represents a marked improvement over standard CT scanning. The helical CT scan continuously obtains images as the patient is passed through the gantry. This produces faster and more accurate images. Because the helical CT can image the abdomen or chest in less than 30 seconds, the entire study can be performed with one breath hold. Therefore breathing and motion misrepresentations are eliminated. Images are improved and scan time is reduced. This is particularly helpful in scanning uncooperative adults or children. Through volume averaging, three-dimensional images can be re-created. Furthermore, when contrast material is used, the entire region can be imaged in just a few seconds after the contrast injection, thereby further improving contrast imaging.

Helical CT scan is very helpful in identifying liver and pancreatic tumors. With the development of multichannel CT helical scans that take as many as 16 "slices" per turn of the x-ray gantry, *virtual colonoscopy* is possible. With no sedation and no discomfort, this is fast becoming a reality in many hospitals. A mechanical bowel prep is still used; however, it is possible to use a "barium contrast" 1 day prior to CT scanning. The barium marks all the stool, and can then be "subtracted," leaving only the virtual "clean" colon to evaluate. Unlike endoscopic colonoscopy, polypectomy or biopsy cannot be performed with virtual testing.

Helical *CT arteriography or angiography* is developing through the use of multichannel helical CT scanning. After IV injection of contrast, CT imaging can demonstrate the arteries in any given organ. With computerized subtraction of the surrounding tissue, the arteries can be even better displayed. Three-dimensional re-creations of the aorta and other abdominal vessels are possible. This is particularly helpful in identifying renal artery stenosis and hepatic vasculature for cancer-related resections. Renal helical arteriography can be used to demonstrate and evaluate each functional phase of urinary excretion.

The CT scan can be used as a guide to aspirate fluid from the abdomen or one of the abdominal organs. This fluid can be sent for cultures and other studies. The CT scan can also be used to guide biopsy needles into areas of abdominal tumors to obtain tissue of study. Catheters for drainage of intraabdominal abscess can be placed with CT guidance.

The CT scan is an important part of staging and monitoring of many tumors before and after therapy. Tumors of the colon, rectum, liver, breast, lung, prostate, ovary, uterus, kidney, lymph, and adrenal commonly recur in the abdomen. Recurrence can be detected early with the CT scan.

Contraindications

- Patients who are allergic to iodinated dye or shellfish
- Patients who are pregnant, unless the benefits outweigh the risks
- Patients whose vital signs are unstable
- Patients who are very obese, usually more than 300 lb
- Patients who are claustrophobic

Potential complications

- Allergic reaction to iodinated dye
  See p. xix for appropriate interventions concerning the care of patients with iodine allergy.
- Acute renal failure from dye infusion
  Adequate hydration before the infusion may reduce this likelihood.
- Hypoglycemia or acidosis may occur in patients who are taking Glucophage and receive iodine dye.

Interfering factors

- Presence of metallic objects (e.g., hemostasis clips)
- Retained barium from previous studies
- Large amounts of fecal material or gas in the bowel

Procedure and patient care

Before

PT Explain the procedure to the patient. The patient's cooperation is necessary, because he or she must lie still during the procedure.
- Obtain informed consent if required by the institution.
- Assess the patient for allergies to iodinated dye or shellfish.

PT Show the patient a picture of the CT machine. Encourage the patient to verbalize his or her concerns because some patients may have claustrophobia. Most patients who are mildly claustrophobic can be scanned after appropriate premedication with antianxiety drugs.

- Keep the patient NPO for at least 4 hours before the test if oral contrast is to be administered; however, this test can be performed on an emergency basis on patients who have recently eaten.

- Note that this procedure is usually performed by a radiologist in less than 30 minutes. If dye is administered, the procedure time may be doubled, because the CT scan is done both with and without contrast dye.

PT Tell the patient that the discomforts associated with this study include lying still on a hard table and the peripheral venipuncture. Mild nausea is a common sensation when contrast dye is used. An emesis basin should be readily available. Some patients may experience a salty taste, flushing, and warmth during the dye injection.

During

- Note the following procedure for the abdominal CT scan:
  1. The patient is taken to the radiology department and placed on the CT scan table.
  2. The patient then is placed in an encircling body scanner (gantry). The x-ray tube travels around the gantry and takes pictures of the various levels of the abdomen and pelvis. Any motion causes blurring and streaking of the final picture. Therefore the patient is asked to remain motionless during x-ray exposure. Television monitoring equipment allows for immediate display of the CT scan image, which is then recorded on an x-ray film. In a separate room the technicians manipulate the CT scan table, affecting the level of the abdomen that is scanned.
  3. Through audio communication, the patient is instructed to hold his or her breath during x-ray exposure.
- Remember that oral and IV iodinated x-ray contrast dye provides better results for this test. One can accurately differentiate the gastrointestinal organs from the other abdominal organs with oral contrast. Likewise, the vessels and ureters are contrasted with the surrounding structures with use of IV dye. Sometimes contrast is given rectally to visualize the pelvic organs.

After

PT Encourage the patient to drink fluids to avoid dye-induced renal failure and promote dye excretion.

PT Inform the patient that diarrhea may occur after ingestion of the oral contrast.

- Evaluate the patient for delayed reaction to dye.

Abnormal findings

Liver
Tumor
Abscess
Bile duct dilation

Pancreas
Tumor
Pseudocyst
Inflammation
Bleeding

Spleen
Hematoma
Fracture
Laceration
Tumor
Venous thrombosis

Gallbladder/biliary system
Gallstones
Tumor
Bile duct dilation

Kidneys
Tumor
Cyst
Ureteral obstruction
Calculi
Congenital abnormalities
Renal artery stenosis

Adrenal
Adenoma
Cancer
Pheochromocytoma
Hemorrhage
Myelolipoma hyperplasia

GI tract
Perforation
Tumor
Inflammatory bowel disease
Diverticulitis
Appendicitis

Uterus, tubes, ovaries
Tumor
Abscess
Infection
Hydrosalpinx
Cyst
Fibroid

Prostate
Hypertrophy
Tumor

Retroperitoneum
Tumor
Lymphadenopathy

Other
Abdominal aneurysm
Ascites, hemoperitoneum
Abscess

computed tomography of the brain (CT scan of the brain, Computerized axial transverse tomography [CATT], Helical/spiral CT scan of the brain)

Type of test X-ray with contrast dye

Normal findings No evidence of pathologic conditions

Test explanation and related physiology

Computed tomography of the brain consists of a computerized analysis of multiple tomographic x-ray films taken of the brain tissue at successive layers, providing a three-dimensional view of the cranial contents. The CT image provides a view of the head as if one were looking down through its top. The variation in density of each tissue allows for variable penetration of the x-ray beam. An attached computer calculates the amount of x-ray penetration of each tissue and displays this as shades of gray. The image is placed on a television screen and photographed. The final result is a series of actual anatomic pictures of coronal sections of the brain.

The CT scan is used in the differential diagnosis of intracranial neoplasms, cerebral infarctions, ventricular displacement or enlargement, cortical atrophy, cerebral aneurysms, intracranial hemorrhage and hematoma, and arteriovenous (AV) malformation. Information about the ventricular system can be obtained by CT scanning. Multiple sclerosis and other degenerative abnormalities can be identified also.

Visualization of a neoplasm, previous infarction, or any pathologic process that destroys the blood-brain barrier may be enhanced by IV injection of an iodinated contrast dye. CT scans may be repeated frequently to monitor the progress of any disease or to monitor the healing process. In many cases, CT scanning has eliminated the need for more invasive procedures such as cerebral arteriography and pneumoencephalography. In many localities, MRI scanning of the brain has replaced the use of CT scans of the brain.

Recently the CT scan has been used to determine *cerebral blood flow (CBF)*. In this study *(xenon CT scan)*, the patient is asked to inhale stable xenon gas (mixed with oxygen) while in the CT scanner. The xenon immediately diffuses into the bloodstream. The blood delivers the xenon to the brain. Uptake of xenon by the brain is almost immediate and is primarily determined by the flow of blood to the brain. Xenon concentration is calculated by the computer based on post-xenon images. The computer almost immediately converts those images to precise CBF measurement in ml per 100 g of brain tissue per minute. Cerebral vascular occlusive disease, increased intracranial pressure, and intracranial bleeding are just a few of the abnormalities associated with reduced CBF. Normal average CBF is about 55 ml per 100 g per minute. Xenon scanning is also used to determine "brain death" (CBF = 0).

Helical (also called spiral, or volume-averaging) *CT scanning* represents a significant improvement over standard CT scanning. The helical CT scan continuously obtains images as the patient is passed through the gantry. This produces faster and more accurate images. Because the helical CT scan images the selected area in less than 30 seconds, the entire study can be performed with one breath hold. Therefore breathing and motion misrepresentations are eliminated. Images are improved and scan time is reduced. This is particularly helpful in scanning uncooperative adults or children. Through volume averaging, three-dimensional images can be re-created. Furthermore, when contrast material is used, the entire region can be imaged in just a few seconds after the contrast injection, thereby further improving contrast imaging.

Helical CT scan is very helpful in re-creation of three-dimensional images to determine accurate localization of brain tumors. Helical CT arteriography is developing. Helical CT scanning is performed immediately after arterial contrast injection. Three-dimensional re-creations of the carotid artery and its branches are also extremely helpful in the evaluation of cerebral vascular disease.

Contraindications

- Patients who are allergic to iodinated dye or shellfish
- Patients who are claustrophobic
- Patients who are pregnant, unless the benefits outweigh the risks
- Patients whose vital signs are unstable
- Patients who are very obese, usually more than 300 lb

Potential complications

- Allergic reaction to iodinated dye
  See p. xix for appropriate interventions concerning the care of patients with iodine allergy.
- Acute renal failure from dye infusion
  Adequate hydration beforehand may reduce this likelihood.

- Hypoglycemia or acidosis may occur in patients who are taking Glucophage and receive iodine dye.
- Apnea if xenon is used as an anesthetic gas

Procedure and patient care

Before

PT Explain the procedure to the patient. The patient's cooperation is necessary, because he or she must lie still during the procedure.

- Obtain informed consent if required by the institution.

PT Show the patient a picture of the CT machine and encourage the patient to verbalize his or her concerns, because some patients may have claustrophobia. Most patients who are mildly claustrophobic can be scanned after appropriate premedication with antianxiety drugs.

- Keep the patient NPO for 4 hours before the study, because contrast dye may cause nausea. It is not usually known before the test if enhanced visualization by dye injection will be indicated. If contrast will not be used, food and fluids may be taken.

PT Instruct the patient that wigs, hairpins, clips, or partial dental plates cannot be worn during the procedure because they hamper visualization of the brain.

- Assess the patient for allergies to iodinated dye or shellfish. Tell the patient that he or she may hear a "clicking" noise as the scanning machine moves around the head.

During

- Note the following procedure for the brain CT scan:
  1. The patient lies in the supine position on an examining table with the head resting on a snug-fitting rubber cap within a water-filled box. The patient's head is enclosed only to the hairline (as in a hair dryer). The face is not covered, and the patient can see out of the machine at all times. Sponges are placed along the side of the head to ensure that the patient's head does not move during the study.
  2. The scanner passes an x-ray beam through the brain from one side to the other. The machine then rotates 1 degree, and the procedure is repeated at each degree through a 180-degree arc. The machine is then moved, and the entire procedure is repeated through a total of three to seven planes.

- Remember that an iodinated dye will usually then be used. A peripheral IV line is started, and the iodinated dye is administered through it. The entire scanning process is repeated.
- If a *xenon scan* is requested, a 26% xenon-oxygen gas is inhaled while CT scanning is repeated. The patient must be closely monitored (respiratory rate, CO_2 levels, and pulse oximetry). Apnea can occur and must be recognized. With verbal encouragement, the patient can usually be stimulated to breathe.
- Note that this procedure is performed by a radiologist in less than 1 hour. If dye is administered, the procedure time is doubled, because the CT scan is done with and without the contrast dye.

PT Tell the patient that the discomforts associated with this study include lying still on a hard table and peripheral venipuncture. Mild nausea is a common sensation when contrast dye is used. An emesis basin should be readily available. Some patients may experience a salty taste, flushing, and warmth during the dye injection.

After

PT Encourage the patient to drink fluids, because dye is excreted by the kidneys and causes diuresis.
- See p. xix for appropriate interventions concerning care of patients with iodine allergy.

Abnormal findings

Intracranial neoplasm
Cerebral infarction
Ventricular displacement
Ventricular enlargement
Cortical atrophy
Cerebral aneurysm
Intracranial hemorrhage
Hematoma
AV malformation
Meningioma
Multiple sclerosis
Hydrocephalus
Abscess

computed tomography of the chest (Chest CT scan, Helical/spiral CT scan of the chest)

Type of test   X-ray with contrast dye

Normal findings   No evidence of pathologic conditions

Test explanation and related physiology

Computed tomography of the chest is a noninvasive yet very accurate x-ray procedure for diagnosing and evaluating pathologic conditions such as tumors, nodules, hematomas, parenchymal coin lesions, cysts, abscesses, pleural effusion, and enlarged lymph nodes affecting the lungs and mediastinum. Tumors, cysts, and fractures of the chest wall and pleura also can be seen. When an IV contrast material is given, vascular structures can be identified, and a diagnosis of aortic or other vascular abnormality can be made. With oral contrast, the esophagus and upper structures can be evaluated for tumor and other conditions. This procedure provides a cross-sectional view of the chest and is especially useful in detecting small differences in tissue densities, demonstrating lesions that cannot be seen with conventional radiology and tomography. The mediastinal structures can be visualized in a manner that cannot be equaled with conventional x-ray and tomographic scans.

The x-ray image results from using a body scanner (x-ray tube held in a circular gantry) to deliver x-rays through the patient's chest at many different angles. The variation in density of each tissue allows for a variable penetration of the x-rays. Each density is given a numeric value called a *coefficient,* which is digitally computed into shades of gray. This is then displayed on a television screen as thousands of dots in various shades of gray. The final display appears as an actual photograph of the anatomic area sectioned by the x-rays.

Helical (also called spiral, or volume-averaging) *CT scanning* represents a significant improvement over standard CT scanning. The helical CT scan continuously obtains images as the patient is passed through the gantry. This produces faster and more accurate images. Because the helical CT can image the abdomen or chest in less than 30 seconds, the entire study can be performed with one breath hold. Therefore breathing and motion misrepresentations are eliminated. Images are improved and scan time is reduced. This is particularly helpful in scanning uncooperative adults or children. Through volume averaging, three-dimensional images can be re-created. Furthermore, when contrast material is used, the entire region can be imaged in just a few seconds after the contrast injection, thereby further improving contrast imaging.

Helical CT scan is now considered the preferred study to identify pulmonary emboli. It can be performed easily and rapidly. Helical CT scanning of the heart can identify tiny calcifications in the coronary arteries. This finding is indicative of increased risk for an ischemic event. Pulmonary nodules are particularly well evaluated with this rapid form of CT scanning because breathing misrepresentations are eliminated.

Contraindications

- Patients who are pregnant, unless the benefits outweigh the risks
- Patients who are allergic to iodinated dye or shellfish
- Patients who are claustrophobic
- Patients who are very obese, usually more than 300 lb
- Patients whose vital signs are unstable

Potential complications

- Allergic reaction to iodinated dye.
  See p. xix for appropriate interventions concerning the care of patients with iodine allergy.
- Acute renal failure from dye infusion
  Adequate hydration beforehand may reduce this likelihood.
- Hypoglycemia or acidosis may occur in patients who are taking Glucophage and receive iodine dye.

Procedure and patient care

Before
PT Explain the procedure to the patient. The patient's cooperation is necessary, because he or she must lie still during the procedure.
- Obtain informed consent if required by the institution.
- Assess the patient for allergies to iodinated dye or shellfish.
PT Show the patient a picture of the CT machine and encourage the patient to verbalize concerns regarding claustrophobia. Most patients who are mildly claustrophobic can tolerate this study after appropriate premedication with antianxiety drugs.
- Keep the patient NPO for 4 hours before the test in the event that contrast dye is administered.

During

- Note the following procedure for the chest CT scan.
  The patient is taken to the radiology department and asked to remain motionless in a supine position, because any motion will cause blurring and streaking of the final picture. An encircling x-ray camera (body scanner) takes pictures at varying intervals and levels over the chest area. Television equipment allows for immediate display, and the image is recorded on Polaroid or x-ray film. Occasionally IV dye is administered to enhance the chest image, and the x-ray studies are repeated.

- Note that this procedure is performed by a radiologist in 30 to 45 minutes. If dye is administered, the procedure time may be doubled because the CT scan is done with and without contrast dye.

PT Tell the patient that the discomforts associated with this study include lying still on a hard table and peripheral venipuncture. Mild nausea is a common sensation when contrast dye is used. An emesis basin should be readily available. Some patients may experience a salty taste, flushing, and warmth during the dye injection.

After

PT Encourage patients who received dye injection to increase their fluid intake, because the dye is excreted by the kidneys and causes diuresis.

- See p. xix for appropriate interventions concerning the care of patients with iodine allergy.

Abnormal findings

Pulmonary tumor
Inflammatory nodules
Granuloma
Cyst
Pleural effusion
Enlarged lymph nodes
Aortic aneurysm
Postpneumonic scanning
Pneumonitis
Esophageal tumor
Hiatal hernia
Mediastinal tumor (e.g., lymphoma, thymoma)
Primary or metastatic chest wall tumor

computed tomography portogram (CT portogram)

Type of test X-ray with contrast dye

Normal findings No evidence of liver abnormalities

Test explanation and related physiology

A CT scan of the abdomen (see p. 295) is inaccurate in identifying tumors in the liver smaller than 2 cm. However, a CT portogram can accurately identify abnormalities in the liver as small as 5 mm. The difference between a CT scan of the liver and a CT portogram is in the manner in which the contrast dye is injected. In a routine CT scan, dye is injected through a peripheral vein. In a CT portogram, dye is injected through a catheter that is placed in the splenic artery. The dye passes through the spleen and into the splenic vein and subsequently into the portal vein and its tributaries. However, hepatic tumors and cysts do not take up dye. These lesions appear as a filling defect (dark spots) in the liver. Therefore, use of this test is limited to identification of suspected smaller neoplasms involved in the liver. It is used in cancer patients who are suspected to have liver metastasis. The number and locations of these metastatic lesions are best visualized with a CT portogram.

Contraindications

- Patients with allergies to shellfish or iodinated dye
- Patients who are uncooperative or agitated
- Patients who are pregnant, unless the benefits outweigh the risks
- Patients with renal disorders, because iodinated contrast is nephrotoxic
- Patients with a bleeding propensity
- Patients with unstable cardiac disorders
- Patients who are dehydrated, because they are especially susceptible to dye-induced renal failure

Potential complications

- Allergic reaction to iodinated dye.
  See p. xix for appropriate interventions concerning the care of patients with iodine allergy.
- Hemorrhage from the arterial puncture site used for arterial access
- Arterial embolism from dislodgment of an arteriosclerotic plaque

- Soft tissue infection around the puncture site
- Renal failure, especially in elderly patients who are chronically dehydrated or have a mild degree of renal failure
- Pseudoaneurysm development as a result of failure of the puncture site to seal
- Hypoglycemia or acidosis may occur in patients who are taking Glucophage and receive iodine dye.

Procedure and patient care

Before

PT Explain the procedure to the patient. Allay any fears and allow the patient to verbalize concerns.

- Ensure that written and informed consent for this procedure is in the patient's chart.
- Determine if the patient has been taking anticoagulants.
- Keep the patient NPO for at least 2 to 4 hours before testing.
- Mark the site of the patient's peripheral pulses with permanent ink before arterial catheterization. This will permit assessment of the peripheral pulses after the procedure.

During

- Note the following preprocedure steps:
  1. The patient may be sedated before being taken to the angiography room, which is usually within the radiology department.
  2. The patient is placed on the x-ray table in the supine position.
  3. If the femoral artery is to be used, the groin is shaved, prepared, and draped in a sterile manner.
  4. The femoral artery is cannulated, and a wire is threaded up that artery and into or near the opening of the splenic artery.
  5. A catheter is placed over that wire and into the splenic artery.
  6. The patient is transferred to the CT scan unit, which is usually also in the x-ray department.
  7. Through the catheter, iodinated contrast material is injected into the splenic artery.
  8. CT scan images are taken subsequent to the injection.
- Note that the placement of the arterial catheter takes about 30 minutes and is minimally uncomfortable. This is done by a physician.

PT Inform the patient that CT scan imaging takes about 15 minutes and is not uncomfortable. This is done by a technician.

After

- After x-rays are completed, the catheter is removed, and a pressure dressing is applied to the puncture site.
- Monitor the patient's vital signs for indications of hemorrhage.
- Assess the peripheral pulse in the extremity used for vascular access and compare it with the preprocedure baseline values.
- Maintain pressure at the puncture site with a 1- to 2-lb sandbag or an IV bag for several hours.
- Keep the patient on bed rest for about 4 to 8 hours after the procedure to allow for complete sealing of the arterial puncture site.
- See p. xix for appropriate interventions concerning the care of patients with iodine allergy.

Abnormal findings

Hepatic tumor
Hepatic cyst
Hepatic hemangioma

notes

Coombs' test, direct (Antiglobulin test, direct)

Type of test Blood

Normal findings Negative; no agglutination

Test explanation and related physiology

This test is performed to identify hemolysis (lysis of RBCs) or to investigate hemolytic transfusion reactions. Most of the antibodies to RBCs are directed against the ABO/Rh blood grouping antigens, such as that which occurs in hemolytic anemia of the newborn (erythroblastosis fetalis) or transfusion of incompatible blood. When a transfusion reaction occurs, the Coombs' test can detect the patient's antibodies coating the transfused RBCs. Therefore the Coombs' test is very helpful in evaluating suspected transfusion reactions.

Non-"blood grouping" antigens can develop on the RBC membrane and stimulate formation of antibodies. Drugs such as levodopa or methyldopa cause this. Also, in some diseases antibodies not originally directed against the patient's RBCs can attach to the RBCs and cause hemolysis that is detected by the direct Coombs' test. Examples include antibodies developed in reaction to drugs such as penicillin, autoantibodies formed in various autoimmune diseases, and antibodies developed in some patients with advanced cancer (e.g., lymphoma). Frequently the inciting factor for the production of these autoantibodies against RBCs is not associated with any identifiable disease, and the resulting hemolytic anemia is called *idiopathic.*

The direct Coombs' test demonstrates if the patient's RBCs have been attacked by antibodies in the patient's own bloodstream. Coombs' serum is a solution containing antibodies to human globulin (antibodies). Coombs' serum is mixed with the patient's RBCs. If the RBCs have antibodies on them, agglutination of the patient's RBCs will occur. The greater the quantity of antibodies against RBCs, the more clumping occurs. This test is read as *positive,* with clumping on a scale of trace to +4. If the RBCs are not coated with autoantibodies against RBCs (immunoglobulins), agglutination will not occur; this is a *negative* test.

Interfering factors

☛ Drugs that may cause false-positive results include ampicillin, captopril, cephalosporins, chlorpromazine (Thorazine), chlorpropamide, hydralazine, indomethacin (Indocin), insulin, isoniazid (INH), levodopa, methyldopa (Aldomet), penicillin, phenytoin (Dilantin), procainamide, quinidine, quinine, rifampin, streptomycin, sulfonamides, and tetracyclines.

Procedure and patient care

Before

PT Explain the procedure to the patient.

PT Tell the patient that no fasting is required.

During

- Collect approximately 5 to 7 ml of venous blood in a red- or lavender-top tube.
- Use venous blood from the umbilical cord to detect the presence of antibodies in the newborn.
- List on the laboratory slip all medications that the patient has taken in the last few days.

After

- Apply pressure to the venipuncture site.

Abnormal findings

Autoimmune hemolytic anemia
Transfusion reaction
Erythroblastosis fetalis
Lymphoma
Lupus erythematosus
Mycoplasmal infection
Infectious mononucleosis

notes

Coombs' test, indirect (Blood antibody screening)

Type of test Blood

Normal findings Negative; no agglutination

Test explanation and related physiology

The indirect Coombs' test detects circulating antibodies against RBCs. The major purpose of this test is to determine if the patient has minor serum antibodies (other than the major ABO/Rh system) to RBCs that he or she is about to receive by blood transfusion. Therefore this test is the "screening" part of the "type and screen" routinely performed for blood compatibility testing (cross-matching in the blood bank). This test is also used to detect other agglutinins, such as cold agglutinins, which are associated with *Mycoplasma* infections.

Unlike the direct Coombs' test that is performed on the patient's RBCs, this test is performed on the patient's serum. In this test a small amount of the recipient's serum is added to donor RBCs containing known antibodies on their surface. This is the first stage. In the second stage of the test, Coombs' serum is added. Coombs' serum is a solution containing antibodies to human globulin (antibodies). If antibodies exist in the patient's serum, agglutination occurs. In blood transfusion screening, visible agglutination indicates that the recipient has antibodies to the donor's RBCs. If the recipient has no antibodies against the donor's RBCs, agglutination will not occur; transfusion should then proceed safely and without any transfusion reaction. Circulating antibodies against RBCs also may occur in an Rh-negative pregnant woman who is carrying an Rh-positive fetus.

Interfering factors

✴ Drugs that may cause false-positive results include antiarrhythmics, antituberculins, cephalosporins, chlorpromazine (Thorazine), insulin, levodopa, methyldopa (Aldomet), penicillins, phenytoin (Dilantin), quinidine, sulfonamides, and tetracyclines.

Procedure and patient care

Before

PT Explain the procedure to the patient.

PT Tell the patient that no fasting is required.

During

- Collect approximately 7 ml of venous blood in a red-top tube.
- List on the laboratory slip all medications that the patient has taken in the last few days.

After

- Apply pressure to the venipuncture site.
- Remember that if this antibody screening test is positive, antibody identification is then done.

Abnormal findings

Incompatible cross-matched blood
Maternal anti-Rh antibodies
Erythroblastosis fetalis
Acquired hemolytic anemia
Presence of specific cold agglutinin antibody

notes

cortisol, blood and urine (Hydrocortisone, Serum cortisol, Free urinary cortisol)

Type of test Blood; urine

Normal findings

Blood

Adult/elderly
   8 AM: 5-23 mcg/dl or 138-635 nmol/L (SI units)
   4 PM: 3-13 mcg/dl or 83-359 nmol/L (SI units)
Child
   8 AM: 15-25 mcg/dl
   4 PM: 5-10 mcg/dl
Newborn: 1-24 mcg/dl

Urine (24-hour)

Adult/elderly: <100 mcg/24 hr or <276 nmol/day (SI units)
Adolescent: 5-55 mcg/24 hr
Child: 2-27 mcg/24 hr

Test explanation and related physiology

An elaborate feedback mechanism for cortisol exists to coordinate the functions of the hypothalamus, pituitary gland, and adrenal glands. Cortisol is a potent glucocorticoid released from the adrenal cortex. This hormone affects the metabolism of carbohydrates, proteins, and fats. It especially has a profound effect on glucose serum levels.

The best method of evaluating adrenal activity is by directly measuring plasma cortisol levels. Normally, cortisol levels rise and fall during the day; this is called the diurnal variation. Cortisol levels are highest around 6 AM to 8 AM and gradually fall during the day to their lowest point around midnight.

Sometimes the earliest sign of adrenal hyperfunction is only the loss of this diurnal variation, even though the cortisol levels are not yet elevated. For example, individuals with Cushing's syndrome often have top-normal plasma cortisol levels in the morning and do not exhibit a decline as the day proceeds. High levels of cortisol indicate Cushing's syndrome, and low levels of plasma cortisol are suggestive of Addison's disease.

For this test, blood is usually collected at 8 AM and again at around 4 PM. One would expect the 4 PM value to be one third to two thirds of the 8 AM value. Normal values may be transposed in individuals who have worked during the night and slept during the day for long periods.

Free or unconjugated cortisol is filtered by the kidneys and excreted into the urine. Free cortisol levels can be evaluated in a 24-hour urine test.

Interfering factors

- Pregnancy is associated with increased levels.
- Physical and emotional stress can artificially elevate cortisol levels.
- Recent radioisotope scans can affect test results.
- ✶ Drugs that may cause *increased* serum levels include estrogen, oral contraceptives, amphetamines, cortisone, and spironolactone (Aldactone).
- ✶ Drugs that may cause *decreased* serum levels include androgens, aminoglutethimide, betamethasone, danazol, lithium, levodopa, metyrapone, and phenytoin (Dilantin).

Procedure and patient care

Before

PT Explain the procedure to the patient to minimize anxiety.

- Assess the patient for signs of physical stress (e.g., infection, acute illness) or emotional stress and report these to the physician.

During

Blood

- Collect approximately 7 to 10 ml of venous blood in a red- or green-top tube in the morning after the patient has had a good night's sleep.
- Collect another blood sample at about 4 PM.
- Indicate on the laboratory slip the time of the venipuncture and any drugs that may affect test results.

Urine

PT Instruct the patient to begin the 24-hour collection after voiding. Discard this specimen.

- Collect all urine passed by the patient during the next 24 hours.
- Note that it is not necessary to measure each urine specimen.

PT Remind the patient to void before defecating so that the urine is not contaminated by feces.

PT Tell the patient not to put toilet paper in the collection container.

PT Encourage the patient to drink fluids during the 24 hours unless this is contraindicated for medical purposes.

PT Instruct the patient to collect the last specimen as close as possible to the end of the 24-hour period. Add this to the collection.

- Place the 24-hour urine collection in a plastic container and keep on ice. Use a preservative.

After
- Apply pressure to the venipuncture site.

Abnormal findings

▲ **Increased levels**

Cushing's disease
Adrenal adenoma or carcinoma
Ectopic ACTH-producing tumors
Hyperthyroidism
Obesity
Stress

▼ **Decreased levels**

Congential adrenal hyperplasia
Addison's disease
Hypopituitarism
Hypothyroidism
Liver disease

notes

C-peptide (Connecting peptide insulin, Insulin C-peptide, Proinsulin C-peptide)

Type of test Blood

Normal findings

Fasting: 0.78-1.89 ng/ml or 0.26-0.62 nmol/L (SI units)
1 hour after glucose load: 5-12 ng/ml

Test explanation and related physiology

In the islet of Langerhans of the pancreas, the chains of proinsulin are broken down to form insulin and C-peptide. Because C-peptide has a longer half-life than insulin, more C-peptide exists in the peripheral circulation. In general, C-peptide levels correlate with insulin levels in the blood. The capacity of the pancreatic beta cells to secrete insulin can be evaluated by directly measuring either insulin or C-peptide. In most cases, direct measurement of insulin is more accurate. C-peptide levels, however, more accurately reflect islet cell function in the following situations:

1. Patients with diabetes who are treated with exogenous insulin and who have antiinsulin antibodies
2. Patients who secretly administer insulin to themselves (factitious hypoglycemia). Insulin levels will be elevated. Direct insulin measurement in these patients tends to be high because the insulin measured is the self-administered exogenous insulin. But C-peptide levels in that same specimen will be low because *exogenously* administered insulin suppresses *endogenous* insulin (and C-peptide) production.
3. Diabetic patients who are taking insulin. This is done to see if the diabetic patient is in remission and may not need exogenous insulin.

Further, C-peptide is used in evaluating patients who are suspected of having an insulinoma. In patients with an autonomous secreting insulinoma, C-peptide levels are high. Further, C-peptide can be used to monitor treatment for insulinoma. A rise in C-peptide levels indicates a recurrence or progression of the insulinoma. Likewise, some clinicians use C-peptide testing as an indicator of the adequacy of therapeutic surgical pancreatectomy in patients with pancreatic tumors. C-peptide also can be used to diagnose "insulin resistance" syndrome.

Interfering factors

- Because the majority of C-peptide is degraded in the kidney, renal failure can cause increased levels.
- ✗ Drugs that may cause *increased* levels of C-peptide include oral hypoglycemic agents (e.g., sulfonylureas).

Procedure and patient care

Before

PT Explain the procedure to the patient.
PT Instruct the patient to fast for 8 to 10 hours before the test. Only water is permitted.

During

- Collect venous blood in one red-top tube.

After

- Apply pressure or a pressure dressing to the venipuncture site.

Abnormal findings

▲ **Increased levels**
    Insulinoma
    Renal failure
    Pancreas transplant

▼ **Decreased levels**
    Factitious hypoglycemia
    Radical pancreatectomy
    Diabetes mellitus

notes

C-reactive protein test (CRP, high sensitivity CRP, hs-CRP)

Type of test Blood

Normal findings <1.0 mg/dl or <10.0 mg/L (SI units)

Cardiac risk
   Low <1.0 mg/dl
   Average 1.0-3.0 mg/dl
   High >3.0 mg/dl

Test explanation and related physiology

C-reactive protein is a nonspecific, acute-phase reactant used to diagnose bacterial infectious disease and inflammatory disorders such as acute rheumatic fever and rheumatoid arthritis. CRP levels do not consistently rise with viral infections. CRP is a protein produced primarily by the liver during an acute inflammatory process and other diseases. A positive test result indicates the presence, but not the cause, of the disease. The synthesis of CRP is initiated by antigen-immune complexes, bacteria, fungi, and trauma. CRP is functionally analogous to immunoglobulin G, except that it is not antigen specific. CRP interacts with the complement system.

The CRP test is a more sensitive and rapidly responding indicator than the erythrocyte sedimentation rate (ESR, see p. 402). In an acute inflammatory change, CRP shows an earlier and more intense increase than ESR; with recovery, the disappearance of CRP precedes the return of ESR to normal. The CRP also disappears when the inflammatory process is suppressed by salicylates or steroids.

This test is also useful in evaluating patients with an acute myocardial infarction. The level of CRP correlates with peak levels of the MB isoenzyme of creatine phosphokinase (see p. 322), but CRP peaks occur 1 to 3 days later. Failure of CRP to normalize may indicate ongoing damage to the heart tissue. Levels are not elevated in patients with angina.

Recent development of a *high sensitivity assay for CRP (hs-CRP)* has enabled accurate assays at even low levels. Atheromatous plaques in diseased arteries typically contain inflammatory cells. Multiple prospective studies also have demonstrated that baseline CRP is a good marker of future cardiovascular events. The C-reactive protein level is a stronger predictor of cardiovascular events than the low-density lipoprotein (LDL) cholesterol level. However, when used together with the lipid profile (see page 262), it adds prognostic information to that conveyed by the Framingham risk score. Because of the individual variability in hs-CRP, two separate measurements are required to classify a person's risk level. In patients with stable coronary disease or acute coronary syndromes, hs-CRP measurement may be useful as an independent marker for assessing the likelihood of recurrent events, including death, myocardial infarction, or restenosis after percutaneous coronary intervention.

This test may also be used after surgery to detect wound infections. CRP levels increase within 4 to 6 hours after surgery and generally begin to decrease after the third postoperative day. Failure of the levels to fall is an indicator of complications such as infection or pulmonary infarction.

Measurement of serum CRP is useful as an adjunct to the history and physical examination for the detection of acute bacterial meningitis in an acutely febrile child. Some studies have shown that the serum CRP test can distinguish gram-negative bacterial meningitis from viral meningitis. The presence of a normal CRP level excludes the diagnosis of bacterial meningitis. In some areas of the world, serum CRP levels are used as a cheap, simple, and reliable prognostic indicator in bacterial meningitis. CRP can also be measured in the cerebrospinal fluid (CSF) (see p. 602).

Interfering factors

- Elevated test results can occur in patients with hypertension, elevated body mass index, metabolic syndrome/diabetes mellitus, chronic infection (gingivitis, bronchitis), chronic inflammation (rheumatoid arthritis), and low HDL/high triglycerides.
- Cigarette smoking can cause increased levels.
- Decreased test levels can result from moderate alcohol consumption, weight loss, and increased activity or endurance exercise.
- ☒ Medications that may cause *increased* test results include estrogens and progesterones.
- ☒ Medications that may cause *decreased* test reults include fibrates, niacin, and statins.

Procedure and patient care

Before

PT Explain the procedure to the patient.

PT Tell the patient that fasting usually is not required; however, some laboratories require a 4- to 12-hour fast. Water is permitted.

During

PT Collect one red-top tube of venous blood.

After

- Apply pressure or a pressure dressing to the venipuncture site.

Abnormal findings

▲   **Increased levels**

Arthritis
Acute rheumatic fever
Reiter's syndrome
Crohn's disease
Vasculitis syndrome
Lupus erythematosus
Tissue infarction or damage
Acute myocardial infarction
Pulmonary infarction
Kidney transplant rejection
Bone marrow transplant rejection
Soft tissue trauma
Bacterial infection
Postoperative wound infection
Urinary tract infection
Tuberculosis
Malignant disease
Bacterial meningitis

notes

creatine kinase (CPK, CP, Creatine phosphokinase [CK])

Type of test Blood

Normal findings

Total CPK

Adult/elderly
   Male: 55-170 units/L or 55-170 units/L (SI units)
   Female: 30-135 units/L or 30-135 units/L (SI units)
Values are higher after exercise.
Newborn: 68-580 units/L (SI units)

Isoenzymes

CPK-MM: 100%
CPK-MB: 0%
CPK-BB: 0%

Test explanation and related physiology

CPK is found predominantly in the heart muscle, skeletal muscle, and brain. Serum CPK levels are elevated whenever injury occurs to these muscle or nerve cells. CPK levels can rise within 6 hours after damage. If damage is not persistent, the levels peak at 18 hours after injury and return to normal in 2 to 3 days (see Figure 13).

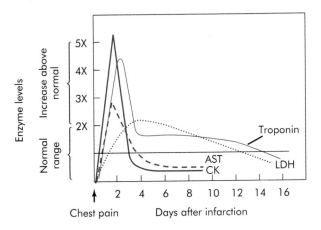

Figure 13 Serum cardiac enzymes in the blood after myocardial infarction. (*AST*, Aspartate aminotransferase; *CK*, creatine kinase; *LDH*, lactic dehydrogenase.)

To test specifically for myocardial muscle injury, electrophoresis is performed to detect the three *CPK isoenzymes*: CPK-BB (CPK1), CPK-MB (CPK2), and CPK-MM (CPK3). The CPK-MB isoenzyme part appears to be specific for myocardial cells. CPK-MB levels rise 3 to 6 hours after infarction occurs. If there is no further myocardial damage, the level peaks at 12 to 24 hours and returns to normal 12 to 48 hours after infarction. CPK-MB levels do not usually rise with transient chest pain caused by angina, pulmonary embolism, or congestive heart failure. One can expect to see a rise in CPK-MB in patients with shock, malignant hyperthermia, myopathies, or myocarditis. Very small amounts of CPK-MB also exist in skeletal muscle. Severe injury to skeletal muscle can be significant enough to raise the CPK-MB isoenzyme above normal. To avoid the misdiagnosis of myocardial injury, a *relative index* is calculated to determine whether myocardial injury has occurred. This relative index is a mathematical calculation of the ratio of CPK-MB to total CPK. A CPK-MB of 3.0 ng/ml with a relative index of ≥2.5 is highly suggestive of myocardial injury. A CPK-MB of >3.0 ng/ml with a relative index of <2.5 is indeterminate for myocardial injury.

The CPK-MB isoenzyme level is helpful in both quantifying the degree of myocardial infarction and timing the onset of infarction. With the more frequent use of thrombolytic therapy for myocardial infarction, the CPK-MB isoenzyme is often used to determine appropriateness of thrombolytic therapy. High CPK-MB levels suggest that significant infarction has already occurred, thereby precluding the benefit of thrombolytic therapy.

Because the CPK-BB isoenzyme is predominantly found in the brain and lung, injury to either of these organs (e.g., cerebrovascular accident, pulmonary infarction) is associated with elevated levels of this isoenzyme.

The CPK-MM isoenzyme normally comprises almost all the circulatory total CPK enzymes in healthy people. When the total CPK level is elevated as a result of increases in CPK-MM, injury to or disease of the skeletal muscle is present. Examples of this include myopathies, vigorous exercise, multiple IM injections, electroconvulsive therapy, cardioversion, chronic alcoholism, or surgery. Because CPK is made only in the skeletal muscle, the normal value of total CPK (and therefore CPK-MM) varies according to a person's muscle mass. Large, muscular people may normally have a CPK level in the high range of normal.

Each isoenzyme has been found to have isoforms. The CPK-MM isoforms MM1 and MM3 are most useful for cardiac disease. An MM3/MM1 ratio of greater than 1 suggests acute myocardial injury. A CPK-MB ratio of MB2/MB1 greater than 1 also indicates acute myocardial injury.

Another commonly performed relative index that was used to indicate myocardial injury was the CK-MB/total CK. If the ratio was >5%, myocardial injury occurred. However, these relative ratios are no longer considered as accurate as the troponin I test (see p. 941). If a borderline high CK-MB is obtained and the clinical picture is not entirely diagnostic of myocardial infarction, it is suggested that a troponin I level be obtained.

Creatine phosphokinase is the main cardiac enzyme studied in patients with heart disease. Because its blood clearance and metabolism are well known, its frequent determination (on admission, at 12 hours and at 24 hours) can accurately reflect timing, quantity, and resolution of a myocardial infarction.

Interfering factors

- IM injections may cause elevated CPK levels.
- Strenuous exercise and recent surgery may cause increased levels.
- Early pregnancy may cause decreased levels.
- Drugs that may cause *increased* levels include amphotericin B, ampicillin, some anesthetics, anticoagulants, aspirin, clofibrate, dexamethasone (Decadron), furosemide (Lasix), captopril, colchicine, alcohol, lovastatin, lithium, lidocaine, propranolol, succinylcholine, and morphine.

Procedure and patient care

Before

PT Explain the procedure to the patient.
PT Discuss with the patient the need and reason for frequent venipuncture in diagnosing myocardial infarction.
- Avoid IM injections in patients with cardiac disease. These injections may falsely elevate the total CPK level.
PT Tell the patient that no food or fluid restrictions are necessary.

During

- Collect a venous blood sample in a red-top tube. This is usually done daily for 3 days and then at 1 week.
- Rotate the venipuncture sites.
- Avoid hemolysis.
- Record the time and date of any IM injection.

- Record the exact time and date of venipuncture on each laboratory slip. This aids in the interpretation of the temporal pattern of enzyme elevations.

After

- Apply pressure to the venipuncture site.

Abnormal findings

▲ **Increased levels of total CPK**

Diseases or injury affecting the heart muscle, skeletal muscle, and brain

▲ **Increased levels of CPK-BB isoenzyme**

Diseases affecting the central nervous system
Adenocarcinoma (especially breast and lung)
Pulmonary infarction

▲ **Increased levels of CPK-MB isoenzyme**

Acute myocardial infarction
Cardiac aneurysm surgery
Cardiac defibrillation
Myocarditis
Ventricular arrhythmias
Cardiac ischemia

▲ **Increased levels of CPK-MM isoenzyme**

Rhabdomyolysis
Muscular dystrophy
Myositis
Recent surgery
Electromyography
IM injections
Crush injuries
Delirium tremens
Malignant hyperthermia
Recent convulsions
Electroconvulsive therapy
Shock
Hypokalemia
Hypothyroidism

notes

creatinine, blood (Serum creatinine)

Type of test Blood

Normal findings

Adult
  Female: 0.5-1.1 mg/dl or 44-97 µmol/L (SI units)
  Male: 0.6-1.2 mg/dl or 53-106 µmol/L (SI units)
Elderly: decrease in muscle mass may cause decreased values
Adolescent: 0.5-1.0 mg/dl
Child: 0.3-0.7 mg/dl
Infant: 0.2-0.4 mg/dl
Newborn: 0.3-1.2 mg/dl

Possible critical values >4 mg/dl (indicates serious impairment in renal function)

Test explanation and related physiology

This test measures the amount of creatinine in the blood. Creatinine is a catabolic product of creatine phosphate, which is used in skeletal muscle contraction. The daily production of creatine, and subsequently creatinine, depends on muscle mass, which fluctuates very little. Creatinine, as with blood urea nitrogen (BUN, see p. 952), is excreted entirely by the kidneys and therefore is directly proportional to renal excretory function. Thus, with normal renal excretory function, the serum creatinine level should remain constant and normal. Only renal disorders such as glomerulonephritis, pyelonephritis, acute tubular necrosis, and urinary obstruction, will cause an abnormal elevation in creatinine. There are slight increases in creatinine levels after meals, especially after ingestion of large quantities of meat. Furthermore, there may be some diurnal variation in creatinine—nadir at 7 AM and peak at 7 PM.

The serum creatinine test, as with the BUN, is used to diagnose impaired renal function. Unlike the BUN, however, the creatinine level is affected very little by hepatic function. The serum creatinine level has much the same significance as the BUN level but tends to rise later. Therefore, elevations in creatinine suggest chronicity of the disease process. In general, a doubling of creatinine suggests a 50% reduction in the glomerular filtration rate. The creatinine level is interpreted in conjunction with the BUN. These tests are referred to as *renal function studies.* The BUN/creatinine ratio is a good measurement of kidney and liver function. The normal adult range is 6-25, with 15.5 being the optimal adult value for this ratio.

Interfering factors

✠ Drugs that may *increase* creatinine values include aminoglycosides (e.g., gentamicin), cimetidine, heavy-metal chemotherapeutic agents (e.g., cisplatin), and other nephrotoxic drugs such as cephalosporins (e.g., cefoxitin).

Procedure and patient care

Before

PT Explain the procedure to the patient.
PT Tell the patient that no fasting is required.

During

- Collect approximately 5 ml of blood in a red-top tube.
- For pediatric patients, blood is usually drawn from a heel stick.

After

- Apply pressure to the venipuncture site.

Abnormal findings

▲ **Increased levels**
Glomerulonephritis
Pyelonephritis
Acute tubular necrosis
Urinary tract obstruction
Reduced renal blood flow
(e.g., shock, dehydration, congestive heart failure, atherosclerosis)
Diabetic nephropathy
Nephritis
Rhabdomyolysis
Acromegaly
Gigantism

▼ **Decreased levels**
Debilitation
Decreased muscle mass
(e.g., muscular dystrophy, myasthenia gravis)

notes

creatinine clearance (CC)

Type of test   Urine (24-hour); blood

Normal findings

Adult (<40 years)
    Male: 107-139 ml/min or 1.78-2.32 ml/s (SI units)
    Female: 87-107 ml/min or 1.45-1.78 ml/s (SI units)
Values decrease 6.5 ml/min/decade of life because of decline in
    glomerular filtration rate (GFR).
Newborn: 40-65 ml/min

Test explanation and related physiology

Creatinine is a catabolic product of creatine phosphate, which is used in skeletal muscle contraction. The daily production of creatinine depends on muscle mass, which fluctuates very little. Creatinine is entirely excreted by the kidneys and therefore is directly proportional to the glomerular filtration rate (GFR; i.e., the number of milliliters of filtrate made by the kidneys per minute). The creatinine clearance (CC) is a measure of the glomerular filtration rate.

The CC depends on the amount of blood present to be filtered and the ability of the glomeruli to act as a filter. The amount of blood present for filtration is decreased in renal artery atherosclerosis, dehydration, or shock. The ability of the glomeruli to act as a filter is decreased by diseases such as glomerulonephritis, acute tubular necrosis, and most other primary renal diseases. Significant bilateral obstruction to urinary outflow affects glomerular filtration only after it is long-standing.

When one kidney alone becomes diseased, the opposite kidney, if normal, has the ability to compensate by increasing its filtration rate. Therefore, with unilateral kidney disease or nephrectomy, a decrease in CC is not expected if the other kidney is normal.

Several nonrenal factors may influence CC. With each decade of age, the CC decreases 6.5 ml/min because of a decrease in the GFR. Urine collections are timed, and incomplete collections will falsely decrease CC. Muscle mass varies among people. Decreased muscle mass will give lower CC values. Likewise, ingestion of large meat meals will temporarily increase CC.

The CC test requires a 24-hour urine collection and a serum creatinine level. Creatinine clearance is then computed using the following formula:

$$\text{Creatinine clearance} = \frac{UV}{P}$$

where

U = Number of milligrams per deciliter of creatinine excreted in the urine over 24 hours

V = Volume of urine in milliliters per minute

P = Serum creatinine in milligrams per deciliter

A 24-hour urine collection for creatinine is often measured along with other urine collections to assess the completeness of other 24-hour collections. In patients with normal creatinine, the CC should indicate whether all the urine has been collected for the 24 hours.

Interfering factors

- Exercise may cause increased creatinine values.
- Incomplete urine collection may give a falsely lowered value.
- Pregnancy increases creatinine clearance.
- A diet high in meat content can transiently cause elevation of the creatinine clearance.
- Drugs that may cause *increased* levels include aminoglycosides (e.g., gentamicin), cimetidine, heavy-metal chemotherapeutic agents (e.g., cisplatin), and nephrotoxic drugs such as cephalosporins (e.g., cefoxitin).

Procedure and patient care

Before

- PT Explain the procedure to the patient.
- PT Tell the patient that no special diet is usually required.
- PT Note that some laboratories instruct the patient to avoid cooked meat, tea, coffee, or drugs on the day of the test. Check with the laboratory.

During

- PT Instruct the patient to begin the 24-hour urine collection after voiding. Discard the initial specimen and start the 24-hour timing as of that point.
- Collect all the urine passed during the next 24 hours.
- PT Show the patient where to store the urine specimen.
- Keep the specimen on ice or refrigerated during the 24 hours.

- Indicate the starting time on the urine container and laboratory slip.
- Post the hours for the urine collection in a noticeable place to prevent accidental discharge of a specimen.

PT Instruct the patient to void before defecating so that urine is not contaminated by feces.

PT Remind the patient not to put toilet paper in the collection container.

PT Encourage the patient to drink fluids during the 24 hours unless this is contraindicated for medical purposes.

PT Instruct the patient to avoid vigorous exercise during the 24 hours, because exercise may cause an increased creatinine clearance.

PT Tell the patient to collect the last specimen as close as possible to the end of the 24-hour period. Add this urine to the container.

- Make sure a venous blood sample is drawn in a red-top tube during the 24-hour collection.
- Mark the patient's age, weight, and height on the requisition sheet.

After

- Transport the urine specimen promptly to the laboratory.
- Apply pressure to the venipuncture site.

Abnormal findings

▲ **Increased levels**

Exercise
Pregnancy
High cardiac output
syndromes

▼ **Decreased levels**

Impaired kidney
function (e.g., renal
artery atherosclerosis,
glomerulonephritis,
acute tubular
necrosis)
Conditions causing
decreased GFR
(e.g., congestive heart
failure, cirrhosis with
ascites, shock,
dehydration)

cryoglobulin

Type of test Blood

C

Normal findings No cryoglobulins detected

Test explanation and related physiology

Cryoglobulins are abnormal globulin protein complexes that exist within the blood of patients with various diseases. These proteins precipitate reversibly at low temperatures and redissolve with rewarming. They can precipitate within the blood vessel of the fingers when exposed to cold temperatures. This precipitation causes sludging of the blood within those blood vessels. These patients may have symptoms of purpura, arthralgia, or Raynaud's phenomenon (pain, cyanosis, coldness of the fingers).

These proteins exist in varying degrees, depending on the disease entity with which they are associated. Serum levels greater than 5 mg/ml are associated with multiple myeloma, macroglobulinemia, and leukemia. Globulin levels between 1 and 5 mg/ml are associated with rheumatoid arthritis. Levels less than 1 mg/ml can be associated with systemic lupus erythematosus, rheumatoid arthritis, infectious mononucleosis, viral hepatitis, endocarditis, cirrhosis, and glomerulonephritis. Idiopathic or primary cryoglobulinemia is not associated with any primary disease process.

For this test, the blood sample is taken to the chemistry laboratory, where it is refrigerated for 72 hours. After that time the specimen is evaluated for precipitation. If precipitation is identified, it is measured and recorded. The tube is then rewarmed, and the specimen is reexamined for dissolution of that precipitation. If precipitation of the refrigerated specimen is identified and dissolved on rewarming, cryoglobulins are present.

Procedure and patient care

Before

PT Explain the procedure to the patient.

PT Inform the patient that an 8-hour fast may be required. This will minimize turbidity of the serum caused by ingestion of a recent (especially fatty) meal. Turbidity may make the detection of precipitation rather difficult.

During
- Collect 10 ml of venous blood in a red-top tube that has been prewarmed to body temperature.

After
- Apply pressure to the venipuncture site.
- PT If cryoglobulins are found to be present, warn the patient to avoid cold temperatures and contact with cold objects to minimize Raynaud's symptoms. Tell the patient to wear gloves in cold weather.

Abnormal findings

Connective tissue disease (e.g., lupus erythematosus, Sjögren's syndrome, rheumatoid arthritis)

Lymphoid malignancies (e.g., multiple myeloma, leukemia, Waldenström's macroglobulinemia, lymphoma)

Acute and chronic infections (e.g., infectious mononucleosis, endocarditis, poststreptococcal glomerulonephritis)

Liver disease (e.g., hepatitis, cirrhosis)

notes

cutaneous immunofluorescence biopsy
(Immunofluorescence skin biopsy, Skin biopsy antibodies, Skin immunohistopathology)

Type of test Microscopic examination of skin tissue

Normal findings Normal skin histology

Test explanation and related physiology

This test of inflamed skin is performed to evaluate and diagnose immunologic-mediated dermatitis. It is indicated when an immunologic source for a skin rash is suspected. For this study, a skin biopsy is obtained and evaluated by immunofluorescence. Deposition of human immunoglobulins and complement components is determined by immunofluorescent patterns. This test is useful in detecting immune complexes, complement, and immunoglobulin deposition in systemic and discoid lupus erythematosus, pemphigus, bullous pemphigoid, and dermatitis herpetiformis. This test is also used to confirm the histopathology of skin lesions and to follow the results of treatment.

Procedure and patient care

Before

- PT Explain the procedure to the patient.
- Obtain an informed consent.

During

- A 4-mm punch biopsy or tissue excision is obtained.

After

- Apply a dry, sterile dressing over the biopsy site.
- PT Tell the patient that results may not be available for several days.
- Deliver the specimen on ice immediately to the laboratory after the biopsy is taken.

Abnormal findings

Systemic lupus erythematosus
Discoid lupus erythematosus
Pemphigus
Bullous pemphigoid
Dermatitis herpetiformis

cystography (Cystourethrography, Voiding cystography, Voiding cystourethrography)

Type of test X-ray with contrast dye

Normal findings Normal bladder structure and function

Test explanation and related physiology

Filling the bladder with radiopaque contrast material provides visualization of the bladder for radiographic study. Either fluoroscopic or x-ray films demonstrate bladder filling and collapse after emptying. Filling defects or shadows within the bladder indicate primary bladder tumors. Extrinsic compression or distortion of the bladder is seen with pelvic tumor (e.g., rectal, cervical) or hematoma (secondary to pelvic bone fractures). Extravasation of the dye is seen with traumatic rupture, perforation, and fistula of the bladder. Vesicoureteral reflux (abnormal backflow of urine from bladder to ureters), which can cause persistent or recurrent pyelonephritis, also may be demonstrated during cystography. Although the bladder is visualized during an intravenous pyelogram (see p. 560), primary pathologic bladder conditions are best studied by cystography.

Contraindications

- Patients with urethral or bladder infection or injury

Potential complications

- Urinary tract infection
  This may result from catheter placement or the instillation of contaminated contrast material.
- Allergic reaction to iodinated dye
  This rarely occurs because the dye is not administered intravenously.

Procedure and patient care

Before

PT Explain the procedure to the patient.
- Obtain informed consent if required by the institution.
- Give clear liquids for breakfast on the morning of the test.
PT Assure the patient that he or she will be draped to prevent unnecessary exposure.
- Insert a Foley catheter if ordered.

During

- Note the following procedural steps:
  1. The patient is taken to the radiology department and placed in a supine or lithotomy position.
  2. Unless the catheter is already present, one is placed.
  3. Through the catheter, approximately 300 ml of air or radiopaque dye (much less for children) is injected into the bladder.
  4. The catheter is clamped.
  5. X-ray films are taken.
  6. If the patient is able to void, the catheter is removed, and the patient is asked to urinate while films are taken of the bladder and urethra (voiding cystourethrogram).
- Ensure that males wear a lead shield over the testes to prevent irradiation of the gonads.
- Remember that female patients cannot be shielded without blocking bladder visualization.
- Note that a radiologist performs the study in approximately 15 to 30 minutes.
- **PT** Tell the patient that this test is moderately uncomfortable if bladder catheterization is required.

After

- Assess the patient for signs of urinary tract infection.
- **PT** Encourage the patient to drink fluids to eliminate the dye and to prevent accumulation of bacteria.

Abnormal findings

Bladder tumor
Pelvic tumor
Hematoma
Bladder trauma
Vesicoureteral reflux

notes

cystometry (Cystometrogram [CMG], Urethral pressure profile [UPP], Urethral pressure measurements)

Type of test Manometric

Normal findings

Normal sensations of fullness and temperature
Normal pressures and volumes
Maximal cystometric capacity
  Male: 350-750 ml
  Female: 250-550 ml
Intravesical pressure when bladder is empty: usually <40 cm H_2O
Detrusor pressure: <10 cm H_2O
Maximal urethral pressures in normal patients (cm H_2O):

Age	Male	Female
<25 years	37-126	55-103
25-44 years	35-113	31-115
45-64 years	40-123	40-100
>64 years	35-105	35-75

Test explanation and related physiology

The purpose of cystometry is to evaluate the motor and sensory functions of the bladder when incontinence is present or neurologic bladder dysfunction is suspected. A graphic recording of pressure exerted at varying phases of the filling of the urinary bladder is produced. A pressure/volume relationship of the bladder is made. This urodynamic study assesses the neuromuscular function of the bladder by measuring the efficiency of the detrusor muscle, intravesical pressure and capacity, and the bladder's response to thermal stimulation.

Cystometry can determine whether bladder pathology is caused by neurologic, infectious, or obstructive diseases. Cystometry is indicated to elucidate the causes for frequency and urgency, especially before surgery on the urologic outflow tract. Cystometry is also part of the evaluation for incontinence, persistent residual urine, vesicoureteral reflux, neurologic disorders, sensory disorders, and the effect of certain drugs on bladder function.

A *urethral pressure profile (UPP)* is often performed during cystometry. The UPP indicates the intraluminal pressure along the length of the urethra with the bladder at rest. Indications for this urodynamic investigation include the following:

1. Assessment of prostatic obstruction
2. Assessment of stress incontinence in females
3. Assessment of postprostatectomy sequelae of incontinence
4. Assessment of the adequacy of external sphincterotomy
5. Analysis of the effects of drugs on the urethra
6. Analysis of the effects of stimulation on urethral flow
7. Assessment of the adequacy of implanted artificial urethral sphincter devices

Contraindications

- Patients with urinary tract infections, because of the possibility of false results and the potential for the spread of infection

Procedure and patient care

Before

- **PT** Explain the purpose and the procedure to the patient.
- **PT** Tell the patient that no fluid or food restrictions are needed.
- **PT** Assure the patient that he or she will be draped to prevent unnecessary exposure.
- Assess the patient for signs and symptoms of urinary tract infection.
- **PT** Instruct the patient not to strain while voiding, because the results can be skewed.
- If the patient has a spinal cord injury, transport him or her on a stretcher. The test will then be performed with the patient on the stretcher.

During

- Note the following procedural steps:
  1. Cystometry, usually performed in a urologist's office or a special procedure room, begins with the patient being asked to void.
  2. The amount of time required to initiate voiding and the size, force, and continuity of the urinary stream are recorded. The amount of urine, the time of voiding, and the presence of any straining, hesitancy, or terminal urine dribbling are also recorded.
  3. The patient is placed in a lithotomy or supine position.
  4. A retention catheter is inserted through the urethra and into the bladder.
  5. Residual urine volume is measured and recorded.

6. Thermal sensation is evaluated by the instillation of approximately 30 ml of room-temperature saline solution into the bladder followed by an equal amount of warm water. The patient reports any sensations.

7. This fluid is withdrawn from the bladder.

8. The urethral catheter is connected to a cystometer (a tube used to monitor bladder pressure).

9. Sterile water, normal saline solution, or carbon dioxide gas is slowly introduced into the bladder at a controlled rate, usually with the patient in a sitting position.

10. Patients are asked to indicate the first urge to void and then when they have the feeling that they must void. The bladder is full at this point.

11. The pressures and volumes are plotted on a graph.

12. The patient is asked to void, and the maximal intravesical voiding pressure is recorded.

13. The bladder is drained for any residual urine.

14. If no additional studies are to be done, the urethral catheter is removed.

15. For urethral pressures, fluid or gas is instilled through the catheter, which is withdrawn while pressures along the urethral wall are obtained.

PT Throughout the study, ask the patient to report any sensations such as pain, flushing, sweating, nausea, bladder filling, and an urgency to void.

■ Note that certain drugs may be administered during the cystometric examination to distinguish between underactivity of the bladder because of muscle failure and underactivity associated with denervation. Cholinergic drugs (e.g., bethanechol [Urecholine]) may be given to enhance the tone of a flaccid bladder. Anticholinergic drugs (e.g., atropine) may be given to promote relaxation of a hyperactive bladder. If these drugs are to be given, the catheter is left in place. The drugs are given, and the examination is repeated 20 to 30 minutes later using the first test as a control value.

■ Note that this test is performed by a urologist in approximately 45 minutes.

PT Explain to the patient that the only discomfort is that associated with the urethral catheterization.

After

- Observe the patient for any manifestations of infection (e.g., elevated temperature, chills).
- Examine the urine for hematuria. Notify the physician if the hematuria persists after several voidings.
- Provide a warm sitz bath or tub bath for the patient's comfort if desired.

Abnormal findings

Neurogenic bladder
Bladder obstruction
Bladder infection
Bladder hypertonicity
Diminished bladder capacity
Prostatic obstruction secondary to benign prostatic hypertrophy or cancer
Urinary incontinence

notes

cystoscopy (Endourology)

Type of test   Endoscopy

Normal findings   Normal structure and function of the urethra, bladder, ureters, and prostate (in males)

Test explanation and related physiology

Cystoscopy provides direct visualization of the urethra and bladder through the transurethral insertion of a cystoscope into the bladder (Figure 14). Cystoscopy is used *diagnostically* to allow:

1. Direct inspection and biopsy of the prostate, bladder, and urethra
2. Collection of a separate urine specimen directly from each kidney by the placement of ureteral catheters

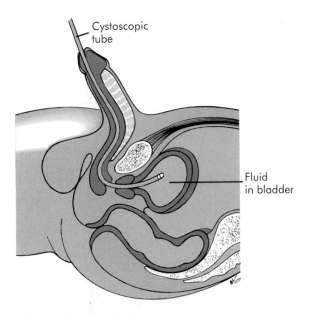

Figure 14 Cystoscopic examination of the male bladder. The cystoscope is passed through the urethra into the bladder. Although shown here as a flexible scope, usually the scope is rigid. Through the scope fluid is instilled to maintain bladder distention.

3. Measurement of bladder capacity and determination of ureteral reflux
4. Identification of bladder and ureteral calculi
5. Placement of ureteral catheters (Figure 15) for retrograde pyelography (see p. 807)
6. Identification of the source of hematuria

Cystoscopy is used *therapeutically* to provide:

1. Resection of small, superficial bladder tumors
2. Removal of foreign bodies and stones
3. Dilation of the urethra and ureters
4. Placement of catheters to drain urine from the renal pelvis
5. Coagulation of bleeding areas
6. Implantation of radium seeds into a tumor

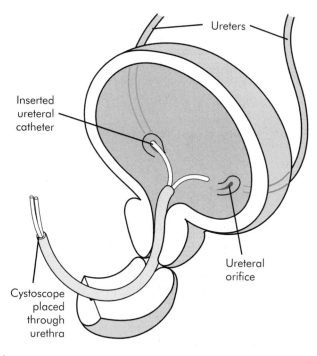

Figure 15 Ureteral catheterization through the cystoscope. Note the ureteral catheter inserted into the right orifice. The left ureteral catheter is ready to be inserted.

7. Resection of hypertrophied or malignant prostate gland overgrowth
8. Placement of ureteral stents for identification of ureters during pelvic surgery

The cystoscope consists primarily of an obturator and a telescope. The obturator is used to insert the cystoscope atraumatically. After the cystoscope is within the bladder, the obturator is removed, and the telescope is passed through the cystoscope. The lens and lighting system of the telescope permit adequate visualization of the lower genitourinary tract. Transendoscopic instruments such as forceps, scissors, needles, and electrodes are used when appropriate. *Endourology* refers to endoscopic surgery performed on the bladder and urethra during cystoscopy.

Cystoscopy is important in the evaluation of hematuria, chronic infection, suspected stones, and radiographic filling defects. On inspection, the urethra may show inflammation or structural causes of obstruction (e.g., stricture, neoplasia, prostatic hypertrophy). If the obstruction is functional rather than structural (e.g., detrusor-bladder neck dyssynergia), no site of obstruction will be demonstrated by endoscopy.

Potential complications

- Perforation of the bladder
- Sepsis by seeding the bloodstream with bacteria from infected urine
- Hematuria
- Urinary retention

Procedure and patient care

Before

PT Explain the procedure to the patient.
- Ensure that an informed consent is obtained.
- If enemas are ordered to clear the bowel, assist the patient as needed and record the results.

PT Encourage the patient to drink fluids several hours before the procedure to maintain a continuous flow of urine for collection and to prevent multiplication of bacteria that may be introduced during this technique.
- If the procedure will be done with the patient under local anesthesia, allow a liquid breakfast.
- If the procedure will be performed with the patient under general anesthesia, follow routine precautions. Keep the

patient NPO after midnight on the day of the test. Fluids may be given intravenously.

- Administer the preprocedure medications as ordered 1 hour before the study. Sedatives decrease the spasm of the bladder sphincter, decreasing the patient's discomfort.

C

During

- Note the following procedural steps:
    1. Cystoscopy is usually performed in the operating room but also can be done in the urologist's office.
    2. The patient is placed in the lithotomy position with his or her feet in stirrups.
    3. The external genitalia are cleansed with an antiseptic solution such as povidone-iodine (Betadine).
    4. A local anesthetic is instilled into the urethra if general anesthesia has not been used.
    5. The cystoscope is inserted, and the desired diagnostic or therapeutic studies are performed.

PT Instruct the patient to lie very still during the entire procedure to prevent trauma to the urinary tract.

PT Tell the patient that he or she will have the desire to void as the cystoscope passes the bladder neck.

- When the procedure is completed, keep the patient on bed rest for a short time.
- Note that if endourology is performed, the urethra will also be evaluated.
- Note that this procedure is performed by a urologist in approximately 25 minutes.

PT When local anesthesia is used, inform the patient of the associated discomfort (much more than with urethral catheterization).

After

PT Instruct the patient not to walk or stand alone immediately after his or her legs have been removed from the stirrups. The orthostasis that may result from standing erect may cause dizziness and fainting.

- Assess the patient's ability to void for at least 24 hours after the procedure. Urinary retention may be secondary to edema caused by instrumentation.
- Note the urine color. Pink-tinged urine is common. The presence of bright red blood or clots should be reported to the physician.

- Monitor the patient for complaints of back pain, bladder spasms, urinary frequency, and burning on urination. Warm sitz baths and mild analgesics may be ordered and given. Sometimes belladonna and opium (B&O) suppositories are given to relieve bladder spasms. Warm, moist heat to the lower abdomen may help relieve pain and promote muscle relaxation.

PT Encourage increased intake of fluids. A dilute urine decreases dysuria. Fluids also maintain a constant flow of urine to prevent stasis and the accumulation of bacteria in the bladder.

- Check and record the patient's vital signs as ordered. Watch for a decrease in blood pressure and an increase in pulse as an indication of hemorrhage.

- Observe for signs and symptoms of sepsis (elevated temperature, flush, chills, decreased blood pressure, increased pulse).

- Note that antibiotics are occasionally ordered 1 day before and 3 days after the procedure to reduce the incidence of bacteremia that may occur with instrumentation of the urethra and bladder.

PT Encourage the patient to use cathartics, especially after cystoscopic surgery. Increases in intraabdominal pressure caused by constipation may initiate severe lower urologic bleeding.

- If postprocedure irrigation is ordered, use an isotonic solution containing mannitol, glycine, or sorbitol to prevent fluid overhydration in the event any of the irrigation is absorbed through opened venous sinuses in the bladder.

PT If a catheter is left in after the procedure, provide catheter care instructions.

🏠 **Home care responsibilities**

- Watch for signs of urinary retention for 24 to 48 hours.
- Watch for signs of bleeding. Pink urine is normal; clots are not.
- Report symptoms of increasing lower abdominal pain immediately.
- Use warm sitz baths or B&O suppositories to reduce bladder spasms.
- Encourage the patient to drink lots of fluids.
- Watch for fever, shaking chills, or prolonged dysuria as possible signs of urinary tract infection.
- If ordered, stress the importance of postprocedure antibiotics.

Abnormal findings

Lower urologic tract tumor
Stones in the ureter or bladder
Prostatic hypertrophy
Prostate cancer
Inflammation of the bladder and urethra
Urethral/ureteral stricture
Prostatitis
Vesical neck contracture

notes

cytokines

Type of test Blood

Normal findings Varies by laboratory and technique

Test explanation and related physiology

Cytokines are a group of proteins that have multiple functions. In general they are produced by immune cells to communicate and orchestrate the immune response. The immune system has many different cells that must act together to effectively protect the body from infection, inflammation, or tumor. The cytokines are made by lymphocytes (T cells, B cells), monocytes, and eosinophils. Some cytokines stimulate each other; some inhibit other cytokines in order to maintain balance. Originally, cytokines were named by their function (T cell growth factor, colony stimulating factor, etc.). As more was learned about this complex group of proteins, it became apparent that a single cytokine might act differently in different cells. Therefore, naming the cytokine by function was confusing and misleading. As more cytokines were identified, they were named *interleukins* and numbered by the sequence of discovery. Interleukins, in general, are made by leukocytes. Lymphokines and monokines are made by lymphocytes and monocytes, respectively. Other cytokines include *interferon* and *growth factors.*

Cytokines have receptors in other cells to which they attach and instigate a series of intracellular activities that may be associated with secretion, motion, or cell division. In general, cytokines act very close to their cells of origin or even on the cell that generated them. Because their effect is so significant over a small area, only small quantities are needed. That makes quantitative assays very difficult. Radioimmunoassay, immunoradiometric assays, enzyme-linked immunosorbent assays (ELISA), and radioreceptor assays are some of the latest laboratory techniques used to measure these proteins accurately.

Cytokines are used therapeutically to stimulate bone marrow production of blood cells in patients with suppression (by chemotherapy) or disease of the bone marrow. They are used as potent antiinflammatory or antineoplastic agents. Some cytokines are produced at increased levels in certain disease states and, therefore, become markers for disease extent, progression, and response to therapy. They act as "tumor markers" in cancers associated with elevated cytokines.

Any table created to list all the cytokines and their functions quickly becomes inaccurate and imperfect. The discovery of new cytokines and new functions changes so frequently that any table is outdated in the delay to publication. Likewise, any listing of normal values will be just as quickly obsolete, as methods of testing change so frequently. It is suggested that reference to "normal values" be directed to the laboratory performing the assay.

At present, cytokine quantitative and qualitative assays are predominantly used for research. Often cytokine testing is done in panels including measurement of cytokine receptor proteins. Clinically, cytokine assays may have the following uses:

- Measurement of AIDS progression
- Measurement of progression of inflammatory diseases such as rheumatoid arthritis (RA) and other autoimmune diseases
- Tumor markers (e.g., breast cancer, lymphoma, and leukemia)
- Determination of disease risk (e.g., risk of developing Kaposi's sarcoma in AIDS patients)
- Determination of treatment of disease (e.g., which patients with rheumatoid arthritis may benefit from cytokine therapy)
- Determination of immune function and response
- Monitoring of patients receiving cytokine therapy or anticytokine therapy

Usually, cytokine testing is performed on serum. However, joint fluid is often tested in the evaluation of the patient with arthritis. Likewise, if inflammatory encephalitis or meningitis is considered, cerebrospinal fluid may be the specimen.

Interfering factors

- Cells can still produce cytokines after specimen collection. It is best to freeze the specimen.
- Cytokines can degrade in the specimen container
- Cytokines can stimulate or inhibit other cytokines while in the specimen container.

Procedure and patient care

Before

PT Explain the procedure to the patient.

PT Tell the patient that no fasting or preparation is required.

During

- Collect about 10 to 20 ml of venous blood in a red-top tube.
- Usually this specimen is sent to a reference laboratory.

After
- Apply pressure to the venipuncture site.

Abnormal findings

Inflammatory disease
AIDS
Various malignancies

notes

cytomegalovirus (CMV)

Type of test Blood

Normal findings No virus isolated

Test explanation and related physiology

Cytomegalovirus (CMV) is part of the viral family that includes herpes simplex, Epstein-Barr, and varicella-zoster viruses. CMV infection is widespread and common. Infections usually occur in the fetus, during early childhood, and in the young adult. Certain populations are at increased risk. Male homosexuals, transplant patients, and AIDS patients are particularly susceptible. Infections are acquired by contact with body secretions or urine. Blood transfusions are a common form of spread for CMV. Most patients with acute disease have no or very few (mononucleosis-like) symptoms.

CMV is the most common congenital infection. Pregnant mothers can get the disease during their pregnancy, or an old previous CMV infection can become reactivated. Approximately 10% of infected newborns exhibit permanent damage, usually mental retardation and auditory damage. Fetal infection can cause microcephaly, hydrocephaly, cerebral palsy, mental retardation, or death. The term TORCH (toxoplasmosis, other, rubella, cytomegalovirus, herpes) has been applied to infections with recognized detrimental effects on the fetus.

Virus culture is the most definitive method of diagnosis. However, a culture cannot differentiate an acute infection from a chronic, inactive infection. Antibodies reveal much more information about the activity of the infection. CMV IgG antibody levels persist for years after infection. Identification of IgM antibodies, however, indicates a relatively recent infection. Three different CMV antigens can be detected immunologically. They are called early, intermediate-early, and late antigens and indicate onset of infection. A fourfold increase in CMV titer in paired sera drawn 10 to 14 days apart is usually indicative of an acute infection.

Procedure and patient care

Before

PT Explain the procedure to the patient.

During

- For culture specimens, a urine, sputum, or mouth swab is the specimen of choice. Fresh specimens are essential.
- The specimens are cultured in a virus laboratory, which takes about 3 to 7 days.
- For antibody or antigen titer, draw 4 to 7 ml of blood in a gold- or red-top tube.
- Collect a specimen from a mother with suspected acute infection as early as possible.
- Collect the convalescent specimen 2 to 4 weeks later.

After

- Apply pressure to the venipuncture site.

Abnormal findings

CMV infection

notes

D-dimer test (Fragment D-dimer, Fibrin degradation fragment)

Type of test Blood

Normal findings

Negative (no D-dimer fragments present)
<250 ng/ml or <250 mcg/L (SI units)

Test explanation and related physiology

The fragment D-dimer test assesses both thrombin and plasmin activity. D-dimer is a fibrin degradation fragment that is made through fibrinolysis. As plasmin acts on the fibrin polymer clot, fibrin degradation products and D-dimer are produced. The D-dimer assay provides a highly specific measurement of the amount of fibrin degradation that occurs. Normal plasma does not have detectable amounts of fragment D-dimer.

This test provides a simple and confirmatory test for disseminated intravascular coagulation (DIC). Positive results of the D-dimer assay correlate with positive results of fibrin degradation products (FDPs) (see p. 908). Although the D-dimer assay is more specific than the FDP assay, it is less sensitive. Therefore, combining the FDP and the D-dimer provides a highly sensitive and specific test for recognizing DIC in a patient.

Levels of D-dimer can also increase when a fibrin clot is lysed by thrombolytic therapy. Thrombotic problems such as deep-vein thrombosis, pulmonary embolism, sickle cell anemia, and thrombosis of malignancy are also associated with high D-dimer levels.

Procedure and patient care

Before

PT Explain the procedure to the patient.
PT Tell the patient that no fasting is required.

During

- Collect a venous blood sample in a blue-top tube.

After

- Apply pressure to the venipuncture site.
- Assess the venipuncture site for bleeding. Remember that if the patient is receiving anticoagulants or has coagulopathies, the bleeding time will be increased.

Abnormal findings

▲ **Increased levels**

Fibrinolysis

During thrombolytic or defibrination therapy with tissue plasminogen activator

Deep-vein thrombosis

Pulmonary embolism

Arterial thromboembolism

DIC

Vasoocclusive crisis of sickle cell anemia

Pregnancy

Malignancy

Surgery

notes

delta-aminolevulinic acid (Aminolevulinic acid [ALA], Delta-ALA)

D

Type of test Urine (24-hour)

Normal findings 1.5-7.5 mg/24 hr or 11-57 μmol/24 hr (SI units)

Possible critical values >20 mg/24 hr

Test explanation and related physiology

As the basic precursor for the porphyrins (see p. 726), delta-ALA is needed for the normal production of porphobilinogen, which ultimately leads to heme synthesis in erythroid cells. Heme is used in the synthesis of hemoglobin. Genetic disorders (porphyria) are associated with a lack of a particular enzyme vital to heme metabolism. These disorders are characterized by an accumulation of porphyrin products in the liver or red blood cells. The liver porphyrias are much more common. Symptoms of liver porphyrias include abdominal pain, neuromuscular signs and symptoms, constipation, and occasionally psychotic behavior. Acute intermittent porphyria (AIP) is the most common form of the liver porphyrias; this is caused by a deficiency in uroporphyrinogen-I-synthase (also called porphobilinogen deaminase).

Most patients with AIP have no symptoms (latent phase) until the acute phase is precipitated by medication or other factors (see uroporphyrinogen). The acute phase is highlighted by symptoms of abdominal and muscular pain, nausea, vomiting, hypertension, mental symptoms (anxiety, insomnia, hallucinations, and paranoia), sensory loss, and urinary retention. Hemolytic anemia also may occur with these acute attacks. These acute symptoms are associated with increased serum and urine levels of porphyrin precursors (aminolevulinic acid, porphyrins, and porphobilinogens).

In lead intoxication, heme synthesis is similarly diminished by the inhibition of ALA dehydrase. This enzyme assists in the conversion of ALA to porphobilinogen. As a result of lead poisoning, ALA accumulates in the blood and urine.

Interfering factors

▼ Drugs that may cause *increased* ALA levels include penicillin, barbiturates, and griseofulvin.

Procedure and patient care

Before

PT Explain the procedure to the patient.

During

PT Instruct the patient to begin a 24-hour urine collection after voiding. Discard the initial specimen and start the 24-hour timing at that point.

- Collect all urine passed during the next 24 hours.

PT Show the patient where to store the urine container.

- Keep the specimen on ice or refrigerated during the 24 hours.
- Keep the urine in a light-resistant container with a preservative.
- Indicate the starting time on the urine container and on the laboratory slip.
- Post the hours for the urine collection in a noticeable place to prevent accidental discarding of the specimen.

PT Instruct the patient to void before defecating so that urine is not contaminated by feces.

PT Remind the patient not to put toilet paper in the collection container.

PT Encourage the patient to drink fluids during the 24 hours unless this is contraindicated for medical purposes.

PT Tell the patient to collect the last specimen as close as possible to the end of the 24-hour period. Add this to the urine collection.

- If the patient has a Foley catheter in place, cover the drainage bag to prevent exposure to light.
- Indicate on the laboratory slip any drugs that may affect test results.

After

- Apply pressure to the venipuncture site.
- Transport the urine specimen promptly to the laboratory.

Abnormal findings

▲ **Increased levels**

Porphyria
Lead intoxication
Chronic alcoholic disorders
Diabetic ketoacidosis

dexamethasone suppression test (DST, Prolonged/rapid DST, Cortisol suppression test, ACTH suppression test)

D

Type of test Blood; urine (24-hour)

Normal findings

Prolonged method

Low dose: >50% reduction of plasma cortisol and
17-hydroxycorticosteroid (17-OCHS) levels
High dose: 50% reduction of plasma cortisol and 17-OCHS
levels

Rapid method

Normal: nearly 0 cortisol levels

Test explanation and related physiology

An elaborate feedback mechanism for cortisol exists to coordinate the function of the hypothalamus, pituitary gland, and adrenal glands. The DST is based on pituitary adrenocorticotropic hormone (ACTH) secretion being dependent on the plasma cortisol feedback mechanism. As plasma cortisol levels increase, ACTH secretion is suppressed; as cortisol levels decrease, ACTH secretion is stimulated. Dexamethasone is a synthetic steroid (similar to cortisol) that normally should suppress ACTH secretion. Under normal circumstances, this results in reduced stimulation to the adrenal glands and ultimately a drop of 50% or more in plasma cortisol and 17-OCHS levels. This important feedback system does not function properly in patients with Cushing's syndrome.

In Cushing's syndrome caused by bilateral adrenal hyperplasia (Cushing's disease), the pituitary gland is reset upward and responds only to high plasma levels of cortisol or its analogues. In Cushing's syndrome caused by adrenal adenoma or cancer (which acts autonomously), cortisol secretion continues, despite a decrease in ACTH. When Cushing's syndrome is caused by an ectopic ACTH-producing tumor (as in lung cancer), that tumor is also considered autonomous and will continue to secrete ACTH despite high cortisol levels. Again, no decrease occurs in plasma cortisol. Knowledge of the following defects in the normal cortisol-ACTH feedback system is the basis for understanding the DST:

Cushing's syndrome caused by:
   Bilateral adrenal hyperplasia
      Low dose: no change
      High dose: >50% reduction of plasma cortisol and
         17-OCHS levels
   Adrenal adenoma or carcinoma
      Low dose: no change
      High dose: no change
   Ectopic ACTH-producing tumor
      Low dose: no change
      High dose: no change
   The DST also may identify depressed persons likely to respond
to electroconvulsive therapy or antidepressants rather than to
psychologic or social interventions. ACTH production will not
be suppressed after administration of low-dose dexamethasone
in these patients.
   The *prolonged* DST can be performed over a 6-day period on an
outpatient basis. The *rapid* DST is easily and quickly performed
and is used primarily as a screening test to diagnose Cushing's syndrome. It is less accurate and informative than the prolonged DST,
but when its results are normal, the diagnosis of Cushing's syndrome can be safely excluded. The ease with which the rapid DST
can be performed makes it useful in clinical medicine.

Interfering factors

- Physical and emotional stress can elevate ACTH release and
  obscure interpretation of test results.
- Drugs that can affect test results include barbiturates,
  estrogens, oral contraceptives, phenytoin (Dilantin),
  spironolactone (Aldactone), steroids, and tetracyclines.

Procedure and patient care

Before
PT Explain the procedure (prolonged or rapid test) to the
   patient.
- Obtain the patient's weight as a baseline for evaluating side
  effects of steroids.

During
Prolonged test
- Obtain a baseline 24-hour urine collection for
  corticosteroids (urine 17-OHCS [see p. 543] or urinary
  cortisol [see p. 314]).

- Collect blood for determination of baseline plasma cortisol levels (see p. 314) if indicated.
- Collect 24-hour urine specimens daily over a 6-day period. Because 6 continuous days of urine collections are needed, no urine specimens are discarded, except for the first voided specimen on day 1, after which the collection begins.
- On day 3 administer a low dose (0.5 mg) of dexamethasone by mouth every 6 hours for a total of 2 mg.
- On day 5 administer a high dose (2 mg) of dexamethasone by mouth every 6 hours for a total of 8 mg.
- Administer the dexamethasone with milk or an antacid to prevent gastric irritation.
- Note that the urine samples for cortisol and 17-OCHS do not need a preservative.
- Note that the creatinine content is measured in all the 24-hour urine collections to demonstrate their accuracy and adequacy.
- Keep the urine specimens refrigerated or on ice during the collection period.

D

Rapid test
- Give the patient 1 mg of dexamethasone by mouth at 11 PM.
- Administer the dexamethasone with milk or an antacid to prevent gastric irritation.
- If ordered, administer a barbiturate to sedate the patient and ensure a good night's sleep.
- At 8 o'clock the next morning, draw blood for determination of the plasma cortisol level before the patient arises.
- If no cortisol suppression occurs after 1 mg of dexa-methasone, at 11 PM, administer a higher dose (8 mg of dexamethasone) and obtain a cortisol level as described above. This is referred to as the *overnight 8-mg dexa-methasone suppression test*. Patients with adrenal hyperplasia will suppress. Patients with adrenal or ectopic tumors will not suppress.

After
- Evaluate the patient for evidence of gastric irritation.
- Assess the patient for steroid-induced side effects by monitoring weight, glucose levels, and potassium levels.
- Send specimens to the laboratory promptly.

Abnormal findings

Cushing's syndrome
Cushing's disease
Ectopic ACTH-producing tumors
Adrenal adenoma or carcinoma
Bilateral adrenal hyperplasia
Mental depression
Hyperthyroidism

notes

diabetes mellitus autoantibody panel (Insulin autoantibody [IAA], Islet cell antibody [ICA], Glutamic acid decarboxylase antibody [GAD Ab])

D

Type of test Blood

Normal findings <1:4 titer; no antibody detected

Test explanation and related physiology

Type 1 diabetes mellitus (DM) is insulin-dependent diabetes (IDDM). It is now becoming increasingly recognized that this disease is an "organ specific" form of autoimmune disease that results in destruction of the pancreatic islet cells and their products. These antibodies are used to differentiate type 1 DM from type 2 non–insulin–dependent DM. Nearly 90% of young diabetics have one or more of these autoantibodies at the time of their diagnosis. Type 2 diabetics have low or negative titers.

These antibodies often appear years before the onset of symptoms. The panel is useful to screen relatives of IDDM patients who are at risk of developing the disease. Sixty percent to 80% of first-degree relatives with both ICA and IAA will develop IDDM within 10 years. GAD Ab provides confirmatory evidence. The presence of these antibodies identifies which gestational diabetic will eventually require insulin permanently. Once recognized, preventive diabetic treatment is instituted. This may include counseling and antibody and glucose monitoring.

Because insulin antibodies appear in nearly all patients with diabetes treated with exogenous (human, bovine, or porcine) insulin, testing for the presence of these antibodies must precede insulin administration. Insulin antibodies develop from impurities in animal insulin or from antigenic stimulation of the insulin molecule. Antiinsulin antibodies reduce the amount of insulin available for glucose metabolism and may contribute to insulin resistance. The presence of insulin antibodies is diagnostic of factitious hypoglycemia from surreptitious administration of insulin. This antibody panel is also used in surveillance of patients who have received pancreatic islet cell transplantation.

Interfering factors

- Radioactive scans within 7 days before the test may interfere with the test result.

Procedure and patient care

Before

PT Tell the patient that no fasting is required.

During

- Collect 4 to 6 ml venous blood in a plain red-top or a blood/serum separator tube.

After

- Apply pressure to the venipuncture site.

Abnormal findings

▲   **Increased levels**

Type 1 DM/IDDM
Insulin resistance
Allergies to insulin
Factitious hypoglycemia

notes

2,3-diphosphoglycerate (2,3-DPG in erythrocytes)

D

Type of test Blood

Normal findings

12.3 ± 1.87 μmol/g of hemoglobin or 0.79 ± 0.12 mol/mol hemoglobin (SI units)

4.2 ± 0.64 μmol/ml of erythrocytes or 4.2 ± 0.64 mmol/L erythrocytes (SI units)

(Levels are lower in newborns and even lower in premature infants.)

Test explanation and related physiology

This test is used in the evaluation of nonspherocytic anemia. 2,3-DPG is a by-product of the glycolytic respiratory pathway of the RBC. A congenital enzyme deficiency in this vital pathway alters the RBC shape and survival significantly. Anemia is the result. Another result of the enzyme deficiency is reduced synthesis of 2,3-DPG. Since 2,3-DPG controls oxygen transport from the RBCs to the tissues, deficiencies of this enzyme result in alterations of the RBC-oxygen dissociation curve that controls release of oxygen to the tissues. Many anemias not due to 2,3-DPG deficiency are associated with increased levels of 2,3-DPG as a compensatory mechanism.

Usually 2,3-DPG levels increase in response to anemia or hypoxic conditions (e.g., obstructive lung disease, congenital cyanotic heart disease, after vigorous exercise). Increases in 2,3-DPG decrease the oxygen binding to hemoglobin so that oxygen is more easily released to the tissues when needed (lower arterial Po_2). Levels of 2,3-DPG are decreased as a result of inherited genetic defects. This genetic defect parallels that of sickle cell anemia and hemoglobin C diseases.

Interfering factors

- Vigorous exercise may cause increased levels.
- High altitudes may increase levels.
- Banked blood has decreased amounts of 2,3-DPG.
- Acidosis decreases levels.

Procedure and patient care

Before
PT Explain the procedure to the patient.
PT Tell the patient that no fasting is required.

During
- Collect a venous blood sample in a red-top tube.

After
- Apply pressure to the venipuncture site.

Abnormal findings

▲ **Increased levels**

Anemia
Hypoxic heart (e.g., cyanotic
   heart disease) or lung
   (e.g., chronic obstructive
   pulmonary disease) diseases
Hyperthyroidism
Chronic renal failure
Pyruvate kinase deficiency

▼ **Decreased levels**

Polycythemia
Acidosis
Post–massive blood
   transfusion
2,3-DPG disease
Respiratory distress
   syndrome

notes

disseminated intravascular coagulation screening
(DIC screening)

Type of test   Blood

Normal findings   No evidence of DIC

Test explanation and related physiology

This is a group of tests used to detect disseminated intravascular coagulation. Many pathologic conditions can instigate or are associated with DIC. The more common ones include bacterial septicemia, amniotic fluid embolism, retention of a dead fetus, malignant neoplasia, liver cirrhosis, extensive surgery (especially on the liver), postextracorporeal heart bypass, extensive trauma, severe burns, and transfusion reactions.

In DIC, the entire clotting mechanism is inappropriately triggered. This results in significant systemic or localized intravascular formation of fibrin clots. Consequences of this futile clotting are intravascular sludging and excessive bleeding caused by consumption of the platelets and clotting factors that have been used in intravascular clotting. The fibrinolytic system is also activated to break down the clot formation and the fibrin involved in the intravascular coagulation. This fibrinolysis results in the formation of fibrin degradation products (FDPs), which by themselves act as anticoagulants; these FDPs serve only to enhance the bleeding tendency.

Organ injury can occur as a result of the intravascular clots, which cause microvascular occlusion in various organs. This may cause serious anoxic injury in affected organs. Also, red blood cells passing through partly plugged vessels are injured and subsequently hemolyzed. The result may be ongoing hemolytic anemia. Figure 16 summarizes DIC pathophysiology and effects.

When a patient with a bleeding tendency is suspected to have DIC, a series of readily performed laboratory tests should be done (Table 12). With these tests, a hematologist can make the appropriate diagnosis confidently. All these tests are discussed separately within this book.

Abnormal findings

DIC

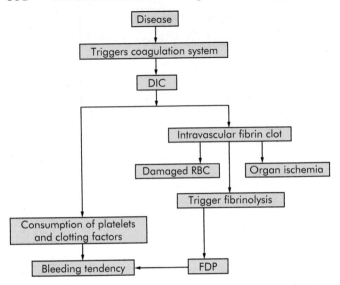

Figure 16 Pathology of disseminated intravascular coagulation *(DIC)*, which may result in bleeding tendency, organ ischemia, and hemolytic anemia. *RBC,* Red blood cell; *FDP,* Fibrin degradation product.

TABLE 12 Disseminated intravascular coagulation screening tests

Test	Result
Bleeding time (p. 169)	Prolonged
Platelet count (p. 714)	Decreased
Prothrombin time (p. 766)	Prolonged
Partial thromboplastin time (p. 654)	Prolonged
Coagulating factors (p. 279)	Decreased factors I, II, V, VIII, X, and XIII
Fibrin degradation products (p. 908)	Increased
Red blood smear (p. 174)	Damaged red blood cells
Euglobulin lysis time (p. 422)	Normal or prolonged
D-dimer (p. 351)	Increased

echocardiography (Cardiac echo, Heart sonogram, Transthoracic echocardiography [TTE])

Type of test   Ultrasound

Normal findings

Normal position, size, and movement of the cardiac valves and heart muscle wall

Normal directional flow of blood within the heart chambers

Test explanation and related physiology

Echocardiography is a noninvasive ultrasound procedure used to evaluate the structure and function of the heart. In diagnostic ultrasonography, a harmless, high-frequency sound wave emitted from a transducer penetrates the heart. Sound waves are bounced off the heart structures and reflected back to the transducer as a series of echoes. These echoes are amplified and displayed on an oscilloscope. Tracings also can be recorded on moving graph paper or videotape. The study usually includes M-mode recordings, two-dimensional recordings, and a Doppler study.

M-mode echocardiography is a linear tracing of the motion of the heart structures over time. This allows the various cardiac structures to be located and studied regarding their movement during a cardiac cycle.

Two-dimensional echocardiography angles a beam within one sector of the heart. This produces a picture of the spatial anatomic relationships within the heart.

A recent addition has been *color Doppler echocardiography.* This test detects the pattern of the blood flow and measures changes in velocity of blood flow within the heart and great vessels. Turbulent blood or altered velocity and direction of blood flow can be identified by changes in color. This is seen in a photograph. In most Doppler ultrasound color flow imaging, blue and red represent the direction of a given stream of blood; the various hues from dull to bright represent varying blood velocities. The most useful application of the color flow imaging is in determining the direction and turbulence of blood flow across regurgitant or narrowed valves. Doppler color flow imaging also may be helpful in assessing proper functioning of prosthetic valves.

E

Echocardiography, in general, is used in the diagnosis of a pericardial effusion, valvular heart disease (e.g., mitral valve prolapse, stenosis, regurgitation), subaortic stenosis, myocardial wall abnormalities (e.g., cardiomyopathy), infarction, and aneurysm. Cardiac tumors (e.g., myxomas) are easily diagnosed with ultrasound. Atrial and ventricular septal defects and other congenital heart diseases are also recognized by ultrasound. Finally, postinfarction mural thrombi are readily apparent with this testing.

Echocardiography is also used in *cardiac stress testing*. It is fast becoming the method of choice in heart imaging for stress testing. During an exercise or chemical cardiac stress test, ischemic muscle areas are evident as hypokinetic areas within the myocardium. Echocardiography is being used with increased frequency in emergent and urgent evaluations of patients with chest pains. If the myocardium is normal and without areas of hypokinesia, no coronary artery occlusive disease is suspected. If, however, a hypokinetic or akinetic area is noted, ischemia or infarction has occurred, and the chest pain is cardiac in origin.

It is now possible to perform echocardiography via the esophagus using a probe mounted on an endoscope. This is referred to as *transesophageal echocardiography* or *TEE* (see p. 933).

Contraindications

- Patients who are uncooperative

Interfering factors

- Chronic obstructive pulmonary disease (COPD)
  Patients who have severe COPD have a significant amount of air and space between the heart and the chest cavity. Air space does not conduct ultrasound waves well.
- Obesity
  In obese patients the space between the heart and the transducer is greatly enlarged; therefore accuracy of the test is decreased.

Procedure and patient care

Before

PT Assure the patient that this is a painless study.
- Complete the request for the echocardiogram, including the pertinent patient history.

During

- Note the following procedural steps:
  1. The patient is placed in the supine position.
  2. Electrocardiographic (ECG) leads are placed (see p. 368).
  3. A gel, which allows better transmission of sound waves, is placed on the chest wall immediately under the transducer.
  4. Ultrasound is directed to the heart, and appropriate tracings are obtained.
- Note that this procedure usually takes approximately 45 minutes and is performed by an ultrasound technician in a darkened room within the cardiac laboratory or radiology department.
- **PT** Tell the patient that no discomfort is associated with this study but that the transmission gel is usually cooler than body temperature.

After

- Remove the gel from the patient's chest wall.
- **PT** Inform the patient that the physician must interpret the study and that the results will be available in a few hours.

Abnormal findings

Valvular stenosis
Valvular regurgitation
Mitral valve prolapse
Pericardial effusion
Ventricular or atrial mural thrombi
Myxoma
Poor ventricular muscle motion
Septal defects
Ventricular hypertrophy
Endocarditis

notes

---

electrocardiography (Electrocardiogram [ECG, EKG])

Type of test Electrodiagnostic

Normal findings Normal heart rate (60-100 beats/min), rhythm, and wave deflections

Test explanation and related physiology

The ECG is a graphic representation of the electrical impulses that the heart generates during the cardiac cycle. These electrical impulses are conducted to the body's surface, where they are detected by electrodes placed on the patient's limbs and chest. The monitoring electrodes detect the electrical activity of the heart from a variety of spatial perspectives. The ECG lead system is composed of several electrodes that are placed on each of the four extremities and at varying sites on the chest. Each combination of electrodes is called a *lead*.

A *12-lead ECG* provides a comprehensive view of the flow of the heart's electrical currents in two different planes. There are six limb leads (combination of electrodes on the extremities) and six chest leads (corresponding to six sites on the chest). Leads I, II, and III are considered the standard *limb* leads. Lead I records the difference in electrical potential between the left arm (LA) and the right arm (RA). Lead II records the electrical potential between the RA and the left leg (LL). Lead III reflects the difference between the LA and the LL. The right leg (RL) electrode is an inactive ground in all leads. There are three *augmented* limb leads: aV_R, aV_L, and aV_F (*a*, augmented; *V*, vector [unipolar]; *R*, right arm; *L*, left arm; *F*, left foot or leg). The augmented leads measure the electrode potential between a calculated center point and the right arm (aV_R), the left arm (aV_L), and the left leg (aV_F). The six standard chest, or precordial, leads (V_1, V_2, V_3, V_4, V_5, V_6) are placed at six different positions on the chest, surrounding the heart.

In general, it is said that leads II, III and aV_F look at the inferior part of the heart. Leads aV_L and I look at the lateral part of the heart, and leads V_2-V_4 look at the anterior part of the heart.

The ECG is recorded on special paper with a graphic background of horizontal and vertical lines for rapid measurement of time intervals (*X* coordinate) and voltages (*Y* coordinate). Time duration is measured by vertical lines 1 mm apart, each representing 0.04 second. Voltage is measured by horizontal lines 1 mm apart. Five 1-mm squares equal 0.5 mV.

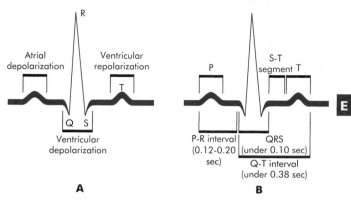

E

Figure 17 Electrocardiography. **A,** Normal ECG deflections during depolarization and repolarization of the atrium and ventricles. **B,** Principal ECG intervals between P, QRS, and T waves.

The normal ECG pattern is composed of waves arbitrarily designated by the letters *P, Q, R, S,* and *T*. The Q, R, and S waves are grouped together and described as the QRS complex. The significance of the waves and time intervals is as follows (Figure 17).

P wave. This represents atrial electrical depolarization associated with atrial contraction. It represents electrical activity associated with the spread of the original impulse from the sinoatrial (SA) node through the atria. If the P waves are absent or altered, the cardiac impulse originates outside the SA node.

PR interval. This represents the time required for the impulse to travel from the SA node to the atrioventricular (AV) node. If this interval is prolonged, a conduction delay exists in the AV node (e.g., a first-degree heart block). If the PR interval is shortened, the impulse must have reached the ventricle through a "shortcut" (as in Wolff-Parkinson-White syndrome).

QRS complex. This represents ventricular electrical depolarization associated with ventricular contraction. This complex consists of an initial downward (negative) deflection (Q wave), a large upward (positive) deflection (R wave), and a small downward deflection (S wave). A widened QRS complex indicates abnormal or prolonged ventricular depolarization time (as in a bundle-branch block), Wolff-Parkinson-White syndrome, or pacemaker rhythms.

ST segment. This represents the period between the completion of depolarization and the beginning of repolarization of the ventricular muscle. This segment may be elevated or depressed in transient muscle ischemia (e.g., angina) or in muscle injury (as in the early stages of myocardial infarction).

T wave. This represents ventricular repolarization (i.e., return to the resting state).

U wave. This deflection follows the T wave and is usually quite small. It represents repolarization of the Purkinje nerve fibers within the ventricles.

Through the analysis of these waveforms and time intervals, valuable information about the heart may be obtained. The ECG is used primarily to identify abnormal heart rhythms (arrhythmias [dysrhythmias]) and to diagnose acute myocardial infarction, conduction defects, and ventricular hypertrophy. It is important to note that the ECG may be normal, even in the presence of heart disease.

For some patients at high risk for malignant ventricular arrhythmias, a *signal-averaged ECG (SAECG)* can be performed. This test averages several hundred QRS waveforms to detect late potentials that are likely to lead to ventricular arrhythmias. SAECGs have been a useful precursor to electrophysiologic studies (see p. 387) because they can identify patients with unexplained syncope who may have ventricular tachycardias induced by the electrophysiologic study. SAECGs can be performed at the bedside in 15 to 20 minutes and must be ordered separately from a standard ECG. This type of ECG uses a non-standard ECG patch placement and is not performed like a standard ECG.

Interfering factors

- Inaccurate placement of the electrodes
- Electrolyte imbalances
- Poor contact between the skin and the electrodes
- Movement or muscle twitching during the test
- ✠ Drugs that can affect results include digitalis, quinidine, and barbiturates.

Procedure and patient care

Before
PT Explain the procedure to the patient.
PT Tell the patient that no food or fluid restriction is necessary.

PT Assure the patient that the flow of electric current is *from* the patient. He or she will feel nothing during this procedure.

- Expose only the patient's chest and arms. Keep the abdomen and thighs adequately covered.

During

- Note the following procedural steps:
  1. The skin areas designated for electrode placement are prepared by using alcohol swabs or sandpaper to remove skin oil or debris. Sometimes the skin is shaved if the patient has a large amount of hair.
  2. Pads with special gel are applied to ensure electrical conduction between the skin and the electrodes.
  3. Electrodes are applied to the four extremities. Many cardiologists recommend that arm electrodes be placed on the upper arm, because fewer muscle tremors are detected there.
  4. The chest leads are applied either one at a time, three at a time, or six at a time, depending on the type of ECG machine. These leads are positioned as follows:
     V_1: in the fourth intercostal space (4ICS) at the right sternal border
     V_2: in 4ICS at the left sternal border
     V_3: midway between V_2 and V_4
     V_4: in 5ICS at the midclavicular line
     V_5: at the left anterior axillary line at the level of V_4 horizontally
     V_6: at the left midaxillary line on the level of V_4 horizontally

- List medications the patient is taking on the ECG request form.
- Note that cardiac technicians, nurses, or physicians perform this procedure in less than 5 minutes at the bedside or in the cardiology clinic.
- **PT** Tell the patient that, although this procedure carries no discomfort, he or she must lie still in the supine position without talking while the ECG is recorded.

After

- Remove the electrodes from the patient's skin and wipe off the electrode gel.
- Indicate on the ECG strip or request slip if the patient was experiencing chest pain during the study. The pain may be correlated to an arrhythmia on the ECG.

E

Abnormal findings

Arrhythmia
Acute myocardial infarction
Myocardial ischemia
Old myocardial infarction
Conduction defects
Conduction system disease
Wolff-Parkinson-White syndrome
Ventricular hypertrophy
Cor pulmonale
Pulmonary embolus
Electrolyte imbalance
Pericarditis

notes

electroencephalography (Electroencephalogram [EEG])

Type of test Electrodiagnostic

Normal findings Normal frequency, amplitude, and characteristics of brain waves

Test explanation and related physiology

The EEG is a graphic recording of the electrical activity of the brain. EEG electrodes are placed on the scalp over multiple areas of the brain to detect and record electrical impulses within the brain. This study is invaluable in the investigation of epileptic states, in which the focus of seizure activity is characterized by rapid, spiking waves seen on the graph. Patients with cerebral lesions (e.g., tumors, infarctions) have abnormally slow EEG waves, depending on the size and location of the lesion. Because this study determines the overall activity of the brain, it can be used to evaluate trauma and drug intoxication and to determine cerebral death in comatose patients.

The EEG also can be used to monitor cerebral blood flow during surgical procedures. For example, during carotid endarterectomy, the carotid vessel must be temporarily occluded. When this surgery is performed with the patient under general anesthesia, the EEG can be used for early detection of cerebral tissue ischemia, which would indicate that continued carotid occlusion will result in a cerebrovascular accident (stroke) syndrome. Temporary shunting of the blood during the surgery is then required.

Interfering factors

- Fasting may cause hypoglycemia, which could modify the EEG pattern.
- Drinks containing caffeine (e.g., coffee, tea, cocoa, cola) interfere with test results.
- Body and eye movements during the test can cause changes in brain wave patterns.
- Drugs that may affect test results include sedatives.

Procedure and patient care

Before

PT Explain the procedure to the patient.

PT Assure the patient that this test cannot "read the mind" or detect senility.

PT Assure the patient that the flow of electrical activity is *from* the patient. He or she will not feel anything during the test.

PT Instruct the patient to wash his or her hair the night before the test. No oils, sprays, or lotion should be used.

■ Check if the physician wants to discontinue any medications before the study. (Anticonvulsants should be taken unless contraindicated by the physician.)

PT Instruct the patient if sleeping time should be shortened the night before the test. Adults may not be allowed to sleep more than 4 or 5 hours, and children not more than 5 to 7 hours if a sleep EEG will be done.

■ *Do not* administer any sedatives or hypnotics before the test because they will cause abnormal waves on the EEG.

PT Inform the patient not to fast before the study. Fasting may cause hypoglycemia, which could alter test results.

PT Instruct the patient not to drink any coffee, tea, cocoa, or cola on the morning of the test because of their stimulating effect.

PT Tell the patient that he or she needs to remain still during the test. Any movement, including opening the eyes, will create interference and alter the EEG recording.

During

■ Note the following procedural steps:
  1. The EEG is usually performed in a specially constructed room that is shielded from outside disturbances.
  2. The patient is placed in a supine position on a bed or reclining on a chair.
  3. Sixteen or more electrodes are applied to the scalp with electrode paste in a uniform pattern over both sides of the head, covering the prefrontal, frontal, temporal, parietal, and occipital areas.
  4. One electrode may be applied to each earlobe for grounding.
  5. After the electrodes are applied, the patient is instructed to lie still with eyes closed.

6. The technician continuously observes the patient during the EEG recording for any movements that could alter results.

7. Approximately every 5 minutes, the recording is interrupted to permit the patient to move if desired.

- In addition to the resting EEG, note that the following *activating procedures* can be performed:

E

1. The patient is *hyperventilated* (asked to breathe deeply 20 times a minute for 3 minutes) to induce alkalosis and cerebral vasoconstriction, which can activate abnormalities.

2. *Photostimulation* is performed by flashing a light over the patient's face with the eyes opened or closed. Photostimulated seizure activity may be seen on the EEG.

3. A *sleep EEG* may be performed to aid in the detection of some abnormal brain waves that are seen only if the patient is sleeping (e.g., frontal lobe epilepsy). The sleep EEG is performed after orally administering methyprylon (Noludar) or chloral hydrate (Noctec). A recording is performed while the patient is falling asleep, while the patient is asleep, and while the patient is waking.

- Note that this study is performed by an EEG technician in approximately 45 minutes to 2 hours.

PT Tell the patient that no discomfort is associated with this study, other than possibly missing sleep.

After

- Help the patient remove the electrode paste. The paste may be removed with acetone or witch hazel.

PT Instruct the patient to shampoo the hair.

- Ensure safety precautions until the effects of any sedatives have worn off. Keep the bed's siderails up.

PT Tell the patient who has had a sleep EEG not to drive home alone.

Abnormal findings

Seizure disorders
  (e.g., epilepsy)
Brain tumor
Brain abscess
Head injury
Cerebral death

Encephalitis
Intracranial hemorrhage
Cerebral infarct
Narcolepsy
Alzheimer's disease

electromyography (EMG)

Type of test Electrodiagnostic

Normal findings No evidence of neuromuscular abnormalities

Test explanation and related physiology

By placing a recording electrode into a skeletal muscle, the electrical activity of a skeletal muscle can be monitored in a way very similar to electrocardiography. The electrical activity is displayed on an oscilloscope as an electrical waveform. An audio-electrical amplifier can be added to the system so that both the appearance and sound of the electrical potentials can be analyzed and compared simultaneously. EMG is used to detect primary muscular disorders, along with muscular abnormalities caused by other system diseases (e.g., nerve dysfunction, sarcoidosis, paraneoplastic syndrome).

Spontaneous muscle movement such as fibrillation and fasciculation can be detected during EMG. When seen, these waves indicate injury or disease of the nerve innervating that muscle, or spastic myotonic muscle disease. Reduced amplitude size of the electrical waveform is indicative of a primary muscle disorder (e.g., polymyositis, muscular dystrophies, various myopathies). A progressive decrease in amplitude of the electrical waveform is a classic sign of myasthenia gravis. A decrease in the number of muscle fibers able to contract is seen with peripheral nerve damage. This study is usually done in conjunction with nerve conduction studies (see p. 381) and also may be called *electromyoneurography*.

Contraindications

- Patients receiving anticoagulant therapy
- Patients with extensive skin infection

Potential complications

- Rarely, hematoma at the needle insertion site

Interfering factors

- Edema, hemorrhage, or thick subcutaneous fat can interfere with test results.
- Patients with excessive pain may have false results.

Procedure and patient care

Before

PT Explain the procedure to the patient. Allay any fears and allow the patient to express concerns.

- Obtain informed consent if required by the institution.

PT Tell the patient that fasting is not usually required; however, some facilities may restrict stimulants (coffee, tea, cocoa, cola, cigarettes) for 2 to 3 hours before the test.

- If serum enzyme tests (e.g., AST [SGOT], CPK, LDH) are ordered, the specimen should be drawn before EMG or 5 to 10 days after the test, because the EMG may cause misleading elevations of these enzymes.

- Premedication or sedation is usually avoided because of the need for patient cooperation.

During

- Note the following procedural steps:
  1. This study is usually done in an EMG laboratory.
  2. The patient's position depends on the muscle being studied.
  3. A needle that acts as a recording electrode is inserted into the muscle being examined.
  4. A reference electrode is placed nearby on the skin surface.
  5. The patient is asked to keep the muscle at rest.
  6. The oscilloscope display is viewed for any evidence of spontaneous electrical activity such as fasciculation or fibrillation.
  7. The patient is asked to contract the muscle slowly and progressively.
  8. The electrical waves produced are examined for their number, form, and amplitude.

- Note that the EMG is performed by a physical therapist, physiatrist, or neurologist in approximately 20 minutes.

PT Tell the patient that this test is moderately uncomfortable. Slight pain may occur with the insertion of the needle electrode.

After

- Observe the needle site for hematoma or inflammation.
- Provide pain medication if needed.

Abnormal findings

Polymyositis
Muscular dystrophy
Myopathy
Traumatic injury
Hyperadrenalism
Hypothyroidism
Paraneoplastic syndrome (e.g., lung cancer)
Sarcoidosis
Guillain-Barré syndrome
Myasthenia gravis
Peripheral nerve injury, entrapment, or compression
Spinal cord injury or disease
Acetylcholine blockers (e.g., curare, snake venom)
Multiple sclerosis
Diabetic neuropathy
Anterior poliomyelitis
Muscle denervation
Amyotrophic lateral sclerosis

notes

electromyography of the pelvic floor sphincter
(Pelvic floor sphincter electromyography, Pelvic floor sphincter EMG, Rectal EMG procedure)

Type of test Electrodiagnostic

Normal findings

Increased EMG signal during bladder filling
Silent EMG signal on voluntary micturition
Increased EMG signal at the end of voiding
Increased EMG signal with voluntary contraction of the anal
    sphincter

Test explanation and related physiology

This test uses the placement of electrodes on or in the pelvic floor musculature to evaluate the neuromuscular function of the urinary or anal sphincter. It is performed most often in patients who have urinary or fecal incontinence. The pathology causing the muscle weakness can be muscular or neurologic. With sphincter EMG, these two causes can be separated.

The main benefit of this study is to evaluate the external sphincter (skeletal muscle) activity during voiding. This test is also used to evaluate the bulbocavernous reflex and voluntary control of external sphincter or pelvic floor muscles. The pelvic floor sphincter EMG also aids in the investigation of "functional" or "psychologic" disturbances of voiding. Fecal incontinence caused by muscular dysfunction can also be evaluated by rectal sphincter EMG.

Recordings may be made from surface or needle electrodes within the muscle; surface electrodes are most often used. These electrodes allow for observation of and change in the muscle activity before and during voiding.

Patient cooperation is essential. If the patient does not cooperate, the interpretation of the test results will be difficult.

Contraindications

■ Patients who cannot cooperate during the procedure

Procedure and patient care

Before
PT Explain the procedure to the patient.
PT Inform the patient that cooperation is essential.

During
- Note the following procedural steps:
  1. Two electrodes are placed at the 2 o'clock and 10 o'clock positions on the perianal skin to monitor the pelvic floor musculature during voiding.
  2. The third electrode is usually placed on the thigh and serves as a ground.
  3. Electrical activity is recorded with the bladder empty and the patient relaxed.
  4. Reflex activity is evaluated by asking the patient to cough and by stimulating the urethra and trigone by gently tugging on an inserted Foley catheter (bulbocavernous reflex).
  5. Voluntary activity is evaluated by asking the patient to contract and relax the sphincter muscle.
  6. The bladder is filled with sterile water at room temperature at a rate of 100 ml/min.
  7. The EMG responses to filling and detrusor hyperreflexia (if present) are recorded.
  8. Finally, when the bladder is full and with the patient in a voiding position, the filling catheter is removed, and the patient is asked to urinate. In the normal patient the EMG signals build during bladder filling and cease promptly on voluntary micturition, remaining silent until the pelvic floor contracts at the end of voiding.
  9. The electrical waves produced are examined for their number and form.
- Note that a urologist performs this study in less than 30 minutes.
- PT Explain to the patient that this study is slightly more uncomfortable than urethral catheterization.

After
- If needle electrodes were used, observe the needle site for hematoma or inflammation.

Abnormal findings

Neuromuscular dysfunction of lower urinary sphincter
Pelvic floor muscle dysfunction of the anal sphincter

electroneurography (ENG, Nerve conduction studies)

Type of test   Electrodiagnostic

Normal findings

No evidence of peripheral nerve injury or disease
(Conduction velocity is usually decreased in the elderly.)

E

Test explanation and related physiology

Electroneurography, or nerve conduction studies, allow for the detection and location of peripheral nerve injury or disease. By initiating an electrical impulse at one site (proximal) of a nerve and recording the time required for that impulse to travel to a second site (distal) of the same nerve, the conduction velocity of any impulse in that nerve can be determined. This study is usually done in conjunction with electromyography (see p. 376) and also may be called *electromyoneurography*.

The normal value for conduction velocity varies from one nerve to another. Variation also exists from person to person. It is always best to compare the conduction velocity of the suspected side with the contralateral nerve conduction velocity. In general, a range of normal conduction velocity will be approximately 50 to 60 m/sec.

Traumatic transection or contusion of a nerve will usually cause maximal slowing of conduction velocity in the affected side as compared with the normal side. Neuropathies, both local and generalized, also will cause a slowing of conduction velocity. A velocity greater than normal does not indicate a pathologic condition.

Because conduction velocity may require contraction of a muscle as an indication of an impulse arriving at the recording electrode, primary muscular disorders may cause a falsely slow nerve conduction velocity. This "muscular" variable is eliminated if one evaluates the suspected pathologic muscle group before performing nerve conduction studies. This muscular factor can be evaluated by measuring *distal latency* (i.e., the time required for stimulation of the distal end of the nerve to cause muscular contraction). Once the distal latency is calculated, the nerve conduction study is then performed normally by stimulating the proximal part of the nerve bundle. Conduction velocity can then be determined by the following equation:

$$\text{Conduction velocity (in meters per second)} = \frac{\text{Distance (in meters)}}{\text{Total latency} - \text{Distal latency}}$$

Interfering factors

- Patients in severe pain may have false results.

Procedure and patient care

Before

PT Explain the procedure to the patient. Allay any fears and allow the patient to express concerns.

- Obtain informed consent if required by the institution.

PT Tell the patient that no fasting or sedation is usually required.

During

- Note the following procedural steps:
  1. This test can be performed in a nerve conduction laboratory or at the patient's bedside.
  2. The patient's position depends on the area of suspected peripheral nerve injury or disease.
  3. A recording electrode is placed on the skin overlying a muscle innervated solely by the relevant nerve.
  4. A reference electrode is placed nearby.
  5. All skin-to-electrode connections are ensured by using electrical paste.
  6. The nerve is stimulated by a shock-emitting device at an adjacent location.
  7. The time between nerve impulse and muscular contraction (distal latency) is measured in milliseconds on an EMG machine.
  8. The nerve is similarly stimulated at a location proximal to the area of suspected injury or disease.
  9. The time required for the impulse to travel from the site of initiation to muscle contraction (total latency) is recorded in milliseconds.
  10. The distance between the site of stimulation and the recording electrode is measured in centimeters.
  11. Conduction velocity is converted to meters per second and is computed as in the previous equation.

- Note that this test takes approximately 15 minutes and is performed by a physiatrist or a neurologist.
PT Tell the patient that this test is uncomfortable in that a mild shock is required for nerve impulse stimulation.

After

- Remove the electrode gel from the patient's skin.

Abnormal findings

Peripheral nerve injury or disease
Carpal tunnel syndrome
Herniated disc disease
Poliomyelitis
Diabetic neuropathy
Myasthenia gravis
Guillain-Barré syndrome

notes

electronystagmography

Type of test Electrodiagnostic

Normal findings

Normal nystagmus response
Normal oculovestibular reflex

Test explanation and related physiology

Electronystagmography is used to evaluate nystagmus (involuntary rapid eye movement) and the muscles controlling eye movement. By measuring changes in the electrical field around the eye, this study can make a permanent recording of eye movement at rest, with a change in head position, and in response to various stimuli. The test delineates the presence or absence of nystagmus, which is caused by the initiation of the oculovestibular reflex. Nystagmus should occur when initiated by positional, visual, or caloric (see p. 224) stimuli. Unlike caloric studies in which nystagmus is usually determined visually, with electronystagmography, the direction, velocity, and degree of nystagmus can be recorded electrically.

If nystagmus does not occur with stimulation, the vestibular-cochlear apparatus, cerebral cortex (temporal lobe), auditory nerve, or brain stem is abnormal. Tumors, infection, ischemia, and degeneration can cause such abnormalities. When put together with the entire clinical picture, the pattern of nystagmus helps in the differentiation between central and peripheral vertigo. This test is used in the differential diagnosis of lesions in the vestibular system, brain stem, and cerebellum.

This study also may help evaluate unilateral hearing loss and vertigo. Unilateral hearing loss may be caused by middle ear problems or nerve injury. If the patient experiences nystagmus with stimulation, the auditory nerve is working, and hearing loss can be blamed on the middle ear.

Contraindications

- Patients with perforated eardrums, who should not have water irrigation
- Patients with pacemakers

Interfering factors

- Blinking of the eyes can alter test results.
- Drugs that can alter results include sedatives, stimulants, and antivertigo agents.

Procedure and patient care

Before

PT Explain the procedure to the patient.

PT Instruct the patient not to apply facial makeup before the test because electrodes will be taped to the skin around the eyes.

- Hold solid food before the test to reduce the likelihood of vomiting.

PT Instruct the patient not to drink caffeine or alcoholic beverages for approximately 24 to 48 hours (as ordered) before the test.

- Check with the physician regarding withholding any medications that could interfere with the test results.

During

- Note the following procedural steps:
  1. This procedure is usually performed in a darkened room with the patient seated or lying down on an examining table.
  2. If there is any wax in the ear, it is removed.
  3. Electrodes are taped to the skin around the eyes.
  4. Various procedures are used to stimulate nystagmus, such as pendulum tracking, changing head position, changing gaze position, and caloric tests (see p. 224).
  5. Several recordings are made with the patient at rest and to demonstrate patient response to various procedures (e.g., blowing air into the ear, irrigating the ear with water).
  6. Nystagmus response is compared with the expected ranges, and the results are recorded as normal, borderline, or abnormal.
- Note that this procedure is performed by a physician or audiologist in approximately 1 hour.

PT Tell the patient that nausea and vomiting may occur during the test.

After

- Consider prescribing bed rest until nausea, vertigo, or weakness subsides.

Abnormal findings

Brain stem lesions
Cerebellum lesions
VIII cranial nerve injury
Vestibular system lesions
Congenital disorder
Demyelinating disease

notes

electrophysiologic study (EPS, Cardiac mapping)

Type of test Electrodiagnostic; manometric

Normal findings Normal conduction intervals, refractive periods, and recovery times

Tilt-table testing

<20 mm Hg decrease in systolic blood pressure and <10 mm Hg increase in diastolic blood pressure. Heart rate increase should be less than 10 beats/min.

Test explanation and related physiology

In this invasive procedure, multiple electrode catheters are fluoroscopically placed through a peripheral vein and into the right atrium and/or ventricle or, less often, through an artery into the left atrium and/or ventricle. With close cardiac monitoring, the electrode catheters are used to pace the heart and potentially induce arrhythmias. Defects in the heart conduction system can then be identified; arrhythmias that are otherwise inapparent also can be induced, identified, and treated. The effectiveness of antiarrhythmic drugs (e.g., lidocaine, phenytoin, quinidine) can be assessed by determining the electrical threshold required to induce arrhythmias.

EPS can also be therapeutic. With the use of radiofrequency, sites with documented low thresholds for inducing arrhythmias can be obliterated to stop the arrhythmias.

The *tilt-table test* is sometimes performed with an electrophysiologic cardiac study and is a provocative test used to diagnose vasopressor syncope syndrome. Patients with this syndrome usually demonstrate symptomatic hypotension and syncope within a few to 30 minutes of being tilted upright by approximately 60 to 80 degrees. The tilt-table test is often used to assess the efficacy of prophylactic pacing in some patients with vasopressor syncope. It is also used to evaluate the impact of posture with some forms of tachyarrhythmias. Normally a minimal drop in systolic blood pressure, rise in diastolic blood pressure, and increase in heart rate occur in the tilted position. Patients with vasopressor syncope demonstrate these changes in an exaggerated fashion and become lightheaded and dizzy on assuming the tilted position.

Contraindications

- Patients who are uncooperative
- Patients with acute myocardial infarction

Potential complications

- Cardiac arrhythmias leading to ventricular tachycardia or fibrillation
- Perforation of the myocardium
- Catheter-induced embolic cerebrovascular accident (stroke) or myocardial infarction
- Peripheral vascular problems
- Hemorrhage
- Phlebitis at the venipuncture site

Interfering factors

- Patients with dehydration or hypovolemia demonstrate similar changes in blood pressure and heart rate with tilt-table testing. This is especially true in elderly patients.
- Patients on antihypertensive medications or diuretics also may demonstrate similar changes when placed in the tilt position.
- Drugs that may interfere with test results include analgesics, sedatives, and tranquilizers.

Procedure and patient care

Before

- **PT** Instruct the patient to fast for 6 to 8 hours before the procedure. Usually fluids are permitted until 3 hours before the test.
- Obtain an informed consent from the patient.
- **PT** Encourage the patient to verbalize any fears regarding this test.
- Shave and prepare the catheter insertion site.
- Collect a blood sample for potassium or drug levels if indicated.
- Obtain peripheral IV access for the administration of drugs.
- Often an arterial line is placed to accurately monitor blood pressure during tilt-table testing.
- Inquire as to whether the patient has had excessive fluid loss (diarrhea or vomiting) in the previous 24 hours.
- Record antihypertensive or diuretic medicines that the patient may be taking.

During

- Note the following procedural steps:

Electrophysiologic study

1. After being transported to the cardiac catheterization laboratory, the patient has electrocardiographic (ECG) leads attached.
2. The catheter insertion site, usually the femoral vein, is prepared and draped in a sterile manner.
3. Under fluoroscopic guidance the catheter is passed to the atrium and ventricle.
4. Baseline surface intracardiac ECGs are recorded.
5. Various parts of the cardiac electroconduction system are stimulated by atrial or ventricular pacing.
6. Mapping of the electroconduction system and its defects is performed.
7. Arrhythmias are identified.
8. Drugs may be administered to assess their efficacy in preventing EPS-induced arrhythmias.
9. Because dangerous arrhythmias can be prolonged, cardioversion must be immediately available.
10. Not only are vital signs and the heart monitored, the patient is constantly engaged in light conversation to assess mental status and consciousness.

Tilt-table test

1. The patient lies supine on a horizontal tilt table.
2. Obtain the patient's blood pressure and pulse as baseline values before tilting is carried out.
3. Monitor these vital signs during the procedure.
4. Question the patient as to the presence of symptoms of dizziness and lightheadedness.
5. The table is progressively tilted to 60 to 80 degrees while the patient is being monitored. Alternatively, the patient is asked to sit or stand.

PT Tell the patient that he or she may experience palpitations, lightheadedness, or dizziness when arrhythmias are induced. Report these sensations to the physician. For most patients this is an anxiety-producing experience.

PT Inform the patient that discomfort from catheter insertion is minimal.

After

- Keep the patient on bed rest for approximately 6 to 8 hours.
- Evaluate the venous/arterial access site for swelling and bleeding.
- Monitor the patient's vital signs for at least 2 to 4 hours for hypotension and arrhythmias. Additional monitoring is especially important for certain medications that the patient received during the test. For example, if the patient received quinidine, monitoring is necessary for hypotension and abdominal cramping.
- Continue cardiac monitoring to identify arrhythmias. Transfer arrangements to a monitored unit may be necessary.
- Cover the area with sterile dressings if the electrical catheter is left in place for subsequent studies.

Abnormal findings

Electroconduction defects
Cardiac arrhythmia
Sinoatrial node defects (e.g., sick sinus syndrome)
Atrioventricular node defects and heart blocks
Vasomotor syncope syndrome

notes

endometrial biopsy

Type of test Microscopic examination of tissue

Normal findings

No pathologic conditions

Presence of a "secretory-type" endometrium 3 to 5 days before normal menses

Test explanation and related physiology

An endometrial biopsy can determine whether ovulation has occurred. A biopsy specimen taken 3 to 5 days before normal menses should demonstrate a "secretory-type" endometrium on histologic examination if ovulation and corpus luteum formation have occurred. If not, only a preovulatory "proliferative-type" endometrium will be seen.

Occasionally an endometrial biopsy is performed to indicate estrogen's effect in patients with suspected ovarian dysfunction or absence. Similarly, adequate circulating progesterone levels can be determined by identifying secretory endometrium. Another major use of endometrial biopsy is to diagnose endometrial cancer, tuberculosis, polyps, or inflammatory conditions and to evaluate uterine bleeding.

Contraindications

- Patients with infections (e.g., trichomonal, candidal, or suspected gonococcal) of the cervix or vagina
- Patients in whom the cervix cannot be visualized (e.g., because of abnormal position or previous surgery)

Potential complications

- Perforation of the uterus
- Uterine bleeding
- Interference with early pregnancy
- Infection

Procedure and patient care

Before

PT Explain the procedure to the patient.
- Ensure that written and informed consent for this procedure is obtained from the patient.
PT Tell the patient that neither fasting nor sedation is usually required.

During

- Note the following procedural steps:
  1. The patient is placed in the lithotomy position, and a pelvic examination is performed to determine the position of the uterus.
  2. The cervix is exposed and cleansed.
  3. A biopsy instrument is inserted into the uterus, and specimens are obtained from the anterior, posterior, and lateral walls. This can be performed as part of a D&C or hysteroscopy (p. 550).
  4. The specimens are placed in a solution containing 10% formalin solution and sent to a pathologist for histologic examination.
- Note that this procedure is performed by an obstetrician/gynecologist in approximately 10 to 30 minutes.
- **PT** Tell the patient that this procedure may cause momentary discomfort (menstrual-type cramping).

After

- Assess the patient's vital signs at regular intervals. Any temperature elevation should be reported to the physician because this procedure may activate pelvic inflammatory disease.
- **PT** Advise the patient to wear a pad because some vaginal bleeding is to be expected. Instruct the patient to call her physician if excessive bleeding (requiring more than one pad per hour) occurs.
- **PT** Inform the patient that douching and intercourse are not permitted for 72 hours after the biopsy specimen removal.
- **PT** Instruct the patient to rest during the next 24 hours and to avoid heavy lifting to prevent uterine hemorrhage.

🏠 Home care responsibilities

- Instruct the patient to report any temperature elevation to her physician because this procedure may activate pelvic inflammatory disease (PID).
- Advise the patient to wear a sanitary pad after this procedure. Tell the patient to call her physician for excessive bleeding (>1 pad per hour).
- Tell the patient to avoid heavy lifting after this procedure to prevent increased intraabdominal pressure and possible uterine bleeding.

Abnormal findings

Anovulation
Tumor
Tuberculosis
Polyps
Inflammatory condition

notes

endoscopic retrograde cholangiopancreatography
(ERCP, ERCP of the biliary and pancreatic ducts)

Type of test Endoscopy

Normal findings

Normal size of biliary and pancreatic ducts
No obstruction or filling defects within the biliary or pancreatic ducts

Test explanation and related physiology

With the use of a fiberoptic endoscope, ERCP provides radiographic visualization of the bile and pancreatic ducts. This is especially useful in patients with jaundice. If a partial or total obstruction of those ducts exists, characteristics of the obstructing lesion can be demonstrated. Stones, benign strictures, cysts, ampullary stenosis, anatomic variations, and malignant tumors can be identified.

Incision of the papillary muscle in the ampulla of Vater can be performed through the scope at the time of ERCP. This incision widens the distal common duct so that common bile duct gallstones can be removed. Stents can be placed through narrowed bile ducts with the use of ERCP, and the bile of jaundiced patients can be internally drained. Pieces of tissue and brushings of the common bile duct can be obtained by ERCP for pathologic review. Manometric studies of the sphincter of Oddi and pancreaticobiliary ducts can be performed at the time of ERCP. These are used to investigate unusual functional abnormalities of these structures.

Other less commonly used methods of visualizing the biliary tree include *oral cholecystography (OCG), IV cholangiography (IVC),* and *percutaneous transhepatic cholangiography (PTHC).* OCG is a method of visualizing the gallbladder in order to identify gallstones. The patient is asked to ingest iopanoic acid tablets, which are then concentrated in the normal gallbladder. X-rays of the abdomen visualize the gallbladder. IVC is another method used to visualize the entire biliary tree by the intravenous administration of contrast that concentrates weakly in the biliary tree. Neither OCG nor IVC will visualize the biliary tree in the jaundiced patient. Only ERCP and PTHC can provide direct visualization of the biliary ducts in the face of jaundice. PTHC is performed by passing a needle through the skin into the liver and into an intrahepatic bile duct. Iodinated x-ray contrast dye is directly injected into the biliary system. The intrahepatic and extrahepatic biliary ducts and occasionally the gallbladder can be visualized. If the jaundice is found to result from extrahepatic obstruction, a catheter can be left in the bile duct and used for external drainage of bile. Furthermore, with the assistance of ERCP, a stent can be placed across a stricture to decompress the biliary system internally. PTHC is an invasive procedure with significant risks of bleeding, and intraabdominal bile leaks; ERCP is associated with much less morbidity but must be performed by an experienced endoscopist.

Contraindications

- Patients who are uncooperative
  Cannulation of the ampulla of Vater requires that the patient lie very still.
- Patients whose ampulla of Vater is not accessible endoscopically because of previous upper gastrointestinal surgery (e.g., gastrectomy patients whose duodenum containing the ampulla is surgically separated from the stomach)
- Patients with esophageal diverticula
  The scope can fall into a diverticulum and perforate its wall.
- Patients with known acute pancreatitis

Potential complications

- Perforation of the esophagus, stomach, or duodenum
- Gram-negative sepsis
  This results from introducing bacteria through the biliary system and into the blood. Usually this occurs in patients who have obstructive jaundice.
- Pancreatitis
  This results from pressure of the dye injection.
- Aspiration of gastric contents into the lungs
- Respiratory arrest as a result of oversedation

Interfering factors

- Barium within the abdomen as a result of a previous upper GI series or barium enema x-ray studies precludes adequate visualization of the biliary and pancreatic ducts.

Procedure and patient care

Before

PT Explain the procedure to the patient.
- Obtain informed consent from the patient.
PT Inform the patient that breathing will not be compromised by the insertion of the endoscope.
- Keep the patient NPO as of midnight the day of the test.

- Administer appropriate premedication (e.g., midazolam [Versed] and atropine) if ordered.

During

- Note the following procedural steps:
    1. A flat plate of the abdomen is taken to ensure that any barium from previous studies will not obscure visualization of the bile duct.
    2. The patient is placed in the supine position or on the left side.
    3. The patient is usually sedated with a narcotic and a sedative/hypnotic.
    4. The pharynx is sprayed with a local anesthetic (lidocaine [Xylocaine]) to inactivate the gag reflex and to lessen the discomfort caused by the passage of the scope.
    5. A side-viewing fiberoptic duodenoscope is inserted through the oral pharynx and passed through the esophagus and stomach and into the duodenum (Figure 18).
    6. Glucagon is often administered intravenously to minimize the spasm of the duodenum and to improve visualization of the ampulla of Vater.
    7. Through the accessory lumen within the scope, a small catheter is passed through the ampulla and into the common bile or pancreatic ducts.
    8. Radiographic dye is injected, and x-ray films are taken.
- Note that the test usually takes approximately 1 hour and is performed by a physician trained in endoscopy. The x-ray films are interpreted by a radiologist.
- **PT** Tell the patient that no discomfort is associated with the dye injection but that minimal gagging may occur during the initial introduction of the scope into the oral pharynx.

After

- Do *not* allow the patient to eat or drink until the gag reflex returns.
- Observe the patient closely for development of abdominal pain, nausea, and vomiting. This may herald the onset of ERCP-induced pancreatitis.
- Observe safety precautions until the effects of the sedatives have worn off.
- Monitor the patient for signs of respiratory depression. Medication (e.g., naloxone [Narcan]) should be available to counteract serious respiratory depression. Resuscitative equipment should also be present.

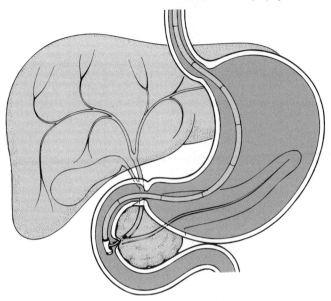

Figure 18 Endoscopic retrograde cholangiopancreatography. The fiberoptic scope is passed into the duodenum. Note the small catheter being advanced into the biliary duct.

- Assess the patient for signs and symptoms of septicemia, which may indicate the onset of ERCP-induced cholangitis.
- **PT** Inform the patient that he or she may be hoarse and have a sore throat for several days. Drinking cool fluids and gargling will help relieve some of this soreness.

🏠 Home care responsibilities

- A sore throat is expected. A soothing mouthwash gargle may help.
- Notify the physician immediately if increasing abdominal pain, nausea, or vomiting occurs. These may be the early signs of pancreatitis or gastroduodenal perforation.
- Notify the physician immediately of fever or shaking chills. This may indicate possible cholangitis.
- Encourage the patient to eat lightly for the next 12 to 24 hours.

Abnormal findings

Tumor, strictures, or gallstones of the common bile duct
Sclerosing cholangitis
Biliary sclerosis
Cysts of the common bile duct
Tumor, strictures, or inflammation of the pancreatic duct
Pseudocyst of the pancreatic duct
Chronic pancreatitis
Anatomic biliary or pancreatic duct variations
Cancer of the duodenum or ampulla

notes

Epstein-Barr virus titer (EBV)

Type of test Blood

Normal findings

Titers ≤1:10 are nondiagnostic.

Titers of 1:10 to 1:60 indicate infection at some undetermined time.

Titers of 1:320 or greater suggest active infection.

Fourfold increase in titer in paired sera drawn 10 to 14 days apart is usually indicative of an acute infection.

Test explanation and related physiology

EBV infects 80% of the U.S. population. Once infection occurs, the virus becomes dormant but can be reactivated later. EBV infection can produce infectious mononucleosis (IM). Mononucleosis is seen most often in children, adolescents, and young adults. Clinical features include those of acute fatigue, fever, sore throat, lymphadenopathy, and splenomegaly. Lymphocytosis, atypical lymphocytes, and the development of transient serum heterophil antibodies are found in patients with acute EBV infection. Most patients with infectious mononucleosis recover uneventfully and return to normal activity within 4 to 6 weeks. In Africa, EBV has been associated with Burkitt's lymphoma. In China, EBV infection has been associated with nasopharyngeal carcinoma.

After recovery from primary EBV infection, a lifelong latent EBV-carrier status is established. In the last several years, specific immunologic tests to identify EBV activity indicate that latent EBV can reactivate and become associated with a constellation of chronic signs and symptoms resembling infectious mononucleosis. Clinical manifestations of chronic EBV are variable and include nonspecific symptoms, such as profound fatigue, pharyngitis, myalgia, arthralgia, low-grade fever, headache, paresthesia, and loss of abstract thinking.

Serologic tests are the only way to make the diagnosis of EBV. The heterophil agglutination slide test (monospot test) is explained on p. 649. Other, more specific immunologic tests indicate more precisely the timing of the infection (Table 13). The viral capsid antigen-antibodies (VCAs) can be IgG or IgM. The EBV nuclear antigen (EBNA) is located in the nuclei of the infected lymphocyte. Another EBV antigen is called the early

TABLE 13 Serologic studies and the timing of infections

Serologic study	Appears/disappears	Clinical significance
Monospot heterophil	5 days/2 weeks	Acute or convalescent infection
VCA-IgM	7 days/3 months	Acute or convalescent infection
VCA-IgG	7 days/exists for life	Acute, convalescent, or old infection
EBNA-IgG	3 weeks/exists for life	Old infection
EA-D	7 days/2 weeks	Acute or convalescent infection

antigen (EA). There are two types of early antigens. One is spread diffusely about the cytoplasm of the infected cell (EA-D), and the other is restricted to only one area of the cytoplasm (EA-R). The EA-D is commonly found in nasopharyngeal cancer. The EA-R is commonly found in Burkitt's lymphoma.

The interpretation of EBV antibody tests is based on the following assumptions:

1. Once a person becomes infected with EBV, the anti-VCA antibodies appear first.
2. Anti-EA (EA-D or EA-R) antibodies appear next or are present with anti-VCA antibodies early in the course of illness. An anti-EA antibody titer greater than 80 in a patient 2 years after acute infectious mononucleosis indicates chronic EBV syndrome.
3. As the patient recovers, anti-VCA and anti-EA antibodies decrease, and anti-EBNA antibodies appear. The anti-EBNA antibody persists for life and reflects a past infection.
4. After the patient is well, anti-VCA and anti-EBNA antibodies are always present but at lower ranges. Occasionally, anti-EA antibodies also may be present after the patient recovers.

If an acute infection is suspected to have occurred more than a few weeks before testing, the monospot may be negative. Detecting anti-VCA-IgG or EBNA will not be helpful because it indicates that an EBV infection has occurred sometime in the patient's life—not necessarily the recent syndrome. But detecting anti-VCA-IgM would indicate that the syndrome of complaint the patient experienced a few weeks earlier was the result of EBV.

Procedure and patient care

Before

PT Explain the procedure to the patient.

PT Tell the patient that no fasting or special preparation is required.

During

- Collect 5 to 10 ml of venous blood in a red-top tube.
- Record the day of onset of illness on the laboratory slip.
- Obtain serum samples as soon as possible after the onset of the illness.
- Obtain a second blood specimen 14 to 21 days later.

After

- Apply pressure to the venipuncture site.

Abnormal findings

Infectious mononucleosis
Chronic fatigue syndrome
Chronic EBV carrier state
Burkitt's lymphoma
Nasopharyngeal cancer

notes

erythrocyte sedimentation rate (ESR, Sed rate test)

Type of test Blood

Normal findings

Westergren method

Male: up to 15 mm/hr
Female: up to 20 mm/hr
Child: up to 10 mm/hr
Newborn: 0-2 mm/hr

Test explanation and related physiology

ESR is a measurement of the rate with which the red blood cells (RBCs) settle in saline or plasma over a specified time period. It is nonspecific and therefore not diagnostic for any particular organ disease or injury. Because acute and chronic infection, inflammation (collagen-vascular diseases), advanced neoplasm, and tissue necrosis or infarction increase the protein (mainly fibrinogen) content of plasma, RBCs have a tendency to stack up on one another, increasing their weight and causing them to descend faster. Therefore, in these diseases the ESR is increased. ESR is considered an "acute-phase" or a "reactant" protein (i.e., it occurs as a reaction to acute illnesses as described previously).

The test can be used to detect occult disease. Many physicians use the ESR test in this way for routine patient evaluation for vague symptoms. Other physicians regard this test as so nonspecific that it is useless as a routine study. The ESR test occasionally can be helpful in differentiating disease entities or complaints. For example, in the patient with chest pain, the ESR will be increased with myocardial infarction but will be normal with angina.

The ESR is a fairly reliable indicator of the course of disease and can be used to monitor disease therapy, especially for inflammatory autoimmune diseases such as temporal arteritis or polymyalgia rheumatica. In general, as the disease worsens, the ESR increases; as the disease improves, the ESR decreases. If the results of the ESR are equivocal or inconsistent with clinical impressions, the C-reactive protein test (see p. 319) is often performed.

Interfering factors

- Artificially low results can occur when the collected specimen is allowed to stand longer than 3 hours before the testing.
- Pregnancy (second and third trimesters) can cause elevated levels.
- Menstruation can cause elevated levels.
- Polycythemia is associated with decreased ESR.
- ✶ Drugs that may cause *increased* ESR levels include dextran, methyldopa (Aldomet), oral contraceptives, penicillamine, procainamide, theophylline, and vitamin A.
- ✶ Drugs that may cause *decreased* levels include aspirin, cortisone, and quinine.

Procedure and patient care

Before
PT Explain the procedure to the patient.
- Hold medications that may affect test results if indicated.

During
- Collect approximately 5 to 10 ml of venous blood in a lavender-top tube.

After
- Apply pressure to the venipuncture site.
- Transport the specimen immediately to the laboratory.

Abnormal findings

▲ **Increased levels**

Chronic renal failure
Malignant diseases
Bacterial infection
Inflammatory diseases
Necrotic tissue diseases
Hyperfibrinogenemia
Macroglobulinemia
Severe anemias such as
    iron deficiency or B_{12}
    deficiency

▼ **Decreased levels**

Sickle cell anemia
Spherocytosis
Hypofibrinogenemia
Polycythemia vera

notes

erythropoietin (EPO)

Type of test Blood

Normal findings 5-35 international units/L

Test explanation and related physiology

Erythropoietin is a hormone produced by the kidney. In response to decreased oxygen, the production of EPO is increased. EPO stimulates the bone marrow to increase RBC production. This improves oxygenation in the kidney, and the stimulus for EPO is reduced. This feedback mechanism is very sensitive to minimal persistent changes in oxygen levels. In patients with normal renal function, EPO levels are inversely proportional to the hemoglobin concentration.

As a hormone, EPO is often administered to patients who experience anemia as a result of chemotherapy. Occasionally athletes, in order to improve oxygen carrying capacity and thereby improve performance, abuse this hormone.

EPO testing is performed to assist in the differential diagnosis of patients with anemia or polycythemia. EPO is elevated in patients who have low hemoglobin due to failure of marrow production or with increased RBC destruction (iron-deficiency or hemolytic anemia, respectively). However, patients with anemia due to renal diseases (or bilateral nephrectomy) do not have elevated EPO levels. The renal cells are damaged by disease. EPO levels fall and these patients develop anemia.

Patients who have polycythemia as an appropriate response to chronic hypoxemia have elevated EPO levels. Yet patients who have malignant marrow causes of polycythemia vera have reduced EPO levels. Some renal cell or adrenal carcinomas can produce elevated EPO levels.

Interfering factors

- Pregnancy is associated with elevated EPO levels.
- The use of transfused blood decreases EPO levels.
- ✘ Drugs that may *increase* EPO levels include steroids, birth control pills, and ACTH.

Procedure and patient care

Before

PT Explain the procedure to the patient.

During

- Collect 5 to 7 ml of blood in a red-top or gel separator tube.
- Indicate on the laboratory slip any drugs that may affect test results.

After

- Apply pressure or a pressure dressing to the venipuncture site.
- Observe the venipuncture site for bleeding.

Abnormal findings

▲   **Increased levels**

    Iron-deficiency anemia
    Megaloblastic anemia
    Hemolytic anemia
    Myelodysplasia
    Chemotherapy
    AIDS
    Pheochromocytoma
    Renal cell carcinoma
    Adrenal carcinoma

▼   **Decreased levels**

    Polycythemia vera
    Renal diseases

notes

esophageal function studies (Esophageal manometry, Esophageal motility studies)

Type of test Manometric

Normal findings

Lower esophageal sphincter pressure: 10-20 mm Hg
Swallowing pattern: normal peristaltic waves
Acid reflux: negative
Acid clearing: <10 swallows
Bernstein test: negative

Test explanation and related physiology

Esophageal function studies include the following:

1. Determination of the *lower esophageal sphincter (LES)* pressure (manometry).
2. Graphic recording of esophageal swallowing waves, or *swallowing pattern* (manometry).
3. Detection of reflux of gastric acid back into the esophagus (acid reflux).
4. Detection of the ability of the esophagus to clear acid (acid clearing).
5. An attempt to reproduce symptoms of heartburn (Bernstein test).

Manometry studies

Two manometry studies are used in assessing esophageal function: (1) measurement of LES pressure, and (2) graphic recording of swallowing waves (motility). The LES is a sphincter muscle that acts as a valve to prevent reflux of gastric acid into the esophagus. Free reflux of gastric acid occurs when sphincter pressures are low. An example of such a disorder in adults is gastroesophageal reflux; in children it is called chalasia (incompetent or relaxed LES).

With increased sphincter pressure, as found in patients with achalasia (failure of the LES to relax normally with swallowing) and diffuse esophageal spasms, food cannot pass from the esophagus into the stomach. Increased LES pressures are noted on manometry. In achalasia, few if any swallowing waves are detected. In contrast, diffuse esophageal spasm is characterized by strong, frequent, asynchronous, and nonpropulsive waves.

Acid reflux with pH probe

Acid reflux is the primary component of gastroesophageal reflux. Patients with an incompetent LES will regurgitate gastric acid into the esophagus. This will then cause a drop in pH testing done by the pH probe. With the newer and smaller catheters, 24-hour pH monitoring can be performed. Episodes of acid reflux are evident. If they coincide with patient symptoms of chest pain, esophagitis can be incriminated.

Acid clearing

Patients with normal esophageal function can completely clear hydrochloric acid from the esophagus in less than 10 swallows. Patients with decreased esophageal motility (frequently caused by severe esophagitis) require a greater number of swallows to clear the acid.

Bernstein test (acid perfusion)

The Bernstein test is simply an attempt to reproduce the symptoms of gastroesophageal reflux. If the patient suffers pain with the instillation of hydrochloric acid into the esophagus, the test is positive and proves that the patient's symptoms are caused by reflux esophagitis. If the patient has no discomfort, a cause other than esophageal reflux must be sought to explain the patient's symptoms.

Contraindications

- Patients who cannot cooperate
- Patients who are medically unstable

Potential complications

- Aspiration of gastric contents

Interfering factors

- Eating shortly before the test may affect results.
- Drugs such as sedatives can alter test results.

Procedure and patient care

Before

- **PT** Explain the procedure to the patient.
- **PT** Instruct the patient not to eat or drink anything for at least 8 hours before the test.
- **PT** Allay any fears and allow the patient to verbalize concerns. Be sensitive to the patient's fears about choking during the procedure.

During

- Note the following procedural steps:
  1. Esophageal studies are usually performed in the endoscopy laboratory.
  2. The fasting, unsedated patient is asked to swallow two or three very tiny tubes. The tubes are equipped so that pressure measurements can be taken at 5-cm intervals (Figure 19).
  3. The outer ends of the tubes are attached to a pressure transducer.
  4. All tubes are passed into the stomach; then three tubes are slowly pulled back into the esophagus. A rapid and extreme increase in the pressure readings indicates the high-pressure zone of the LES.
  5. The LES pressure is recorded.

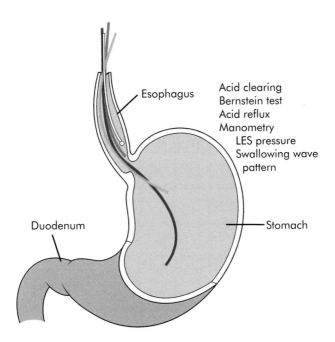

Figure 19 Esophageal function studies demonstrating placement of manometry tubes and a pH probe within the esophagus. *LES*, lower esophageal sphincter.

6. With all tubes in the esophagus, the patient is asked to swallow. Motility wave patterns are recorded.

7. The pH indicator probe is placed in the esophagus.

8. The patient's stomach is filled with approximately 100 ml of 0.1-N hydrochloric acid. A decrease in the pH of the esophageal pH probe indicates gastro-esophageal reflux.

9. Hydrochloric acid is instilled into the esophagus, and the patient is asked to swallow. The number of swallows is counted to determine acid clearing. More than 10 swallows to clear the acid (as determined by the pH probe) indicates decreased esophageal motility.

10. Finally, 0.1-N hydrochloric acid and saline solution are alternately instilled into the esophagus for the Bernstein test. The patient is not told which solution is being infused. If the patient volunteers symptoms of discomfort while the acid is running, the test is considered positive. If no discomfort is recognized, the test is negative.

- Note that these tests are performed by an esophageal technician in approximately 30 minutes.

PT Inform the patient that the test results are interpreted by a physician and will be available in a few hours.

PT Tell the patient that, except for some initial gagging when swallowing the tubes, these tests are not uncomfortable.

After

PT Inform the patient that it is not unusual to have a mild sore throat after placement of the tubes.

Abnormal findings

Presbyesophagus
Diffuse esophageal spasm
Chalasia
Achalasia
Gastroesophageal reflux
Reflux esophagitis

notes

esophagogastroduodenoscopy (EGD, Upper gastrointestinal [UGI] endoscopy, Gastroscopy)

Type of test   Endoscopy

Normal findings   Normal esophagus, stomach, and duodenum

Test explanation and related physiology

Endoscopy enables direct visualization of the upper gastrointestinal (GI) tract by means of a long, flexible, fiberoptic-lighted scope. The esophagus, stomach, and duodenum are examined for tumors, varices, mucosal inflammations, hiatal hernias, polyps, ulcers, and obstructions. The endoscope has one to three channels. The first channel is used for viewing, the second for insufflation of air and aspiration of fluid, and the third for passing cable-activated instruments to perform a biopsy of suspected pathologic tissue. Probes also can be passed through the third channel to allow for coagulation or injection of sclerosing agents to areas of active GI bleeding. A laser beam can pass through the endoscope to perform endoscopic surgery (e.g., obliteration of tumors or polyps, control of bleeding), and the fiberoptics of endoscopy are so refined that video images and "still pictures" can be taken.

This test is used to visualize the lumen of the esophagus, stomach, and duodenum. It is used to evaluate patients with dysphagia, weight loss, early satiety, upper abdominal pain, "ulcer symptoms," or dyspepsia. It is also used to detect esophageal varices in alcoholics. Suspicious barium swallow or upper GI x-ray findings can be corroborated by EGD.

With endoscopy, one can also visualize and perform a biopsy of tissue in the upper small intestinal tract, using an extralong fiberoptic endoscope. This procedure is referred to as *enteroscopy*. Abnormalities of the small intestine such as arteriovenous (AV) malformations, tumors, enteropathies (e.g., celiac disease), and ulcerations can be diagnosed with enteroscopy.

Besides being much more sensitive and specific than an upper GI series in diagnosing diseases of the esophagus, stomach, and duodenum, EGD also can be used therapeutically. An experienced endoscopist often can control active GI bleeding by electrocoagulation, laser coagulation, or the injection of sclerosing agents such as alcohol. Also, with the endoscope, benign and malignant strictures can be dilated to reestablish patency of the upper GI tract. Biliary stents and a percutaneous gastrostomy can be placed with the use of EGD. The role of endoscopic surgery is expanding in light of its dramatic success and minimal morbidity.

Contraindications

- Patients with severe upper GI bleeding
  The viewing lens will become covered with blood clots, preventing adequate visualization. If the stomach can be lavaged and aspirated to clear the blood clots, however, EGD can be performed.
- Patients with esophageal diverticula
  The scope can easily fall into the diverticulum and perforate the wall of the esophagus.
- Patients with suspected perforation
  The perforation can be worsened by the insufflation of pressurized air into the GI tract.
- Patients who have had recent GI surgery
  The anastomosis may not be able to withstand the pressure of the required air insufflation. This may lead to anastomotic disruption.

Potential complications

- Perforation of the esophagus, stomach, and duodenum
- Bleeding from a biopsy site
- Pulmonary aspiration of gastric contents
- Oversedation from the medication administered during the test
- Hypotension induced by the sedative medication
  Usually, however, the patient already has some significant element of hypovolemia or dehydration.
- Local IV phlebitic reaction to the injection of sclerosing sedative medication

Interfering factors

- Food in the stomach
- Excessive GI bleeding

Procedure and patient care

Before

PT Explain the procedure to the patient.
- Obtain informed consent if required by the institution.

PT Instruct the patient to abstain from eating as of midnight the day of the test.

PT Reassure the patient that this test is not painful. Tell the patient that the throat will be anesthetized with a spray to depress the gag reflex.

■ Encourage the patient to verbalize fears. Provide support.

■ Remove the patient's dentures and eyewear before testing.

PT Remind the patient that he or she will not be able to speak during the test but that respiration will not be affected.

PT Instruct the patient not to bite down on the endoscope.

PT Instruct the patient as to appropriate oral hygiene, because the tube will be passed through the mouth.

During

■ Note the following procedural steps:
1. The patient is placed on the endoscopy table in the left lateral decubitus position.
2. The throat is topically anesthetized with viscous lidocaine (Xylocaine) or another anesthetic spray. This is to decrease the gag reflex caused by passage of the endoscope.
3. The patient is usually sedated. This minimizes anxiety and allows the patient to experience a "light" sleep.
4. The endoscope is gently passed through the mouth and finally into the esophagus; once in the esophagus, visualization can be performed.
5. Air is insufflated to distend the upper GI tract for adequate visualization.
6. The esophagus, stomach, and duodenum are evaluated.
7. During *enteroscopy* the upper small bowel is visualized, and a biopsy is performed if needed.
8. Biopsy or any endoscopic surgery is performed with direct visualization.
9. On completion of direct inspection and surgery, the excess air and GI secretions are aspirated through the scope.

■ Note that the test is performed in the endoscopy laboratory by a physician trained in GI endoscopy and takes approximately 20 to 30 minutes.

PT Tell the patient that the test is mildly uncomfortable.

After

PT Inform the patient that he or she may have hoarseness or a sore throat after the test.

■ Withhold any fluids until the patient is completely alert and the swallowing reflex returns to normal, usually 2 to 4 hours.

- Observe the patient's vital signs. Evaluate the patient for bleeding, fever, abdominal pain, dyspnea, or dysphagia.
- Observe safety precautions until the effects of the sedatives have worn off.

🏠 Home care responsibilities

- A sore throat is expected after EGD. A soothing mouthwash may help.
- Notify the doctor immediately if bleeding, fever, abdominal pain, dyspnea, or dysphagia occurs.
- Inform the patient that it is normal to have some bloating, belching, and flatulence after the procedure.
- Inform the patient that the sedation may cause some retrograde and antegrade amnesia for a few hours.

Abnormal findings

Tumor (benign or malignant) of the esophagus, stomach, or duodenum
Esophageal diverticula
Hiatal hernia
Esophagitis, gastritis, duodenitis
Gastroesophageal varices
Peptic ulcer
Peptic stricture and subsequent scarring
Extrinsic compression by a cyst or tumor outside the upper GI tract
Source of upper GI bleeding
Helicobacter pylori infection

notes

estrogen fractions (Estriol excretion)

Type of test Urine (24-hour); blood
Normal findings

	Serum	*Urine mcg/24 hours*
Estradiol		
Child <10 years old	<15 pg/ml	0-6
Adult male	10-50 pg/ml	0-6
Adult female		
Follicular phase	20-350 pg/ml	0-13
Midcycle peak	150-750 pg/ml	4-14
Luteal phase	30-450 pg/ml	4-10
Postmenopause	≤20 pg/ml	0-4
Estriol		
Male or child		
<10 years old	N/A	1-11
Female, adult		
Follicular phase	N/A	0-14
Ovulatory phase	N/A	13-54
Luteal phase	N/A	8-60
Postmenopausal	N/A	0-11
Female, pregnant		
1st trimester	<38 ng/ml	0-800
2nd trimester	38-140 ng/ml	800-12,000
3rd trimester	31-460 ng/ml	5000-12,000
Total estrogen		
Male or child		
<10 years old	N/A	4-25
Female, nonpregnant	N/A	4-60
Female, pregnant		
1st trimester	N/A	0-800
2nd trimester	N/A	800-5000
3rd trimester	N/A	5000-50,000

Possible critical values Values 40% below the average of two previous values demand immediate evaluation of fetal well-being.

Test explanation and related physiology

There are three major estrogens. E_2 (estradiol), the most potent estrogen, is produced predominantly in the ovary. In females, there is a feedback mechanism for the secretion of E_2. Low levels of E_2 stimulate the hypothalamus to produce gonadotropin-releasing factors. These hormone factors stimulate the pituitary to produce follicle-stimulating hormone (FSH) and luteinizing hormone (LH). LH and FSH stimulate the ovary to produce E_2, which peaks during the ovulatory phase of the menstrual cycle. This hormone is measured most often to evaluate menstrual and fertility problems, menopausal status, sexual maturity, gynecomastia, and feminization syndromes, or as a tumor marker for patients with certain ovarian tumors.

E_1 (estrone) is also secreted by the ovary, but most is converted from androstenedione in peripheral tissues. Estrone is a more potent estrogen than estriol but is less potent than estradiol. Estrone is the major circulating estrogen after menopause.

E_3 (estriol) is the major estrogen in the pregnant female. Serial urine and blood studies for estriol excretion provide an objective means of assessing placental function and fetal normality in high-risk pregnancies. Excretion of estriol increases around the eighth week of gestation and continues to rise until shortly before delivery. Estriol is produced in the placenta from estrogen precursors, which are made by the fetal adrenal gland and liver. The measurement of excreted estriol is an important index of fetal well-being. Rising values indicate an adequately functioning fetoplacental unit. Decreasing values suggest fetoplacental deterioration (failing pregnancy, dysmaturity, preeclampsia/eclampsia, complicated diabetes mellitus, anencephaly, fetal death) and require prompt reassessment of the pregnancy. If the estriol levels fall, early delivery of the fetus may be indicated.

Serial studies usually begin at approximately 28 to 30 weeks of gestation and are then repeated weekly. The frequency of these estriol determinations can be increased as needed to evaluate a high-risk pregnancy. Collection may be done daily. Although the first collection is the baseline value, all collection results are compared with previous ones, because decreasing values suggest fetal deterioration. Some physicians suggest using an average of three previous values as a control value.

Estriol excretion studies can be done using 24-hour urine tests or blood studies. A serially increasing estriol/creatinine ratio is a favorable sign in pregnancy. Plasma estriol determinations also can be used to evaluate the fetoplacental unit. The blood estriol is an accurate reflection of the current status of the placenta and fetus. The advantage of the plasma estriol determination is that it is more easily obtained than a 24-hour urine specimen and less affected by medications.

Unfortunately, only severe placental distress will decrease urinary estriol sufficiently to reliably predict fetoplacental stress. Furthermore, plasma and urinary estriol levels are normally associated with significant daily variation, which may confuse serial results. Maternal illnesses such as hypertension, preeclampsia, anemia, and impaired renal function can also factitiously decrease urinary estriol levels. Because these problems create a high number of false-positive and false-negative findings, most clinicians now use nonstress fetal monitoring (see p. 446) to indicate fetal-placental health.

Interfering factors

- Recent administration of radioisotopes may alter test results.
- Glycosuria and urinary tract infections can increase urine estriol levels.
- Drugs that may *increase* levels include adrenocorticosteroids, ampicillin, estrogen-containing drugs, phenothiazines, and tetracyclines.
- Drugs that may *decrease* levels include clomiphene.

Procedure and patient care

Before

PT Explain the procedure to the patient.
- If the patient is going to collect the 24-hour urine specimen at home, give her the collection bottle (with a preservative) and instruct her to keep the urine refrigerated.
PT Tell the patient that no food or fluid restrictions are needed.

During

Blood

- Collect approximately 5 ml of venous blood in a red-top tube.

24-hour urine

PT Instruct the patient to begin the 24-hour urine collection after voiding. Discard the initial specimen and start the 24-hour timing at that point.
PT Collect all urine passed during the next 24 hours. Make sure the patient knows where to store the urine container.

- Keep the specimen on ice or refrigerated during the 24-hour collection period.
- Indicate the starting time on the urine container and laboratory slip.
- Post the hours for the urine collection in a prominent place to prevent accidental discarding of the specimen.
- **PT** Instruct the patient to void before defecating so that the urine is not contaminated by feces.
- **PT** Remind the patient not to put toilet paper in the collection container.
- **PT** Encourage the patient to drink fluids during the 24 hours.
- **PT** Tell the patient to collect the last specimen as close as possible to the end of the 24-hour period. Add this urine to the collection.
- List any drugs that may affect test results on the laboratory slip.

After

- Apply pressure to the venipuncture site.
- Transport the 24-hour urine specimen promptly to the laboratory.
- **PT** Inform the patient how and when to obtain the results of this study.

Abnormal findings

▲ **Increased levels**

Feminization syndromes
Precocious puberty
Ovarian tumor
Testicular tumor
Adrenal tumor
Normal pregnancy
Hepatic cirrhosis
Necrosis of the liver
Hyperthyroidism

▼ **Decreased levels**

Failing pregnancy
Turner's syndrome
Hypopituitarism
Primary and secondary
  hypogonadism
Stein-Leventhal
  syndrome
Menopause
Anorexia nervosa

notes

estrogen receptor assay (ER assay, ERA, Estradiol receptor)

Type of test Microscopic examination

Normal findings

Negative: <5% of the cells stain for receptors
Positive: >5% of the cells stain for receptors

Test explanation and related physiology

The ER assay is useful in determining the prognosis and treatment of breast cancer. The assay is used to determine whether a tumor is likely to respond to endocrine therapy. Tumors with a positive ER assay are more than twice as likely to respond to endocrine therapy than ER-negative tumors. Hormone receptor assay should be performed on all primary breast cancers. Where possible, the test should be performed on metastatic breast cancers. Breast tumors in postmenopausal women tend to be positive more often than in premenopausal women. In general, ER-positive tumors have a better prognosis than ER-negative tumors. ER status is now being evaluated on other gynecologic tumors, but its exact role in these patients has yet to be defined.

Slightly more than 50% of patients with breast carcinoma who are ER positive respond to endocrine therapy (e.g., tamoxifen, estrogens, androgens, oophorectomy, adrenalectomy). The response is greater when the progesterone receptors (see p. 748) are also positive. Patients whose breast cancers lack these hormone receptors (i.e., are ER negative) have a much lower chance of tumor response to hormone therapy and may not be candidates for this form of treatment.

Specimens are obtained from surgical specimens by a pathologist. ER assays are performed by immunohistochemical methods on fixed, paraffin-embedded tissue. Positive reactivity by immunohistochemistry is observed in the nuclei of the tumor cells. Routinely positive and negative controls are performed with the specimen testing in order to avoid false-positive and false-negative results. This method of measuring ER receptors is considered very accurate. The testing is usually performed in a reference laboratory. Only a small portion of the paraffin-embedded tissue is required for testing. Results are usually available in about 1 week. Only cancerous tissue is evaluated for ER receptors. Normal tissue usually contains ER receptors.

Interfering factors

- Delay in tissue fixation may cause deterioration of receptor proteins and produce lower values.
- Hormones should be discontinued before breast biopsy is performed. Antiestrogen preparations (e.g., tamoxifen [Nolvadex]) during the past 2 months may cause false-negative ER assays.
- Exogenous hormones that are taken for contraceptive purposes or menopausal estrogens may produce lower receptor values.

Procedure and patient care

Before

- **PT** Explain the procedure to the patient.
- **PT** Instruct the patient to discontinue hormones before breast biopsy is performed.
- Before biopsy, a gynecologic history is obtained, including menopausal status and exogenous hormone use.

During

- The surgeon obtains tumor tissue.
- This tissue should be placed on ice or in formalin.
- Part of the tissue is used for routine histology. A portion of the paraffin block is sent to a reference laboratory.

After

- Results are usually available in 1 week.

Abnormal findings

Nonapplicable

notes

ethanol (Ethyl alcohol, Blood alcohol, Blood EtOH)

Type of test Blood; urine; gastric; breath

Normal findings None

Possible critical values >300 mg/dl or >65 mmol/L (SI units)

Test explanation and related physiology

Ethanol depresses the central nervous system and may lead to coma and death. This test is usually performed to evaluate alcohol-impaired driving or overdose. Proper collection, handling, and storage of blood alcohol are important for medicolegal cases involving sobriety. The blood test is the specimen of choice. Blood is taken from a peripheral vein in living patients and from the aorta in cadavers. Ethanol can also be detected in the urine, in gastric contents, and by breath analyzer. Conversion tables are available to calculate blood levels based on alcohol levels identified in the various nonblood specimens.

Blood alcohol levels greater than 80 mg/dl (>17 mmol/L, SI units) may cause flushing, slowing of reflexes, and impaired visual activity. Most courts do not consider this level definite proof of intoxication. Persons with alcohol levels less than 0.05% weight/volume are not considered under the influence of alcohol. Levels greater than 0.10% are considered in most states to be illegal and definite evidence of intoxication. Depression of the CNS occurs with levels over 100 mg/dl, and fatalities are reported with levels greater than 400 mg/dl. Levels of blood alcohol greater than 100 mg/dl can cause hypotension, although this is rare. This is especially important to recognize in the trauma patient in shock.

Interfering factors

- Elevated blood ketones (as with diabetic ketoacidosis) can cause false elevation of blood and breath test results.

Procedure and patient care

Before

PT Explain the procedure to the patient.

- Follow the institution's protocol if the specimen will be used for legal purposes.

During

- Use a povidone-iodine wipe instead of an alcohol wipe for cleansing the venipuncture site.
- Collect a venous blood sample in a gray- or red-top tube according to the agency's protocol.
- If a gastric or urine specimen is indicated, approximately 20 to 50 ml of fluid is necessary.
- Breath analyzers are taken at the end of expiration after a deep inspiration.

After

- Apply pressure to the venipuncture site.
- Follow the agency's protocol regarding specimen collection.
- The exact time of specimen collection should be indicated. Also, in some instances signatures of the collector and a witness may be needed for legal evidence.

Abnormal findings

Alcohol intoxication or overdose

notes

euglobulin lysis time (Euglobulin clot lysis, Fibrinolysis/euglobulin lysis)

Type of test   Blood

Normal findings   >2 hours

Possible critical values   <1 hour, indicating excessive fibrinolytic activity (danger of bleeding)

Test explanation and related physiology

The euglobulin lysis test is used to identify systemic fibrinolysis. Fibrinolysis is an important part of normal hemostasis. Clots are constantly being made and dissolved. The fibrinolytic system is responsible for clot dissolution. When this system is abnormally activated by drugs or protein fibrinolysins, a fibrin clot that had been formed will be dissolved immediately, resulting in a bleeding tendency. Primary fibrinolysins are abnormal proteins that are associated with disease such as malignancy, shock, or sepsis. Secondary fibrinolysins, on the other hand, are a normal part of hemostasis and clot dissolution. However, they can be abnormally activated during disseminated intravascular coagulation. Plasmin is the main secondary fibrinolysin normally active in clot dissolution (see Figure 11, p. 282). Drugs such as streptokinase and urokinase, used in therapeutic clot lysis (thrombolytic therapy of coronary, cerebral, and other organ arterial/venous blood clots), are also considered secondary fibrinolysins. Euglobulin lysis time can detect either primary or secondary fibrinolysis.

Euglobulin lysis time is performed by adding the patient's plasma to a blood clot of a normal person. The clot is observed for up to 24 hours. The time measured from clot formation to clot lysis is referred to as the *euglobulin lysis time*. The occurrence of clot lysis before 1 hour is considered abnormal. This test also may be used to monitor streptokinase, urokinase, and tissue plasminogen activator (tPA) therapy in patients with acute myocardial infarction.

Interfering factors

- Vigorous exercise, increasing age, and hyperventilation may cause increased fibrinolysis.
- Postmenopausal women and normal newborns may have decreased fibrinolysis.

- Decreased fibrinogen levels may result in a falsely shortened lysis time because of the reduced amount of fibrin to be lysed.
- Patients who are obese may have decreased fibrinolysis.
- Drugs that may cause *increased* fibrinolysis include steroids and adrenocorticotropic hormone.

Procedure and patient care

Before

PT Explain the procedure to the patient.

PT Instruct the patient not to exercise before the blood sample is collected.

PT Tell the patient that no fasting is required.

During

- Collect approximately 5 ml of blood in a blue-top tube.
- Avoid excessive agitation of the blood sample.
- Deliver the blood specimen to the laboratory immediately on ice.

After

- Apply pressure to the venipuncture site.

Abnormal findings

▲ **Increased fibrinolysis (shortened euglobulin lysis time)**

Incompatible blood transfusion

Cirrhosis

Obstetric complications (e.g., antepartum hemorrhage, septic abortion, hydatidiform mole, amniotic embolism)

Malignancies (e.g., leukemia, cancer of the prostate or pancreas)

Shock (hemorrhagic or septic)

Streptokinase or urokinase administration for thrombolytic therapy

Extensive vascular trauma or surgery

Disseminated intravascular coagulation

▼ **Decreased fibrinolysis (increased lysis time)**

Prematurity

Diabetes

evoked potential studies (EP studies, Evoked brain
potentials, Evoked responses, Visual-evoked potentials,
Auditory brain stem–evoked potentials, Somatosensory-evoked
responses)

Type of test Electrodiagnostic

Normal findings No neural conduction delay

Test explanation and related physiology

EP studies are indicated for patients who are suspected of having a sensory deficit but are unable to or cannot reliably indicate recognition of a stimulus. These may include infants, comatose patients, or patients with inability to communicate. These tests are also used to evaluate specific areas of the cortex that receive incoming stimulus from the eyes, ears, and lower/upper extremity sensory nerves. They are used to monitor natural progression or treatment of deteriorating neurologic diseases. Finally, they also are used to identify histrionic or malingering patients who have sensory deficit complaints.

EP studies focus on changes and responses in brain waves that are evoked from stimulation of a sensory pathway. The study of EPs grew out of early work with the electroencephalogram (EEG) (see p. 373). The EEG measures "spontaneous" brain electrical activity, whereas the sensory EP study measures minute voltage changes produced in response to a specific stimulus such as a light pattern, a click, or a shock. In contrast to the EEG, which records signals that reach amplitudes of up to 50 to 100 millivolts (mV), EP signals are usually less than 5 mV. Because of this, they can be detected only with an averaging computer. The computer averages out (or cancels) unwanted random waves to sum the evoked response that occurs at a specific time after a given stimulus.

Evoked potential studies allow one to measure and assess the entire sensory pathway from the peripheral sensory organ all the way to the brain cortex (recognition of the stimulus). These tests are also used to monitor progressive neurologic diseases (e.g., multiple sclerosis).

Clinical abnormalities are usually detected by an increase in *latency*, which refers to the delay between the stimulus and the wave response. Normal latency times are calculated depending on body size, position of the body where the stimulus is applied, conduction velocity of axons in the neural pathways, number of synapses in the system, location of nerve generators of EP components (brain stem or cortex), and presence of central nervous system pathology. Conduction delays indicate damage or disease anywhere along the neural pathway from the sensory organ to the cortex. Sensory stimuli used for the EP study can be visual, auditory, or somatosensory. The sensory stimulus chosen depends on which sensory system is suspected to be pathologic (e.g., questionable blindness, deafness, or numbness). Also, the sensory stimulus chosen may depend on the area of brain where pathology is suspected (auditory stimuli check the brain stem and temporal lobes of the brain; visual stimuli test the optic nerve, central neural visual pathway, and occipital parts of the brain; and somatosensory stimuli check the peripheral nerves, spinal cord, and parietal lobe of the brain). Increased latency (i.e., abnormally prolonged time span from the time of stimulus to the time of brain EEG recognition) indicates pathology of the sensory organ or the specific neural pathway as described earlier.

Visual-evoked responses (VERs) are usually stimulated by a strobe light flash, reversible checkerboard pattern, or retinal stimuli. Ninety percent of patients with multiple sclerosis show abnormal latencies of VERs, a phenomenon attributed to demyelination of nerve fibers. In addition, patients with other neurologic disorders (e.g., Parkinson's disease) show an abnormal latency of VERs. The degree of latency seems to correlate with the severity of the disease. Abnormal results also may be seen in patients with lesions of the optic nerve, optic tract, visual center, and the eye itself. Absence of binocularity, which is a neurologic developmental disorder in infants, can be detected and evaluated by VERs. Eyesight problems or blindness can be detected in infants through VERs or *electroretinography*. This test can also be used during eye surgery to provide a warning of possible damage to the optic nerve. The gross visual acuity of infants can even be checked via VERs.

Auditory brain stem–evoked potentials (ABEPs) are usually stimulated by clicking sounds to evaluate the central auditory pathways of the brain stem. Either ear can be evoked to detect lesions in the brain stem that involve the auditory pathway without affecting hearing. One of the most successful applications of ABEPs has been screening low–birth-weight newborns and other infants for hearing disorders. Recognition of deafness enables infants to be fitted with corrective devices as soon as possible before learning to speak (to prevent speech pathology).

ABEPs also have great therapeutic implications in the early detection of posterior fossa brain tumors.

Somatosensory-evoked responses (SERs) are usually stimulated by sensory stimulus to an area of the body. The time is then measured for the current of the stimulus to travel along the nerve to the cortex of the brain. SERs are used to evaluate patients with spinal cord injuries and to monitor spinal cord functioning during spinal surgery. They are also used to monitor treatment of diseases (e.g., multiple sclerosis), to evaluate the location and extent of areas of brain dysfunction after head injury, and to pinpoint tumors at an early stage. These tests can also be used to identify malingering or hysterical numbness, for example, that latency is normal in these patients, despite the fact that patients indicate numbness.

One of the main benefits of EPs is their objectivity, because voluntary patient response is not needed. This objectivity makes EPs useful with nonverbal and uncooperative patients. It permits the distinction of organic from psychogenic problems. This is invaluable in settling lawsuits concerning worker's compensation insurance.

Procedure and patient care

Before
PT Explain the procedure to the patient.
PT Instruct the patient to shampoo his or her hair before the test.
PT Tell the patient that no fasting or sedation is required.

During
- Note that the position of the electrode depends on the type of EP study to be done:
  1. *VERs* are measured using electrodes placed on the scalp along the vertex and the cortex lobes. Stimulation occurs by using a strobe light, checkerboard pattern, or retinal stimuli.
  2. *ABEPs* are stimulated with clicking noises or tone bursts delivered via earphones. The responses are detected by scalp electrodes placed along the vertex and on each earlobe.
  3. *SERs* are stimulated using electrical stimuli applied to nerves at the wrist (medial nerve) or knee (peroneal nerve). The response is detected by electrodes placed over the sensory cortex of the opposite hemisphere on the scalp.

- Note that this study is performed by a physician in less than 30 minutes.
- **PT** Tell the patient that little discomfort is associated with this study.

After

- Remove the gel used for the adherence of the electrodes.

Abnormal findings

E

Prolonged latency for ABEP

Demyelinating diseases (e.g., multiple sclerosis)
Tumor—acoustic neuroma
Cerebrovascular accident (stroke)
Auditory nerve damage
Deafness

Abnormal latency for SER

Spinal cord injury
Cervical disk disease
Spinal cord demyelinating diseases
Peripheral nerve injury, transection, or disease
Parietal cortical tumor or CVA

Prolonged latency for VER

Parkinson's disease
Demyelinating diseases (e.g., multiple sclerosis)
Optic nerve damage
Ocular disease or injury
Blindness
Optic tract disease
Occipital lobe tumor or CVA
Absence of binocularity
Visual field defects

notes

fecal fat (Fat absorption, Quantitative stool fat determination)

Type of test Stool

Normal findings

Fat: 2-6 g/24 hr or 7-21 mmol/day (SI units)
Retention coefficient: ≥95%

Test explanation and related physiology

This test is performed to confirm the diagnosis of steatorrhea. Steatorrhea occurs when fat content in the stool is high. It is suspected when the patient has large, greasy, and foul-smelling stools. Determining an abnormally high fecal fat content confirms the diagnosis. Short-gut syndrome and any condition that may cause malabsorption (e.g., spruc, Crohn's disease, Whipple's disease) or maldigestion (e.g., bile duct obstruction, pancreatic duct obstruction secondary to tumor or gallstones) are also associated with increased fecal fat. Children with cystic fibrosis may have steatorrhea. Mucous plugs obstruct their pancreatic ducts; thus the pancreatic enzymes (amylase, lipase, trypsin, and chymotrypsin) cannot be mixed with food to assist with fat digestion.

The fecal fat test measures fat content in the stool. The total output of fecal fat per 24 hours in a 3-day stool collection provides the most reliable measurement.

Interfering factors

- Drugs that may alter test results include enemas and laxatives, especially mineral oil.
- Drugs that may *decrease* levels of fecal fat include Metamucil and barium.

Procedure and patient care

Before

PT Explain the procedure to the patient.
PT Give the patient instructions regarding the appropriate diet (a diet diary may be requested by the laboratory):
  1. For adults, usually 100 g of fat per day is suggested for 3 days before and throughout the collection period.

2. Children, and especially infants, cannot ingest 100 g of
    fat. Therefore a *fat retention coefficient* is determined by
    measuring the difference between ingested fat and fecal
    fat and then expressing that difference (the amount of fat
    retained) as a percentage of the ingested fat:

$$\frac{\text{Ingested fat} - \text{Fecal fat}}{\text{Ingested fat}} \times 100\% = \text{Fat retention coefficient}$$

- Note that the fat retention coefficient in normal children
  and adults is 95% or greater. A low value indicates
  steatorrhea.
- **PT** Instruct the patient to defecate in a dry, clean container.
- Occasionally, a tongue blade is required to transfer the stool
  to the specimen container.
- **PT** Tell the patient not to urinate in the stool container.
- **PT** Inform the patient that even diarrheal stools should be
  collected.
- **PT** Instruct the patient that toilet paper should not be placed in
  the stool container.
- **PT** Tell the patient not to take any laxatives or enemas during
  this test because they will interfere with intestinal motility
  and alter test results.

During

- Collect each stool specimen and send immediately to the
  laboratory during the 24- to 72-hour testing period. Label
  each specimen and include the time and date of collection.
- If the specimen is collected at home, give the patient a large
  stool container to keep in the freezer.

After

- **PT** Inform the patient that a normal diet can be resumed.

Abnormal findings

▲   **Increased levels**

Cystic fibrosis

Malabsorption secondary to sprue, celiac disease, Whipple's
disease, Crohn's disease (regional enteritis), or radiation
enteritis

Maldigestion secondary to obstruction of the pancreaticobiliary tree (e.g., cancer, stricture, gallstones)

Short-gut syndrome secondary to surgical resection,
surgical bypass, or congenital anomaly

ferritin

Type of test Blood

Normal findings

Male: 12-300 ng/ml or 12-300 mcg/L (SI units)
Female: 10-150 ng/ml or 10-150 mcg/L (SI units)
Children
    Newborn: 25-200 ng/ml
    1 month: 200-600 ng/ml
    2-5 months: 50-200 ng/ml
    6 months-15 years: 7-142 ng/ml

Test explanation and related physiology

The serum ferritin study is a good indicator of available iron stores in the body. Ferritin, the major iron storage protein, is normally present in the serum in concentrations directly related to iron storage. In normal patients, 1 ng/ml of serum ferritin corresponds to approximately 8 mg of stored iron. Ferritin levels rise with age in males and postmenopausal females. In premenopausal females, levels stay about the same. Decreases in ferritin levels indicate a decrease in iron storage associated with iron deficiency anemia. A ferritin level less than 10 ng/100 ml is diagnostic of iron deficiency anemia. The decrease in serum ferritin level often precedes other signs of iron deficiency such as decreased iron levels or changes in red blood cell size, chromasia, and number. Only when protein depletion is severe can ferritin be decreased by malnutrition. Pregnancy is also associated with decreased ferritin levels. Increased levels are a sign of iron excess, as seen in hemochromatosis, hemosiderosis, iron poisoning, or recent blood transfusions. Increased ferritin is also noted in patients with megaloblastic anemia, hemolytic anemia, and chronic hepatitis. Further, ferritin is factitiously elevated in patients with chronic disease states such as neoplasm, alcoholism, uremia, collagen diseases, or chronic liver diseases. Ferritin is also used in patients with chronic renal failure to monitor iron stores.

A limitation of this study is that ferritin levels also can act as an "acute phase" reactant protein and may be elevated in conditions not reflecting iron stores (e.g., acute inflammatory diseases, infections, metastatic cancer, lymphomas). Elevations in ferritin occur 1 to 2 days after onset of the acute illness and peak at 3 to 5 days. If iron deficiency were to coexist in patients with these diseases, it may not be recognized because the levels of ferritin would be factitiously elevated by the concurring disease.

When combined with the serum iron level and total iron-binding capacity (TIBC, see p. 565), this test is useful in differentiating and classifying anemias. For example, in patients with iron deficiency anemia, the ferritin, iron, and transferrin saturation levels are low, whereas the TIBC and transferrin levels are high.

F

Interfering factors

- Recent transfusions and recent ingestion of a meal with high iron content may cause elevated ferritin levels.
- Recent administration of a radionuclide can cause abnormal levels if testing is performed by radioimmunoassay.
- Hemolytic diseases may be associated with an artificially high iron content.
- Disorders of excessive iron storage (e.g., hemochromatosis, hemosiderosis) are associated with high ferritin levels.
- Menstruating women may have decreased ferritin levels.
- Drugs that may *increase* ferritin levels include iron preparations.

Procedure and patient care

Before
- **PT** Explain the procedure to the patient.
- **PT** Tell the patient that no fasting is required.

During
- Collect approximately 5 to 7 ml of venous blood in a red-top tube.

After
- Apply pressure to the venipuncture site.

Abnormal findings

▲ **Increased levels**

Hemochromatosis

Hemosiderosis

Megaloblastic anemia

Hemolytic anemia

Alcoholic/inflammatory
  hepatocellular disease

Inflammatory disease

Advanced cancers

Chronic illnesses
  (e.g., leukemias, cirrhosis,
  chronic hepatitis)

Collagen vascular diseases

▼ **Decreased levels**

Severe protein deficiency

Iron deficiency anemia

Hemodialysis

notes

fetal biophysical profile (Biophysical profile [BPP])

Type of test Ultrasound; fetal activity study

Normal findings Score of 8-10 points (if amniotic fluid volume is adequate)

Possible critical values Less than 4 may necessitate immediate delivery.

F

Test explanation and related physiology

The BPP is a method of evaluating fetal status during the antepartal period based on five variables originating within the fetus: fetal heart rate, fetal breathing movement, gross fetal movements, fetal muscle tone, and amniotic fluid volume. Fetal heart rate reactivity is measured by the nonstress test (see p. 446), and the other four parameters are measured by ultrasound scanning.

The major premise behind the BPP is that variable assessments of fetal biophysical activity are more reliable than an examination of a single parameter (such as fetal heart rate). Indications for this test include factors such as postdate pregnancy, maternal hypertension, diabetes mellitus, vaginal bleeding, maternal Rh sensitization, maternal history of stillbirth, and premature rupture of membranes. The BPP is probably more useful in identifying a fetus in jeopardy than in predicting future fetal well-being.

The five parameters are briefly described here. Each parameter is scored and contributes either a 2 or a 0 to the score. Therefore, 10 is the perfect score, and 0 is the lowest score.

1. *Fetal heart rate reactivity*. This is measured and interpreted in the same way as the nonstress test (see p. 446). The fetal heart rate is considered reactive when there are movement-associated fetal heart rate accelerations of at least 15 beats/min above baseline, and 15 seconds in duration over a 20-minute period. A score of 2 is given for reactivity, and a score of 0 indicates that the fetal heart rate is nonreactive.

2. *Fetal breathing movements*. This parameter is assessed based on the assumption that fetal breathing movements indicate fetal well-being and their absence may indicate hypoxemia. Fetal breathing becomes increasingly regular

in frequency and uniformity after the 36th week of gestation. To earn a score of 2, the fetus must have at least one episode of fetal breathing lasting at least 60 seconds within a 30-minute observation. Absence of this breathing pattern is scored a 0 on the BPP. It is important to note that several factors can alter fetal breathing movements. For example, fetal breathing movements increase during the second and third hours after maternal meals and at night. Fetal breathing movements may decrease in conditions such as hypoxemia, hypoglycemia, nicotine use, and alcohol ingestion.

3. *Fetal body movements.* Fetal activity is a reflection of neurologic integrity and function. The presence of at least three discrete episodes of fetal movements within a 30-minute observation period is given a score of 2. A score of 0 is given with two or fewer fetal movements in this time period. It is important to note that fetal activity is greatest 1 to 3 hours after the mother has consumed a meal. For this reason, it is often suggested that this test be arranged in relation to mealtime.

4. *Fetal tone.* In the uterus the fetus is normally in a position of flexion. However, the fetus also stretches, rolls, and moves in the uterus. The arms, legs, trunk, and head may be flexed and extended. A score of 2 is earned when there is at least one episode of active extension with return to flexion. An example of this would be the opening and closing of a hand. A score of 0 is given for slow extension with a return to only partial flexion; fetal movement not followed by return to flexion; limbs or spine in extension; and an open fetal hand.

5. *Amniotic fluid volume.* Amniotic fluid volume has been demonstrated to be an effective method of predicting fetal distress. Oligohydramnios (too little amniotic fluid) has been associated with fetal anomalies, uterine growth retardation, and postterm pregnancy. A score of 2 is given for this parameter when there is at least one pocket of amniotic fluid that measures 1 cm in two perpendicular planes. A score of 0 indicates either that fluid is absent in most areas of the uterine cavity or that the largest pocket measures 1 cm or less in the vertical axis.

A score of 8 or 10 with a normal amount of amniotic fluid indicates a healthy fetus. A score of 8 with oligohydramnios or a score of 4 to 6 is equivocal. An equivocal test result is interpreted as possibly abnormal. Some clinicians may recommend repeating the test within 24 hours. However, others may advocate extending testing after any equivocal or abnormal test result. A score of 0 or 2 is abnormal and indicates the need for assessment of immediate delivery.

Although the BPP is fairly new, it has already been modified. Some physicians omit the nonstress test if the ultrasound parameters are normal. Some physicians have added placental grading as a sixth parameter.

Another measure of fetal well-being is the *amniotic fluid index (AFI)*. Ultrasound is used to measure the largest collection of amniotic fluid in each of the four quadrants within the uterus. The numbers are added together and the sum is the AFI. The normal range for the AFI is 8-18 cm. The sum is plotted on a graph where the age of gestation also is taken into account. If the AFI is less than the 2.4 percentile, oligohydramnios is present. If AFI exceeds the 97th percentile, polyhydramnios exists. An abnormal amniotic fluid index observed in antepartum testing is associated with an increased risk of intrauterine growth restriction and overall adverse perinatal outcome. Some suggest that patients with a borderline amniotic fluid index have this test performed twice weekly. Yet other studies have shown AFI to be so weak a predictor of poor neonatal outcome as to be useless. The percentile value seems to be a better indicator than an absolute fluid volume. Oligohydramnios is associated with placental failure or fetal renal problems. Polyhydramnios is associated with maternal diabetes or fetal upper gastrointestinal malformation/obstruction.

Doppler ultrasound evaluations of the placenta and the *umbilical artery velocity* can recognize alterations in umbilical artery flow and direction that may indicate fetal stress or illness.

Interfering factors

- Central nervous system stimulants such as catecholamine can increase BPP activities.
- Occasionally no movement is noted. If no eye movement or respiratory movement is noted, the fetus may be sleeping.

Procedure and patient care

Before

PT Explain the procedure to the patient.
PT Inform the patient that no fasting is required.

During

- Fetal heart rate reactivity is measured and interpreted from a nonstress test (see p. 446).

- Fetal breathing movements, fetal body movements, fetal tone, and amniotic fluid volume are determined by ultrasound imaging (see obstetric ultrasonography, p. 694)

After

- If the test results are abnormal or equivocal, support the patient in the next phase of the fetal evaluation process.

Abnormal findings

Fetal asphyxia
Congenital anomalies
Oligohydramnios
Intrauterine growth retardation
Postterm pregnancy
Fetal stress
Fetal death

notes

fetal contraction stress test (contraction stress test [CST], Oxytocin challenge test [OCT])

Type of test Electrodiagnostic

Normal findings Negative

Test explanation and related physiology

CST is used to evaluate the viability of a fetus. It documents the function of the placenta in its ability to supply adequate blood to the fetus.

The CST, frequently called the *oxytocin challenge test (OCT)*, is a relatively noninvasive test of fetoplacental adequacy used in the assessment of high-risk pregnancy. For this study, a temporary stress in the form of uterine contractions is applied to the fetus after the IV administration of oxytocin. The reaction of the fetus to the contractions is assessed by an external fetal heart monitor. Uterine contractions cause transient impediment of placental blood flow. If the placental reserve is adequate, the maternal-fetal oxygen transfer is not significantly compromised during the contractions, and the fetal heart rate (FHR) remains normal (a *negative* test). The fetoplacental unit can then be considered adequate for the next 7 days.

If the placental reserve is inadequate, the fetus does not receive enough oxygen during the contraction. This results in intrauterine hypoxia and late deceleration of the FHR. The test is considered to be *positive* if consistent, persistent, late decelerations of the FHR occur with two or more uterine contractions. False-positive results caused by uterine hyperstimulation can occur in 10% to 30% of patients. Thus, positive test results warrant a complete review of other studies (e.g., amniocentesis) before the pregnancy is terminated by delivery.

The test is considered to be *unsatisfactory* if the results cannot be interpreted (e.g., because of hyperstimulation of the uterus, excessive movement of the mother, or deceleration of unknown meaning). In the case of unsatisfactory results, other means of management should be considered.

Two advantages of the CST are that it can be done at any time and that its results are available shortly afterward. Although this test can be performed reliably at 32 weeks of gestation, it usually is done after 34 weeks. CST can induce labor, and a fetus at 34 weeks is more likely to survive an unexpectedly induced delivery than a fetus at 32 weeks. Nonstress testing (see p. 446) of the fetus is the preferred test in almost every instance and can be performed more safely at 32 weeks; it can then be followed 2 weeks later by CST if necessary. The CST may be performed weekly until delivery terminates pregnancy.

A noninvasive method of performing the CST is called the *breast stimulation* or *nipple stimulation technique*. Stimulation of the nipple causes nerve impulses to the hypothalamus that trigger the release of oxytocin into the mother's bloodstream. This causes uterine contractions and may eliminate the need for IV administration of oxytocin. Uterine contractions are usually satisfactory after 15 minutes of nipple stimulation (gentle twisting of the nipples). Advantages of this technique include the ease of performing the test; shorter duration of the study; and elimination of the need to start, monitor, and stop IV infusions.

Contraindications

- Patient pregnant with multiple fetuses, because the myometrium is under greater tension and is more likely to be stimulated to premature labor
- Patient with a prematurely ruptured membrane, because labor may be stimulated by the CST
- Patient with placenta previa, because vaginal delivery may be induced
- Patient with abruptio placentae, because the placenta may separate from the uterus as a result of the oxytocin-induced uterine contractions
- Patient with a previous hysterotomy, because the strong uterine contractions may cause uterine rupture
- Patient with a previous vertical or classic cesarean section, because the strong uterine contractions may cause uterine rupture (The test can be performed, however, if it is carefully monitored and controlled.)
- Patient with pregnancy of less than 32 weeks, because early delivery may be induced by the procedure

Potential complications

- Premature labor

Interfering factors

- Hypotension may cause false-positive results.

Procedure and patient care

Before

PT Explain the procedure to the patient.
- Obtain informed consent for the procedure.

PT Teach the patient breathing and relaxation techniques.
- Record the patient's blood pressure and FHR before the test as baseline values.
- If the CST is performed on an elective basis, the patient may be kept NPO in case labor occurs.

During
- Note the following procedural steps:
  1. After the patient empties her bladder, place her in a semi-Fowler's position and tilted slightly to one side to avoid vena caval compression by the enlarged uterus.
  2. Check her blood pressure every 10 minutes to avoid hypotension, which may cause diminished placental blood flow and a false-positive test result.
  3. Place an external fetal monitor over the patient's abdomen to record the fetal heart tones. Attach an external tokodynamometer to the abdomen at the fundal region to monitor uterine contractions.
  4. Record the output of the fetal heart tones and uterine contractions on a two-channel strip recorder.
  5. Monitor baseline FHR and uterine activity for 20 minutes.
  6. If uterine contractions are detected during this pretest period, withhold oxytocin and monitor the response of the fetal heart tone to spontaneous uterine contractions.
  7. If no spontaneous uterine contractions occur, administer oxytocin (Pitocin) by IV infusion pump.
  8. Increase the rate of oxytocin infusion until the patient is having moderate contractions, then record the FHR pattern.
  9. After the oxytocin infusion is discontinued, continue FHR monitoring for another 30 minutes until the uterine activity has returned to its preoxytocin state. The body metabolizes oxytocin in approximately 20 to 25 minutes.
- Note that the CST is performed safely on an outpatient basis in the labor and delivery unit, where qualified nurses and necessary equipment are available. The test is performed by a nurse with a physician available.
- Note that if sufficient contractions do not result from the *nipple stimulation technique,* the standard CST procedure is followed.

- Note that the duration of this study is approximately 2 hours.

PT Tell the patient that the discomfort associated with the CST may consist of mild labor contractions. Usually, breathing exercises are sufficient to control any discomfort. Administer analgesics if needed.

After

- Monitor the patient's blood pressure and FHR.
- Discontinue the IV line and assess the site for bleeding.

Abnormal findings

Fetoplacental inadequacy

notes

fetal fibronectin (fFN)

Type of test Fluid analysis

Normal findings

Negative: ≤0.05 mcg/ml

Test explanation and related physiology

F

Fibronectin may help with implantation of the fertilized egg into the uterine lining. Normally, fibronectin cannot be identified in vaginal secretions after 22 weeks of pregnancy. However, concentrations are very high in the amniotic fluid. If fibronectin is identified in vaginal secretions after 24 weeks, the patient is at high risk for preterm (premature) delivery within the next 2 weeks. fFN's use is limited to women whose membranes are intact and with cervical dilatation of less than 3 cm.

Procedure and patient care

Before

PT Explain the procedure to the patient.

PT Tell the patient that no fasting is required.

During

Note the following procedural steps:

1. The patient is placed in the lithotomy position.
2. A vaginal speculum is inserted to expose the cervix.
3. Vaginal secretions are collected from the posterior vagina and paracervical area with a dacron swab that comes with the fibronectin laboratory kit.
4. The slide is labeled with the patient's name, age, and estimated date of confinement.

PT Tell the patient that no discomfort, except for insertion of the speculum, is associated with this procedure.

After

PT Inform the patient that usually the result will be available the next day.

PT Educate the patient about the signs of preterm labor: cramps, uterine contractions, pelvic pressure, or the rupture of membranes.

■ Encourage the patient to express concerns regarding the plans for preterm delivery.

Abnormal findings

High risk for preterm premature delivery

notes

fetal hemoglobin testing (Kleihauer-Betke test)

Type of test Blood

Normal findings

<1% of RBCs

Test explanation and related physiology

F

Fetal hemoglobin may be present in the mother's blood because of fetal-maternal hemorrhage (FMH), which causes leakage of fetal cells into the maternal circulation. When large volumes of fetal blood are lost in this way, neonatal outcomes can be serious and potentially fatal. Massive FMH may cause about one in every 50 stillbirths. No historical or clinical features allow antecedent identification of those in whom FMH may cause an intrauterine death. Therefore, a large proportion of patients with FMH will remain undetected.

Leakage of fetal red blood cells can begin any time after the middle of the first trimester. It presumably results from a breach in the integrity of the placental circulation. As pregnancy continues, more women will show evidence of fetal red cells in their circulation so that by term, about 50% will have detectable fetal cells. Most of these, however, are the result of very small leaks. In 96% to 98% of pregnancies the total fetal blood volume lost in this way is 2 ml or less. Small leaks are not implicated in intrauterine death.

Risk factors correlated with the increasing risk of massive FMH include maternal trauma, placental abruption, placental tumors, third trimester amniocentesis, fetal hydrops, pale fetal organs, antecedent sinusoidal fetal heart tracing, and twinning. Having one or more of these features should be an indication for fetal hemoglobin testing.

The standard method of detecting FMH is the *Kleihauer-Betke test*. This takes advantage of the differential resistance of fetal hemoglobin to acid. A standard blood smear is prepared from mother's blood. An acid bath is then used to remove all adult hemoglobin; however, it does not remove fetal hemoglobin. Subsequent staining makes fetal cells (containing fetal hemoglobin) rose-pink, whereas the mother's cells are only seen as "ghosts." A large number of cells (e.g., 5000) are counted under the microscope and the ratio of fetal to maternal cells is generated. The *flow cytometric method* for fetal hemoglobin determination offers several advantages over the traditional Kleihauer-Betke method. This more objective method has been shown to improve sensitivity, precision, and linearity over traditional methods.

FMH becomes of even greater significance when the mother is Rh−, as this is the mechanism through which Rh sensitization could develop if the fetus has paternal Rh+ blood cells. If this is known to exist, RhoGAM (RhIG) antibodies directed to Rh+ fetal cells are given to the pregnant mother at the time any invasive procedure is performed when the mother may be exposed to the blood of the fetus or upon delivery. The RhoGAM antibodies kill the fetal RBCs in the maternal bloodstream before the mother can develop antibodies to fetal Rh+ RBCs. This precludes more aggressive antifetal RBC occurrences in the future. By determination of the amount and volume of fetal blood loss, a dose of RhoGAM can be calculated using the following formula:

$$\text{Vials of RhIG} = \frac{\text{ml of fetal blood}}{30}$$

This test is often performed on women who have delivered a stillborn baby, to see if FMH was a potential cause of fetal death.

Interfering factors

- Any maternal condition (such as sickle cell disease) that involves persistence of fetal hemoglobin in the mother will cause a false positive.
- If the blood is drawn after C-section, a false positive could occur. Vaginal delivery results in higher frequency of detection of FMH.

Procedure and patient care

Before

PT Explain the procedure to the patient.

During

- Collect approximately 7 to 10 ml of venous blood in a red-top tube for serum testing.
- Avoid hemolysis.

After

- Apply pressure to the venipuncture site.
PT Emphasize to the patient the importance of antepartal health care.

- Provide emotional support in the event this test is performed after a stillborn delivery.

Abnormal findings

Feto-maternal hemorrhage
Hereditary persistence of fetal hemoglobin
Intrachorionic thrombi

notes

F

fetal nonstress test (Nonstress test, NST, Fetal activity determination)

Type of test Electrodiagnostic

Normal findings "Reactive" fetus (heart rate acceleration associated with fetal movement)

Test explanation and related physiology

The NST is a method of evaluating the viability of a fetus. It documents the function of the placenta in its ability to supply adequate blood to the fetus. The NST can be used to evaluate any high-risk pregnancy in which fetal well-being may be threatened.

The NST is a noninvasive study that monitors acceleration of the fetal heart rate (FHR) in response to fetal movement. This FHR acceleration reflects the integrity of the central nervous system and fetal well-being. Fetal activity may be spontaneous, induced by uterine contraction, or induced by external manipulation. Oxytocin stimulation is not used. Fetal response is characterized as "reactive" or "nonreactive." The NST indicates a *reactive fetus* when, with fetal movement, two or more FHR accelerations are detected, each of which must be at least 15 beats/min for 15 seconds or more within any 10-minute period. The test is 99% reliable in indicating fetal viability and negates the need for the contraction stress test (CST, see p. 437). If the test detects a *nonreactive fetus* (i.e., no FHR acceleration with fetal movement) within 40 minutes, the patient is a candidate for the CST. A 40-minute test period is used because this is the average duration of the sleep-wake cycle of the fetus. The cycle may vary considerably, however.

The NST is useful in screening high-risk pregnancies and in selecting patients who may require the CST. An NST is now routinely performed before the CST to avoid the complications associated with oxytocin administration. No complications are associated with the NST.

Procedure and patient care

Before

PT Explain the procedure to the patient.

- Encourage verbalization of the patient's fears. The necessity for the study usually raises realistic fears in the expectant mother.

PT If the patient is hungry, instruct her to eat before the NST is begun. Fetal activity is enhanced with a high maternal serum glucose level.

During

- After the patient empties her bladder, place her in Sims' position.
- Place an external fetal monitor on the patient's abdomen to record the FHR. The mother can indicate fetal movement by pressing a button on the fetal monitor whenever she feels the fetus move. FHR and fetal movement are concomitantly recorded on a two-channel strip graph.
- Observe the fetal monitor for FHR accelerations associated with fetal movement.
- If the fetus is quiet for 20 minutes, stimulate fetal activity by external methods such as rubbing or compressing the mother's abdomen, ringing a bell near the abdomen, or placing a pan on the abdomen and hitting the pan.
- Note that a nurse performs the NST in approximately 20 to 40 minutes in the physician's office or a hospital unit.

PT Tell the patient that no discomfort is associated with NST.

After

- If the results detect a nonreactive fetus, inform the patient that she is a candidate for the CST.

Abnormal findings

Fetal stress

Fetal death

notes

fetal scalp blood pH (Fetal oxygen saturation monitoring)

Type of test Blood

Normal findings

pH: 7.25-7.35
O_2 saturation: 30%-50%
PO_2: 18-22 mm Hg
PCO_2: 40-50 mm Hg
Base excess: 0 to −10 mEq/L

Test explanation and related physiology

Measurement of fetal scalp blood pH provides valuable information on fetal acid-base status. This screening test is useful clinically for diagnosing fetal distress.

Although the oxygen partial pressure (PO_2), carbon dioxide partial pressure (PCO_2), and bicarbonate ion concentration can be measured with a fetal scalp blood sample, the pH is the most useful clinically. The pH normally ranges from 7.25 to 7.35 during labor; a mild decline within the normal range is noted with contractions and as labor progresses.

Fetal hypoxia causes anaerobic glycolysis, resulting in excess production of lactic acid. This causes an increase in hydrogen ion concentration (acidosis) and a decrease in pH. Acidosis reflects the effect of hypoxia on cellular metabolism. A high correlation exists between low pH levels and low Apgar scores.

Fetal oxygen saturation monitoring (FSpo₂) also is available to assist the monitoring of fetal well-being during delivery. When the FHR becomes significantly abnormal (nonreassuring), C-section is often performed because of concern for fetal well-being. However, with $FSpo_2$, an accurate measure of fetal oxygen saturation can be determined. The technology is based on the same principle as adult pulse oximetry, except that the machine is far more sensitive and able to accurately read saturations of less than 70%. After membranes are ruptured, and if the baby is in vertex position with good cervical dilatation, a specialized probe can be placed on the temple or cheek of the fetus for $FSpo_2$ monitoring. Expertise is required for appropriate placement of the sensor. The oxygen saturation is displayed on a monitor screen as a percentage. The normal oxygen saturation for a baby in the womb receiving oxygenated blood from the placenta is usually between 30% and 70%. When $FSpo_2$ is less than 30% for several minutes, there is marked and progressive deterioration in fetal well-being as hypoxia and acidemia progress.

Contraindications

- Patients with premature membrane rupture
- Patients with active cervical infection (e.g., gonorrhea, herpes, HIV)

Potential complications

- Continued bleeding from the puncture site
- Hematoma
- Ecchymosis
- Infection

Procedure and patient care

Before

PT Explain the procedure to the patient.
- Obtain informed consent for this procedure.
PT Tell the patient that no fasting or sedation is required.

During

- Note the following procedural steps for fetal scalp pH:
  1. Amnioscopy is performed with the mother in the lithotomy position.
  2. The cervix is dilated, and the endoscope (amnioscope) is introduced into the cervical canal.
  3. The fetal scalp is cleansed with an antiseptic and dried with a sterile cotton ball.
  4. A small amount of petroleum jelly is applied to the fetal scalp to cause droplets of fetal blood to bead.
  5. After the skin on the scalp is pierced with a small metal blade, beaded droplets of blood are collected in long, heparinized capillary tubes.
  6. The tube is sealed with wax and placed on ice to retard cellular respiration, which can alter the pH.
  7. The physician performing the procedure applies firm pressure to the puncture site to retard bleeding.
  8. Scalp blood sampling can be repeated as necessary.
- Note that this study is performed by a physician in approximately 10 to 15 minutes.
PT Tell the patient that she may be uncomfortable during the cervical dilation.

After

PT Inform the patient that she may have vaginal discomfort and
menstrual-type cramping.

After delivery

- Assess the newborn and identify and document the puncture
  site(s).
- Cleanse the fetal scalp puncture site with an antiseptic
  solution and apply an antibiotic ointment.

Abnormal findings

Fetal distress

notes

fetoscopy

Type of test Endoscopy

Normal findings No fetal distress

Test explanation and related physiology

Fetoscopy is an endoscopic procedure that allows direct visualization of the fetus via the insertion of a tiny, telescope-like instrument through the abdominal wall and into the uterine cavity (Figure 20). Direct visualization may lead to diagnosis of a severe malformation such as a neural tube defect. During the procedure, fetal blood samples to detect congenital blood disorders (e.g., hemophilia, sickle cell anemia) can be drawn from a blood vessel in the umbilical cord for biochemical analysis. Fetal skin biopsies also can be done to detect primary skin disorders.

Fetoscopy is performed at approximately 18 weeks of gestation. At this time the vessels of the placental surface are of adequate size, and the fetal parts are readily identifiable. A therapeutic abortion would not be as hazardous at this time as it would be if it were done later in the pregnancy. An ultrasound is usually performed the day after the procedure to confirm the adequacy of the amniotic fluid and fetal viability.

Potential complications

- Spontaneous abortion
- Premature delivery
- Amniotic fluid leak
- Intrauterine fetal death
- Amnionitis

Procedure and patient care

Before

PT Explain the procedure to the patient.
- Obtain informed consent.
- Assess the fetal heart rate before the test to serve as a baseline value.
- Administer meperidine (Demerol) if ordered before the test because it crosses the placenta and quiets the fetus. This prevents excessive fetal movement, which would make the procedure more difficult.

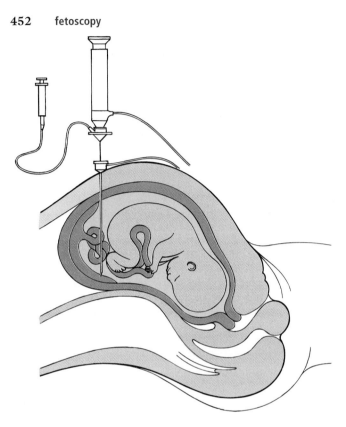

Figure 20 Fetoscopy for fetal blood sampling.

During
- Note the following procedural steps:
  1. The woman is placed in the supine position on an examining table.
  2. The abdominal wall is anesthetized locally.
  3. Ultrasonography is performed to locate the fetus and the placenta.
  4. The endoscope is inserted.
  5. Biopsies and blood samples may be obtained.
- Note that this procedure is performed by a physician in 1 to 2 hours.

PT Tell the patient that the only discomfort associated with this study is the injection of the local anesthetic.

After

- Assess the FHR and compare with the baseline value to detect any side effects related to the procedure.
- Monitor the mother and fetus carefully for alterations in blood pressure, pulse, uterine activity, and fetal activity; vaginal bleeding; and loss of amniotic fluid.
- Administer RhoGAM to mothers who are Rh negative unless the fetal blood is found to be Rh negative.
- Note that a repeat ultrasound is usually performed the day after the procedure to confirm the adequacy of the amniotic fluid and fetal viability.
- If ordered, administer antibiotics prophylactically after the test to prevent amnionitis.

🏠 Home care responsibilities

- Instruct the mother to avoid strenuous activity for 1 to 2 weeks after the procedure.
- Advise the mother to report any pain, bleeding, amniotic fluid loss, or fever.

Abnormal findings

Developmental defects (e.g., neural tube defects)
Congenital blood disorders (e.g., hemophilia, sickle cell anemia)
Primary skin disorders

notes

fibrinogen (Factor I, Quantitative fibrinogen)

Type of test Blood

Normal findings

Adult: 200-400 mg/dl or 2-4 g/L (SI units)

Newborn: 125-300 mg/dl

Possible critical values <100 mg/dl

Test explanation and related physiology

Fibrinogen is essential to the blood-clotting mechanism. It is part of the "common pathway" in the coagulation system. Fibrinogen is converted to fibrin by action of thrombin during the coagulation process. (See discussion of coagulating factors, p. 279.) Fibrinogen, which is produced by the liver, is also an acute-phase protein reactant. It rises sharply during instances of tissue inflammation or necrosis. High levels of fibrinogen have been associated with an increased risk of coronary heart disease, stroke, myocardial infarction, and peripheral arterial disease. This makes fibrinogen an important risk factor for cardiovascular disease.

Reduced levels of fibrinogen can be seen in patients with liver disease, malnourished states, and consumptive coagulopathies (e.g., disseminated intravascular coagulation). Large-volume blood transfusions are also associated with low levels, because banked blood does not contain fibrinogen. Reduced levels of fibrinogen will cause a prolonged pro-time and partial thromboplastin time.

Interfering factors

- Blood transfusions within the past month may affect test results.
- Fibrinolysins can attack fibrinogen and reduce the serum levels.
- Diets rich in omega-3 and omega-6 fatty acids reduce fibrinogen levels.
- Drugs that may cause *increased* levels include estrogens and oral contraceptives.
- Drugs that may cause *decreased* levels include anabolic steroids, androgens, asparaginase, phenobarbital, streptokinase, urokinase, and valproic acid.

Procedure and patient care

Before
PT Explain the procedure to the patient.
PT Tell the patient that no fasting is required.

During
- Collect one tube of venous blood in a blue-top tube.

After
- Apply pressure to the venipuncture site.

F

Abnormal findings

▲ **Increased levels**

Acute inflammatory
reactions (e.g., rheumatoid
arthritis, glomerulonephritis)
Trauma
Acute infection such as
pneumonia
Coronary heart disease
Cigarette smoking
Pregnancy
Stroke
Myocardial infarction
Peripheral arterial disease

▼ **Decreased levels**

Liver disease
(e.g., hepatitis,
cirrhosis)
Consumptive
coagulopathy
Fibrinolysins
Congenital
afibrinogenemia
Advanced carcinoma
Malnutrition
Large-volume blood
transfusion

notes

folic acid (Folate)

Type of test   Blood

Normal findings   5-25 ng/ml or 11-57 nmol/L (SI units)

Test explanation and related physiology

Folic acid, one of the B vitamins, is necessary for normal function of red and white blood cells (RBCs, WBCs) and for the adequate synthesis of certain purines and pyrimidines, which are precursors for deoxyribonucleic acid (DNA). As with vitamin B_{12} (see p. 821), folate depends on normal function of the intestinal mucosa.

Folic acid blood levels are performed to evaluate hemolytic disorders and to detect anemia caused by folic acid deficiency (in which the RBCs are abnormally large, causing a megaloblastic anemia). These RBCs have a shortened life span and impaired oxygen-carrying capacity.

The main causes of folic acid deficiency include dietary deficiency, malabsorption syndrome, pregnancy, and certain anticonvulsant drugs. Decreased folic acid levels are seen in patients with folic acid deficiency anemia (megaloblastic anemia), hemolytic anemia, malnutrition, malabsorption syndrome, malignancy, liver disease, sprue, and celiac disease. Some drugs (e.g., anticonvulsants, antimalarials, alcohol, aminopterin, and methotrexate) are folic acid antagonists and interfere with nucleic acid synthesis.

Elevated levels of folic acid may be seen in patients with pernicious anemia. The folic acid test may be done in conjunction with tests for vitamin B_{12} levels (see p. 821). This test for folate is often done in the workup for alcoholic patients to assess nutritional status. One must be depleted of folate for at least 5 months before megaloblastic anemia occurs.

Interfering factors

- Because radioimmunoassay is the method of choice for folic acid determination, radionuclide administration should be avoided for at least 24 hours.
- Drugs that may cause *decreased* folic acid levels include alcohol, aminopterin, aminosalicylic acid (PAS), ampicillin, antimalarials, chloramphenicol, erythromycin, estrogens, methotrexate, oral contraceptives, penicillin, phenobarbital, phenytoin, and tetracyclines.

Procedure and patient care

Before

PT Explain the procedure to the patient.
PT Tell the patient that usually no fasting is required. (However, some laboratories prefer an 8-hour fast.)
PT Instruct the patient not to consume alcoholic beverages before the test.
- Draw the specimen before starting folate therapy.

F

During
- Collect approximately 7 to 10 ml of venous blood in a red-top tube.
- Avoid hemolysis.
- Indicate on the laboratory slip any medications that may affect test results.

After
- Apply pressure to the venipuncture site.
- Transport the blood immediately to the laboratory after collection.

Abnormal findings

▲ **Increased levels**

Pernicious anemia
Vegetarianism
Recent massive blood
  transfusion

▼ **Decreased levels**

Folic acid deficiency
  anemia
Hemolytic anemia
Malnutrition
Malabsorption syn-
  drome (e.g., sprue,
  celiac disease)
Malignancy
Liver disease
Pregnancy
Alcoholism
Anorexia nervosa
Chronic renal disease

notes

fungal antibody tests (Antifungal antibodies)

Type of test Blood

Normal findings No antibodies detected

Test explanation and related physiology

Fungal infections can be superficial, subcutaneous, or systemic (deep). The systemic fungal infections (mycoses) are the most important, for which serologic antibody testing is performed. Generally mycoses are caused by the inhalation of airborne fungal spores. In the United States, the most serious fungal infections are coccidioidomycosis, blastomycosis, histoplasmosis, and paracoccidioidomycosis. These infections start out as primary pulmonary infections. *Aspergillus, Candida,* and *Cryptococcus* systemic infections usually affect only those with compromised immunity.

Fungal antibody testing is not highly reliable. Antibodies are present in only about 70% to 80% of infected patients. When positive, they merely indicate that the person has an active or has had a recent fungal infection. These antibodies can also be identified in the cerebrospinal fluid. They can be tested singularly or as a fungal panel. Cross-reactions can occur (e.g., antibodies to blastomycosis can cross-react with histoplasmosis antigens).

Procedure and patient care

Before
PT Explain the procedure to the patient.
PT Tell the patient that no fasting or preparation is required.

During
- Collect 7 ml of venous blood in a red-top or any serum separator tube.
- Indicate on the laboratory slip the particular antibody or panel of antibodies that are to be tested.

After
- Apply pressure or a pressure dressing to the venipuncture site.

Abnormal findings

▲   **Increased levels**
Acute fungal infection
Previous systemic exposure to fungal disease

gallbladder nuclear scanning (Hepatobiliary scintigraphy, Hepatobiliary imaging, Biliary tract radionuclide scan, Cholescintigraphy, DISIDA scanning, HIDA scanning, IDA gallbladder scanning)

Type of test Nuclear scan

Normal findings Gallbladder, common bile duct, and duodenum visualize within 60 minutes after radionuclide injection. (This confirms patency of the cystic and common bile ducts.)

G

Test explanation and related physiology

Through the use of iminodiacetic acid analogues (IDAs) labeled with technetium-99m (^{99m}Tc), the biliary tract can be evaluated in a safe, accurate, and noninvasive manner. These radionuclide compounds are extracted by the liver and excreted into the bile. Gamma rays emitted from the bile are detected by a scintillator, and a realistic image of the biliary tree is apparent.

Failure to visualize the gallbladder 60 to 120 minutes after injection of the radionuclide dye is virtually diagnostic of an obstruction of the cystic duct (acute cholecystitis). Delayed filling of the gallbladder is associated with chronic or acalculus cholecystitis. The identification of the radionuclide in the biliary tree, but not in the bowel, is diagnostic of common bile duct obstruction.

With cholescintigraphy, gallbladder function can be numerically determined by calculating the capability of the gallbladder to eject its contents. It is believed that an ejection fraction below 35% indicates chronic cholecystitis or functional obstruction of the cystic duct.

Occasionally, morphine sulfate is given intravenously during nuclear scanning. The morphine causes increased ampullary contraction. This reproduces the patient's symptoms of biliary colic and forces the bile containing the radionuclide into the gallbladder, shortening the expected time of visualization of the gallbladder. If no radionuclide is seen in the gallbladder with the use of morphine within 15 to 30 minutes, the diagnosis of acute cholecystitis is nearly certain.

Contraindications

- Patients who are pregnant, because of the risk of fetal damage

Interfering factors

- If the patient has not eaten for more than 24 hours, the radionuclide may not fill the gallbladder. This would produce a false-positive result.

Procedure and patient care

Before

PT Explain the procedure to the patient.

PT Assure the patient that he or she will not be exposed to large amounts of radioactivity.

PT Instruct the patient to fast for at least 2 hours before the test. This fasting is preferable but not mandatory.

During

- Note the following procedural steps:
  1. After IV administration of a ^{99m}Tc-labeled IDA analogue (e.g., DISIDA, PIPIDA, HIDA), the right upper quadrant of the abdomen is scanned.
  2. Serial images are obtained over 1 hour.
  3. Subsequent images can be obtained at 15- to 30-minute intervals.
  4. If the gallbladder, common bile duct, or duodenum is not visualized within 60 minutes after injection, delayed images are obtained up to 4 hours later.
  5. When an *ejection fraction* is to be determined, the patient is given a fatty meal or cholecystokinin to evaluate emptying of the gallbladder. The gallbladder is continually scanned to measure the percentage of isotope ejected.
- Note that a radiologist performs this study in 1 to 4 hours in the nuclear medicine department.

PT Tell the patient that the only discomfort associated with this procedure is the IV injection of radionuclide.

After

- Obtain a meal for the patient if indicated.

Abnormal findings

Acute cholecystitis

Chronic cholecystitis

Acalculus cholecystitis

Common bile duct obstruction secondary to gallstones, tumor, or stricture

Cystic duct syndrome

gallium scan

Type of test Nuclear scan

Normal findings

Diffuse, low level of gallium uptake, especially in the liver and spleen

No increased gallium uptake within the body

Test explanation and related physiology

A gallium scan of the total body is usually performed 24, 48, and 72 hours after an IV injection of radioactive gallium. Gallium is a radionuclide that is concentrated by areas of inflammation and infection, abscesses, and benign and malignant tumors. However, not all types of tumors will concentrate gallium. Lymphomas are particularly gallium avid. Other tumors that can be detected by a gallium scan include sarcomas, hepatomas, and carcinomas of the gastrointestinal tract, kidney, uterus, stomach, and testicle.

This test is useful in detecting metastatic tumor, especially lymphoma, even when other diagnostic imaging tests are normal. The gallium scan also is useful in demonstrating a source of infection in patients with a fever of unknown origin. Gallium can be used to identify noninfectious inflammation within the body in patients who have an elevated sedimentation rate. Unfortunately, this test is not specific enough to differentiate among tumor, infection, inflammation, or abscess.

Contraindications

- Pregnancy, unless the benefits outweigh of the risk of fetal damage

Procedure and patient care

Before

PT Explain the procedure to the patient.

- Usually, administer a cathartic or enema to the patient to minimize increased gallium uptake within the bowel.

During

- Note the following procedural steps:
  1. The unsedated patient is injected with gallium.
  2. A total-body scan may be performed 4 to 6 hours later by slowly passing a radionuclide detector over the body.

3. Additional scans are usually taken 24, 48, and 72 hours later.
4. During the scanning process the patient is positioned in the supine, prone, and lateral positions.

- Note that a nuclear medicine technologist performs each scan in approximately 30 to 60 minutes. Repeated scanning is required. Repeated injections are not necessary.

PT Inform the patient that test results are interpreted by a physician trained in nuclear medicine and are usually available 72 hours after the injection.

After

PT Assure the patient that only tracer doses of radioisotopes have been used and that no precautions against radioactive exposure to others are necessary.

Abnormal findings

Tumor
Noninfectious inflammation
Infection
Abscess

notes

gamma-glutamyl transpeptidase (GGTP, γ-GTP, Gamma-glutamyl transferase [GGT])

Type of test Blood

Normal findings

Male and female age 45 and older: 8-38 units/L or
   8-38 international units/L (SI units)
Female younger than age 45: 5-27 units/L or 5-27 international
   units/L (SI units)
Elderly: slightly higher than adult level
Child: similar to adult level
Newborn: 5 times higher than adult level

Test explanation and related physiology

The enzyme GGTP participates in the transfer of amino acids and peptides across the cellular membrane and possibly participates in glutathione metabolism. Highest concentrations of this enzyme are found in the liver and biliary tract. Lesser concentrations are found in the kidney, spleen, heart, intestine, brain, and prostate gland. This test is used to detect liver cell dysfunction, and it very accurately indicates even the slightest degree of cholestasis. This is the most sensitive liver enzyme in detecting biliary obstruction, cholangitis, or cholecystitis. As with leucine aminopeptidase and 5-nucleotidase, the elevation of GGTP generally parallels that of alkaline phosphatase; however, GGTP is more sensitive. Also, as with 5-nucleotidase and leucine aminopeptidase, GGTP is not increased in bone diseases as is alkaline phosphatase. A normal GGTP level with an elevated alkaline phosphatase level implies skeletal disease. Elevated GGTP and alkaline phosphatase levels imply hepatobiliary disease. GGTP is also not elevated in childhood or pregnancy.

Another important clinical aspect of GGTP is that it can detect chronic alcohol ingestion. Therefore, it is very useful in the screening and evaluation of alcoholic patients. GGTP is elevated in approximately 75% of patients who chronically drink alcohol.

Why this enzyme is elevated after an acute myocardial infarction is not clear. It may represent the associated hepatic insult (if elevation occurs in the first 7 days) or the proliferation of capillary endothelial cells in the granulation tissue that replaces the infarcted myocardium. The elevation usually occurs 1 to 2 weeks after infarction.

Interfering factors

- Values may be decreased in late pregnancy.
- Drugs that may cause *increased* GGTP levels include alcohol, phenytoin (Dilantin), and phenobarbital.
- Drugs that may cause *decreased* levels include clofibrate and oral contraceptives.

Procedure and patient care

Before

PT Explain the procedure to the patient.

PT Tell the patient that an 8-hour fast is recommended. Only water is permitted.

During

- Collect approximately 7 to 10 ml of venous blood in a red-top tube.
- Indicate on the laboratory slip any medications the patient is taking that may affect test results.

After

- Apply pressure to the venipuncture site. Patients with liver dysfunction often have prolonged clotting times.

Abnormal findings

▲ **Increased levels**

Hepatitis
Cirrhosis
Hepatic necrosis
Hepatic tumor or metastasis
Hepatotoxic drugs
Cholestasis
Jaundice
Myocardial infarction
Alcohol ingestion
Pancreatitis
Cancer of the pancreas
Epstein-Barr (infectious mononucleosis)
Cytomegalovirus infections
Reye's syndrome

gastrin

Type of test Blood

Normal findings

0-180 pg/ml or 0-180 ng/L (SI units)
Levels are higher in elderly patients.

Test explanation and related physiology

Gastrin is a hormone produced by the G cells located in the distal part of the stomach (antrum). Gastrin is a potent stimulator of gastric acid. In normal gastric physiology an alkaline environment (created by food or antacids) stimulates the release of gastrin. Gastrin then stimulates the parietal cells of the stomach to secrete gastric acid. The pH environment in the stomach is thereby reduced. By negative feedback this low-pH environment suppresses further gastrin secretion.

Zollinger-Ellison (ZE) syndrome (gastrin-producing pancreatic tumor) and G-cell hyperplasia (overfunctioning of G cells in the distal stomach) are associated with high serum gastrin levels. Patients with these tumors have aggressive peptic ulcer disease. Unlike a patient with routine peptic ulcers, a patient with ZE syndrome or G-cell hyperplasia has a high incidence of complicated and recurrent peptic ulcers. It is important to identify this latter group of patients to institute more appropriate, aggressive medical and surgical therapy. The serum gastrin level is normal in patients with routine peptic ulcer and greatly elevated in patients with ZE syndrome or G-cell hyperplasia.

It is important to note that patients who are taking antacid peptic ulcer medicines, have had peptic ulcer surgery, or have atrophic gastritis will have a high serum gastrin level. However, levels usually are not as high as in patients with ZE syndrome or G-cell hyperplasia.

Not all patients with ZE syndrome exhibit increased levels of serum gastrin. Some may have "top" normal gastrin levels, which makes these patients difficult to differentiate from patients with routine peptic ulcer disease. ZE syndrome or G-cell hyperplasia can be diagnosed in these "top" normal patients by *gastrin stimulation tests* using calcium or secretin. Patients with these diseases have greatly increased serum gastrin levels associated with the infusion of these drugs.

Interfering factors

- Peptic ulcer surgery creates a persistent alkaline environment, which is the strongest stimulant to gastrin.
- Ingestion of high-protein food can result in an increase in serum gastrin two to five times the normal level.
- ✗ Patients with diabetes who take insulin may have falsely elevated levels.
- ✗ Drugs that may *increase* serum gastrin levels include antacids, H_2-blocking agents (e.g., cimetidine [Tagamet], ranitidine [Zantac], and hydrogen pump inhibitors (e.g., omeprazole [Prilosec]).
- ✗ Drugs that may *decrease* levels include anticholinergics and tricyclic antidepressants.

Procedure and patient care

Before

- PT Explain the procedure to the patient.
- PT Usually instruct the patient to fast for 12 hours. Water is permitted.
- PT Tell the patient to avoid alcohol for at least 24 hours.

During

- Collect approximately 5 to 7 ml of venous blood in a red-top tube.
- For the *calcium infusion test*, administer calcium gluconate intravenously for 3 hours. A preinfusion serum gastrin level is then compared with specimens taken every 30 minutes for 4 hours.
- For the *secretin test*, administer secretin intravenously. Preinjection and postinjection serum gastrin levels are taken at 15-minute intervals for 1 hour after injection.

After

- Apply pressure to the venipuncture site.

Abnormal findings

▲ **Increased levels**

ZE syndrome
G-cell hyperplasia
Pernicious anemia
Atrophic gastritis
Gastric carcinoma

Chronic renal failure
Pyloric obstruction or gastric outlet obstruction
Retained antrum after gastric surgery

gastroesophageal reflux scan (GE reflux scan, Aspiration scan)

Type of test Nuclear scan

Normal findings No evidence of gastroesophageal reflux

Test explanation and related physiology

GE reflux scans are used to evaluate patients with symptoms of heartburn, regurgitation, vomiting, and dysphagia. They are also used to evaluate the medical or surgical treatment of patients with GE reflux. Finally, *aspiration scans* may be used to detect aspiration of gastric contents into the lungs.

Contraindications

- Patients who cannot tolerate abdominal compression
- Patients who are pregnant or lactating, unless the benefits outweigh the risks

Procedure and patient care

Before

PT Explain the procedure to the patient.

PT Assure the patient that no pain is associated with this test.

PT Instruct the patient to eat a full meal just before the study.

During

- Note the following procedural steps:

GE reflux scan

1. The patient is placed in the supine position and asked to swallow a tracer cocktail (e.g., orange juice, diluted hydrochloric acid, and technetium-99m–labeled colloid).
2. Images are taken of the patient over the esophageal area.
3. The patient is asked to assume other positions to determine whether GE reflux occurs and, if so, in what position.
4. A large abdominal binder that contains an air-inflatable cuff is placed on the patient's abdomen. This is insufflated to increase abdominal pressure.
5. Images are again taken over the esophageal area to determine if any GE reflux occurs.

Aspiration scans

1. These scans may be performed by adding a radionuclide to the patient's evening meal and keeping the patient in the supine position until the next morning.

2. Images are made over the lung fields to detect esophagotracheal aspiration of the tracer.

- Note that this procedure is performed in the nuclear medicine department in approximately 30 minutes.

PT Remind the patient that no discomfort is associated with this test.

- In infants being evaluated for chalasia, note that the tracer is added to the feeding or formula. Nuclear tracer films are then taken over the next hour, with delayed films as needed.

After

PT Assure the patient that he or she has ingested only a small dose of nuclear material. No radiation precautions need to be taken against the patient or his or her bodily secretions.

Abnormal findings

Gastroesophageal reflux
Pulmonary aspiration

notes

gastrointestinal bleeding scan (Abdominal scintigraphy, GI scintigraphy)

Type of test Nuclear scan

Normal findings No collection of radionuclide in GI tract

Test explanation and related physiology

The GI bleeding scan is a test used to localize the site of bleeding in patients who are having active GI hemorrhage. The scan also can be used in patients who have suspected intraabdominal (nongastrointestinal) hemorrhage from an unknown source. Localization of the source of GI or other bleeding can be difficult. When surgery is required under these circumstances, it is difficult, cumbersome, and prolonged. The surgeon may have extreme difficulty finding the source of bleeding. The bleeding scan helps localize the bleeding for the surgeon.

Arteriography has limitations in its evaluation of GI bleeding. Arteriography can determine the site of bleeding only if the rate of bleeding exceeds 0.5 ml/min for detection. The GI bleeding scan has several advantages over arteriography. It can detect bleeding if the rate is greater than 0.05 ml/min. Also, with the use of Tc-labeled red blood cells, delayed films (as long as 24 hours) can be obtained indicating the site of an intermittent or extremely slow intestinal bleed.

A GI scintigram is much more sensitive in locating the area of GI bleeding; however, it is not very specific in pinpointing the site or cause of bleeding. Usually, when positive, it cannot localize the exact source of bleeding any more accurately than to indicate the affected quadrant of the abdomen (e.g., right upper, left lower). This test is usually performed by injecting sulfur colloid labeled with technetium-99m (^{99m}Tc) or ^{99m}Tc-labeled red blood cells (RBCs) into the patient. If the patient is bleeding at a rate in excess of 0.05 ml/min, pooling of the radionuclide will ultimately be detected in the abnormal segment of the intestine. Few false-positive results occur. Again, it is important to recognize that the test only localizes the bleeding; it does not indicate the exact pathologic condition causing the bleeding. With this test result, if surgery is required, the surgeon is directed to the abnormal area and hopefully can detect and resect the pathologic bleeding source.

It is important to realize that this test can take at least 1 to 4 hours to obtain useful information. Unstable patients should

G

not leave the intensive care environment for that long a period. Further, an unstable patient may need to go to surgery in minutes, and several hours may not be available to determine the region of active bleeding.

Contraindications

- Patients who are pregnant or lactating, unless the benefits outweigh the risks
- Medically unstable patients whose stay in the nuclear medicine department may be risky

Interfering factors

- Barium within the GI tract may mask a small source of bleeding.

Procedure and patient care

Before

PT Explain the procedure to the patient.
- Assess the patient's vital signs to ensure that they are stable for the patient's transfer to and from the nuclear medicine department.
- Accompany the patient to the nuclear medicine department if vital signs are unstable.

PT Assure the patient that only a small amount of nuclear material will be administered.

PT Instruct the patient to notify the nuclear medicine technologist if he or she has a bowel movement during the test. Blood in the GI tract can act as a cathartic.

PT Inform the patient that no pretest preparation is required.
- Inform the nuclear medicine technologist to notify the nurse of all bloody bowel movements that occur while the patient is in the nuclear medicine department.

During

- Note the following procedural steps:
  1. Ten millicuries of freshly prepared ^{99m}Tc-labeled sulfur colloid is administered intravenously to the patient. If ^{99m}Tc-labeled RBCs are to be used, 3 to 5 ml of the patient's own blood is combined with the ^{99m}Tc and reinjected into the patient.
  2. Immediately after administration of the radionuclide, the patient is placed under a scintillation camera.
  3. Multiple images of the abdomen are obtained at short intervals (5 to 15 minutes). Scintigrams are recorded on Polaroid or x-ray film.

4. Detection of radionuclide in the abdomen indicates the site of bleeding. If no bleeding sites are noted in the first hour, the scan is repeated at hourly intervals for as long as 24 hours.

- Note that areas of the bowel hidden by the liver or spleen may not be adequately evaluated by this procedure. Also, the rectum cannot be easily evaluated, because other pelvic structures (e.g., the bladder) obstruct the view. If the initial study is negative and subsequent films give evidence of active bleeding, a repeat scan may be performed.

- Note that this test is usually performed in approximately 60 minutes by a technologist in the nuclear medicine department.

PT Tell the patient that the only discomfort associated with this study is the injection of the radioisotope.

After

- Reevaluate the patient's vital signs on return to the nursing unit.

PT Assure the patient that only tracer doses of radioisotopes have been used and that no precautions against radioactive exposure to others are necessary.

Abnormal findings

Ulcer
Tumor
Angiodysplasia
Polyps
Diverticulosis
Inflammatory bowel disease
Aortoduodenal fistula

notes

genetic testing (Breast cancer and ovarian cancer [BRCA], Colon cancer, Cardiovascular disease, Tay-Sachs disease, Cystic fibrosis, Paternity [Parentage analysis], and Forensic genetic testing)

Type of test Miscellaneous

Normal findings No genetic mutation

Test explanation and related physiology

Tests for defective genes known to be associated with certain diseases are now commonly used in screening populations of people who have certain phenotypes and a family history compatible with a genetic mutation. A family history is not always reliable, accurate, or available; however, genetic testing is very accurate in its determination of risks. Preventive medicine or surgery can be provided to eliminate disease development. Reproductive counseling and pregnancy prevention can preclude the conception of children who are likely to suffer the consequence of disease. Paternity and forensic genetic testing can accurately determine responsibility, guilt, and innocence.

This testing may be expensive and not covered by insurance. The information obtained by testing may cause great emotional turmoil in affected individuals or their family. Voluntary genetic testing should always be associated with aggressive counseling and support. Because of the potential changes in life for other family members, each person receiving the genetic information must be counseled separately.

Breast cancer and ovarian cancer genetic testing

BRCA (BReast CAncer) genes indicate an increased susceptibility for development of breast cancer. Two genes have been identified: BRCA 1 and BRCA 2. The BRCA 1 gene, the more common defect, exists on chromosome 17. BRCA 2 is on chromosome 13. These genes are responsible for the synthesis of tumor suppression proteins. More than half of women with mutations of this gene will develop breast cancer by the age of 50, as compared with less than 2% of women without the genetic defect.

The BRCA gene also confers an increased susceptibility for ovarian cancer. In the normal population, less than 2% of women develop ovarian cancer by age 70. Of women with mutations of the BRCA gene, 44% develop ovarian cancer by that age. Furthermore, a woman who has already had breast cancer and who has a BRCA genetic mutation has a 65% chance of developing a contralateral breast cancer in her lifetime (compared with less than 15% of women without the genetic defect). The woman with breast cancer and a BRCA genetic defect has a 10 times greater risk of developing ovarian cancer as a second primary cancer when compared with similar women without the mutated form of the gene.

This genetic defect is an autosomal dominant gene, indicating that women with just one genetic defect can develop the phenotypic cancers. Although men with a BRCA genetic mutation may not necessarily develop breast cancer, their risk of developing prostate and colon cancer is significantly higher. In addition, they can pass the defective gene to their daughters. Because BRCA is an autosomal dominant gene, 50% of the children are at risk.

Colon cancer genetic testing

Two common forms of colon cancer are associated with a strong familial link. The first is familial adenomatous polyposis (FAP). These patients present with hundreds of polyps in their colon—one or more of which may degenerate into cancer. The second type is hereditary nonpolyposis colorectal cancer (HNPCC). HNPCC is also known as Lynch syndrome. These patients are more difficult to recognize because they do not have polyps; colon cancers develop de novo.

FAP is caused by a genetic mutation in the 5q 21-22 (APC) gene on chromosome 5. Like BRCA genes, these genes are responsible for the synthesis of tumor-suppressor proteins. HNPCC is associated with mutations of MLH 1 and MLH 2 genes. These genes are on chromosome 5 and are important for genome stability (prevention of chromosomal breakage and exchange). HNPCC is associated with several other cancers (endometrial, gastric, and ovarian). These genetic defects are autosomal dominant.

Cardiovascular disease genetic testing

Because half of all patients with cardiovascular disease (CVD) do not have the traditional risk factors (cholesterol, obesity, diabetes, and high blood pressure), these factors alone may fall short in the identification of patients at high risk for cardiac disease. Although a family history is helpful in identifying families at risk for CVD, genetic testing is more accurate and, if confirmed, more predictive among individuals in such a family. The angiotensinogen (AGT) gene demonstrates the strongest and most consistent associations with CVD. This gene is on chromosome 1. This is an autosomal recessive gene. When a patient has just one AGT mutation, the risk of CVD is moderately elevated. When an individual has two AGT genetic mutations, the risk of CVD is nearly triple that of the general population. These patients have early-age onset of hypertension, myocardial infarction, and hypertrophic cardiomyopathy. With genetic testing of individuals in families in which CVD is predominant, early therapeutic interventions (e.g., aggressive lipid-lowering agents and aggressive use of antihypertensives) may preclude disease.

Tay-Sachs disease genetic testing

Tay-Sachs disease is characterized by the onset of severe mental and developmental retardation in the first few months of life. Affected children become totally debilitated by 2 to 5 years of age and die by ages 5 to 8. Another form of the same disease is "late-onset Tay-Sachs" or chronic GM2, also known as gangliosidosis. The basic defect in affected patients is a mutation in the hexosaminidase gene, which is on chromosome 15. This gene is responsible for the synthesis of hexosaminidase [HEX], an enzyme that normally breaks down a fatty substance called GM2 gangliosides (see p. 527). Ashkenazi (Eastern European) Jews and non-Jewish French Canadians, particularly those in the Cajun population in Louisiana, are affected most. This gene is an autosomal recessive gene. Carriers have one defective gene. Affected individuals have both defective genes. A "carrier couple" has a 25% chance of having a child affected with the disease.

At present, there is no treatment for the disease so it is important to identify carriers so that reproductive counseling can be provided. Hexosaminidase protein testing (p. 527) has been extremely effective for identification of carriers and affected individuals. However, sometimes the results of HEX protein tests are inconclusive or uncertain. Both the test for the protein and that for the gene mutation are performed on a blood sample or on chorionic villus samples obtained during amniocentesis (p. 54).

Cystic fibrosis genetic testing

Cystic fibrosis (CF) is caused by a mutation in the cystic fibrosis transmembrane conductance regulator (CFTR) gene. This gene encodes the synthesis of a protein that serves as a channel through which chloride enters and leaves cells. A mutation in this gene alters the cell's capability to regulate the chloride transport (see p. 260).

Currently six different genetic mutations can be recognized to cause CF, and these account for 90% of the cases. However, the most common mutation that accounts for 70% of the CF cases is known as the Delta AF508.

The CFTR gene is an autosomal recessive gene located on chromosome 7. A carrier has one mutated gene. The person affected by CF has both defective genes. Genetic testing is now used to identify both carriers of CF and neonates with the disease, as well as to detect fetal disease during pregnancy. The sweat chloride test (p. 886) is a more easily performed and cheaper way to diagnose the disease in affected children. The use of genetic testing for CF is often limited to those with a family history of CF, partners of CF patients, and pregnant couples with a family history of CF. The main purpose of CF genetic testing is to identify carriers who could conceive a child with CF.

It is important to recognize that not all patients who have the CF genetic mutation will develop the disease. Further, because only a few mutations that may cause CF can be detected, a negative test does not necessarily eliminate the possibility of being affected by the diseases. Genetic testing can be performed on blood samples or on samples taken during chorionic villus sampling (CVS) (p. 269) or during amniocentesis (p. 54).

Paternity genetic testing (parentage analysis)

DNA testing is the most accurate form of testing to prove or exclude paternity when the identity of the biological father of a child is in doubt. By comparing DNA characteristics of the mother and child, it is possible to determine characteristics that the child inherited from the biological mother. Thus any remaining DNA must have come from the biological father. If the DNA from the tested man is found to contain these paternal characteristics, then the probability of paternity can be determined. Testing is 99% accurate.

Testing is so reliable that it is admissible in court. Testing can be done on a mouth swab, blood, or CVS samples. Results are usually available in 1 to 3 weeks.

Many parents are given misinformation at the time of twin births as to whether the twins are identical or fraternal. DNA samples from siblings can be analyzed to indicate twinship with an accuracy of 99%.

Forensic genetic testing

Forensic DNA testing is used with increasing frequency in today's courtrooms because of its accuracy. In a courtroom, the reliability of the evidence can protect the individual and society as a whole. Further, DNA testing can be so conclusive that it often motivates plea-bargaining and thereby reduces court time. It can quickly establish guilt or innocence beyond a reasonable doubt. Because DNA does not change or deteriorate even after death, testing can be performed on any body part, cadaver, or live person. Specimens considered adequate for DNA testing include blood, teeth, semen, saliva, bone, nails, skin scrapings, and hair. Forensic testing is also used for body identification.

Contraindications

- Patients who are not emotionally able to deal with the results

Procedure and patient care

Before

- PT Explain the procedure to the patient.
- PT Tell the patient that no fasting is required.
- It is recommended that all patients who undergo testing should receive genetic counseling.
- PT Indicate to the patient the time it will take to have the results back.
- PT Ensure that the patient is well aware of the high costs of genetic testing and that it may not be covered by all medical insurance plans.

During

- Obtain the specimen in a manner provided by the specialized testing laboratory.

Blood: (collected in a lavender-top tube)
Adult: 0.5 to 7 ml
Child: 0.5 to 3 ml
Infant: 0.5 ml. This can be cord blood.

Buccal swab: A cotton swab is placed between the lower cheek and gums. It is twisted and then placed on a special paper or in a special container. Usually two to four swabs are requested.

Amniotic fluid: At least 20 ml of fluid is preferred.

Chorionic villus sampling: 10 mg of cleaned villi are sent as prescribed by the testing laboratory.

Product of conception: 10 mg of placental tissue is preserved in a sterile medium.

Other body parts: As much tissue as is available is sent for testing.

After

- Apply pressure or a pressure dressing to the venipuncture site.
- Make sure that the patient has an appointment scheduled for obtaining the results. It is very upsetting for a patient and family to wait for the results. They should have a definite appointment made at a time that the results will be assuredly available.
- Arrangements should be made to ensure genetic and emotional counseling after results are obtained.

Abnormal findings

Genetic carrier state
Affected state

notes

gliadin antibodies, endomysial antibodies

Type of test Blood

Normal findings

	Age	Normal
Gliadin IgA/IgG	0-2 years	<20 EU
	3 years and older	<25 EU
Endomysial IgA	All	negative

Test explanation and related physiology

Gliadin and gluten are proteins found in wheat and wheat products. Patients with celiac disease and celiac sprue cannot tolerate ingestion of these proteins or any products containing wheat. These proteins are toxic to the mucosa of the small intestine and cause characteristic pathologic lesions. These patients experience severe intestinal malabsorption symptoms. The only treatment is for the patient to abstain from wheat and wheat-containing products.

When an affected patient ingests wheat-containing foods, gluten and gliadin build up in the intestinal mucosa. These gliadin and gluten proteins (and their metabolites) cause direct mucosal damage. Furthermore, immunoglobulins (particularly IgG and IgA) are made and they appear in the gut mucosa and in the serum of severely affected patients. The identification of these antibodies in the blood of patients with malabsorption is helpful in supporting the diagnosis of celiac sprue. However, a definitive diagnosis of celiac disease or celiac sprue can be made only when a patient with malabsorption is found to have the pathologic intestinal lesions characteristic of celiac disease and is improved with a gluten-free diet.

In patients with known celiac disease, these antibodies can be used to monitor disease status and dietary compliance. Not all patients with celiac disease have IgG, and fewer still have IgA antibodies. Patients with dermatitis herpetiformis have celiac disease and dermatitis.

Endomysial antibodies are even more accurate in identifying patients with celiac disease. About 70% of patients with dermatitis herpetiformis and 100% of patients with celiac disease will have IgA endomysial antibodies. Furthermore, these antibodies identify successful treatment, as they will become negative in patients on a gluten-free diet. Both the gliadin and endomysial antibodies are measured with the enzyme-linked immunosorbent assay (ELISA).

Interfering factors

- Other GI diseases such as Crohn's disease, colitis, and severe lactose intolerance can cause elevated gliadin antibodies.

Procedure and patient care

Before
PT Explain the procedure to the patient.
PT Tell the patient that no fasting is required.
- Obtain a list of foods that have been ingested in the last 48 hours.
- Assess how many malabsorption symptoms the patient has been experiencing in the last few weeks.

During
- Draw 5 to 7 ml of venous blood in a red-top tube.

After
- Apply pressure to the venipuncture site.
- Assess the venipuncture site for bleeding.

Abnormal findings

Celiac disease
Celiac sprue
Nontropical sprue
Dermatitis herpetiformis

notes

glucagon

Type of test Blood

Normal findings 50-100 pg/ml or 50-100 ng/L (SI units)

Test explanation and related physiology

Glucagon is a hormone secreted by the alpha cells of the pancreatic islets of Langerhans. It is secreted in response to hypoglycemia and increases the blood glucose. As serum glucose levels rise in the blood, glucagon is inhibited by a negative feedback mechanism.

Elevated glucagon levels may indicate the diagnosis of a *glucagonoma* (i.e., an alpha islet cell neoplasm). Glucagon deficiency occurs with extensive pancreatic resection or with burned-out pancreatitis. Arginine is a potent stimulator of glucagon. If glucagon levels fail to rise even with arginine infusion, a diagnosis of glucagon deficiency as a result of pancreatic insufficiency is confirmed.

In an insulin-dependent patient with diabetes, glucagon stimulation caused by hypoglycemia does not occur. To differentiate the causes of glucagon insufficiency (between pancreatic insufficiency and diabetes), *arginine stimulation* is performed. Patients with diabetes will have an exaggerated elevation of glucagon with arginine. In pancreatic insufficiency, glucagon is not stimulated with arginine. Further, in patients with diabetes, hypoglycemia fails to stimulate glucagon release as would occur in a nondiabetic person.

Because glucagon is thought to be metabolized by the kidneys, renal failure is associated with high glucagon and, as a result, high glucose levels. When rejection of a transplanted kidney occurs, one of the first signs of rejection may be increased serum glucagon levels.

Interfering factors

- Test results may be invalidated if a patient has undergone a radioactive scan within the previous 48 hours.
- Levels may be elevated after prolonged fasting or moderate to severe exercise.
- ✶ Drugs that may cause *increased* levels include some amino acids (e.g., arginine), danazol, glucocorticoids, gastrin, insulin, and nifedipine.

♦ Drugs that may cause *decreased* levels include atenolol, propranolol, and secretin.

Procedure and patient care

Before

PT Explain the procedure to the patient.
PT Tell the patient that fasting is necessary for 10 to 12 hours before the test. Only water is permitted.

During

- Collect a venous blood sample in a lavender-top tube.

After

- Apply pressure to the venipuncture site.
- Place the specimen on ice and send it immediately to the laboratory.

Abnormal findings

▲ **Increased levels**

Familial hyperglucagonemia
Glucagonoma
Diabetes mellitus
Chronic renal failure
Severe stress including
  infection, burns, surgery,
  and acute hypoglycemia
Acromegaly
Hyperlipidemia
Acute pancreatitis
Pheochromocytoma

▼ **Decreased levels**

Idiopathic glucagon
  deficiency
Cystic fibrosis
Chronic pancreatitis
Postpancreatectomy
Cancer of the pancreas

notes

glucose, blood (Blood sugar, Fasting blood sugar [FBS])

Type of test   Blood

Normal findings

Cord: 45-96 mg/dl or 2.5-5.3 mmol/L (SI units)
Premature infant: 20-60 mg/dl or 1.1-3.3 mmol/L
Neonate: 30-60 mg/dl or 1.7-3.3 mmol/L
Infant: 40-90 mg/dl or 2.2-5.0 mmol/L
Child <2 years: 60-100 mg/dl or 3.3-5.5 mmol/L
Child >2 years to adult: 70-105 mg/dl or 3.9-5.8 mmol/L
Elderly: increase in normal range after age 50 years

Possible critical values

Adult male: <50 and >400 mg/dl
Adult female: <40 and >400 mg/dl
Infant: <40 mg/dl
Newborn: <30 and >300 mg/dl

Test explanation and related physiology

Through an elaborate feedback mechanism, glucose levels are controlled by insulin and glucagon. In the fasting state, glucose levels are low. In response, glucagon is secreted. Glucagon causes glucose levels to rise.

After eating, glucose levels are elevated. Insulin is secreted. Insulin drives glucose into the cells to be metabolized to glycogen, amino acids, and fatty acids. Blood glucose levels diminish. Many other hormones such as adrenocorticosteroids, adrenocorticotropic hormone, epinephrine, and thyroxine can also affect glucose metabolism.

Serum glucose levels must be evaluated according to the time of day they are performed. For example, a glucose level of 135 mg/dl may be abnormal if the patient is in the fasting state, but this level would be within normal limits if the patient had eaten a meal within the last hour.

In general, true glucose elevations indicate diabetes mellitus; however, one must be aware of many other possible causes of hyperglycemia. Similarly, hypoglycemia has many causes. The most common cause is inadvertent insulin overdose in patients with brittle diabetes. If diabetes is suspected by elevated fasting blood levels, glycosylated hemoglobin (p. 496) or glucose tolerance tests (p. 492) can be performed.

Glucose determinations must be performed frequently in new patients with diabetes to monitor closely the insulin dosage to be administered. Fingerstick blood glucose determinations are often performed before meals and at bedtime. Results are compared with a sliding-scale insulin chart ordered by the physician to provide coverage with SQ Regular insulin.

Interfering factors

- Many forms of stress (e.g., general anesthesia, cerebrovascular accident, myocardial infarction) can cause increased serum glucose levels.
- Most IV fluids contain dextrose, which is quickly converted to glucose. Therefore, most patients receiving IV fluids will have increased glucose levels.
- Many pregnant women experience some degree of glucose intolerance. If significant, it is called gestational diabetes.
- Drugs that may cause *increased* levels include antidepressants (tricyclics), beta-adrenergic–blocking agents, corticosteroids, dextrose IV infusion, dextrothyroxine, diazoxide, diuretics, epinephrine, estrogens, glucagon, isoniazid, lithium, phenothiazines, phenytoin, salicylates (acute toxicity), and triamterene.
- Drugs that may cause *decreased* levels include acetaminophen, alcohol, anabolic steroids, clofibrate, disopyramide, gemfibrozil, insulin, monoamine oxidase inhibitors, pentamidine, propranolol, tolazamide, and tolbutamide.

Procedure and patient care

Before

PT Explain the procedure to the patient.
- For FBS, keep the patient fasting at least 8 hours. Water is permitted.
- To prevent starvation, which may artificially raise the glucose levels, the patient should not fast longer than 16 hours.
- Withhold insulin or oral hypoglycemics until after blood is obtained.

During

- Collect approximately 7 ml of venous blood in a red- or gray-top tube.
- Glucose levels also can be evaluated by performing a fingerstick and using either a visually read or a reflectance meter. The advantage of the *visually read* test is that it does

not require an expensive machine. However, the patient must be able to visually interpret the color of the reagent strip. Using *reflectance meters* (e.g., Glucometer, Accu Check bG, Stat Tek) improves the accuracy of the blood glucose determination. However, this method is more complex because it requires machine calibration and control testing.

After
- Apply pressure to the venipuncture site.
- Be certain that the patient receives a meal after fasting blood work.

Abnormal findings

▲ **Increased levels (hyperglycemia)**

Diabetes mellitus
Acute stress response
Cushing's syndrome
Pheochromocytoma
Chronic renal failure
Glucagonoma
Acute pancreatitis
Diuretic therapy
Corticosteroid therapy
Acromegaly

▼ **Decreased levels (hypoglycemia)**

Insulinoma
Hypothyroidism
Hypopituitarism
Addison's disease
Extensive liver disease
Insulin overdose
Starvation

notes

glucose, postprandial (2-hour postprandial glucose [2-hour PPG], 2-hour postprandial blood sugar, 1-hour glucose screen for gestational diabetes mellitus, O'Sullivan test)

Type of test Blood

Normal findings

2-hour PPG

0-50 years: <140 mg/dl or <7.8 mmol/L (SI units)
50-60 years: <150 mg/dl
60 years and older: <160 mg/dl

1-hour glucose screen for gestational diabetes

<140 mg/dl

Test explanation and related physiology

For this study a meal acts as a glucose challenge to the body's metabolism. Normally, insulin is secreted immediately after a meal in response to the elevated blood glucose level, causing the level to return to the premeal range within 2 hours. In patients with diabetes, the glucose level usually is still elevated 2 hours after the meal. The PPG is an easily performed screening test for diabetes mellitus. If the results are greater than 140 mg/dl and less than 200 mg/dl, a glucose tolerance test (see p. 492) may be performed to confirm the diagnosis. If the 2-hour PPG is greater than 200 mg/dl, a diagnosis of diabetes mellitus is confirmed.

The *1-hour glucose screen* is used to detect gestational diabetes mellitus (GDM). GDM affects 3% to 8% of pregnant women, with up to half of these women developing overt diabetes later in life. The detection and treatment of GDM may reduce the risk for several adverse perinatal outcomes (such as excessive fetal growth and birth trauma, fetal death, or neonatal morbidity).

Screening for GDM is performed with a 50-g oral glucose load, followed by a glucose level determination 1 hour later. This is called the *O'Sullivan test*. Screening is done between weeks 24 and 28 of gestation. However, patients with risk factors, such as a previous history of GDM, may benefit from earlier screening. Patients whose serum glucose level equals or exceeds 140 mg/dl should be evaluated by a 3-hour glucose tolerance test (GTT) (see p. 492).

Interfering factors

- Stress can increase glucose levels.

- If the patient is not able to eat the entire test meal, or vomits some or all of the meal, levels will be falsely decreased.

Procedure and patient care

Before

PT For the *2-hour PPG*, instruct the patient to eat the entire meal (with at least 75 g of carbohydrates) and then not to eat anything else until the blood is drawn.

- For the *1-hour glucose screen for GDM*, give the fasting or nonfasting patient a 50-g oral glucose load.

PT Instruct the patient not to smoke during the testing. Smoking may increase glucose levels.

PT Inform the patient that he or she should rest during the 1- or 2-hour interval.

During

- Collect approximately 7 ml of blood in a red- or gray-top tube 1 or 2 hours after the patient has eaten the test meal.

After

- Apply pressure to the venipuncture site.

Abnormal findings

▲ Increased levels	▼ Decreased levels
Diabetes mellitus	Insulinoma
Gestational diabetes mellitus	Hypothyroidism
Malnutrition	Hypopituitarism
Hyperthyroidism	Addison's disease
Acute stress response	Insulin overdose
Cushing's syndrome	Malabsorption or
Pheochromocytoma	maldigestion
Chronic renal failure	
Glucagonoma	
Diuretic therapy	
Corticosteroid therapy	
Acromegaly	
Extensive liver disease	

notes

glucose, urine (Urine sugar, Urine glucose)

Type of test Urine

Normal findings

Random specimen: negative
24-hour specimen: <0.5 g/day or <2.78 mmol/day (SI units)

Test explanation and related physiology

A qualitative glucose test is usually part of a routine urinalysis. This screening test for the presence of glucose within the urine may indicate the likelihood of diabetes mellitus or other causes of glucose intolerance (see glucose, p. 482). This diagnosis must be confirmed by other tests (e.g., glucose tolerance test). Urine glucose tests are also used to monitor the effectiveness of diabetes therapy; however, today this is largely supplanted by finger-stick determinations of blood glucose levels.

Glucose is filtered from the blood by the glomeruli of the kidney. Normally, all of the glucose is resorbed in the proximal renal tubules. When the blood glucose level exceeds the capability of the renal threshold to resorb the glucose (normally, around 180 mg/dl), it begins to spill over into the urine (glycosuria). As the blood glucose level increases further, greater amounts of glucose are spilled into the urine.

Glucosuria is not always abnormal. It may occur immediately after eating a high-carbohydrate meal. It can also occur in patients receiving dextrose-containing IV fluids. In patients who do not have diabetes, glucosuria can occur with a normal serum glucose level when kidney diseases affect the renal tubule. The renal threshold for glucose becomes abnormally low, and glucosuria occurs.

Interfering factors

- Any substance that can reduce the copper in Clinitest can produce positive results. This may include other sugars such as galactose, fructose, or lactose.
- Drugs that may cause false-positive tests with Clinitest but not with Clinistix or Tes-Tape include acetylsalicylic acid, aminosalicylic acid, ascorbic acid, cephalothin, chloral hydrate, nitrofurantoin, streptomycin, and sulfonamides.
- Drugs that may cause false-negative tests include ascorbic acid (Clinistix, Tes-Tape), levodopa (Clinistix), and phenazopyridine (Clinistix, Tes-Tape).

☙ Drugs that may cause *increased* urine glucose levels include aminosalicylic acid, cephalosporins, chloral hydrate, chloramphenicol, dextrothyroxine, diazoxide, diuretics (loop and thiazide), estrogens, glucose infusions, isoniazid, levodopa, lithium, nafcillin, nalidixic acid, and nicotinic acid (large doses).

Procedure and patient care

Before

PT Explain the procedure to the patient.

- Read the directions on the bottle or container of the reagent strips.
- Check the expiration date on the bottle before use.

PT Inform the patient that urine tests for glucose may be performed at specified times during the day, generally before meals and at bedtime, and that test results may be used to determine insulin requirements.

During

- Because accuracy is necessary, collect a "fresh" urine specimen. Stagnant urine that has been in the bladder for several hours will not accurately reflect the serum glucose level at testing.
- Preferably, obtain a *double-voided specimen*:
  1. Collect a urine specimen 30 to 40 minutes before the time the urine specimen is actually needed.
  2. Discard this first specimen.
  3. Give the patient a glass of water to drink.
  4. At the required time, obtain a second specimen, which is tested for glucose.

PT Inform the patient that testing for glucose can be performed easily using enzyme tests such as Clinistix, Diastix, or Tes-Tape.

- Remember that urine glucose also can be determined using the Clinitest method (a copper-reducing approach).
- If a 24-hour specimen is required, refrigerate the urine during the collection period.

After

- Record the urine glucose results on the patient's chart.

Abnormal findings

▲   **Increased levels**

Diabetes mellitus

Pregnancy

Renal glycosuria

Hereditary defects in metabolism of other reducing
substance (e.g., galactose, fructose, pentose)

Nephrotoxic chemicals (e.g., carbon monoxide, mercury,
lead)

G

notes

glucose-6-phosphate dehydrogenase (G-6-PD screen)

Type of test Blood

Normal findings

Negative (screening test)

12.1 ± 2 international units/g of hemoglobin

Test explanation and related physiology

Glucose-6-phosphate dehydrogenase (G-6-PD) is an enzyme used in glucose metabolism. In the red blood cell a G-6-PD deficiency causes precipitation of hemoglobin and cellular membrane changes. This may result in hemolysis of variable severity. This disease is a sex-linked trait carried on the X chromosome. Affected males inherit this abnormal gene from their mothers, who are usually asymptomatic. In these males the disease consequence is most severe. Heterozygous women have variable expressions of the disease, from no symptoms to moderate symptoms if under a significant degree of stimulation.

In patients with G-6-PD deficiency, oxidizing drugs such as antimalarials, sulfa, aspirin, phenacetin, antipyretics, quinidine, sulfonamides, thiazide diuretics, tolbutamide (Orinase), and others can cause red blood cell destruction and hemolysis. Hemolysis may start as early as the first day and usually by the fourth day after drug ingestion. Infections or acidosis can also precipitate a hemolytic process in these patients. Certain foods (e.g., fava beans) are oxidizing and therefore are harmful to the G-6-PD–deficient patient. This test is used to diagnose G-6-PD deficiency in suspected individuals.

Interfering factors

- With the dye reduction and glutathione screening test, reticulocytosis (often associated with a hemolytic episode) may be associated with false high levels of G-6-PD.

Procedure and patient care

Before

PT Explain the procedure to the patient.

PT Tell the patient that no fasting is required.

During

- Collect approximately 5 ml of venous blood in a lavender- or green-top tube.
- Avoid hemolysis.

After

- Apply pressure to the venipuncture site.
- **PT** If the test indicates a G-6-PD deficiency, give the patient a list of drugs that may precipitate hemolysis. Instruct patients with the Mediterranean type of this disease not to eat fava beans. Teach patients to read labels on any over-the-counter drugs for the presence of agents (e.g., aspirin, phenacetin) that may cause hemolytic anemia.

Abnormal findings

▲ **Increased levels**

   Pernicious anemia

   Megaloblastic anemia

   Chronic blood loss

   Myocardial infarction

   Hepatic coma

   Hyperthyroidism

▼ **Decreased levels**

   G-6-PD deficiency

   Hemolytic anemia

   Unusual nonspherocytic anemias

notes

glucose tolerance test (GTT, Oral glucose tolerance test [OGTT])

Type of test   Blood; urine

Normal findings

Serum test

Fasting: 70-115 mg/dl or <6.4 mmol/L (SI units)
30 minutes: <200 mg/dl or <11.1 mmol/L
1 hour: <200 mg/dl or <11.1 mmol/L
2 hours: <140 mg/dl or <7.8 mmol/L
3 hours: 70-115 mg/dl or <6.4 mmol/L
4 hours: 70-115 mg/dl or <6.4 mmol/L

Urine test

Negative

Test explanation and related physiology

A normal fasting blood glucose, but a GTT peak and 2-hour value of greater than 200 mg/100 ml on more than one occasion, is one of the criteria of the National Diabetes Data Group (NDDG) for the diagnosis of DM. The GTT is used when diabetes is suspected (retinopathy, neuropathy, diabetic-type renal diseases). It is also suggested for the following:

Patients with a family history of diabetes
Patients who are massively obese
Patients with a history of recurrent infections
Patients with delayed healing of wounds (especially on the lower legs or feet)
Women who have a history of delivering large babies, stillbirths, or neonatal births
Patients who have transient glycosuria or hyperglycemia during pregnancy, or following myocardial infarction, surgery, or stress

In the GTT, the patient's ability to tolerate a standard oral glucose load is evaluated by obtaining serum and urine specimens for glucose level determinations before glucose administration and then at 30 minutes, 1 hour, 2 hours, 3 hours, and sometimes 4 hours afterward. Normally, there is a rapid insulin response to the ingestion of a large oral glucose load. This response peaks in 30 to 60 minutes and returns to normal in about 3 hours. Patients with an appropriate insulin response are able to tolerate the glucose load quite easily, with only a minimal and transient rise in serum glucose levels within 1 to 2 hours after ingestion. In normal patients, glucose does not spill over into the urine.

Patients with diabetes will not be able to tolerate this load. As a result, their serum glucose levels will be greatly elevated from 1 to 5 hours (Figure 21). Also, glucose can be detected in their urine. It is important to note that intestinal absorption may vary among individuals. For this reason, some centers prefer the glucose load to be administered intravenously.

The American Diabetes Association recommends that pregnant women who have not previously had an abnormal GTT should be tested at the 24th and 28th weeks of gestation with a 50-g dose of glucose. This is called the *O'Sullivan test.* A glucose level of more than 140 mg/100 ml one hour later suggests that these women should be retested with a nonpregnant GTT 6 weeks or more after delivery.

Glucose intolerance also may exist in patients with oversecretion of hormones that have an ancillary effect on glucose, such as in patients with Cushing's syndrome, pheochromocytoma, acromegaly, aldosteronism, or hyperthyroidism. Patients with chronic renal failure, acute pancreatitis, myxedema, type IV lipoproteinemia, infection, or cirrhosis can also have an abnormal GTT. Certain drugs mentioned in the following paragraphs can also cause abnormal GTT results.

The GTT also is used to evaluate patients with reactive hypoglycemia. This may occur as late as 5 hours after the initial glucose load.

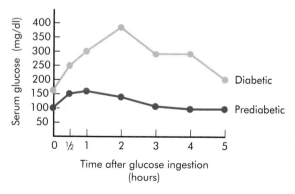

Figure 21 Glucose tolerance test curve for a diabetic and a pre-diabetic patient.

Contraindications

- Patients with serious concurrent infections or endocrine disorders, because glucose intolerance will be observed even though these patients may not have diabetes

Potential complications

- Dizziness, tremors, anxiety, sweating, euphoria, or fainting during testing
  If these symptoms occur, a blood specimen is obtained. If the glucose level is too high, the test may need to be stopped and insulin administered.

Interfering factors

- Smoking during the testing period stimulates glucose production because of the nicotine.
- Stress (e.g., from surgery, infection) can increase glucose levels.
- Exercise during the testing can affect glucose levels.
- Fasting or reduced caloric intake before GTT can cause glucose intolerance.
- ⚕ Drugs that may cause glucose intolerance include antihypertensives, antiinflammatory drugs, aspirin, beta-blockers, furosemide, nicotine, oral contraceptives, psychiatric drugs, steroids, and thiazide diuretics.

Procedure and patient care

Before

- **PT** Explain the procedure to the patient.
- **PT** Educate the patient about the importance of having adequate food intake with adequate carbohydrates (150 g) for at least 3 days before the test.
- **PT** Instruct the patient to fast for 12 hours before the test.
- **PT** Instruct the patient to discontinue drugs (including tobacco) that could interfere with the test results. This should be done in consultation with the physician.
- **PT** Give the patient written instructions explaining the pretest dietary requirement.
- Obtain the patient's weight to determine the appropriate glucose loading dose (especially in children).

During

- Obtain fasting blood and urine specimens.
- Administer the oral glucose solution, usually a 75- to 100-g carbohydrate load.

- Give pediatric patients a carbohydrate load of 1.75 g/kg body weight, up to a maximum of 75 g.
- **PT** Instruct the patient to ingest the entire glucose load.
- **PT** Tell the patient that he or she cannot eat anything until the test is completed. However, encourage the patient to drink water. No other liquids should be taken.
- **PT** Inform the patient that tobacco, coffee, and tea are not allowed because they cause physiologic stimulation.
- Collect approximately 5 ml of venous blood in a gray-top tube at 30 minutes and at hourly periods. Apply pressure or a pressure dressing to the sites.
- Collect urine specimens at hourly periods.
- Mark on the tubes the time that the specimens are collected.
- Assess the patient for reactions such as dizziness, sweating, weakness, and giddiness. (These are usually transient.)
- For the IV-GTT, administer the glucose load intravenously over 3 to 4 minutes.
- Indicate on the laboratory slip any drugs that may affect test results.

G

After
- Send all specimens promptly to the laboratory.
- Allow the patient to eat and drink normally.
- Administer insulin or oral hypoglycemics if ordered.
- Apply pressure to the venipuncture site.

Abnormal findings

Diabetes mellitus
Acute stress response
Cushing's syndrome
Pheochromocytoma
Chronic renal failure
Glucagonoma
Acute pancreatitis
Diuretic therapy
Corticosteroid therapy
Acromegaly
Myxedema
Somogyi response to hypoglycemia
Postgastrectomy

notes

glycosylated hemoglobin (GHb, GHB, Glycohemoglobin, Glycolated hemoglobin, Hemoglobin [Hb] A$_{1c}$, Diabetic control index)

Type of test   Blood

Normal findings

Vary with laboratory method used

Nondiabetic adult: 2.2%-4.8%

Nondiabetic child: 1.8%-4%

Good diabetic control: 2.5%-5.9%

Fair diabetic control: 6%-8%

Poor diabetic control: >8%

Test explanation and related physiology

This test is used to monitor diabetes treatment. It measures the amount of hemoglobin A$_{1c}$ (HbA$_{1c}$) in the blood and provides an accurate long-term index of the patient's average blood glucose level. In adults, about 98% of the hemoglobin in the red blood cells (RBCs) is hemoglobin A. About 7% of hemoglobin A consists of a type of hemoglobin (HbA$_1$) that can combine strongly with glucose in a process called "glycosylation." Once glycosylation occurs, it is not easily reversible.

Hemoglobin A$_1$ is actually made up of three components: HbA$_{1a}$, A$_{1b}$, and A$_{1c}$. Hemoglobin A$_{1c}$ is the component that combines most strongly with glucose. Therefore, HgA$_{1c}$ is the most accurate measurement because it contains the majority of glycosylated hemoglobin. If the total HgbA$_1$ is measured, its value is 2% to 4% higher than the HgA$_{1c}$ component.

The amount of glycosylated hemoglobin (glycohemoglobin [GHb]) depends on the amount of glucose available in the bloodstream over the RBC's 120-day life span. Therefore, determination of the GHb value reflects the average blood sugar level for the 100- to 120-day period before the test. The more glucose the RBC was exposed to, the greater the GHb percentage. One important advantage of this test is that the sample can be drawn at any time because it is not affected by short-term variations (e.g., food intake, exercise, stress, hypoglycemic agents, patient cooperation).

As mentioned, the average life span of an RBC is 120 days, so the GHb may not reflect more recent changes in glucose levels. Because the turnover rate of proteins is much faster than hemoglobin, the measurement of serum *glycated proteins* (such as *glycated albumin* or *fructosamine*) provides more recent information about glucose levels. Glycated proteins reflect an average blood glucose level of the past 15 to 20 days. Although an initial single glycated protein result may not separate good glucose control from poor control, serial testing provides a much better indication of glucose control.

The GHb or glycated protein tests are particularly beneficial for the following:

1. Evaluating the success and patient compliance of diabetic treatment
2. Comparing and contrasting the success of past and new forms of diabetic therapy
3. Determining the duration of hyperglycemia in patients with newly diagnosed diabetes
4. Providing a sensitive estimate of glucose imbalance in patients with mild diabetes
5. Individualizing diabetic control regimens
6. Providing a feeling of reward for many patients when the test shows achievement of good diabetic control
7. Evaluating the diabetic patient whose glucose levels change significantly day to day (brittle diabetic)
8. Differentiating short-term hyperglycemia in patients who do not have diabetes (e.g., recent stress or myocardial infarction) from those who have diabetes (where the glucose has been persistently elevated)

Interfering factors

- Hemoglobinopathies can affect results because the quantity of hemoglobin A (and, as a result, HbA_1) varies considerably in these diseases.
- Falsely elevated values occur when the RBC life span is lengthened because the hemoglobin A_1 has a longer period available for glycosylation.
- Abnormally low levels of proteins may falsely indicate normal glycated protein levels, despite the reality of high glucose levels.

Procedure and patient care

Before

PT Explain the procedure to the patient.
PT Tell the patient that fasting is not indicated.

During
- Collect approximately 5 ml of venous blood in a gray- or lavender-top tube.

After
- Apply pressure to the venipuncture site.

Abnormal findings

▲ **Increased levels**

Newly diagnosed diabetic
  patient
Poorly controlled diabetic
  patient
Nondiabetic hyperglycemia
  (e.g., acute stress response,
  Cushing's syndrome,
  pheochromocytoma,
  glucagonoma, corticosteroid
  therapy, or acromegaly)
Splenectomized patients
Pregnancy

▼ **Decreased levels**

Hemolytic anemia
Chronic blood loss
Chronic renal failure

notes

growth hormone (GH, Human growth hormone [HGH], Somatotropin hormone [SH])

Type of test Blood

Normal findings

Men: <5 ng/ml or <5 mcg/L (SI units)
Women: <10 ng/ml or <10 mcg/L
Children: 0-10 ng/ml or 0-10 mcg/L
Newborn: 10-40 ng/ml or 10-40 mcg/L

G

Test explanation and related physiology

This test is used to identify growth hormone (GH) deficiency in adolescents who have short stature, delayed sexual maturity, or other growth deficiencies. It is also used to document the diagnosis of GH excess in gigantic or acromegalic patients. Finally, it is often used as a screening test for pituitary hypofunction.

GH, or somatotropin, is secreted by the acidophilic cells in the anterior pituitary gland and plays a central role in modulating growth from birth until the end of puberty. GH exerts its effects on many tissues through a group of peptides called somatomedins. The most commonly tested somatomedin is somatomedin C, which is produced by the liver and has its major effect on cartilage.

If GH secretion is insufficient during childhood, limited growth and dwarfism may result. Also, a delay in sexual maturity may be a result in adolescents with reduced GH levels. Conversely, overproduction of GH during childhood results in gigantism, with the person reaching nearly 7 to 8 feet in height. An excess of GH during adulthood (after closure of long bone end plates) results in acromegaly, which is characterized by an increase in bone thickness and width but no increase in height.

GH tests are also used to confirm hypopituitarism or hyperpituitarism.

Normal GH levels overlap significantly with deficient levels. Low GH levels may indicate deficiency or may be normal for certain individuals at certain times of the day. To negate time variables in GH testing, GH can be drawn 1 to 1½ hours after deep sleep has occurred. Levels increase during sleep. Also, strenuous exercise can be performed for 30 minutes in an effort to stimulate GH production.

To negate the common variations in GH secretion, screening for *insulin-like growth factor (IGF-1)* or *somatomedin C* (see p. 868) provides a more accurate reflection of the mean plasma concentration of growth hormone. These proteins are not affected by the time of day or food intake as is GH. A GH stimulation test (see p. 502) can be performed to evaluate the body's ability to produce growth hormone. *Growth hormone suppression testing* is used to identify gigantism in children or acromegaly in the adult.

Interfering factors

- Random measurements of growth hormone are not adequate determinants of GH deficiency, because hormone secretion is episodic.
- A radioactive scan performed within the week before the test may affect test results because levels are determined by radioimmunoassay.
- GH secretion is increased by stress, exercise, and low blood glucose levels.
- ✗ Drugs that may cause *increased* levels include amphetamines, arginine, dopamine, estrogens, glucagon, histamine, insulin, levodopa, methyldopa, and nicotinic acid.
- ✗ Drugs that may cause *decreased* levels include corticosteroids and phenothiazines.

Procedure and patient care

Before
PT Explain the procedure to the patient.
- The patient should not be emotionally or physically stressed because this can increase GH levels.
- It is preferred that the patient be fasting and well rested. Water is permitted.
- For *GH suppression testing*, the patient is kept NPO after midnight.

During
- Collect one red-top tube of venous blood.
- Because approximately two thirds of the total production of GH occurs during sleep, GH secretion also can be measured during hospitalization by obtaining blood samples while the patient is sleeping.

Growth hormone suppression test
- Obtain peripheral venous access with NSS.
- Obtain baseline GH and glucose levels as described above.
- Administer 75 to 100 g of glucose (Glucola) over 5 minutes.
- Obtain GH and glucose levels at 30, 60, 90, and 120 minutes after glucose ingestion.

After
- Indicate the patient's fasting status and the time the blood is collected on the laboratory slip. Include the patient's recent activity (e.g., sleeping, walking, eating).
- Send the blood to the laboratory immediately after collection because the half-life of GH is only 20 to 25 minutes.

Abnormal findings

▲ **Increased levels**

Gigantism
Acromegaly
Diabetes mellitus
Anorexia nervosa
Stress
Major surgery
Hypoglycemia
Starvation
Deep-sleep state
Exercise

▼ **Decreased levels**

Pituitary insufficiency
Dwarfism
Hyperglycemia
Failure to thrive
Growth hormone
  deficiency

notes

growth hormone stimulation test (GH provocation test, Insulin tolerance test [ITT], Arginine test)

Type of test Blood

Normal findings Growth hormone levels >10 ng/ml or >10 mcg/L (SI units)

Test explanation and related physiology

Because growth hormone (GH) (see p. 499) secretion is episodic, a random measurement of plasma GH is not adequate to make a diagnosis of GH deficiency. To diagnose GH deficiency, GH stimulation tests are needed. One of the most reliable GH stimulators is insulin-induced hypoglycemia, in which the blood glucose declines to less than 40 mg/dl. Other GH stimulants include vigorous exercise and drugs (such as arginine, glucagon, levodopa, and clonidine).

Usually a *double-stimulated test* is performed using an arginine infusion followed by insulin-induced hypoglycemia. A GH concentration more than 10 mcg/L after stimulation effectively excludes the diagnosis of GH deficiency.

Contraindications

- Patients with epilepsy
- Patients with cerebrovascular disease
- Patients with myocardial infarction
- Patients with low basal plasma cortisol levels

Potential complications

- Hypoglycemia so significant and severe as to cause ketosis, acidosis, and shock.
  With close observation this is unlikely.

Interfering factors

- A radioactive scan performed within 1 week before the test may affect test results.

Procedure and patient care

Before
PT Explain the procedure very carefully to the patient and, if appropriate, to the parents.
PT Instruct the patient to remain NPO after midnight on the morning of the test. Water is permitted.

During

- Note the following procedural steps:
  1. A heparin lock IV line is inserted for the administration of medications and the withdrawal of frequent blood samples.
  2. Baseline blood levels are obtained for GH, glucose, and cortisol.
  3. Venous samples for GH are obtained at 0, 60, and 90 minutes after injection of arginine and/or insulin.
  4. Blood glucose levels are monitored at 15- to 30-minute intervals with the glucometer. The blood sugar should drop to less than 40 mg/dl for effective measurement of GH reserve.

- Monitor the patient for signs of hypoglycemia, postural hypotension, somnolence, diaphoresis, and nervousness. Ice chips are often given during the test for patient comfort.
- This procedure is usually performed by a nurse with a physician in proximity.
- This test takes approximately 2 hours to perform.
- **PT** Tell the patient that the minor discomfort associated with this test results from the insertion of the IV line and the hypoglycemic response induced by the insulin injection.
- GH also can be stimulated by vigorous exercise. This entails running or stair-climbing for 20 minutes. Blood samples of GH are obtained at 0, 20, and 40 minutes.

After

- Observe the venipuncture site for bleeding.
- Send the blood to the laboratory immediately after collection, because the half-life of GH is only 20 to 25 minutes.
- Give the patient cookies and punch or an IV glucose infusion.
- **PT** Inform the patient and family that results may not be available for approximately 7 days. Many laboratories run GH tests only once per week.

Abnormal findings

GH deficiency
Pituitary deficiency

Ham's test (Acid serum test for paroxysmal nocturnal hemoglobinuria [PNH])

Type of test Blood

Normal findings No hemolysis of red blood cells

Test explanation and related physiology

Ham's test is used to diagnose paroxysmal nocturnal hemoglobinuria (PNH). PNH is an acquired bone marrow stem cell defect. It affects the white blood cells (WBCs), red blood cells (RBCs), and platelets. Patients with this defect have evidence of hemolysis. When the WBCs, RBCs, and platelets are affected, the patient can develop aplastic anemia.

In patients with PNH, intravascular hemolysis of RBCs intermittently occurs during sleep. The RBCs of patients with PNH are more likely to lyse in an acid pH than are the RBCs of normal patients.

Contraindications

- Patients with recent blood transfusions

Procedure and patient care

Before
PT Explain the procedure to the patient.
PT Tell the patient that no fasting is required.

During
- Collect approximately 5 to 7 ml of venous blood in a lavender-top tube.
- Indicate if the patient has had a recent blood transfusion.

After
- Apply pressure or a pressure dressing to the venipuncture site.

Abnormal findings

▲ **Increased levels**
   PNH
   Type II congenital dyserythropoietic anemia

notes

haptoglobin

Type of test Blood

Normal findings

Adult: 50-220 mg/dl or 0.5-2.2 g/L (SI units)
Newborn: 0-10 mg/dl or 0-0.1 g/L (SI units)

Possible critical values <40 mg/dl

Test explanation and related physiology

The serum haptoglobin test is used to detect intravascular destruction (lysis) of red blood cells (RBCs), also called hemolysis. Haptoglobins are glycoproteins produced by the liver. These haptoglobins are powerful, free hemoglobin–binding proteins. In hemolytic anemias associated with the hemolysis of RBCs, the released hemoglobin is quickly bound to haptoglobin, and the new complex is quickly catabolized. This results in a diminished amount of free haptoglobin in the serum; this decrease cannot be quickly compensated for by normal liver production. As a result, the patient demonstrates a transient, reduced level of haptoglobin in the serum.

Haptoglobins are also decreased in patients with primary liver disease not associated with hemolytic anemias. This occurs because the diseased liver is unable to produce these glycoproteins. Hematoma can reduce haptoglobin levels by the absorption of hemoglobin into the blood and binding with haptoglobin.

Elevated haptoglobin concentrations are found in many inflammatory diseases and can be used as a nonspecific "acute-phase" protein in much the same way as a sedimentation rate test (see p. 402). That is, levels of haptoglobin increase with severe infection, inflammation, tissue destruction, acute myocardial infarction, burns, and some cancers.

Interfering factors

- Ongoing infection can cause falsely elevated test results.
- Drugs that may cause *increased* haptoglobin levels include androgens and steroids.
- Drugs that may cause *decreased* levels include chlorpromazine, diphenhydramine, indomethacin, isoniazid, nitrofurantoin, oral contraceptives, quinidine, and streptomycin.

Procedure and patient care

Before
PT Explain the procedure to the patient.
PT Tell the patient that no fasting is required.

During
- Collect at least 2 ml of venous blood in a red-top tube.
- Avoid hemolysis, which may alter test results.

After
- Apply pressure to the venipuncture site.

Abnormal findings

▲ **Increased levels**

Collagen disease
Infection
Tissue destruction
Biliary obstruction
Nephritis
Pyelonephritis
Ulcerative colitis
Peptic ulcer
Myocardial infarction
Acute rheumatic disease
Neoplasia

▼ **Decreased levels**

Hemolytic anemia
Transfusion reactions
Prosthetic heart valves
Systemic lupus
  erythematosus
Primary liver disease
  not associated with
  hemolytic anemia
Erythroblastosis fetalis
Hematoma
Tissue hemorrhage
Chronic liver disease

notes

Helicobacter pylori antibodies test (*Campylobacter pylori*, Anti–*Helicobacter pylori* immunoglobulin G [IgG] antibody, *Campylobacter*-like organism [CLO] test, Rapid urease test, *H. pylori* breath test, *H. pylori* stool test)

Type of test Blood, microscopic examination of antral or duodenal biopsy specimen, breath test, stool

Normal findings Not present

Test explanation and related physiology

H. pylori, a bacterium found in the mucus overlying the gastric mucosa and in the mucosa (cells that line the stomach), is a risk factor for gastric and duodenal ulcers, chronic gastritis, or even ulcerative esophagitis. This gram-negative bacillus is also a class I gastric carcinogen. Gastric colonization by this organism has been reported in about 90% to 95% of patients with a duodenal ulcer, in 60% to 70% of patients with a gastric ulcer, and in about 20% to 25% of patients with gastric cancer.

Approximately 10% of healthy persons younger than age 30 have gastric colonization with *H. pylori*. Gastric colonization increases with age, with people older than age 60 having rates at a percentage similar to their age. Most patients with gastric colonization by *H. pylori* remain asymptomatic and never develop ulceration.

There are several methods of detecting the presence of this organism. The organism can be cultured from a specimen of mucus obtained through a gastroscope (see p. 410). Cultures are performed at very few laboratories and are used only for research or in patients in whom first-line treatment of *H. pylori* infection seems to have failed. The organism can also be detected on a gastric mucosal biopsy (from the antrum and greater curvature of the corpus). This is slightly more accurate than culture technique and is considered the gold standard for detecting *H. pylori*.

It often takes several weeks before the results from cultures are available. It is preferable to start treatment before that time on a patient with symptomatic or active ulcer disease. For that reason, *rapid urease testing* for *H. pylori* has been developed. *H. pylori* can break down large quantities of urea because of its ability to produce great amounts of an enzyme called urease, which can be found in the lining of the stomach of infected patients. In one such test *(CLO test)*, a small piece of gastric mucosa (obtained through gastroscopy) is inserted into testing gel. Within a few hours, if *H. pylori* organisms are present in the gastric mucosa, the urease (made by the *H. pylori*) will turn the gel orange or red. If the color change does not occur, *H. pylori* is not present. Another rapid urease test uses specially prepared paper on which the gastric mucosa specimen is laid. If *H. pylori* organisms are present, the paper will change color. A third rapid urease test uses a specially prepared tablet that is dissolved in a small test tube. When the gastric mucosa of an infected patient is added, the solution changes color. These tests are nearly 95% accurate.

Although *H. pylori* does not survive in the stool, an enzyme-linked immunosorbent assay (ELISA) using a polyclonal anti–*H. pylori* capture antibody can detect the presence of *H. pylori* antigen in a fresh stool specimen.

A *breath test* is also available for the detection of *H. pylori*. It is the noninvasive test of choice for diagnosis of *H. pylori* infection. It is based on the capability of *H. pylori* to metabolize urea to CO_2 because of the organism's capability to produce urease as discussed previously. In the breath test, radioactive carbon (^{13}C) is administered orally. The urea is absorbed through the gastric mucosa where, if *H. pylori* is present, the urea will be converted to $^{13}CO_2$ (where the carbon is radiolabeled). The $^{13}CO_2$ is then taken up by the capillaries in the stomach wall and delivered to the lungs. There the $^{13}CO_2$ is exhaled. One half to 2 hours later, expired air is tested for radioactivity in the CO_2.

Serologic testing is the most common method of noninvasive diagnosis of *H. pylori* infection. It is the easiest test to perform, and no preparation or abstinence from antacids is required. Immunoassays of antibodies to *H. pylori* have been developed and are very accurate in detecting the presence of the organism. The IgG anti–*H. pylori* antibody is most commonly used. It becomes elevated 2 months after infection and stays elevated for more than a year after treatment. The IgA anti–*H. pylori* antibody, like IgG, becomes elevated 2 months after infection but decreases 3 to 4 weeks after treatment. The IgM anti–*H. pylori* antibody is the first to become elevated (about 3 to 4 weeks after infection) and is not detected 2 to 3 months after treatment. These antibody titers are fast becoming the gold standard for *H. pylori* detection. The most commonly performed laboratory methods used for immunotesting include ELISA and immunochromatography (IMC). Accuracy exceeds 85% with these methods. These antibodies can be detected using a small amount of blood obtained by fingerstick. Serologic testing is often used several months after treatment in order to document cure of *H. pylori* infection. Serologic testing is also used to corroborate the finding of other *H. pylori* testing methods.

Contraindications

- Children and patients who are pregnant
  The breath tests use radioactive carbon to which children should not be exposed.

Interfering factors

- *H. pylori* can be transmitted by contaminated endoscopic equipment during endoscopic procedures.
- Rapid urease tests can be falsely negative if the patient uses antacid therapy within the week prior to testing.

Procedure and patient care

Before

- **PT** Explain the procedure to the patient.
- **PT** Tell the patient that no fasting is required for the blood test.
- If a biopsy or culture will be obtained by endoscopy, see discussion of esophagogastroduodenoscopy (EGD) (p. 410).
- If culture is to be performed, be sure the patient has not had any antibiotic, antacid, or bismuth treatment for 5 to 14 days prior to the endoscopy.

During

- Collect a venous blood sample according to the protocol of the laboratory performing the test.
- A gastric or duodenal biopsy can be obtained by endoscopy. Keep the specimen moist by the addition of approximately 5 ml of sterile saline.
- For the *breath test*, a dose of radioactive ^{14}C or nonradioactive ^{13}C urea is given by mouth.

After

- Apply pressure to the venipuncture site.
- If endoscopy was used to obtain a culture, see procedure for EGD (p. 410). The specimen should be transported to the laboratory within 30 minutes after collection.

Abnormal findings

▲ **Increased levels**

Acute and chronic gastritis
Duodenal ulcer
Gastric ulcer
Gastric carcinoma

notes

hematocrit (Hct, Packed red blood cell volume, Packed cell volume [PCV])

Type of test Blood

Normal findings

Male: 42%-52% or 0.42-0.52 volume fraction (SI units)
Female: 37%-47% or 0.37-0.47 volume fraction (SI units)
Pregnant female: >33%
Elderly: values may be slightly decreased
Children (%)
  Newborn: 44-64
  2-8 weeks: 39-59
  2-6 months: 35-50
  6 months-1 year: 29-43
  1-6 years: 30-40
  6-18 years: 32-44

Possible critical values <15% or >60%

Test explanation and related physiology

The Hct is a measure of the percentage of the total blood volume that is made up by the red blood cells (RBCs). The height of the RBC column is measured after centrifugation. It is compared to the height of the column of the total whole blood (Figure 22). The ratio of the height of the RBC column compared to the original total blood column is multiplied by 100%. This is the Hct value. It is routinely performed as part of a complete blood count. The Hct closely reflects the hemoglobin (Hgb) and RBC values. The Hct in percentage points usually is approximately three times the Hgb concentration in grams per deciliter when RBCs are of normal size and contain normal amounts of Hgb.

Abnormal values indicate the same pathologic states as abnormal RBC counts and Hgb concentrations (see pp. 782 and 514). Decreased levels indicate anemia (reduced number of RBCs). Increased levels can indicate erythrocytosis. Like other RBC values, the Hct can be altered by many factors such as hydration status and RBC morphology.

Interfering factors

- Abnormalities in RBC size may alter Hct values.
- Extremely elevated white blood cell counts may affect values.

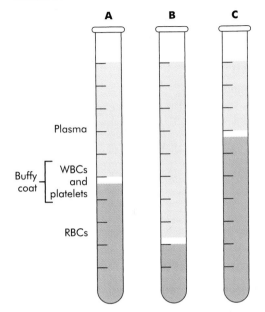

Figure 22 Tubes showing hematocrit levels of normal blood, blood with evidence of anemia, and blood with evidence of polycythemia. Note the buffy coat located between the packed red blood cells (RBCs) and the plasma. **A,** A normal percentage of RBCs. **B,** Anemia (low percentage of RBCs). **C,** Polycythemia (high percentage of RBCs).

- Hemodilution and dehydration may affect the Hct level.
- Pregnancy usually causes slightly decreased values because of hemodilution.
- Living in high altitudes causes increased values.
- Values may not be reliable immediately after hemorrhage.
- Drugs that may cause *decreased* levels include chloramphenicol and penicillin.

Procedure and patient care

Before

PT Tell the patient that no fasting is required.

During

- Collect approximately 5 to 7 ml of venous blood in a lavender-top tube; however, only 0.5 ml is required when using capillary tubes.
- Avoid hemolysis.

After

- Apply pressure to the venipuncture site.

Abnormal findings

▲ **Increased levels**

Congenital heart disease
Polycythemia vera
Severe dehydration
Erythrocytosis
Severe diarrhea
Eclampsia
Burns
Dehydration
Chronic obstructive
  pulmonary disease

▼ **Decreased levels**

Anemia
Hyperthyroidism
Cirrhosis
Hemolytic reaction
Hemorrhage
Dietary deficiency
Bone marrow failure
Normal pregnancy
Rheumatoid arthritis
Multiple myeloma
Malnutrition
Leukemia
Hemoglobinopathy

notes

hemoglobin (Hb, Hgb)

Type of test Blood

Normal findings

Male: 14-18 g/dl or 8.7-11.2 mmol/L (SI units)
Female: 12-16 g/dl or 7.4-9.9 mmol/L (SI units)
Pregnant female: >11 g/dl
Elderly: values are slightly decreased
Children
   Newborn: 14-24 g/dl
   0-2 weeks: 12-20 g/dl
   2-6 months: 10-17 g/dl
   6 months-1 year: 9.5-14 g/dl
   1-6 years: 9.5-14 g/dl
   6-18 years: 10-15.5 g/dl

Possible critical values <5.0 g/dl or >20 g/dl

Test explanation and related physiology

The Hgb concentration is a measure of the total amount of Hgb in the peripheral blood, which reflects the number of red blood cells (RBCs) in the blood. The test is normally performed as part of a complete blood count. Hgb serves as a vehicle for oxygen and carbon dioxide transport.

The hematocrit (Hct) in percentage points usually is approximately three times the Hgb concentration in grams per deciliter when RBCs are of normal size and contain normal amounts of Hgb. Abnormal values indicate the same pathologic states as abnormal RBC counts and Hct concentrations (see pp. 782 and 511). Decreased levels indicate anemia (reduced number of RBCs). Increased levels can indicate erythrocytosis. In addition, however, changes in plasma volume are more accurately reflected by the Hgb concentration. Slight decreases in the values of Hgb and the hematocrit during pregnancy reflect both the expanded blood volume due to a chronic state of overhydration and an increased number of RBCs. Hemoglobinopathies such as sickle cell disease and Hgb C disease are also associated with reduced hemoglobin levels.

Interfering factors

- Slight Hgb decreases normally occur during pregnancy because of the expanded blood volume.

- Living in high-altitude areas causes high Hgb values.
- Drugs that may cause *increased* levels include gentamicin and methyldopa (Aldomet).
- Drugs that may cause *decreased* levels include antibiotics, antineoplastic drugs, aspirin, indomethacin (Indocin), rifampin, and sulfonamides.

Procedure and patient care

Before
PT Explain the procedure to the patient.
PT Tell the patient that no fasting is required.

During
- Collect approximately 5 to 7 ml of venous blood in a lavender-top tube.
- Avoid hemolysis.
- List on the laboratory slip any drugs that may affect test results.

After
- Apply pressure to the venipuncture site.

Abnormal findings

▲ **Increased levels**

Congenital heart disease
Polycythemia vera
Hemoconcentration of the blood
Chronic obstructive pulmonary disease
Congestive heart failure
High altitudes
Severe burns
Dehydration

▼ **Decreased levels**

Anemia
Severe hemorrhage
Hemolysis
Hemoglobinopathies
Cancer
Nutritional deficiency
Lymphoma
Systemic lupus erythematosus
Sarcoidosis
Kidney disease
Chronic hemorrhage
Splenomegaly
Sickle cell anemia
Neoplasia

hemoglobin electrophoresis (Hgb electrophoresis)

Type of test   Blood

Normal findings

Adult/elderly: percentage of total hemoglobin

Hgb A_1: 95%-98%
Hgb A_2: 2%-3%
Hgb F: 0.8%-2%
Hgb S: 0%
Hgb C: 0%

Children: Hgb F

Newborn: 50%-80%
<6 months: <8%
>6 months: 1%-2%

Test explanation and related physiology

Hgb electrophoresis is a test that identifies abnormal forms of Hgb (hemoglobinopathies). Although many different Hgb variations have been described, the more common types are A_1, A_2, F, S, and C. Each major Hgb type is electrically charged to varying degrees. When hemoglobin from lysed RBCs is placed on electrophoresis paper and placed in an electromagnetic field, the Hgb variants migrate at different rates and spread apart from each other. The migrations of the various forms of Hgb make up a series of bands on the paper. The bands correspond to the various forms of hemoglobin present. The pattern of bands is compared with normal and other well-known abnormal patterns. Further, each band can be quantitated as a percentage of the total Hgb, indicating the severity of any recognized abnormality.

The form *Hgb A_1* constitutes the major component of Hgb in the normal red blood cell (RBC). *Hgb A_2* is only a minor component (2% to 3%) of the normal Hgb total. *Hgb F* is the major hemoglobin component in a fetus but normally exists in only minimal quantities in a normal adult. Levels of Hgb F greater than 2% in patients older than age 3 are considered abnormal. Hgb F is able to transport oxygen when only small amounts of oxygen are available (as in fetal life). In patients requiring compensation for prolonged chronic hypoxia (as in congenital cardiac abnormalities), Hgb F may be found in increased levels to assist in the transport of the available oxygen.

Hgb S and *Hgb* C are abnormal forms of Hgb that occur predominantly in American blacks. The Hgb contents of some common hemoglobinopathies, as determined by electrophoresis, are indicated in Table 14 (p. 518).

Interfering factors

- Blood transfusions within the previous 12 weeks may alter test results.

Procedure and patient care

Before

PT Explain the procedure to the patient.
PT Tell the patient that no fasting is required.

During

- Collect approximately 7 ml of venous blood in a lavender-top tube.

After

- Apply pressure to the venipuncture site.

Abnormal findings

Sickle cell disease
Sickle cell trait
Hemoglobin C disease
Hemoglobin H disease
Thalassemia major
Thalassemia minor

notes

TABLE 14 Hemoglobin contents of some common hemoglobinopathies

				Percentage range			
	Hgb A_1	Hgb A_2	Hgb F	Hgb S	Hgb H	Hgb C
Sickle cell disease	0	2	2	80-100	0	0
Sickle cell trait	60-80	2-3	2	20-40	0	0
Hemoglobin C disease	0	2-3	2	0	0	90-100
Hemoglobin H disease	65-90	2-3	0	0	5-30	0
Thalassemia major	5-20	2-3	65-100	0	0	0
Thalassemia minor	50-85	4-6	1-3	0	0	0

hepatitis virus studies (Hepatitis-associated antigen [HAA], Australian antigen)

Type of test Blood

Normal findings Negative

Test explanation and related physiology

Hepatitis is an inflammation of the liver caused by viruses, alcohol ingestion, drugs, toxins, or overwhelming bacterial sepsis. The three common viruses now recognized to cause disease are hepatitis A, hepatitis B, and hepatitis C (also called non-A/non-B) viruses. Hepatitis D and E viruses are much less common in the United States. Hepatitis D can infect the liver only by entering into a hepatitis B virus, which it uses as a carrying vehicle. Therefore hepatitis D cannot cause disease unless patients have hepatitis B virus in their bloodstream in the active, chronic, or carrier forms. The various types of hepatitis cannot be differentiated on the basis of their clinical presentation. The clinical presentations are similar in that they all include low-grade fever, malaise, anorexia, and fatigue. Most often they are all associated with elevations of hepatocellular enzymes such as aspartate aminotransferase (AST), alanine aminotransferase (ALT), and lactic dehydrogenase (LDH).

Hepatitis A virus (HAV) was originally called *infectious hepatitis.* It has a short incubation period of 2 to 6 weeks and is highly contagious. During active infection, HAV is excreted in the stool and transmitted via oral-fecal contamination of food and drink. About half the individuals tested in United States have had this form of hepatitis. Most infections are not associated with symptoms severe enough to warrant medical evaluation. Although immunologic tests are not yet available to detect HAV antigen, two types of antibodies to HAV can be detected by the radioimmunoassay (RIA) and enzyme-linked immunosorbent assay (ELISA) methods.

The first type of antibody to HAV is IgM antibody (HAV-Ab/IgM), which appears approximately 3 to 4 weeks after exposure or just before hepatocellular enzyme elevations occur. These IgM levels usually return to normal in approximately 8 weeks. The second type of antibody to HAV is IgG (HAV-Ab/IgG), which appears approximately 2 weeks after the IgM begins to increase and slowly returns to normal levels. The IgG antibody can remain detectable for more than 10 years after the infection. If the IgM antibody is elevated in the absence of the IgG antibody, acute hepatitis is suspected. If, however, IgG is elevated in the absence of IgM elevation, a convalescent or chronic stage of HAV viral infection is indicated.

Hepatitis B virus (HBV) is commonly known as *serum hepatitis.* It has a long incubation period of 5 weeks to 6 months. HBV is most frequently transmitted by blood transfusion; however, it also can be contracted via exposure to other body fluids. HBV may cause a severe and unrelenting form of hepatitis culminating in liver failure and death. The incidence is increased among blood transfusion recipients, male homosexuals, dialysis patients, transplant patients, IV drug abusers, and patients with leukemia or lymphoma. Hospital personnel are also at increased risk of infection mostly due to needlestick contamination.

HBV, also called the *Dane particle*, is made up of an inner core surrounded by an outer capsule. The outer capsule contains the hepatitis B surface antigen (HBsAg), formerly called Australian antigen. The inner core contains HBV core antigen (HBcAg). The hepatitis B e-antigen (HBeAg) is also found within the core. Antibodies to these antigens are called HBsAb, HBcAb, and HBeAb. The tests used to detect these antigens and antibodies include (Table 15):

1. *Hepatitis B surface antigen (HBsAg).* This is the most frequently and easily performed test for hepatitis B, and it is the first test to become abnormal. HBsAg rises before the onset of clinical symptoms, peaks during the first week of symptoms, and returns to normal by the time jaundice subsides. HBsAg generally indicates active infection by HBV. If the level of this antigen persists in the blood, the patient is considered to be a carrier.

2. *Hepatitis B surface antibody (HBsAb).* This antibody appears approximately 4 weeks after the disappearance of the surface antigen and signifies the end of the acute infection phase. HBsAb also signifies immunity to subsequent infection. Concentrated forms of this agent constitute the hyperimmunoglobulin given to patients who have come in contact with HBV-infected patients (e.g., contact by an inadvertent needle prick from a needle previously used on a patient with HBV infection). HBsAb is the antibody that denotes immunity after administration of hepatitis B vaccine.

TABLE 15 Hepatitis testing

Serologic findings	Appearance/disappearance	Application
HAV-Ab/IgM	4-6 weeks/3-4 months	Acute HAV infection
HAV-Ab/IgG	8-12 weeks/10 years	Previous HAV exposure/immunity
HBeAg	1-3 weeks/6-8 weeks	Acute HBV infection
HBeAb	4-6 weeks/4-6 years	Acute HBV infection ended
HBsAg	4-12 weeks/1-3 months	Acute HBV infection
HBsAb total	3-10 months/6-10 years	Previous HBV infection/immunity indicated
HBVc-Ab/IgM	2-12 weeks/3-6 months	Acute HBV infection
HBVc-Ab total	3-12 weeks/life	Previous HBV infection/convalescent stage
HCV-Ab/IgG	3-4 months/2 years	Previous HCV infection
HDV Ag	1-3 days/3-5 days	Acute HDV infection
HDV-Ab/IgM	10 days/1-3 months	Acute HDV infection
HDV-Ab total	2-3 months/7-14 months	Chronic HDV infection

3. *Hepatitis B core antigen (HBcAg)*. No tests are currently available to detect this antigen.

4. *Hepatitis B core antibody (HBcAb)*. This antibody appears approximately 1 month after infection with HBsAg and declines (although it remains elevated) over several years. HBcAb is also present in patients with chronic hepatitis. The HBcAb level is elevated during the time lag between the disappearance of HBsAg and the appearance of HBsAb. This interval is called the "core window." During the core window, HBcAb is the only detectable marker of a recent hepatitis infection.

5. *Hepatitis B e-antigen (HBeAg)*. This antigen generally is not used for diagnostic purposes but rather as an index of infectivity. The presence of HBeAg correlates with early and active disease, as well as with high infectivity in acute HBV infection. The persistent presence of HBeAg in the blood predicts the development of chronic HBV infection.

6. *Hepatitis B e-antibody (HBeAb)*. This antibody indicates that an acute phase of HBV infection is over, or almost over, and that the chance of infectivity is greatly reduced.

Hepatitis C (HCV) (non-A/non-B [NANB] hepatitis) is transmitted in a manner similar to HBV. Most cases of hepatitis are caused by blood transfusion. HCV is found in as many as 8% of blood donors worldwide. The incubation period is 2 to 12 weeks after exposure. The clinical manifestations of the illness parallel those of HBV. However, unlike with HBV, HCV infection is chronic in more than 60% of infected persons. Although the disease course is variable, it is slowly progressive. Twenty percent of HCV patients develop cirrhosis and hepatocellular cancers associated with this chronic infection.

The main screening test for detecting anti-HCV antibodies is the enzyme immunoassay (EIA). The most recent EIA (EIA3) can detect antibodies to HCV recombinant core antigen, NS3 gene, NS4 antigen, and NS5 antigen. The antibodies can be detected within 4 weeks of infection. Supplemental recombinant immunoblot assay is performed to improve specificity. No vaccine is available for treatment of this disease.

Because the course of HCV infection and response to treatment are so variable, researchers are attempting to determine the genetic variations that occur in HCV. Based on *HCV genotype testing*, six different "types," with several subtypes, of the virus have been identified. Some types are particularly endemic in one or another geographic area. Some types (2 and 3) are more sensitive to antiviral treatment (interferon-alpha) than others. Type 1 most commonly progresses to cirrhosis. Through genotyping, researchers are hoping to understand the manner in which this virus causes disease.

Hepatitis D virus (HDV) is known to cause "delta hepatitis." As stated, the HDV must enter the HBV to gain access to the liver and be infective. The patient must have HBV in the blood from a past or synchronously occurring infection. In the United States this is most commonly transmitted through tainted blood. The HDV antigen can be detected by immunoassay within a few days after infection. The IgM and total antibodies to HDV are detected early in the disease also. A persistent elevation of these antibodies indicates a chronic or carrier state.

Hepatitis E virus (HEV) was initially included in the non-A/non-B virus group but was isolated several years ago as an etiologic virus of short incubation. No antigen or antibody tests are currently widely available and accurate for the serologic identification of this infecting agent.

Procedure and patient care

Before

PT Tell the patient that no fasting is required.

During

- Collect approximately 5 to 7 ml of venous blood in a red-top tube.
- Note that most of the testing for hepatitis is done by radioimmunoassay. Usually a hepatitis profile that includes several HBV antigens and antibodies is performed.

After

- Apply pressure to the venipuncture site.
- Handle the specimen as if it were capable of transmitting hepatitis.
- Immediately discard the needle in the appropriate receptacle.
- Send the specimen promptly to the laboratory.

Abnormal findings

▲ **Increased levels**

Hepatitis A
Hepatitis B
Hepatitis C
Chronic carrier state, hepatitis B
Chronic hepatitis B

herpes simplex (Herpes virus type 2, Herpes simplex virus type 2 [HSV 2], Herpes genitalis)

Type of test Blood; microscopic

Normal findings

No virus present
No HSV antigens or antibodies present

Test explanation and related physiology

Herpes simplex virus can be classified as either type 1 or type 2. *Type 1 (HSV 1)* is primarily responsible for oral lesions (blisters on the lips called "cold sores") or even corneal lesions. *Type 2 (HSV 2)* is a sexually transmitted viral infection of the urogenital tract. Vesicular lesions may occur on the penis, scrotum, vulva, perineum, perianal region, vagina, or cervix.

Because most infants become infected if they pass through a birth canal containing HSV, determining its presence at delivery is necessary. Congenital infections may result in problems such as microcephaly, chorioretinitis, and mental retardation in the newborn. Disseminated neonatal herpesvirus infections carry a high incidence of infant mortality. A vaginal delivery is possible if no virus is present, and birth by cesarean section is needed if HSV is present. Viral testing can be performed on males or females to determine the risk of sexual transmission.

Culture is still the gold standard for HSV detection and can identify HSV in 90% of infected patients. Serologic tests are more easily and conveniently available for detection of HSV 1 and HSV 2 antigen. Unfortunately, accuracy is not great. Only about 85% of patients who are culture positive have positive serologies. The advantage of antigen tests is that results can be available in a day. Serologic tests for antibodies are cumbersome because they require repeated blood tests during the acute and convalescent phases of an acute viral outbreak (about 2 weeks apart). A fourfold rise in titer is expected to diagnose acute initial herpes infection. Recurrent infections are far less likely to demonstrate titer elevations. Furthermore, perhaps more than 50% of people in the United States have positive herpes antibodies.

Procedure and patient care

Before

PT Explain the procedure to the patient.

PT Tell the female patient to refrain from douching and tub bathing before the cervical culture is performed.

- Obtain the urethral specimen from the male patient before voiding.
- Blood can be diagnostic in either sex.

During

- Obtain cultures as follows:

Urethral culture

1. A culture is taken by inserting a sterile swab gently into the anterior urethra (see Figure 38, p. 843) or genital skin lesion of the male patient.
2. It is advisable to place the male patient in the supine position to prevent falling if vasovagal syncope occurs during introduction of the cotton swab or wire loop into the urethra.
3. The patient is observed for hypotension, bradycardia, pallor, sweating, nausea, and weakness.

Cervical culture

1. The female patient is placed in the lithotomy position, and a vaginal speculum is inserted.
2. Cervical mucus is removed with a cotton ball.
3. A sterile cotton-tipped swab is inserted into the endocervical canal and moved from side to side to obtain the culture. If a genital lesion is present, swabs from that area will be more sensitive in indicating infection.

- For pregnant women with herpes genitalis, note that the cervix is cultured weekly for the herpesvirus, beginning 4 to 6 weeks before the due date. Vaginal delivery is possible if the following criteria are met:

1. The two most recent cultures are negative.
2. The woman is not experiencing any symptoms.
3. No lesions are visible on inspection of the vagina and vulva.
4. Throughout pregnancy, the woman has not had more than one positive culture, during which she was symptom free.

Blood for serology

- Obtain 5 to 7 ml of blood in a red-top tube.

After

PT Inform the patient how to obtain the test results.

Abnormal findings

Herpes virus infection

notes

hexosaminidase (Hexosaminidase A, Hex A, Total hexosaminidase, Hexosaminidase A and B)

Type of test Blood

Normal findings

Hexosaminidase A: 7.5-9.8 units/L (SI units)

Total hexosaminidase: 9.9-15.9 units/L (SI units)

(Check with the lab due to wide variety of testing methods.)

Test explanation and related physiology

Tay-Sachs disease (TSD) is a lysosomal storage disease (GM2 gangliosidoses), which, in infancy and early childhood, is characterized by loss of motor skills. Death usually occurs by age 4. TSD is a result of a mutation in an autosomal recessive gene. Thus the affected person must have inherited a mutated gene from each parent in order to have TSD. One of 25 Ashkenazi (Eastern European) Jews is a carrier for a mutation. Eighty different mutations inhibit the function of this important gene. This gene encodes the synthesis of an enzyme called hexosaminidase. Without this enzyme, lyosomes of GM2 accumulate, particularly in the central nervous system.

Two clinically important isoenzymes of hexosaminidase have been detected in the serum: hexosaminidase A (made up of 1 alpha subunit and 1 beta subunit), and hexosaminidase B (made up of 2 beta subunits). Any genetic mutation that affects the alpha unit will cause a deficiency of hexosaminidase A, resulting in TSD. A mutation that affects the beta unit will cause a deficiency in hexosaminidase A and B. Sandhoff's disease, an uncommon variant of Tay-Sachs, occurs with deficiency of both of these enzymes.

Because TSD is uniformly untreatable and fatal, significant effort has gone into the development of biochemical testing to identify carriers of the genetic mutation (persons who carry one of the recessive genetic defective genes). Hex A has been found to be abnormally low in carriers, whereas hex B is high. Therefore testing for total hexosaminidase is not useful. A carrier has a 25% chance of having a child with TSD if the other biological parent is also a carrier. Pregnancy should occur only with significant genetic counseling. In communities where the Ashkenazi Jewish population is high, hex A screening has been very effective for identifying carriers. Further, Hex A is used to diagnose TSD in infants, young children, and adults. Genetic testing (p. 472) is useful to corroborate the identification of an affected person or a carrier.

Interfering factors

- Hemolysis of the blood sample can cause inaccurate test results.
- Pregnancy can cause markedly increased values. For this reason, blood tests are not done during pregnancy.
- ⚡ Oral contraceptives can falsely *increase* levels.

Procedure and patient care

Before

PT Explain the procedure to the patient. Emphasize the importance of this test to Jewish couples of Eastern European ancestry who plan to have children. Explain that both must carry the defective gene to transmit TSD to their offspring.

- Professional genetic counseling should be provided to every person considering undergoing this test.

PT Patients should be made aware of the possible effects on their lives if the test Hex A levels are reduced.

- Check with the lab regarding withholding contraceptives.

During

- Collect venous blood in a red-top tube. Avoid hemolysis.
- Note that pregnant women can be evaluated by amniocentesis (see p. 54) or chorionic villus biopsy (see p. 269).
- Note that infants may have blood obtained by heel sticks. Neonates often have blood drawn through the umbilical cord.

After

PT If only one partner is a carrier, reassure the couple that their offspring cannot inherit TSD.

- Arrange genetic counseling if both partners are carriers of TSD and pregnancy is desired.

Abnormal findings

▼   **Decreased hexosaminidase A**
Tay-Sachs disease

▼   **Decreased hexosaminidase A and B**
Sandhoff's disease

HIV viral load (HIV RNA)

Type of test Blood

Normal findings Undetected

Test explanation and related physiology

Measurement of human immunodeficiency virus (HIV) viral load in the blood of HIV-infected patients is increasingly being used as a marker for progression of acquired immunodeficiency syndrome (AIDS) (Table 16). It is also being used to determine prognosis and as an indicator for recommending the initiation of antiviral treatment (Table 17). HIV viral load reflects a patient's response to antiviral therapy and indicates the course of the disease more accurately than any other tests, including CD4 T-cell counts (see p. 626). HIV viral load testing is also used to monitor the effectiveness of treatment. Finally, viral load testing can predict patient survival (Table 16).

Quantification of HIV viral load is most accurately determined by quantifying the amount of genetic material of the virus in the blood. There are several different laboratory methods of measuring HIV viral load. The same method must be used to monitor the course of the disease. Because results vary according to the testing methods, it is important to know which method is used when considering whether to initiate treatment.

In general it is recommended to determine the baseline viral load by obtaining two measurements 2 to 4 weeks apart after serology is positive. Monitoring should continue with testing every 3 to 4 months in conjunction with CD4 counts. Both data are used to determine when to start antiviral treatment. The test should be repeated every 4 to 6 weeks after starting or changing antiviral therapy. However, the determination of the frequency of performing HIV viral load testing must take into account the cost of the test ($200 on average). Usually, antiviral treatment is continued until the HIV viral load is less than 500 copies/ml. A significant rise of viral load should warrant consideration of alteration of therapy.

Interfering factors

- Incorrect handling and processing of the specimen can cause inconsistent results.
- Recent vaccinations may affect viral levels.
- Concurrent infections can cause inconsistent results.
- Variable compliance to therapy may alter test results.

TABLE 16 Using the viral load to predict disease course

	HIV RNA viral load, copies/ml				
	<500	501-3000	3001-10,000	10,001-30,000	>30,000
% Developing AIDS	5.4	16.6	31.7	55.2	80
% Dying of AIDS	0.9	6.3	18.1	34.9	69.5

TABLE 17 Recommendations for antiretroviral therapy based on viral load and CD4 count

CD 4 count, ×10⁵/L	HIV RNA viral load, copies/ml		
	<5000	5000–30,000	>30,000
<350	Recommend therapy	Recommend therapy	Recommend therapy
350-500	Consider therapy	Recommend therapy	Recommend therapy
>500	Defer therapy	Consider therapy	Recommend therapy
Symptomatic		Recommend therapy	

H

Procedure and patient care

Before

PT Explain the procedure to the patient.

PT Tell the patient that no fasting or preparation is required.

- Maintain a nonjudgmental attitude toward the patient's sexual practices. Allow the patient ample time to express his or her concerns regarding the results.

During

- Observe universal body and blood precautions. Wear gloves when handling blood products from all patients.
- Obtain 7 ml of blood in a lavender (EDTA) tube.
- Never recap needles. Dispose of needles and syringes required for obtaining the blood specimen in a puncture-proof container designed for this purpose.
- Do not give results over the telephone. Increasing viral load may have devastating consequences.

After

- Immediately transport the specimen to the laboratory.
- Most specimens are sent to a central laboratory.
- Apply pressure to the venipuncture site.

PT Instruct the patient to observe the venipuncture site for infection. Patients with AIDS are immunocompromised and susceptible to infection.

PT Encourage the patient to discuss his or her concerns regarding the prognostic information that may be obtained by these results.

🏠 **Home care responsibilities**

- Do not give test results over the phone. Increasing viral load results can have devastating consequences.
- Because test results vary according to the laboratory test method, it is important to use the same laboratory method for monitoring the course of the disease.
- Viral loads are usually repeated after starting or changing antiviral therapy. A significant rise in viral load should warrant immediate reevaluation of therapy.

Abnormal findings

HIV infection

Holter monitoring (Ambulatory monitoring, Ambulatory electrocardiography, Event recorder)

Type of test Electrodiagnostic

Normal findings Normal sinus rhythm

Test explanation and related physiology

Holter monitoring is a continuous recording of the electrical activity of the heart. This can be performed for periods of up to 72 hours. With this technique, an electrocardiogram (ECG) is recorded continuously on magnetic tape during unrestricted activity, rest, and sleep. The Holter monitor is equipped with a clock that permits accurate time monitoring on the ECG tape. The patient is asked to carry a diary and record daily activities, as well as any cardiac symptoms that may develop during the period of monitoring.

Most units in present use are equipped with an "event marker." This is a button the patient can push when symptoms such as chest pain, syncope, or palpitations are experienced. This type of monitor is referred to as an *event recorder*.

The Holter monitor is used primarily to identify suspected cardiac rhythm disturbances and to correlate these disturbances with symptoms such as dizziness, syncope, palpitations, or chest pain. The monitor is also used to assess pacemaker function and the effectiveness of antiarrhythmic medications.

After completion of the determined time period—usually 24 to 72 hours—the Holter monitor is removed from the patient, and the record tape is played back at high speeds. The ECG tracing is usually interpreted by computer, which can detect any significant abnormal waveform patterns that occurred during the testing.

Contraindications

- Patients who are unable to cooperate with maintaining the lead placement from the monitor to the body
- Patients who are unable to maintain an accurate diary of significant activities or events

Interfering factors

- Interruption in the electrode contact with the skin

Procedure and patient care

Before
PT   Explain the procedure to the patient.

PT   Instruct the patient about care of the Holter monitor.

PT   Inform the patient about the necessity of ensuring good contact between the electrodes and the skin.

PT   Teach the patient how to maintain an accurate diary. Stress the need to record significant symptoms.

PT   Instruct the patient to note in the diary if any interruption in Holter monitoring occurs.

PT   Assure the patient that the electrical flow is coming from the patient and that he or she will not experience any electrical stimulation from the machine.

PT   Instruct the patient not to bathe during the period of cardiac monitoring.

PT   Tell the patient to minimize the use of electrical devices (e.g., electric toothbrushes, shavers), which may cause artificial changes in the ECG tracing.

During
- Prepare the sites for electrode placement with alcohol. (This is usually done in the cardiology department by a technologist.)
- Place the gel and electrodes at the appropriate sites. Usually the chest and abdomen are the most appropriate locations for limb-lead electrode placement. The precordial leads also may be placed.
- Usually do not use the extremities for electrode placement to minimize alterations in tracing that occur with normal physical activity.

PT   Encourage the patient to call if he or she has any difficulties.

After
- Gently remove the tape and other paraphernalia securing the electrodes.
- Wipe the patient clean of electrode gel.

PT   Inform the patient that the Holter monitoring interpretation will be available in a few days.

Abnormal findings
Cardiac arrhythmia (dysrhythmia)
Ischemic changes

homocysteine (Hcy)

Type of test Blood

Normal findings 4-14 μmol/L
(Levels may increase with age.)

Test explanation and related physiology

Homocysteine is an intermediate amino acid formed during the metabolism of methionine. Increasing evidence suggests that elevated blood levels of homocysteine may act as an independent risk factor for ischemic heart disease, cerebrovascular disease, peripheral arterial disease, and venous thrombosis. Homocysteine appears to promote the progression of atherosclerosis by causing endothelial damage, promoting low-density lipoprotein (LDL) deposition, and promoting vascular smooth muscle growth. Screening for hyperhomocystinemia (levels >15 μmol/L) should be considered in individuals with progressive and unexplained atherosclerosis despite normal lipoproteins and in the absence of other risk factors. It is also recommended in patients with an unusual family history of atherosclerosis, especially at a young age.

Dietary deficiency of vitamins B_6, B_{12}, or folate is the most common cause of elevated homocysteine. These vitamins are essential for the enzymatic metabolism of homocysteine to methionine. Because of the relationship of homocysteine to these vitamins, homocysteine blood levels are helpful in the diagnosis of deficiency syndromes associated with these vitamins. Homocysteine levels are elevated in patients with megaloblastic anemia. Homocysteine levels may be elevated before the more traditional tests become abnormal. This may result in earlier treatment and improvement of symptoms in patients with these vitamin deficiencies. Some practitioners recommend homocysteine testing in patients with known poor nutritional status (alcoholics, drug abusers) and the elderly.

Some researchers believe that elevated levels of homocysteine can be treated by administration of vitamins B_6, B_{12}, and folate. Several research reports recommend this vitamin therapy for homocysteine levels greater than 14 μmol/L. Whether or not this treatment will reduce the incidence of heart attacks remains to be seen.

Both fasting and postmethionine loading levels of homocysteine can be measured. In most laboratories, total homocysteine concentrations are measured. A major disadvantage in homocysteine testing is that methods are not standardized. With the more recent development of *enzyme immunoassay (EIA)*, results will be more standardized. In general, homocysteine levels less than 12 are considered optimal, levels from 12 to 15 are borderline, and levels greater than 15 are associated with high risk of vascular disease.

Contraindications

- Patients whose creatinine levels exceed 1.5 mg/dl are not candidates for methionine loading
  Elevated creatinine levels indicate malfunctioning kidneys that cannot effectively filter methionine (a protein).

Interfering factors

- Patients with renal impairment have elevated levels of homocysteine due to poor excretion of the protein.
- Men usually have higher levels of homocysteine than women. Most likely, this is due to higher creatinine values and greater muscle mass.
- Patients with a low intake of B vitamins have higher levels of homocysteine. The B vitamins help to break down and recycle homocysteine.
- Smoking is associated with increased homocysteine levels.
- ⚕ Drugs that may cause *increased* levels include azaribine, carbamazepine, methotrexate, nitrous oxide, and phenytoin.
- ⚕ Oral contraceptives containing estrogen may alter the metabolism of homocysteine.

Procedure and patient care

Before

PT Explain the procedure to the patient.
PT Instruct the patient to fast for 10 to 12 hours before the test. Meats contain elevated levels of homocysteine.

During

- Obtain the fasting blood sample in a collection tube that contains EDTA, heparin, or sodium citrate (blue/purple).
- For *methionine loading,* the patient ingests 100 mg/kg of methionine after fasting for 10 to 12 hours. A blood sample is obtained. Repeat blood samples are collected at 2, 4, 8, 12, and 24 hours to compare levels of B vitamins and amino acids in the plasma.

After

- In the laboratory, the blood should be spun down within 30 minutes in order to avoid false elevation caused by release of homocysteine from red blood cells (RBCs).
- Apply pressure to the venipuncture site.

Abnormal findings

▲ **Increased levels**

Cardiovascular disease
Cerebrovascular disease
Peripheral vascular disease
Cystinuria
Vitamin B_6 or B_{12} deficiency
Folate deficiency

notes

human lymphocyte antigen B27 (HLA-B27 antigen, Human leukocyte A antigen, White blood cell antigens, Histocompatibility A antigen)

Type of test Blood

Normal findings Negative

Test explanation and related physiology

The HLA antigens exist on the surface of white blood cells and on the surface of all nucleated cells in other tissues. These antigens can be detected most easily on the cell surface of lymphocytes. The presence or absence of these antigens is determined genetically. Each gene controls the presence or absence of HLA A, B, C, or D.

The HLA system of antigens has been used to indicate tissue compatibility with tissue transplantation. If the HLA antigens of the donor are not compatible with the recipient, the recipient will make antibodies to those antigens and accelerate rejection. Transplant survival of the tissue is increased if HLA matching is compatible. In contrast, prior HLA sensitization causes antibodies to form in the blood recipient, which will shorten the survival of blood cells (red blood cells or platelets) when transfused.

The HLA system has also been used to assist in the diagnosis of certain other diseases, as HLAs are often associated with these diseases. For example, HLA-B27 is present in 80% of patients with Reiter's syndrome. When a patient has recurrent and multiple arthritic complaints, the presence of HLA-B27 supports the diagnosis of Reiter's syndrome. HLA-B27 is found in 5% to 7% of normal patients. Other HLA-disease associations are mentioned in "Abnormal findings."

Because HLA antigens are genetically determined, they are useful in *paternity investigations*. This is particularly helpful if the father or child has an unusual HLA genotype. A common HLA genotype in either the father or child increases the likelihood that there are many potential "fathers" of that child.

Procedure and patient care

Before

PT Explain the procedure to the patient.

PT Tell the patient that no fasting or special preparation is required.

During
- Collect at least 10 ml of venous blood in a heparinized solution.

After
- Apply pressure to the venipuncture site.

Abnormal findings

▲ **Increased levels (HLA antigens present)**

Ankylosing spondylitis
Reiter's syndrome
Yersinia enterocolitica arthritis
Anterior uveitis
Graves' disease
Celiac disease/gluten enteropathy
Chronic active hepatitis
Multiple sclerosis
Myasthenia gravis
Dermatitis herpetiformis
Psoriasis
Juvenile diabetes
Hemochromatosis
Rheumatoid arthritis

notes

human placental lactogen (hPL, Human chorionic somatomammotropin [HCS])

Type of test Blood

Normal findings

Weeks of pregnancy	hPL concentration (mg/l = mcg/ml)
up to 20	0.05-1
up to 22	1.5-3
up to 26	2.5-5
up to 30	4-6.5
up to 34	5-8
up to 38	5.5-9.5
up to 42	5-7

Test explanation and related physiology

The human placenta produces several hormones that are homologous to hormones of the anterior pituitary. Human placental lactogen (hPL), whose task is to maintain the pregnancy, is structurally similar to both human prolactin and growth hormone. Not surprisingly, hPL demonstrates both lactogenic and growth-stimulating activity. Serum levels of hPL rise very early in normal pregnancy and continue to increase until a plateau is reached at about the 35th week after conception. Assays for maternal serum levels of hPL are useful in monitoring placental function. Measurements of hPL also are used in pregnancies complicated by hypertension, proteinuria, edema, post-maturity, placental insufficiency, or possible miscarriage.

A decreased serum concentration of hPL is pathognomonic for a malfunction of the placenta, which may cause intrauterine growth retardation, intrauterine death of the fetus, or imminent miscarriage. Pregnant women with hypertonia also show low serum concentrations of hPL. Because of the short biological half-life of hPL in serum, the determination of hPL always gives a very accurate picture of the present situation.

Increased serum concentrations of hPL are found in women with diabetes mellitus and, because of the higher placental mass, in multiple pregnancies. In contrast to estriol, the hPL concentration only depends on the placental mass and not on fetal function. The simultaneous determination of hPL and estriol can be helpful in the differential evaluation of placental function.

Interfering factors

- Prior nuclear medicine scans, because they can interfere with interpretation of test results.

Procedure and patient care

Before

PT Explain the procedure to the patient.

PT Tell the patient that no fasting is required.

During

- Collect approximately 5 to 7 ml of venous blood in a red-top tube.
- Indicate the date of the patient's last menstrual period on the laboratory slip.

After

- Apply pressure to the venipuncture site.
- Explain the possibility that serial testing is often required.

Abnormal findings

▲ **Increased levels**

Multiple pregnancies
Placental site trophoblastic
   tumor
Intact molar pregnancy
Diabetes
Rh incompatibility

▼ **Decreased levels**

Placental insufficiency
Toxemia
Preeclampsia
Hydatidiform mole
Choriocarcinoma

notes

human T-cell lymphotrophic virus (HTLV) I/II antibody

Type of test Blood

Normal findings Negative

Test explanation and related physiology

Several forms of HTLV, a human retrovirus, affect humans. HTLV-I is associated with adult T-cell leukemia/lymphoma. HTLV-II is associated with adult hairy-cell leukemia and neurologic disorders such as tropical spastic paraparesis. Humans can be infected with these viruses, however, and not develop any malignancy or diseases.

The human immunodeficiency viruses (HIVs), which are known to be the cause of acquired immunodeficiency syndrome (AIDS), are also retroviruses; however, HTLV infection is not associated with AIDS. HTLV transmission is similar, though, to HIV transmission (e.g., body fluid contamination, intravenous drug use, sexual contact, breast-feeding).

Procedure and patient care

Before

PT Explain the procedure to the patient.

PT Tell the patient that no fasting is required.

During

- Collect approximately 7 ml of venous blood in a red-top tube.

After

- Apply pressure to the venipuncture site.

Abnormal findings

Acute HTLV infection
Adult T-cell leukemia
Hairy-cell leukemia
Tropical spastic paraparesis

notes

17-hydroxycorticosteroids (17-OCHS)

Type of test Urine (24-hour)

Normal findings

Adult
    Male: 3-10 mg/24 hr or 8.3-27.6 μmol/day (SI units)
    Female: 2-8 mg/24 hr or 5.2-22.1 μmol/day (SI units)
Elderly: values slightly lower than adult
Children
    <8 years: <1.5 mg/24 hr
    8-12 years: <4.5 mg/24 hr

Test explanation and related physiology

Elevated levels of 17-OCHS are seen in patients with hyperfunctioning of the adrenal gland (Cushing's syndrome), whether this condition is caused by a pituitary or adrenal tumor, bilateral adrenal hyperplasia, or ectopic tumors producing adrenocorticotropic hormone (ACTH). Low levels of 17-OCHS are seen in patients who have a hypofunctioning adrenal gland (Addison's disease) as a result of destruction of the adrenals (by hemorrhage, infarction, metastatic tumor, or autoimmunity), surgical removal of an adrenal gland, congenital enzyme deficiency, hypopituitarism, or adrenal suppression after prolonged exogenous steroid ingestion.

Testing the urine for this hormone metabolite is only an indirect measure of adrenal function. Urine and plasma levels of cortisol (see p. 314) provide a much more accurate measurement of adrenal function. Because the excretion of cortisol metabolites follows a diurnal variation, a 24-hour collection is necessary.

Interfering factors

- Emotional and physical stress (e.g., infection) and licorice ingestion may cause increased adrenal activity.
- Drugs that may cause *increased* 17-OCHS levels include acetazolamide, chloral hydrate, chlorpromazine, colchicine, erythromycin, meprobamate, paraldehyde, quinidine, quinine, and spironolactone.
- Drugs that may cause *decreased* levels include estrogens, oral contraceptives, phenothiazines, and reserpine.

H

Procedure and patient care

Before

PT Explain the procedure to the patient.

- Note that drugs are usually withheld several days before the urine collection. Check with the physician and laboratory for specific guidelines.
- Assess the patient for signs of stress and report these to the physician.

During

- Do not administer to the patient any drugs that may interfere with test results.

PT Instruct the patient to begin the 24-hour urine collection after voiding. Discard this urine and note this as the start time of the test.

- Collect all urine passed by the patient during the next 24 hours.
- Post the hours for the urine collection in a prominent spot.
- Note that it is not necessary to measure each urine specimen.

PT Tell the patient to void before defecating so that the urine is not contaminated by feces.

PT Inform the patient that toilet paper should not be placed in the collection container.

PT Encourage the patient to drink fluids during the 24 hours, unless this is contraindicated for medical purposes.

PT Instruct the patient to collect the last specimen as close as possible to the end of the 24-hour collection. Add this to the container.

- Keep the urine specimen refrigerated or on ice during the entire collection.

After

- Send the urine to the chemistry laboratory as soon as the test is completed.
- List on the laboratory slip any medications the patient may be taking that can affect test results.

Abnormal findings

▲ **Increased levels**

Cushing's disease

Ectopic ACTH-producing
tumors

Stress

Adrenal adenoma or
carcinoma

Hyperthyroidism

Obesity

▼ **Decreased levels**

Adrenal hyperplasia
(adrenogenital
syndrome)

Addison's disease

Adrenal suppression
from steroid therapy

Hypopituitarism

Hypothyroidism

notes

5-hydroxyindoleacetic acid (5-HIAA)

Type of test Urine (24-hour)

Normal findings

2-8 mg/24 hr or 10-40 µmol/day (SI units)
Female levels lower than male levels

Test explanation and related physiology

Quantitative analysis of urine levels of 5-HIAA is used to detect and follow the clinical course of patients with carcinoid tumors. Carcinoid tumors are serotonin-secreting tumors that may grow in the appendix, intestine, lung, or any tissue derived from the neuroectoderm. These tumors contain *argentaffin-staining (enteroendocrine)* cells, which produce serotonin and other powerful neurohormones that are metabolized by the liver to 5-HIAA and excreted in the urine. These powerful neurohormones are responsible for the clinical presentation of carcinoid syndrome (bronchospasm, flushing, diarrhea). This test is used not only to identify patients with carcinoid tumor but also to reevaluate those with known tumor by using serial levels of urinary 5-HIAA. Rising levels of 5-HIAA indicate progression of tumor; falling levels of 5-HIAA indicate a therapeutic response of the tumor to antineoplastic therapy.

Interfering factors

- Bananas, plantains, pineapples, kiwifruit, walnuts, plums, pecans, eggplant, tomatoes, and avocados can factitiously elevate 5-HIAA levels.
- Drugs that may cause *increased* 5-HIAA levels include acetanilid, acetophenetidin (phenacetin), glyceryl guaiacolate (guaifenesin [Robitussin]), methocarbamol, acetaminophen, and reserpine.
- Drugs that may cause *decreased* levels include chlorpromazine, ethyl alcohol, heparin, imipramine (Tofranil), isoniazid (INH), levodopa, MAO inhibitors, methenamine, methyldopa (Aldomet), phenothiazines, promethazine (Phenergan), aspirin, and tricyclic antidepressants.

Procedure and patient care

Before

PT Explain the procedure to the patient.

PT Instruct the patient to refrain from eating foods containing serotonin (e.g., plums, pineapples, bananas, eggplant, tomatoes, avocados, walnuts, plantains, kiwifruit, and pecans) for several days (usually 3) before and during testing.

During

PT To begin the 24-hour urine collection, tell the patient to discard the initial specimen and start the timing at that point.

- Collect all urine passed during the next 24 hours.

PT Show the patient where to store the urine specimen.

- Keep the specimen on ice or in a refrigerator during the 24-hour collection. A preservative is needed to keep the specimen at an appropriate pH.

- Post the hours for urine collection in a noticeable place to prevent accidental discarding of the specimen.

PT Instruct the patient to void before defecating so that urine is not contaminated by stool.

PT Tell the patient not to put toilet paper in the urine container.

PT Instruct the patient to collect the last specimen as close as possible to the end of the 24-hour collection. Add this urine to the container.

After

- Send the urine specimen to the laboratory promptly.

- List on the laboratory slip any medications that may affect the test results.

Abnormal findings

▲ **Increased levels**

Carcinoid tumors
Noncarcinoid illness
Cystic fibrosis
Intestinal malabsorption

▼ **Decreased levels**

Depression
Migraine headaches

notes

hysterosalpingography (Uterotubography, Uterosalpingography, Hysterogram)

Type of test X-ray with contrast dye

Normal findings

Patent fallopian tubes
No defects in uterine cavity

Test explanation and related physiology

In hysterosalpingography, the uterine cavity and fallopian tubes are visualized radiographically after the injection of contrast material through the cervix. Uterine tumors, intrauterine adhesions, and developmental anomalies can be seen. Tubal obstruction caused by internal scarring, tumor, or kinking also can be detected. A possible therapeutic effect of this test is that passage of dye through the tubes may clear mucous plugs, straighten kinked tubes, or break up adhesions. This test also may be used to document adequacy of surgical tubal ligation.

Contraindications

- Patients with infections of the vagina, cervix, or fallopian tubes, because there is risk of extending the infection
- Patients with suspected pregnancy, because contrast material might induce abortion

Potential complications

- Infection of the endometrium (endometritis)
- Infection of the fallopian tubes (salpingitis)
- Uterine perforation
- Allergic reaction to iodinated dye
  This rarely occurs because the dye is not administered intravenously.

Procedure and patient care

Before

PT Explain the procedure to the patient.
- Determine pregnancy status of the patient.
- Administer sedatives (e.g., midazolam [Versed]) or antispasmodics, if ordered, before the test.

PT Tell the patient that no food or fluid restrictions are needed.

During
- Note the following procedural steps:
  1. After voiding, the patient is placed on the fluoroscopy table in the lithotomy position.
  2. With a speculum in the vagina, contrast material is injected through the cervix. The dye fills the entire upper genital tract (uterus and tubes).
  3. Fluoroscopy is performed, and x-ray films are taken.
- Note that this procedure is performed by a physician in approximately 15 to 30 minutes.
- **PT** Tell the patient that she may feel occasional, transient menstrual-type cramping and that she may have shoulder pain caused by subphrenic irritation from the dye as it leaks into the peritoneal cavity.

After
- **PT** Inform the patient that a vaginal discharge (sometimes bloody) may be present for 1 to 2 days after the test.
- **PT** Instruct the patient as to signs and symptoms of infection (e.g., fever, increased pulse rate, pain).

Abnormal findings

Uterine tumor (e.g., leiomyoma, cancer)
Developmental anomaly (e.g., uterus bicornis) of the uterus
Intrauterine adhesions
Uterine fistula
Obstruction, kinking, or twisting of the fallopian tubes
Extrauterine pregnancy
Tumor of the fallopian tubes

notes

hysteroscopy

Type of test Endoscopy

Normal findings Normal structure and function of the uterus

Test explanation and related physiology

Hysteroscopy is an endoscopic procedure that provides direct visualization of the uterine cavity by inserting a hysteroscope (a thin, telescope-like instrument) through the vagina and cervix and into the uterus (Figure 23). Hysteroscopy can be used to identify the cause of abnormal uterine bleeding, infertility, and repeated miscarriages. It is also used to identify, evaluate, and perform biopsies of uterine adhesions (Asherman's syndrome), polyps, cancer, fibroids, and displaced intrauterine devices (IUDs).

In addition to diagnosing and evaluating uterine problems, hysteroscopy can also correct uterine problems. For example, uterine adhesions and small fibroids can be removed through the hysteroscope, thus avoiding open abdominal surgery. Hysteroscopy can also be used to perform endometrial ablation, which destroys the uterine lining to treat some cases of heavy dysfunctional uterine bleeding.

Contraindications

- Patients with pelvic inflammatory disease
- Patients with vaginal discharge

Potential complications

- Uterine perforation
- Infection

Procedure and patient care

Before

PT Explain the procedure to the patient.
- Obtain informed consent for this procedure.
- Assess the pregnancy status of the patient.
PT Instruct the patient to be NPO for at least 8 hours before the test.

During

- Note the following procedural steps:
    1. Hysteroscopy may be performed in the operating room or the doctor's office. Local, regional, general, or no anesthesia may be used. (The type of anesthesia depends on other procedures that may be done at the same time.)

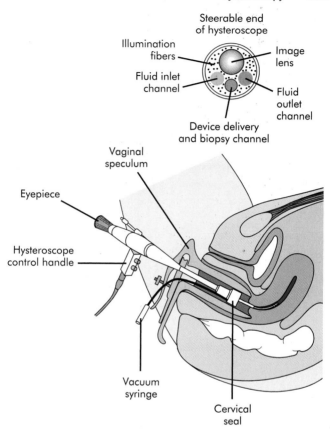

Figure 23 Hysteroscopy.

2. The patient is placed in the lithotomy position. The vaginal area is cleansed with an antiseptic solution.
3. The cervix may be dilated before this procedure.
4. The hysteroscope is inserted through the vagina and cervix and into the uterus.
5. A liquid or gas is released through the hysteroscope to expand the uterus for better visualization.
6. If minor surgery is to be performed, small instruments will be inserted through the hysteroscope.

7. For more detailed or complicated procedures, a laparo-scope may be used (see p. 579) to concurrently view the outside of the uterus.

- Note that hysteroscopy is performed by a physician in approximately 30 minutes.

After

PT Tell the patient that it is normal to have slight vaginal bleeding and cramps for a day or two after the procedure.

PT Inform the patient that signs of fever, severe abdominal pain, or heavy vaginal discharge or bleeding should be reported to her physician.

Abnormal findings

Endometrial cancer, polyps, or hyperplasia
Uterine fibroids
Asherman's syndrome
Septate uterus
Displaced IUD

notes

immunofixation electrophoresis (IFE)

Type of test Blood; urine

Normal findings

No monoclonal immunoglobulins identified

Test explanation and related physiology

This test is used to identify more clearly whether a spike on the serum protein electrophoresis (see p. 758) is monoclonal or when quantitative immunoglobins are elevated. Further it is able to determine whether the monoclonal spike is caused by light chain or heavy chain components.

With this technique, a monospecific antibody is placed in contact with the gel after the proteins have been separated by electrophoresis. The resulting protein-antibody complexes are subsequently specifically stained for visualization after being precipitated out. The pathologist can then identify and classify specific immunoglobulin spikes. For example, multiple myeloma (MM), and Waldenström's macroglobulinemia are associated with monoclonal immunoglobulin spikes. Furthermore, both diseases are associated with light chains in the urine IFE. However, some patients with MM do have heavy chains in the urine. Polyclonal immunoglobulins are noted in chronic inflammatory processes, chronic liver diseases, and in patients with ongoing chronic infections.

This test is also used to follow the course of the disease or treatment in patients with known monoclonal immunoglobulinopathies. For example, with successful treatment for neoplastic gammopathies, IFE, upon repetition, can demonstrate reduction in the specific immunoglobulin. Finally, this test is helpful to define more clearly the immune status of a patient whose immune status may be compromised.

Procedure and patient care

Before

PT Explain the procedure to the patient.

PT Tell the patient that no fasting or special preparation is required.

During

Blood

- Collect 7 to 10 ml of venous blood in a red-top tube. The blood used for immunoglobulin electrophoresis can be reused.
- Indicate on the laboratory slip if the patient has received any vaccinations or immunizations within the past 6 months. Also, list any drugs that may affect test results.

Urine

PT Instruct the patient to begin the 24-hour collection after voiding. Discard this specimen.

- Collect all urine passed by the patient during the next 24 hours.
- Note that it is not necessary to measure each urine specimen.

PT Remind the patient to void before defecating so that the urine is not contaminated by feces.

PT Tell the patient not to put toilet paper in the collection container.

PT Encourage the patient to drink fluids during the 24 hours unless this is contraindicated for medical purposes.

PT Instruct the patient to collect the last specimen as close as possible to the end of the 24-hour period. Add this to the collection.

- Place the 24-hour urine collection in a plastic container and keep on ice. Use a preservative.

After

- Apply pressure to the venipuncture site.

Abnormal findings

▲ **Increased blood monoclonal immunoglobulins**

Multiple myeloma
Waldenström's macroglobulinemia

▲ **Increased blood polyclonal immunoglobulins**

Amyloidosis
Autoimmune diseases
Chronic infection/inflammation
Chronic liver disease

▲ **Increased urine monoclonal immunoglobulins**

Multiple myeloma
Waldenström's macroglobulinemia

immunoglobulin electrophoresis (Gamma globulin electrophoresis)

Type of test Blood

Normal findings

IgG (mg/dl)
  Adults: 565-1765
  Children: 250-1600

IgA (mg/dl)
  Adults: 85-385
  Children: 1-350

IgM (mg/dl)
  Adult: 55-375
  Children: 20-200

IgD and IgE: minimal

Test explanation and related physiology

Proteins within the blood are made up of albumin and globulin. Several types of globulin exist, one of which is gamma globulin. Antibodies are made up of gamma globulin protein and are called *immunoglobulins*. There are many classes of immunoglobulins (antibodies). *Immunoglobulin G (IgG)* constitutes approximately 75% of the serum immunoglobulins; therefore it constitutes the majority of circulating blood antibodies. *IgA* constitutes approximately 15% of the immunoglobulins within the body and is present primarily in secretions of the respiratory and gastrointestinal tracts, in saliva, colostrum, and tears. IgA is also present to a smaller degree in the blood. *IgM* is an immunoglobulin primarily responsible for ABO blood grouping and rheumatoid factor; it is also involved in the immunologic reaction to many other infections (e.g., hepatitis, gram-negative sepsis). IgM does not cross the placenta, so an elevation of IgM in a newborn indicates in utero infection such as rubella, cytomegalovirus (CMV), or sexually transmitted disease (STD). *IgE* often mediates an allergic response and is measured to detect allergic diseases. *IgD*, which constitutes the smallest part of the immunoglobulins, is rarely evaluated or detected.

Serum immunoelectrophoresis is used to detect and monitor the course of diseases, including hypersensitivity diseases, immune deficiencies, autoimmune diseases, chronic infections, multiple myeloma, chronic viral infections, and intrauterine fetal infections. For this test the serum is placed on a slide containing agar gel, and an electric current is passed through this gel. Immunoglobulins are separated out and electrophoresed according to the quantity and difference in electrical charge. Specific antisera are placed alongside the slide to identify the specific type of immunoglobulin present. *Immunofixation electrophoresis (IFE)* (see p. 553) is now being used to identify pathology related to immunoglobulins.

Interfering factors

☤ Drugs that may cause *increased* immunoglobulin levels include therapeutic gamma globulin, hydralazine, isoniazid (INH), phenytoin (Dilantin), procainamide, and tetanus toxoid and antitoxin.

Procedure and patient care

Before
PT Explain the procedure to the patient.
PT Tell the patient that no fasting or special preparation is required.

During
■ Collect 7 to 10 ml of venous blood in a red-top tube.
■ Indicate on the laboratory slip if the patient has received any vaccinations or immunizations within the past 6 months. Also, list any drugs that may affect test results.

After
■ Apply pressure to the venipuncture site.

Abnormal findings

▲ Increased IgA levels
Chronic liver diseases (e.g., primary biliary cirrhosis)
Chronic infections
Inflammatory bowel disease

▼ Decreased IgA levels
Ataxia/telangiectasia
Congenital isolated deficiency
Hypoproteinemia (e.g., nephrotic syndrome or protein-losing enteropathies)
Immunosuppressive drugs (e.g., steroids, dextran)

▲ **Increased IgG levels**

Chronic granulomatous infections (e.g., TB, Wegener's granulomatosis, sarcoidosis)

Hyperimmunization reactions

Chronic liver disease

Multiple myeloma (monoclonal IgG type)

Autoimmune diseases (e.g., rheumatoid arthritis, Sjögren's disease, and SLE)

IUD devices

▼ **Decreased IgG levels**

Wiskott-Aldrich syndrome

Agammaglobulinemia

AIDS

Hypoproteinemia (e.g., nephrotic syndrome or protein-losing enteropathies)

Drug immunosuppression (e.g., steroids, dextran)

Non-IgG multiple myeloma

Leukemia

▲ **Increased IgM levels**

Waldenström's macroglobulinemia

Chronic infections (e.g., hepatitis, mononucleosis, sarcoidosis)

Autoimmune diseases (e.g., SLE or rheumatoid arthritis)

Acute infections

Chronic liver disorders (e.g., biliary cirrhosis)

▼ **Decreased IgM levels**

Agammaglobulinemia

Acquired immunodeficiency syndrome

Hypoproteinemia (e.g., nephrotic syndrome or protein-losing enteropathies)

Drug immunosuppression (e.g., steroids, dextran)

IgG or IgA multiple myeloma

Leukemia

▲ **Increased IgE levels**

Allergy reactions (e.g., hay fever, asthma, eczema, or anaphylaxis)

Allergic infections such as aspergillosis or parasites

▼ **Decreased IgE levels**

Agammaglobulinemia

notes

insulin assay

Type of test Blood

Normal findings

6-26 µU/ml or 43-186 pmol/L (SI units)

Newborn: 3-20 µU/ml

Possible critical values >30 µU/ml

Test explanation and related physiology

Insulin assay is used to diagnose insulinoma (tumor of the islets of Langerhans). It is also used in the evaluation of patients with fasting hypoglycemia.

Some investigators believe that measuring the ratio of the blood sugar and insulin on the same specimen obtained during the oral glucose tolerance test (GTT, see p. 492) is more reliable than measuring insulin levels alone. Combined with the oral GTT, the insulin assay can show characteristic curves. For example, patients with juvenile diabetes have low fasting insulin levels and display flat GTT insulin curves because of little or no increase in insulin levels. Patients who have mild cases of diabetes have normal fasting insulin levels and display GTT curves with a delayed rise.

When combined with a fasting blood sugar, insulin assay is very accurate in detecting insulinoma. After the patient fasts 12 to 14 hours, the insulin/glucose ratio should be less than 0.3. Patients with insulinoma have ratios greater than this. To increase the sensitivity and specificity of these combined tests for insulinoma, Turner and others have proposed the "amended" insulin/glucose ratios using variable mathematic "fudge" factors:

$$\frac{\text{Serum insulin level} \times 100}{\text{Serum glucose} - 30 \text{ mg/100 ml}}$$

A Turner amended ratio of more than 50 suggests insulinoma.

Interfering factors

- Anti-insulin antibodies can interfere with insulin radioimmunoassay.
- Food intake and obesity may cause increased insulin levels.
- Recent administration of radioisotopes may affect test results.

✦ Drugs that may cause *increased* insulin levels include corticosteroids, levodopa, and oral contraceptives.

Procedure and patient care

Before
PT Explain the procedure to the patient.
- Keep the patient NPO for 8 hours.

During
- Collect approximately 5 ml of venous blood in a red-top tube and pack it in ice.
- Avoid hemolysis.
- If the serum insulin level will be measured during the GTT, collect the blood sample before oral ingestion of the glucose load and often at designated intervals after glucose ingestion.

After
- Apply pressure to the venipuncture site.
- Transport the specimen immediately to the laboratory.

Abnormal findings

▲ **Increased levels**
Insulinoma
Cushing's syndrome
Acromegaly
Obesity
Fructose or galactose intolerance

▼ **Decreased levels**
Diabetes
Hypopituitarism

notes

intravenous pyelography (IVP, Excretory urography [EUG], Intravenous urography [IUG, IVU])

Type of test X-ray with contrast dye

Normal findings

Normal size, shape, and position of the kidneys, renal pelvis, ureters, and bladder

Normal kidney excretory function as evidenced by the length of time for passage of contrast material through the kidneys

Test explanation and related physiology

IVP is an x-ray study that uses radiopaque contrast material to visualize the kidneys, renal pelvis, ureters, and bladder. It is indicated on patients with:

Pain compatible with urinary stones

Blood in the urine

Proposed pelvic surgery to locate the ureters

Trauma to the urinary system

Urinary outlet obstruction

A suspected kidney tumor

Dye is injected intravenously, filtered out at the kidney by the glomeruli, and then passed through the renal tubules. X-ray films taken at set intervals over the next 30 minutes will show passage of the dye material through the kidneys and ureters and into the bladder.

If the artery leading to one of the kidneys is blocked, the dye cannot enter that part of the renal system, and that kidney or part thereof will not be visualized. If the artery is partially blocked, the length of time required for the appearance of the contrast material will be prolonged.

With primary glomerular disease (e.g., glomerulonephritis), the glomerular filtrate is reduced, which causes a reduction in the quantity of dye filtered. Therefore it requires more time for enough dye to enter the kidney filtrate and allow for renal opacification. As a result, kidney visualization is delayed. This indicates an estimate of renal function.

Defects in dye filling of the kidney can indicate renal tumors or cysts. Often intrinsic tumors, stones, extrinsic tumors, and scarring can partially or completely obstruct the flow of dye through the collecting system (pelvis, ureters, bladder). If the obstruction has been of sufficient duration, the collecting system proximal to the obstruction will be dilated (hydronephrosis). Retroperitoneal and pelvic tumors, aneurysms, and enlarged lymph nodes also can produce extrinsic compression and distortions of the opacified collecting system.

IVP is also used to assess the effect of trauma on the urinary system. Renal hematomas distort the renal contour. Renal artery laceration is suggested by nonopacification of one kidney. Laceration of the kidneys, pelvis, ureters, or bladder often causes urine leaks, which are identified by dye extravasation from the urinary system.

Further, IVP is used to assess a patient for congenital absence or malposition of the kidneys. Horseshoe kidneys (connection of the two kidneys), double ureters, and pelvic kidneys are typical congenital abnormalities.

Nephrotomography provides radiographic visualization of the kidney using tomographic technique following the IV injection of a radiopaque dye. Tomography permits examination of a single layer or plane of the organ that would otherwise be obscured by the surrounding structures.

Helical CT scanning (see p. 296) has became the method of choice in many medical centers for diagnosing urolithiasis.

Contraindications

- Patients who are allergic to shellfish or iodinated dyes
- Patients who are severely dehydrated, because this can cause renal shutdown and failure (Geriatric patients are particularly vulnerable.)
- Patients with renal insufficiency, as evidenced by a blood urea nitrogen value greater than 40 mg/dl, because the iodinated nephrotoxic dye can worsen kidney function
- Patients with multiple myeloma, because the iodinated nephrotoxic dye can worsen renal function
- Patients who are pregnant, unless the benefits outweigh the risk of radiation exposure to the fetus

Potential complications

- Allergy to iodine dye
- Infiltration of contrast dye
- Renal failure
  This occurs most often in elderly patients who are chronically dehydrated before the dye injection.
- Hypoglycemia or acidosis may occur in patients who are taking metformin (Glucophage) and receive iodine dye.

Interfering factors

- Fecal material, gas, or barium in the bowel may obscure visualization of the renal system.
- Abnormal renal function studies may prevent adequate visualization of the urinary tract.
- Retained barium from previous studies may obscure visualization. Studies using barium (e.g., barium enema) should be scheduled after an IVP.

Procedure and patient care

Before

PT Explain the procedure to the patient. Inform the patient that several x-ray films will be taken over 30 minutes.
- Obtain informed consent if required by the institution.
- Check the patient for allergies to iodinated dye and shellfish.
- Give the patient a laxative (e.g., castor oil) or a cathartic, as ordered, the evening before the test.
PT Inform the patient of the required food and fluid restrictions. Some institutions prefer abstinence from solid foods for 8 hours before testing. Some allow a clear-liquid breakfast on the test day.
- Ensure adequate hydration for the patient (IV or oral) before and after the test to avoid dye-induced renal failure.
- Note that pediatric patients will have decreased fasting times, as ordered on an individual basis.
- Note that elderly and debilitated patients should have fasting times indicated specifically for them.
- Note that patients receiving high rates of IV fluids may have infusion rates decreased for several hours before the study to increase the concentration of the dye within the urinary system.
- Assess the patient's blood urea nitrogen and creatinine levels. Abnormal renal function could deteriorate as a result of the dye injection.
- Schedule any barium studies after completion of the IVP.
- Give the patient an enema or suppository on the morning of the study, if ordered.

During

- Note the following procedural steps:
  1. The patient is taken to the radiology department and placed in the supine position.

2. A plain film of the abdomen (KUB) is taken to ensure that no residual stool obscures visualization of the renal system. This also screens for calculi in the renal collecting system.

3. Skin testing for iodine allergy is often done.

4. A peripheral IV line is started (if not in place), and a contrast dye (e.g., Hypaque, Renografin) is given.

5. X-ray films are taken at specific times, usually at 1, 5, 10, 15, 20, and 30 minutes, and sometimes longer, to follow the course of the dye from the cortex of the kidney to the bladder.

6. Tomography may be performed to identify a mass.

7. The patient is taken to the bathroom and asked to void.

8. A postvoiding film is taken to visualize the empty bladder.

- Note that occasionally it is necessary to partially occlude the ureters temporarily to obtain a better film of the collecting system in the upper part of the ureters. This is done by compressing the abdomen with an inflatable rubber tube, which is wrapped tightly around the abdomen slightly below the umbilicus.

- Note that this test is performed by a radiologist in approximately 45 minutes.

PT Inform the patient that the dye injection often causes a transitory flushing of the face, a feeling of warmth, a salty taste in the mouth, or even transient nausea. Initial IV needle placement and lying on a hard x-ray table are the only other discomforts associated with IVP.

After

- Maintain the patient on adequate oral or IV hydration for several hours after the IVP to counteract fluid depletion caused by the test preparation.

- Assess the patient's urinary output. A decreased output may be an indication of renal failure.

- Evaluate elderly and debilitated patients for weakness because of the combination of fasting and catharsis necessary for test preparation. Instruct these patients to ambulate only with assistance.

- See p. xix for appropriate interventions concerning care for patients with iodine allergy.

🏠 **Home care responsibilities**

- After this test, patients must be encouraged to drink a lot of fluids to reestablish their normal state of hydration.
- Instructions to patients regarding urinary output are crucial. A decreased urine output may be an indication of impending renal failure.

Abnormal findings

Pyelonephritis
Glomerulonephritis
Kidney tumor (benign or malignant)
Renal hematoma
Renal laceration
Cyst or polycystic disease of the kidney
Congenital abnormality of the urologic tract
Renal or ureteral calculi
Trauma to the kidneys, ureters, or bladder
Tumor of the collecting system
Hydronephrosis
Extrinsic compression of the collecting system (e.g., caused by tumor, aneurysm)
Bladder tumor
Prostate enlargement (male)

notes

iron level and total iron-binding capacity (Fe and TIBC, Transferrin saturation, Transferrin)

Type of test Blood

Normal findings

Iron:

    Male: 80-180 mcg/dl or 14-32 µmol/L (SI units)

    Female: 60-160 mcg/dl or 11-29 µmol/L (SI units)

    Newborn: 100-250 mcg/dl

    Child: 50-120 mcg/dl

TIBC:

    250-460 mcg/dl or 45-82 µmol/L (SI units)

Transferrin:

    Adult male: 215-365 mg/dl or 2.15-3.65 g/L (SI units)

    Adult female: 250-380 mg/dl or 2.50-3.80 g/L (SI units)

    Newborn: 130-275 mg/dl

    Child: 203-360 mg/dl

Transferrin saturation:

    Male: 20%-50%

    Female: 15%-50%

Test explanation and related physiology

Serum iron

Abnormal levels of iron are characteristic of many diseases, including iron deficiency anemia and hemochromatosis. Seventy percent of iron in the body is found in the hemoglobin of red blood cells (RBCs). The other 30% is stored iron in the form of *ferritin* (see p. 430) and hemosiderin. Iron is supplied by the diet. Iron is bound to a globulin protein called *transferrin*. The serum iron determination is a measurement of the quantity of iron bound to transferrin.

Iron deficiency anemia is a result of reduced serum iron. Iron deficiency anemia has many causes, including the following:

1. Insufficient iron intake
2. Inadequate gut absorption
3. Increased requirements (as in growing children and late pregnancy)
4. Loss of blood (as in menstruation, bleeding peptic ulcer, and colon neoplasm)

Iron deficiency results in decreased production of hemoglobin, which in turn results in small, pale (microcytic, hypochromic)

RBCs. A decreased serum iron level, elevated TIBC, and low transferrin saturation (TS) value are characteristic of iron deficiency anemia.

Iron overload or poisoning is called hemochromatosis or hemosiderosis. Excess iron is usually deposited in the brain, liver, and heart and causes severe dysfunction of these organs. Massive blood transfusions also may cause elevated serum iron levels, although only transiently. Transfusions should be avoided before serum iron level blood specimens are obtained in the evaluation of anemia. Because serum iron levels may vary significantly during the day, the blood specimen should be drawn in the morning, especially when the results are used to monitor iron replacement therapy.

Total iron-binding capacity and transferrin

TIBC is a measurement of all proteins available for binding mobile iron. *Transferrin* represents the largest quantity of iron-binding proteins. Therefore TIBC is an indirect yet accurate measurement of transferrin. Ferritin is not included in TIBC because it binds only stored iron. TIBC is increased in 70% of patients with iron deficiency.

Transferrin is a *negative* acute phase reactant protein. That is, in various acute inflammatory reactions, transferrin levels diminish. Transferrin also is diminished in the face of chronic illnesses such as malignancy, collagen vascular diseases, or liver diseases. Hypoproteinemia is also associated with reduced transferrin levels. Pregnancy and estrogen therapy are associated with increased transferrin levels.

TIBC varies minimally according to iron intake and is more of a reflection of liver function (transferrin is produced by the liver) and nutrition than of iron metabolism. Transferrin values often are used to monitor the course of patients receiving hyperalimentation.

Total iron-binding capacity and transferrin saturation

The percentage of transferrin and other mobile iron-binding proteins saturated with iron is calculated by dividing the serum iron level by the TIBC:

$$\text{TS (\%)} = \frac{\text{Serum iron level}}{\text{TIBC}} \times 100\%$$

The normal value for TS is 20% to 50%. TS is decreased to less than 15% in patients with iron deficiency anemia. It is increased in patients with hemolytic, sideroblastic, or megaloblastic anemias.

TS is also increased in patients with iron overload or poisoning. Increased intake or absorption of iron (as in hemochromatosis) leads to elevated iron levels. In such cases TIBC is unchanged; as a result, the percentage of transferrin saturation is very high.

Chronic illness (e.g., infections, neoplasia, cirrhosis) is characterized by a low serum iron level, decreased TIBC, and normal TS. Pregnancy is marked by high levels of protein, including transferrin. Because iron requirements are high, it is not unusual to find low serum iron levels, high TIBC, and a low percentage of TS in late pregnancy.

Contraindications

- Patients with hemolytic diseases, because they may have an artificially high iron content

Interfering factors

- Recent blood transfusions may affect test results.
- Recent ingestion of a meal containing high iron content may affect test results.
- Hemolytic diseases may be associated with an artificially high iron content.
- ✘ Drugs that may cause *increased* iron levels include chloramphenicol, dextran, estrogens, ethanol, iron preparations, methyldopa, and oral contraceptives.
- ✘ Drugs that may cause *decreased* iron levels include adrenocorticotropic hormone (ACTH), cholestyramine, chloramphenicol, colchicine, deferoxamine, methicillin, and testosterone.
- ✘ Drugs that may cause *increased* TIBC levels include fluorides and oral contraceptives.
- ✘ Drugs that may cause *decreased* TIBC levels include ACTH and chloramphenicol.

Procedure and patient care

Before

PT Keep the patient fasting for 12 hours before the blood test. Water is permitted.

During

- Collect approximately 5 to 7 ml of venous blood in a red-top tube. The specimen should always be obtained using a 20-gauge or larger needle.
- Avoid hemolysis, because the iron contained in the RBCs will pour out into the serum and cause artificially high iron levels.

- Indicate on the laboratory slip any drugs that may affect test results.

After
- Apply pressure to the venipuncture site.

Abnormal findings

▲ **Increased serum iron levels**

Hemosiderosis
Hemochromatosis
Hemolytic anemia
Hepatitis
Hepatic necrosis
Lead toxicity
Iron poisoning
Massive transfusion
Lead toxicity

▼ **Decreased serum iron levels**

Insufficient dietary iron
Chronic blood loss
Inadequate absorption of iron
Pregnancy (late)
Iron deficiency anemia
Neoplasia
Chronic gastrointestinal blood loss
Chronic hematuria
Chronic heavy physiologic or pathologic menstruation

▲ **Increased TIBC levels**

Oral contraceptives
Pregnancy (late)
Polycythemia vera
Iron deficiency anemia

▼ **Decreased TIBC levels**

Hypoproteinemia
Inflammatory diseases
Cirrhosis
Hemolytic anemia
Pernicious anemia
Sickle cell anemia

notes

17-ketosteroids (17-KS)

Type of test   Urine (24-hour)

Normal findings

Male: 6-20 mg/24 hr or 20-70 μmol/day (SI units)
Female: 6-17 mg/24 hr or 20-60 μmol/day (SI units)
Elderly: values decrease with age
Child
    Younger than 12 years: <5 mg/24 hr
    12-15 years: 5-12 mg/24 hr

Test explanation and related physiology

17-KS are metabolites of the testosterone and nontestosterone androgenic sex hormones that are secreted from the adrenal cortex and the testes. The principal 17-KS is dehydroepiandrosterone (DHEA). In men, approximately one third of the hormone metabolites come from testosterone that is made in the testes, and two thirds come from nontestosterone androgens made in the adrenal cortex; in women and children, almost all the 17-KS are metabolites from nontestosterone androgenic hormones derived from the adrenal cortex. Therefore this test is very useful in diagnosing adrenocortical dysfunction. It is important to note that 17-KS are not metabolites of cortisol and do not reflect levels of cortisol production. Elevated 17-KS levels are frequently seen in patients with congenital adrenal hyperplasia and androgenic tumors of the adrenal glands. In these diseases, excess steroid synthesis is of the "noncortisol" androgenic sterols. These diseases frequently cause virilization syndromes. Low levels of 17-KS have little clinical significance.

Interfering factors

- Drugs that may cause *increased* levels include antibiotics, chloramphenicol, chlorpromazine, dexamethasone, meprobamate, phenothiazines, quinidine, secobarbital, and spironolactone (Aldactone).
- Drugs that may cause *decreased* levels include estrogen, oral contraceptives, probenecid, promazine, reserpine, salicylates (prolonged use), and thiazide diuretics.

Procedure and patient care

Before
- **PT** Explain the procedure to the patient.
- Withhold all drugs (with physician approval) for several days beforehand.
- Assess the patient for signs of stress and report these to the physician.

During
- **PT** Instruct the patient to begin the 24-hour urine collection after urinating; discard this specimen.
- Collect all urine passed by the patient during the next 24 hours.
- Post the hours for the urine collection in a prominent spot.
- Remember that it is not necessary to measure each urine specimen.
- **PT** Tell the patient to void before defecating so that the urine is not contaminated by feces.
- **PT** Inform the patient that toilet paper should not be placed in the collection container.
- **PT** Encourage the patient to drink fluids during the 24 hours, unless this is contraindicated for medical purposes.
- Remember that the urine collection needs a preservative.
- Refrigerate the urine throughout the collection.
- **PT** Instruct the patient to collect the last specimen as close as possible to the end of the 24-hour period. Add this to the urine collection.

After
- Indicate on the laboratory slip the start and end times of the specimen collection.
- List on the laboratory slip any medications that may affect test results.
- Send the specimen to the laboratory as soon as the test is completed.

Abnormal findings

▲ **Increased levels**

Congenital adrenal
hyperplasia
Pregnancy
Adrenocorticotropic
hormone administration
Cushing's syndrome
Testosterone- or estrogen-
secreting tumors of the
adrenals, ovaries, or testes
Severe stress or infection
Hyperpituitarism
Ovarian neoplasia
Stein-Leventhal syndrome

▼ **Decreased levels**

Addison's disease
Hypogonadism
(Klinefelter's
syndrome)
Hypopituitarism
Myxedema
Severe debilitating
disease
Nephrosis
Gout
Castration
Thyrotoxicosis
Severe stress or
infection
Chronic illnesses

K

notes

lactate dehydrogenase (Lactic dehydrogenase [LDH])

Type of test　Blood

Normal findings

Adult/elderly: 100-190 units/L at 37° C (lactate → pyruvate)
　or 100-190 units/L (SI units)

Isoenzymes
　Adult/elderly:
　　LDH-1: 17%-27%
　　LDH-2: 27%-37%
　　LDH-3: 18%-25%
　　LDH-4: 3%-8%
　　LDH-5: 0%-5%
　Child: 60-170 units/L (30° C)
　Infant: 100-250 units/L
　Newborn: 160-450 units/L

Test explanation and related physiology

LDH is found in the cells of many body tissues, especially the heart, liver, red blood cells, kidneys, skeletal muscle, brain, and lungs. Because LDH is widely distributed through the body, the total LDH level is not a specific indicator of any one disease affecting any one organ. When disease or injury affects the cells that contain LDH, the cells lyse, and LDH is spilled into the bloodstream, where it is identified in higher than normal levels. The LDH test is a measure of total LDH. There are actually five separate fractions (isoenzymes) that make up the total LDH. Each tissue contains a predominance of one or more LDH enzymes.

In general, isoenzyme LDH-1 comes mainly from the heart; LDH-2 comes primarily from the reticuloendothelial system; LDH-3 comes from the lungs and other tissues; LDH-4 comes from the kidney, placenta, and pancreas; and LDH-5 comes mainly from the liver and striated muscle. In normal persons, LDH-2 makes up the greatest percentage of total LDH.

With myocardial injury, the serum LDH level rises within 24 to 48 hours after a myocardial infarction (MI), peaks in 2 to 3 days, and returns to normal in approximately 5 to 10 days. Newer cardiac markers have replaced the indications for LDH in the MI patient.

LDH is also measured in other body fluids. Elevated urine levels of total LDH indicate neoplasm or injury to the urologic system. When the LDH in an effusion (pleural, cardiac, or peritoneal) is >60% of the serum total LDH (i.e., effusion LDH/serum LDH ratio is greater than 0.6), the effusion is said to be an *exudate* and not a transudate.

Interfering factors

- Strenuous exercise may cause an elevation of total LDH and specifically LDH-1, -2, and -5.
- Hemolysis of blood will cause false-positive LDH levels.
- ✶ Drugs that may cause *increased* LDH levels include alcohol, anesthetics, aspirin, clofibrate, fluorides, mithramycin, narcotics, and procainamide.
- ✶ Drugs that may cause *decreased* levels include ascorbic acid.

Procedure and patient care

Before
PT Explain the procedure to the patient.
PT Tell the patient that no fasting is required.

During
- Collect approximately 7 to 10 ml of venous blood in a red-top tube.
- Because many diseases cause an increased LDH level, identify disease conditions on the laboratory slip.
- Record the date and time when blood was drawn on the laboratory slip for an accurate evaluation of the temporal pattern of enzyme elevations.

After
- Apply pressure to the venipuncture site.

Abnormal findings

▲   **Increased values**

Myocardial infarction

Pulmonary disease (e.g., embolism, infarction, pneumonia, congestive heart failure)

Hepatic disease (e.g., hepatitis, active cirrhosis, neoplasm)

Red blood cell disease (e.g., hemolytic or megaloblastic anemia or red blood cell destruction from prosthetic heart valves)

Skeletal muscle disease and injury (e.g., muscular dystrophy, recent very strenuous exercises, or muscular trauma)

Renal parenchymal disease (e.g., infarction, glomerulonephritis, acute tubular necrosis, kidney transplantation rejection)

Intestinal ischemia and infarction

Testicular tumors (seminoma or dysgerminomas)

Lymphoma and other reticuloendothelial system tumors

Advanced solid tumor malignancies

Pancreatitis

Diffuse disease or injury (e.g., heatstroke, collagen disease, shock, hypotension)

notes

lactic acid (Lactate)

Type of test Blood

Normal findings

Venous blood: 5-20 mg/dl or 0.6-2.2 mmol/L (SI units)
Arterial blood: 3-7 mg/dl or 0.3-0.8 mmol/L (SI units)

Test explanation and related physiology

Under conditions of normal oxygen availability to tissues, glucose is metabolized to CO_2 and H_2O for energy. When oxygen to the tissues is diminished, anaerobic metabolism of glucose occurs, and lactate (lactic acid) is formed instead of CO_2 and H_2O. To compound the problem of lactic acid buildup, when the liver is hypoxic, it fails to clear the lactic acid. Lactic acid levels accumulate, causing lactic acidosis (LA). Therefore, blood lactate is a fairly sensitive and reliable indicator of tissue hypoxia. The hypoxia may be caused by local tissue hypoxia (e.g., mesenteric ischemia, extremity ischemia) or generalized tissue hypoxia such as exists in shock. Lactic acid blood levels are used to document the presence of tissue hypoxia, determine the degree of hypoxia, and monitor the effect of therapy.

Type I LA is caused by diseases that increase lactate but are not hypoxic related, such as glycogen storage diseases, liver diseases, or drugs. LA caused by hypoxia is classified as type II. Shock, convulsions, and extremity ischemia are the most common causes of type II LA. Type III LA is idiopathic and is most commonly seen in nonketotic patients with diabetes. The pathophysiology of lactic acid accumulation in type III is not known.

Interfering factors

- The prolonged use of a tourniquet or clenching of hands increases lactate levels.
- Drugs that *increase* levels include cyanide, ethanol (chronic use), aspirin, phenformin, and nalidixic acid.

Procedure and patient care

Before
PT Explain the procedure to the patient.
PT Tell the patient that no fasting is required.

During

PT Instruct the patient to avoid making a fist before and while blood is being withdrawn.

- Avoid the use of a tourniquet if possible.
- Collect approximately 7 ml of venous blood or 4 to 7 ml of arterial blood in a red-top tube.

After

- Apply pressure to the venipuncture site.

Abnormal findings

▲ **Increased levels**

Shock

Tissue ischemia

Carbon monoxide poisoning

Severe liver disease

Genetic errors of metabolism

Diabetes mellitus (nonketotic)

notes

lactose tolerance test

Type of test Blood

Normal findings

Blood: Adult/elderly: rise in plasma glucose levels >20 mg/dl
No abdominal cramps or diarrhea
Breath: <50 ppm hydrogen increase over baseline

Test explanation and related physiology

This test is performed to detect lactose intolerance. Lactose is a disaccharide typically found in dairy products. Because lactose-intolerant patients have an absence of lactase, lactose digestion will not occur. Thus the small bowel is flooded with a high lactose load. Bacterial metabolism of the lactose occurs within the intestine. This creates a strong cathartic effect. Symptoms of lactose intolerance include abdominal cramping, flatus, abdominal bloating, and diarrhea.

Although all adults have some degree of lactase reduction, severe lactose intolerance can occur in patients with inflammatory bowel disease, short-gut syndrome, and other malabsorption syndromes. Lactase deficiency can be congenital and become apparent in the newborn. These infants present with vomiting, diarrhea, malabsorption, and failure to thrive.

In the test, the patient is provided a lactose load. If lactase is not present in sufficient quantities, lactose is not metabolized to glucose and galactose. Plasma levels of glucose do not rise as expected. Therefore, lower-than-expected serum glucose levels suggest intestinal lactase deficiency. Patients who have malabsorption without lactase deficiency will also fail to elevate the blood glucose levels. They will also fail to have a glucose rise with an oral glucose load.

There is also a breath test part to this test in which exhaled air is analyzed for hydrogen content. The hydrogen content is directly proportional to the amount of lactose not broken down and absorbed.

Interfering factors

- Enterogenous steatorrhea
- Strenuous exercise
- Smoking may increase blood glucose levels.

- Patients with diabetes may have glucose levels that exceed 20 mg/dl despite lactase insufficiency.

Procedure and patient care

Before

PT Explain the procedure to the patient. Inform the patient that four blood samples will be needed.

PT Instruct the patient to fast 8 hours before testing.

PT Instruct the patient to avoid strenuous exercise for 8 hours before testing. This may factitiously affect the blood glucose level.

PT Inform the patient that smoking is prohibited for approximately 8 hours before testing. This may falsely increase the blood glucose level.

During

- Obtain 5 to 7 ml of venous blood in a gray-top tube from the fasting patient.
- Provide a specified dose of lactose for the patient. Usually dilute 100 g of lactose with 200 ml of water for ingestion in adults.
- Note that pediatric doses of lactose are based on weight.
- Collect three more blood samples at 30, 60, and 120 minutes after the ingestion of lactose.

PT Tell the patient that the only discomfort is the venipuncture; however, patients with lactase deficiency will have the symptoms previously described.

- If the breath test is being done, the exhaled air is evaluated for hydrogen content at 30, 60, and 120 minutes after the ingestion of lactose.

After

- Apply pressure to the venipuncture site.
- Note that patients with abnormal test results may receive a monosaccharide tolerance test (e.g., glucose or galactose tolerance test).

Abnormal findings

▼ **Decreased levels**

Lactase insufficiency
Enterogenous diarrhea

laparoscopy (Pelvic endoscopy, Gynecologic video laparoscopy)

Type of test Endoscopy

Normal findings Normal-appearing abdominal and pelvic organs

Test explanation and related physiology

Laparoscopy is used to visualize directly the abdominal and pelvic organs when pathology is suspected. It is used to evaluate patients with:

Acute abdominal/pelvic pain

Chronic abdominal/pelvic pain

Suspected advanced cancer

Abdominal mass of uncertain etiology

During laparoscopy the abdominal organs can be visualized by inserting a scope through the abdominal wall and into the peritoneum (Figure 24). Usually a television camera is applied to the scope, and the view of the scope is seen on color monitors. This is particularly helpful in diagnosing abdominal and pelvic adhesions, tumors and cysts affecting any abdominal organ, and tubal and uterine causes of infertility. Endometriosis, ectopic pregnancy, ruptured ovarian cyst, and salpingitis can be detected during an

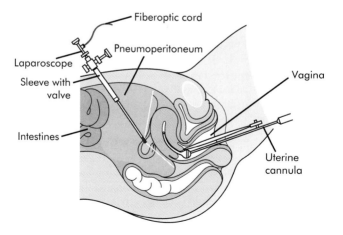

Figure 24 Laparoscopy directed to the pelvis.

evaluation for pelvic pain. This procedure is also used to stage cancers and determine their resectability. Surgical procedures (e.g., cholecystectomy, appendectomy, hernia repair, tubal ligation, oophorectomy, hiatal hernia repair, and bowel resection) can be performed with the laparoscope. Laparoscopy affords many advantages to patients in comparison with an open laparotomy, including reduced pain, length of stay, and time off from work.

Contraindications

- Patients who have had multiple surgical procedures, because adhesions may have formed between the viscera and the abdominal wall
- Patients with suspected intraabdominal hemorrhage, because visualization through the scope is obscured by the blood

Potential complications

- Perforation of the bowel, with spilling of intestinal contents into the peritoneum
- Hemorrhage

Interfering factors

- Adhesions or extreme obesity may obstruct the field of vision.

Procedure and patient care

Before

PT Explain the procedure to the patient.

PT Ensure that an informed consent for this procedure is obtained. Because of the possibility of intraabdominal injury, an open laparotomy may be required. Be sure the patient is aware of that.

- If enemas are ordered to clear the bowel, assist the patient as needed and record the results.
- Because the procedure is usually performed with the patient under general anesthesia, follow routine general anesthesia precautions.
- Shave and prepare the patient's abdomen as ordered.
- Keep the patient NPO after midnight on the day of the test. IV fluids may be given.

PT Instruct the patient to void before going to the operating room because a distended bladder can be easily penetrated.

During

- After general anesthesia is induced, a catheter and nasogastric tube are inserted to minimize the risk of penetrating a distended stomach or bladder with the initial needle placement.
- Note the following procedural steps:
  1. Laparoscopy is performed in the operating room. The patient is initially placed in the supine position. Other positions may be assumed to maximize visibility.
  2. After the abdominal skin is cleansed, a blunt-tipped (Verres) needle is inserted through a small incision in the periumbilical area and into the peritoneal cavity. Alternatively, a slightly larger incision is placed in the skin, and the abdominal wall is separated under direct vision. The peritoneal cavity is entered directly. Adhesions can be lysed under direct vision.
  3. The peritoneal cavity is filled with approximately 3 to 4 L of carbon dioxide to separate the abdominal wall from the intraabdominal viscera, enhancing visualization of pelvic and abdominal structures.
  4. A laparoscope is inserted through a trocar to examine the abdomen (Figure 24). Other trocars can be placed as conduits for other instrumentation.
  5. After the desired procedure is completed, the laparoscope is removed, and the carbon dioxide is allowed to escape.
  6. The incision(s) is closed with a few skin stitches and covered with an adhesive bandage.
- Note that laparoscopy is performed by a surgeon.
- **PT** Inform patients who will be under general anesthesia that they will feel no discomfort during the procedure. Most patients will have mild incisional pain later, and also may complain of shoulder or subcostal discomfort from pneumoperitoneum.

After

- Assess the patient frequently for signs of bleeding (increased pulse rate, decreased blood pressure), perforated viscus (abdominal tenderness, guarding, decreased bowel sounds). Report any significant findings to the physician.
- If patients have shoulder or subcostal discomfort from pneumoperitoneum, assure them that this usually lasts only 24 hours. Minor analgesics usually relieve this discomfort.
- If a surgical procedure has been performed laparoscopically, provide appropriate specific postsurgical care.

🏠 Home care responsibilities

- Observe for increasing abdominal pain, which may indicate bowel perforation.
- Note that fever and chills may indicate a bowel perforation.
- Inform the patient that discomfort in the shoulder area or under the ribs may result from the carbon dioxide inserted into the peritoneal cavity during the procedure.

Abnormal findings

Abdominal adhesions
Ovarian tumor or cyst
Endometriosis
Ectopic pregnancy
Pelvic inflammatory disease
Uterine fibroids
Abscess or infection
Cancer
Ascites
Portal hypertension
Other abdominal pathology

notes

Legionnaires' disease antibody test

Type of test Blood

Normal findings No *Legionella* antibody titer

Test explanation and related physiology

Legionnaires' disease was originally described as a fulminating pneumonia caused by *Legionella pneumophila*, a tiny gram-negative rod-shaped bacterium. This organism can also cause an influenza-type illness called *Pontiac fever*.

The diagnosis of legionnaires' disease can be made by culturing this organism from suspected infected fluids such as blood, sputum, lung tissue, or pleural fluid. Sputum for this test is best obtained by transtracheal aspiration or from bronchial washings. However, growth of this organism in culture is difficult. A negative culture does not mean that the patient does not have legionnaires' disease. Another method of diagnosis is by directly identifying the organism in a microscopic smear of infected fluid with the use of direct fluorescent antibody methods. If positive, this allows for a rapid diagnosis of *Legionella*. However, this is difficult also because the concentration of the bacteria may not be high enough to see the bacterium in the specimen.

The most common and easiest method for diagnosis is detection of the antibody directed against the *Legionella* bacterium in the patient's blood. A presumptive diagnosis of Legionnaires' disease can be made in a symptomatic person when a single antibody titer is 1:256 or greater. A fourfold rise in titer to at least 1:128 between the acute (1-week) and the convalescent (3-week) phase convalescent titer is diagnostic.

Procedure and patient care

Before

PT Explain the procedure to the patient.

PT Tell the patient that no fasting is required.

During

- For blood: Collect approximately 5 to 7 ml of blood in a red-top tube.
- For culture: Obtain sputum as indicated in sputum culture, p. 872.

After

- Apply pressure to the venipuncture site.

Abnormal findings

▲ **Increased levels**

Legionnaires' disease

notes

leucine aminopeptidase (LAP)

Type of test Blood; urine (24-hour)

Normal findings

Blood

Male: 80-200 units/ml or 19.2-48.0 units/L (SI units)
Female: 75-185 units/ml or 18.0-44.4 units/L (SI units)
Urine: 2-18 units/24 hr

Test explanation and related physiology

LAP is an intracellular enzyme that exists in the hepatobiliary system and to a much smaller degree in the pancreas and small intestine. When disease or injury affects these organs, the cells lyse, and LAP is spilled out into the bloodstream. LAP is mainly used in diagnosing liver disorders and in the differential diagnosis of increased levels of alkaline phosphatase (ALP, see p. 36). LAP levels tend to parallel ALP levels in hepatic disease. LAP is a sensitive indicator of cholestasis; however, unlike ALP, LAP remains normal in bone disease. LAP can be detected in both blood and urine. Patients with elevated serum LAP levels will always show elevations in urine levels. When the urine LAP level is elevated, however, the blood level may have already returned to normal.

This enzyme was originally thought to be elevated during pregnancy and to be an indication of the viability of the fetal-placental unit. However, it has been found that the enzyme found in pregnancy is immunochemically different than LAP.

Interfering factors

- Pregnancy may cause increased values.
- Drugs that may cause *increased* LAP levels include estrogens and progesterones.

Procedure and patient care

Before

PT Explain the procedure to the patient.
PT Tell the patient that no fasting is required.

During

- Collect approximately 7 to 10 ml of venous blood in a red-top tube.

- If a urine sample is needed, follow the procedure for a 24-hour urine collection (see p. 416).
- Indicate on the laboratory slip any medications the patient is taking that may affect test results.

After
- Apply pressure to the venipuncture site. Patients with liver dysfunction often have prolonged clotting times.

Abnormal findings

▲   **Increased levels**

Hepatitis
Cirrhosis
Hepatic necrosis
Hepatic ischemia
Hepatic tumor
Hepatotoxic drugs
Cholestasis
Gallstones

notes

leukoagglutinin test

Type of test Blood

Normal findings

Negative for leukoagglutinins

Test explanation and related physiology

Leukoagglutinins are antibodies directed to white blood cells (WBCs). They develop during blood transfusions. Patients who experience a transfusion reaction despite complete compatibility testing before blood administration should have a leukoagglutinin test to see if WBC incompatibility is the source of the reaction. Most commonly, the patient has antibodies to the donor WBCs and will experience a fever during transfusion. More severe, however, is the reaction when the donor plasma contains antibodies to the patient's WBCs. This nonhemolytic reaction can lead to severe transfusion reactions, including pulmonary failure and multiorgan system failure.

L

Procedure and patient care

Before

PT Explain the procedure to the patient.

PT Tell the patient that no fasting is required.

During

- Collect approximately 5 to 7 ml of venous blood in a red- or lavender-top tube.
- Indicate on the request slip that the patient has had a blood transfusion reaction.

After

- Apply pressure to the venipuncture site.

Abnormal findings

Blood transfusion reaction

notes

lipase

Type of test Blood

Normal findings 0-160 units/L or 0-160 units/L (SI units)
(Values are method dependent.)

Test explanation and related physiology

The most common cause of an elevated serum lipase level is acute pancreatitis. Lipase is an enzyme secreted by the pancreas into the duodenum to break down triglycerides into fatty acids. As with amylase (see p. 60), lipase appears in the bloodstream following damage to or disease affecting the pancreatic acinar cells.

Because lipase was thought to be produced only in the pancreas, elevated serum levels were considered to be specific to pathologic pancreatic conditions. It is now apparent that other conditions can be associated with elevated lipase levels. Lipase is excreted through the kidneys. Therefore, elevated lipase levels are often found in patients with renal failure. Intestinal infarction or obstruction also can be associated with lipase elevation. However, the lipase elevations in nonpancreatic diseases are less than 3 times the upper limit of normal, as compared with pancreatitis, where they are often 5 to 10 times normal values. Still other conditions, such as cholangitis, mumps, cholecystitis, or peptic ulcer, are more rarely associated with elevated lipase levels.

In acute pancreatitis, elevated lipase levels usually parallel serum amylase levels. The lipase levels usually rise a little later than amylase (24 to 48 hours after the onset of pancreatitis) and remain elevated for 5 to 7 days. Because lipase peaks later and remains elevated longer than serum amylase, it is more useful in the diagnosis of acute pancreatitis later in the course of the disease. Lipase levels are less useful in more chronic pancreatic diseases (e.g., chronic pancreatitis, pancreatic carcinoma).

Interfering factors

- ✠ Drugs that may cause *increased* lipase levels include bethanechol, cholinergics, codeine, indomethacin, meperidine, methacholine, and morphine.
- ✠ Drugs that may cause *decreased* levels include calcium ions.

Procedure and patient care

Before

PT Explain the procedure to the patient.

PT Instruct the patient to remain NPO, except for water, for 8 to 12 hours before the test.

During

- Collect 5 to 7 ml of venous blood in a red-top tube.
- Indicate on the laboratory slip drugs that may affect test results.

After

- Apply pressure to the venipuncture site.

Abnormal findings

Acute pancreatitis
Chronic relapsing pancreatitis
Pancreatic cancer
Pancreatic pseudocyst
Acute cholecystitis
Cholangitis
Extrahepatic duct obstruction
Renal failure
Bowel obstruction or infarction
Salivary gland inflammation or tumor
Peptic ulcer disease

notes

lipoprotein electrophoresis (Lipid fractionation, Lipoprotein phenotyping)

Type of test Blood

Normal findings

Electrophoretic component	Lipoprotein	Normal percentage of total
Chylomicrons	Triglycerides	0-2
Beta lipoprotein	Low-density lipoprotein (LDL)	33-52
Pre-beta lipoprotein	Very low-density lipoprotein (VLDL)	7-28
Alpha lipoprotein	High-density lipoprotein (HDL)	10-30

Test explanation and related physiology

Lipoproteins are the single most accurate predictor of coronary arteriosclerotic heart disease (CAHD). The World Health Organization adopted the Fredrickson classification of lipid disorders to identify particular lipoprotein patterns (phenotypes) that are associated with certain inherited or acquired diseases or syndromes. Fredrickson's classification, through the use of electrophoresis, simply identifies which lipoproteins are raised. More recently, with recognition of HDL (see p. 592) as the most important predictor of CAHD, the use of lipoprotein electrophoresis is limited to patients with rare lipid profiles.

Interfering factors

- Dietary changes may affect phenotyping.
- Phenotyping is unreliable in patients with diabetes mellitus or renal failure.
- ⚔ Statin drugs alter phenotyping.

Procedure and patient care

Before

PT Instruct the patient to continue a normal diet for the 2 weeks prior to the test to get reliable phenotyping.

PT Instruct the patient to fast for 12 to 14 hours before blood is drawn.

During

- Obtain 5 to 7 ml of blood in a serum or plasma separator tube (red top or green top).
- The blood is refrigerated overnight and observed for turbidity or creamy layer.

After

PT Upon return of test results, instruct the patient regarding any dietary changes that may improve lipid profile.

Abnormal findings

Classification	Elevated lipoprotein	Associated clinical disorders
I	Chylomicrons	Lipoprotein lipase deficiency, apolipoprotein C II deficiency, uncontrolled diabetes mellitus (DM)
Iia	LDL	Familial hypercholesterolemia, nephrosis, hypothyroidism, familial combined hyperlipidemia
Iib	LDL, VLDL	Familial combined hyperlipidemia
III	Intermediate density lipoproteins	Dysbetalipo-proteinemia DM, alcoholism
IV	VLDL	Familial hypertriglyceridemia, familial combined hyperlipidemia, DM
V	Chylomicrons, VLDL	Diabetes, nephrosis, malnutrition

notes

lipoproteins (High-density lipoprotein [HDL], High-density lipoprotein cholesterol [HDL-C], Low-density lipoprotein [LDL], Low-density lipoprotein cholesterol [LDL-C], Very low-density lipoprotein [VLDL])

Type of test Blood

Normal findings

HDL
    Male: >45 mg/dl or >0.75 mmol/L (SI units)
    Female: >55 mg/dl or >0.91 mmol/L (SI units)
LDL: 60-180 mg/dl or <3.37 mmol/L (SI units)
VLDL: 7-32 mg/dl

Test explanation and related physiology

Lipoproteins are considered to be an accurate predictor of coronary heart disease (CHD). As part of the "lipid profile," these tests are performed to indicate persons at risk for developing heart disease and to monitor therapy if abnormalities are found.

Lipoproteins are proteins in the blood whose main purpose is to transport cholesterol, triglycerides, and other insoluble fats. They are used as markers to indicate the levels of lipids within the bloodstream. The "lipid profile" usually includes total cholesterol, triglycerides, HDL, LDL, and VLDL.

HDLs are carriers of cholesterol. They are produced in the liver and to a smaller degree in the intestines. It is suspected that the purpose of HDLs is to remove cholesterol from the peripheral tissues and transport it to the liver for excretion. Also, HDLs may have a protective effect by preventing cellular uptake of cholesterol and lipids. These potential actions may be the source of the protective cardiovascular characteristics associated with HDLs ("good cholesterol") within the blood. Clinical and epidemiologic studies have shown that HDL cholesterol is an independent inverse risk factor for coronary artery disease (CAD). Low levels (<35 mg/dl) are believed to increase a person's risk for CAD, whereas high levels (>60 mg/dl) are considered protective.

Both HDL and total cholesterol are independent variables of risk of CHD. When combined in a ratio fashion, the accuracy of prediction is increased. The total cholesterol/HDL ratio should be at least 5:1, with 3:1 being ideal (see Table 9, p. 263).

LDLs are cholesterol rich. Cholesterol carried by LDLs can be deposited into the peripheral tissues and is associated with an increased risk of arteriosclerotic heart and vascular disease. Therefore high levels of LDL ("bad cholesterol") are atherogenic. The LDL level should be less than 100 mg/dl (and possibly lower than 70 mg/dl) in high risk patients. For patients at moderately high risk, the LDL should be less than 130 mg/dl, although in some circumstances, a target of 100 mg/dl may be recommended. In the past, LDL was very difficult to isolate and measure. It was most usually derived by the Friedwald formula. In this formula, LDL is derived by subtracting the HDL plus one fifth of the triglycerides from the total cholesterol:

$$\text{LDL} = \text{Total cholesterol} - (\text{HDL} + \text{triglycerides}/5)$$

There are other formulas for deriving LDL, which may account for different sets of normal values. LDL can now be directly measured accurately and cheaply.

VLDLs, although carrying a small amount of cholesterol, are the predominant carriers of blood triglycerides. To a lesser degree, VLDLs are also associated with an increased risk of arteriosclerotic occlusive disease. The VLDL value is usually expressed as a percentage of total cholesterol. Levels in excess of 25% to 50% are associated with increased risk of coronary disease. Like LDL, there are now laboratory methods to accurately directly measure VLDL.

Interfering factors

- Smoking and alcohol ingestion decrease HDL levels.
- Binge eating can alter lipoprotein values.
- HDL values are age and sex dependent.
- HDL values, like cholesterol, tend to significantly decrease for as long as 3 months after myocardial infarction.
- HDL is elevated in hypothyroid patients and diminished in hyperthyroid patients.
- Drugs that may cause *increased* lipoprotein levels include aspirin, oral contraceptives, phenothiazines, steroids, and sulfonamides.

Procedure and patient care

Before

- PT Instruct the patient to fast for 12 to 14 hours before testing. Only water is permitted.
- PT Inform the patient that dietary indiscretion within the previous few weeks may influence lipoprotein levels.

During

- Collect 5 to 10 ml of venous blood in a red-top tube.
- Indicate on the laboratory slip any drugs that may affect test results.

After

- Apply pressure to the venipuncture site.
- **PT** Instruct patients with high lipoprotein levels regarding diet, exercise, and appropriate body weight.

Abnormal findings

▲ **Increased HDL levels**

Familial HDL lipoproteinemia
Excessive exercise

▼ **Decreased HDL levels**

Familial low HDL
Hepatocellular disease (e.g., hepatitis or cirrhosis)
Hypoproteinemia (e.g., nephrotic syndrome or malnutrition)

▲ **Increased LDL and VLDL**

Familial LDL lipoproteinemia
Nephrotic syndrome
Glycogen storage diseases (e.g., von Gierke's disease)
Hypothyroidism
Alcohol consumption
Chronic liver disease (e.g., hepatitis or cirrhosis)
Hepatoma
Gammopathies (e.g., multiple myeloma)
Familial hypercholesterolemia type IIa
Cushing's syndrome
Apoprotein CII deficiency

▼ **Decreased LDL and VLDL**

Familial hypolipoproteinemia
Hypoproteinemia (e.g., malabsorption, severe burns, or malnutrition)
Hyperthyroidism

liver biopsy

Type of test Microscopic examination of tissue

Normal findings Normal liver histology

Test explanation and related physiology

Liver biopsy is a safe, simple, and valuable method of diagnosing pathologic liver conditions. For this study, a specially designed needle is inserted through the abdominal wall and into the liver (Figure 25). A piece of liver tissue is removed for microscopic examination. Percutaneous liver biopsy is used in the diagnosis of various liver disorders such as cirrhosis, hepatitis, drug reaction, granuloma, and tumor. Biopsy is indicated for the following:

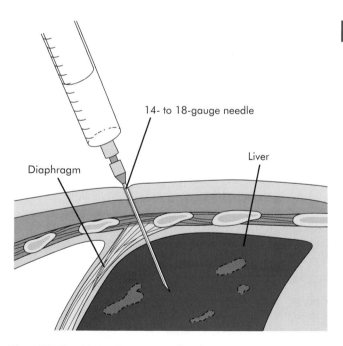

14- to 18-gauge needle

Liver

Diaphragm

Figure 25 Liver biopsy. Percutaneous liver biopsy requires the patient's cooperation. The patient must be able to lie quietly and hold his or her breath after exhaling.

1. Patients with unexplained hepatomegaly
2. Patients with persistently elevated liver enzymes
3. Patients with suspected primary or metastatic tumor, as determined by other studies
4. Patients with unexplained jaundice
5. Patients with suspected hepatitis
6. Patients with suspected infiltrative diseases (e.g., sarcoidosis, amyloidosis)

The biopsy may be performed by a "blind" stick or directed with the use of a computed tomography (CT) or magnetic resonance imaging (MRI) scan. Directed scans are used if there is a specific area of the liver that is suspicious and from which tissue must be obtained (e.g., a metastatic tumor). The "blind" stick is used if the liver is diffusely involved.

Contraindications

- Uncooperative patients who cannot remain still and hold their breath during sustained exhalation
- Patients with impaired hemostasis
- Patients with anemia who could not tolerate major blood loss associated with inadvertent puncture of an intrahepatic blood vessel
- Patients with infections in the right pleural space or right upper quadrant, because the biopsy may spread the infection
- Patients with obstructive jaundice
  In these patients, bile within the ducts is under pressure and may subsequently leak into the abdominal cavity after needle penetration.
- Patients with a hemangioma
  This is a very vascular tumor, and bleeding after a biopsy may be severe.

Potential complications

- Hemorrhage caused by inadvertent puncture of a blood vessel within the liver
- Chemical peritonitis caused by inadvertent puncture of a bile duct, with subsequent leakage of bile into the abdominal cavity
- Pneumothorax (collapsed lung) caused by improper placement of the biopsy needle into the adjacent chest cavity

Procedure and patient care

Before
- **PT** Explain the procedure to the patient. Many patients are apprehensive about it.
- Obtain an informed consent.
- Ensure that all coagulation tests are normal.
- **PT** Instruct the patient to keep NPO after midnight on the day of the test.
- Administer any sedative medications as ordered.

During
- Note the following procedural steps:
  1. The patient is placed in the supine or left lateral position.
  2. The skin area used for puncture is anesthetized locally.
  3. The patient is asked to exhale and hold the exhalation. This causes the liver to descend and reduces the possibility of a pneumothorax. Often, the patient may be instructed to practice exhalation two or three times before insertion of the needle.
  4. During the patient's sustained exhalation, the physician rapidly introduces the biopsy needle into the liver and obtains liver tissue.
     a. Several types of needles are available.
     b. Occasionally the biopsy needle is inserted under CT guidance. This is especially useful when tissue from a specific area of the liver is needed.
  5. The needle is withdrawn from the liver.
- Note that this test is performed by a physician in approximately 15 minutes.
- **PT** Inform the patient that he or she may have minor discomfort during injection of the local anesthetic and needle insertion.

After
- Place the tissue sample into a specimen bottle containing formalin and send it to the pathology department.
- Apply a small dressing over the needle insertion site.
- Place the patient on his or her right side for approximately 1 to 2 hours. In this position, the liver capsule is compressed against the chest wall, thereby decreasing the risk of hemorrhage or bile leak.
- Assess the patient's vital signs frequently for evidence of hemorrhage (increased pulse, decreased blood pressure) and peritonitis (increased temperature).

L

- Evaluate the rate, rhythm, and depth of respirations. Assess breath sounds. Report chest pain and signs of dyspnea, cyanosis, and restlessness, which may be indicative of pneumothorax.

🏠 Home care responsibilities

- Instruct the patient to report signs of bleeding (increased pulse and decreased BP) and peritonitis (increased temperature).
- Tell the patient to avoid coughing or straining that may cause increased intraabdominal pressure. Strenuous activities and heavy lifting should be avoided for 1 to 2 weeks.

Abnormal findings

Benign tumor
Malignant tumor (primary or metastatic)
Abscess
Cyst
Hepatitis
Infiltrative diseases (e.g., amyloidosis, hemochromatosis, cirrhosis)

notes

liver/spleen scanning (Liver scanning)

Type of test Nuclear scan

Normal findings Normal size, shape, and position of the liver and spleen

Test explanation and related physiology

This radionuclide procedure is used to outline and detect structural changes of the liver and spleen. A radionuclide, usually technetium sulfur-labeled albumin colloid, is administered intravenously. Later, a gamma ray scintillator is placed over the right and left upper quadrants of the patient's abdomen. This records the distribution of the radioactive particles emitted from the liver and spleen. Images are obtained comparable to the gamma ray emission and are recorded on film.

Because the scan can demonstrate only filling defects greater than 2 cm in diameter, false-negative results may occur in patients with space-occupying lesions (e.g., tumors, cysts, granulomas, abscesses) smaller than 2 cm. The liver scan can detect tumors, cysts, granulomas, abscesses, and diffuse infiltrative processes affecting the liver (e.g., amyloidosis, sarcoidosis).

Single-photon emission computed tomography (SPECT) has significantly improved the quality and accuracy of liver scanning. With SPECT scanning, the radionuclide is injected, and the scintillator is placed to receive images from multiple angles (around the circumference of the patient). This greatly increases the accuracy of nuclear liver scanning. With the use of radioactive carbon, nitrogen, or oxygen, anatomic and biochemical changes can be visualized within the liver. This method of liver scanning is called PET scanning (p. 729).

This scan can also identify portal hypertension. Normally, most of the radionuclide administered during a liver scan is taken up by the liver. If the liver-to-spleen ratio is reversed (i.e., the spleen takes up more of the radionuclide), reversal of hepatic blood flow exists as a result of portal hypertension.

Splenic hematoma, abscess, cyst, tumor, infarction, and infiltrate processes such as granulomas also can be detected.

Contraindications

- Patients who are pregnant or lactating, unless the benefits of testing outweigh the risk of damage to the fetus or infant

Interfering factors

- Barium in the GI tract overlying the liver or spleen will produce defects on the scan that may be mistaken for masses.

Procedure and patient care

Before

PT Explain the procedure to the patient.

PT Tell the patient that no fasting or premedication is required.

PT Assure the patient that he or she will not be exposed to large amounts of radiation, because only tracer doses of isotopes are used.

During

- Note the following procedural steps:
  1. The patient is taken to the nuclear medicine department, where the radionuclide is administered intravenously.
  2. Thirty minutes after injection, a gamma ray detector is placed over the right upper quadrant of the patient's abdomen.
  3. The patient is placed in supine, lateral, and prone positions so that all surfaces of the liver can be visualized.
  4. The radionuclide image is recorded on x-ray film.
- Note that this procedure is performed by a trained technologist in approximately 1 hour. A physician trained in nuclear medicine interprets the results.

PT Tell the patient that the only discomfort associated with this procedure is the IV injection of the radionuclide.

After

PT Because only tracer doses of radioisotopes are used, inform the patient that no precautions need to be taken by others against radiation exposure.

Abnormal findings

Primary or metastatic tumor of the liver or spleen
Abscess of the liver or spleen
Hematoma of the liver or spleen
Hepatic or splenic cyst
Hemangioma
Lacerations of the liver or spleen
Infiltrative processes (e.g., sarcoidosis, amyloidosis, tuberculosis, or granuloma of the liver or spleen)
Cirrhosis
Portal hypertension
Accessory spleen
Splenic infarction

notes

lumbar puncture and cerebrospinal fluid examination (LP and CSF examination, Spinal tap, Spinal puncture, Cerebrospinal fluid analysis)

Type of test   Fluid analysis

Normal findings

Pressure: <20 cm H_2O
Color: clear and colorless
Blood: none
Cells:
  RBC: 0
  WBC
  Total
    Neonate: 0-30 cells/μl
    1-5 years: 0-20 cells/μl
    6-18 years: 0-10 cells/μl
    Adult: 0-5 cells/μl
  Differential
    Neutrophils: 0%-6%
    Lymphocytes: 40%-80%
    Monocytes: 15%-45%
Culture and sensitivity: no organisms present
Protein: 15-45 mg/dl CSF (up to 70 mg/dl in elderly adults
  and children)
Protein electrophoresis
  Prealbumin: 2%-7%
  Albumin: 56%-76%
  Alpha$_1$ globulin: 2%-7%
  Alpha$_2$ globulin: 4%-12%
  Beta globulin: 8%-18%
  Gamma globulin: 3%-12%
  Oligoclonal bands: none
  IgG: 0-4.5 mg/dl
Glucose: 50-75 mg/dl CSF or 60%-70% of blood glucose
  level
Chloride: 700-750 mg/dl
Lactate dehydrogenase (LDH): <2-7.2 units/ml
Lactic acid: 10-25 mg/dl
Cytology: no malignant cells
Serology for syphilis: negative
Glutamine: 6-15 mg/dl

Test explanation and related physiology

By placing a needle in the subarachnoid space of the spinal column, one can measure the pressure of that space and obtain CSF for examination and diagnosis. Lumbar puncture may also be used therapeutically to inject therapeutic or diagnostic agents and to administer spinal anesthetics.

Examination of the CSF includes evaluation for the presence of blood, bacteria, and malignant cells, along with quantification of the amount of glucose and protein present. Color is noted, and various other tests such as a serologic test for syphilis (see p. 888) are performed.

Pressure

By attaching a sterile manometer to the needle used for LP, the pressure within the subarachnoid space can be measured. A pressure greater than 20 cm H_2O is considered abnormal and indicative of increased spinal pressure. Because the subarachnoid space surrounding the brain is freely connected to the subarachnoid space of the spinal cord, any increase in intracranial pressure will be directly reflected as an increase at the lumbar site. Tumors, infection, hydrocephalus, and intracranial bleeding can cause increased intracranial and spinal pressure. Intracranial pressure is related to the volume of CSF fluid. Also, because the cranial venous sinuses are connected to the jugular veins, obstruction of those veins or the superior vena cava increases intracranial pressure.

Pressures are routinely measured at the beginning and end of an LP. If there is a significant difference in these values, one must suspect a spinal cord obstruction (tumor). Large differences in opening and closing pressures are also seen in patients with hydrocephalus. One must be aware that children who are crying and holding their breath may have transient elevations of pressure that reduce as the child relaxes.

Color

Normal CSF is clear and colorless. Color differences can occur with hyperbilirubinemia, hypercarotenemia, melanoma, or elevated proteins. A cloudy appearance may indicate an increase in the white blood cell (WBC) count or protein. A red tinge to the CSF indicates the presence of blood.

Blood

Normally, CSF contains no blood. Blood may be present because of bleeding into the subarachnoid space or because the needle used in the LP has inadvertently penetrated a blood vessel on the way into the subarachnoid space. With a "traumatic puncture," the blood within the CSF will clot. No clotting occurs in a patient with subarachnoid hemorrhage. Also, with a traumatic tap, the fluid clears toward the end of the procedure as successive CSF samples are obtained. This clearing does not occur with a subarachnoid hemorrhage.

Cells

The number of red blood cells is merely an indication of the amount of blood present within the CSF. Except for a few lymphocytes, the presence of WBCs in the CSF is abnormal. The presence of polymorphonuclear leukocytes (neutrophils) is indicative of bacterial meningitis or cerebral abscess. When mononuclear leukocytes are present, viral or tubercular meningitis or encephalitis is suspected. Leukemia or other primary or metastatic malignant tumors may cause elevated WBCs. Pleocytosis is a term used to indicate turbidity of CSF caused by an increased number of cells within the fluid.

Culture and sensitivity

The organisms that cause meningitis or brain abscess can be cultured from the CSF. Organisms found also may include atypical bacteria, fungi, or *Mycobacterium tuberculosis.* A Gram stain (p. 872) of the CSF may give the clinician preliminary information about the causative infectious agent. This may allow appropriate antibiotic therapy to be initiated before the 24 to 72 hours necessary to complete the culture and sensitivity report.

Protein

Normally, very little protein is found in CSF because proteins are large molecules that do not cross the blood-brain barrier. Normally, the proportion of albumin to globulin is higher in CSF than in blood plasma (see p. 758) because albumin is smaller than globulin and can pass more easily through the blood-brain barrier. Diseases such as meningitis, encephalitis, or myelitis can alter the permeability of the blood-brain barrier, allowing protein to leak into the CSF. Furthermore, central nervous system (CNS) tumors may produce and secrete protein into the CSF.

CSF protein electrophoresis is very important in the diagnosis of CNS diseases. Patients with multiple sclerosis, neurosyphilis, or other immunogenic degenerative central neurologic diseases have elevated immunoglobulins in their CSF. The detection of *oligoclonal gamma globulin bands* is highly suggestive of inflammatory and autoimmune diseases of the CNS, especially multiple sclerosis (MS). Myelin-basic protein, a component of myelin (substance that surrounds normal nerve tissue) is elevated when demyelinating diseases such as MS or amyotrophic lateral sclerosis occur.

Glucose

The glucose level is decreased when bacteria or cells within the CSF increase in number and catabolize the glucose. The cells may be inflammatory cells in response to infection or inflammation or cells that are shed by tumors. A blood sample for glucose (see p. 482) is usually drawn before the spinal tap is performed. A CSF glucose level less than 60% of the blood glucose may indicate meningitis or neoplasm.

Chloride

The chloride concentration in CSF may be decreased in patients with meningeal infections, tubercular meningitis, and conditions of low blood chloride levels. An increase in the chloride level in CSF is not neurologically significant; it correlates with the blood levels of chloride (see p. 260). CSF is not routinely evaluated for chloride; this test is done only if specifically requested.

Lactate dehydrogenase

Quantification of lactate dehydrogenase (LDH) (specifically, fractions 4 and 5; see p. 572) is helpful in diagnosing bacterial meningitis. The source of LDH is the neutrophils that fight the invading bacteria. When the LDH level is elevated, infection or inflammation is suspected. The elevated WBC count associated with CNS leukemia is also associated with elevated LDH levels. The nerve tissue in the CNS is also high in LDH (isoenzymes 1 and 2). Therefore, disease directly affecting the brain or spinal cord (e.g., stroke) is associated with elevated LDH levels.

Lactic acid

Elevated levels indicate anaerobic metabolism associated with decreased oxygenation of the brain. CSF lactic acid is increased in both bacterial and fungal meningitis but not in viral meningitis.

Cytology

Examination of cells found in the CSF can determine if they are malignant. Tumors in the CNS may shed cells from their surface. These cells can float freely in CSF. Their presence suggests neoplasm as the cause of any neurologic symptoms.

Tumor markers

Increased levels of tumor markers such as carcinoembryonic antigen, alpha-fetoprotein, or human chorionic gonadotropin may indicate metastatic tumor.

Serology for syphilis

Latent syphilis is diagnosed by performing one of many presently available serologic tests on CSF. These include the Wasserman test, the Venereal Disease Research Laboratory test (see p. 888), and the fluorescent treponemal antibody (FTA) test (see p. 888). The FTA test is considered to be the most sensitive and specific. When test results are positive, the diagnosis of neurosyphilis is made, and appropriate antibiotic therapy is initiated.

Glutamine

Elevated glutamine levels are helpful in the detection and evaluation of hepatic encephalopathy and hepatic coma. The glutamine is made by increased levels of ammonia, which are commonly associated with liver failure. See serum ammonia (p. 52). Levels of glutamine are also often increased in patients with Reye's syndrome.

C-reactive protein

As noted on p. 319, C-reactive protein (CRP) is a nonspecific, acute-phase reactant used in the diagnosis of bacterial infections and inflammatory disorders. Elevated CSF levels of CRP have been useful in the diagnosis of bacterial meningitis. Failure to find elevated CSF levels of CRP appears to be strong evidence against bacterial meningitis. Some research studies have shown that CSF levels of CRP have been valuable in distinguishing bacterial meningitis from viral encephalitis, tuberculosis, meningitis, febrile convulsions, and other CNS disorders. Serum levels of CRP (see p. 319) are more frequently used in the diagnosis of bacterial meningitis.

Contraindications

- Patients with increased intracranial pressure
  The LP may induce cerebral or cerebellar herniation through the foramen magnum.
- Patients who are anticoagulated
  Because of the risk of epidural hematoma, these patients need to have normal coagulation function prior to this procedure.

- Patients who have severe degenerative vertebral joint disease
  It is very difficult to pass the needle through the degenerated arthritic interspinal space.
- Patients with infection near the LP site
  Meningitis can result from contamination of CSF with infected material.

Potential complications

- Persistent CSF leak, causing severe headache
- Puncture of subcutaneous blood vessel during the procedure
- Introduction of bacteria into CSF, causing suppurative meningitis
- Herniation of the brain through the tentorium cerebelli or herniation of the cerebellum through the foramen magnum
  In patients with increased intracranial pressure, the quick reduction of pressure in the spinal column by the LP may induce herniation of the brain, causing compression of the brain stem. This results in deterioration of the patient's neurologic status and death.
- Inadvertent puncture of the spinal cord caused by inappropriately high puncture of the spinal caral
- Puncture of the aorta or vena cava, causing serious retroperitoneal hemorrhage
- Transient back pain and pain or paresthesia in the legs

Procedure and patient care

Before

PT Explain the procedure to the patient. Many patients have misconceptions regarding LP. Allay the patient's fears and allow time to verbalize concerns.
- Obtain informed consent if required by the institution.
- Perform a baseline neurologic assessment of the legs by assessing the patient's strengths, sensation, and movement.
PT Tell the patient that no fasting or sedation is required.
PT Instruct the patient to empty the bladder and bowels before the procedure.
PT Explain to the patient that he or she must lie very still throughout this procedure. Movement may cause traumatic injury. Encourage the patient to relax and take deep, slow breaths with the mouth open.

During

- Note the following procedural steps:
  1. This study is a sterile procedure that can be easily performed at the bedside. The patient is usually placed in the lateral decubitus (fetal) position (Figure 26).
  2. The patient is instructed to clasp the hands on the knees to maintain this position. Someone usually helps the patient maintain this position. (A sitting position also may be used.)
  3. A local anesthetic is injected into the skin and subcutaneous tissues after the site has been aseptically cleaned.
  4. A spinal needle containing an inner obturator is placed through the skin and into the spinal canal.
  5. The subarachnoid space is entered.
  6. The insert (obturator) is removed, and CSF can be seen slowly dripping from the needle.
  7. The needle is attached to a sterile manometer, and the pressure (opening pressure) is recorded.
  8. Before the pressure reading is taken, the patient is asked to relax and straighten the legs to reduce the intraabdominal pressure, which causes an increase in CSF pressure.

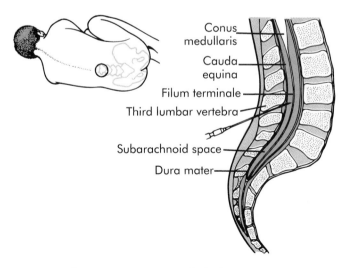

Conus medullaris
Cauda equina
Filum terminale
Third lumbar vertebra
Subarachnoid space
Dura mater

Figure 26 Patient position for lumbar puncture.

   9. Three sterile test tubes are filled with 5 to 10 ml of CSF.
  10. The pressure (closing pressure) is measured.

- Note that if blockage in CSF circulation in the spinal sub-arachnoid space is suspected, a *Queckenstedt-Stookey* test may be performed. For this test the jugular vein is occluded either manually by digital pressure or by a medium-sized blood pressure cuff inflated to approximately 20 mm Hg. Within 10 seconds after jugular occlusion, CSF pressure should increase from 15 to 40 cm H_2O and then promptly return to normal within 10 seconds after release of the pressure. A sluggish rise or fall of CSF pressure suggests partial blockage of CSF circulation. No rise after 10 seconds suggests a complete obstruction within the spinal canal.

- Note that this procedure is performed by a physician in approximately 20 minutes.

PT Inform the patient that this procedure is described as uncomfortable or painful by most patients. Some patients complain of feeling pressure from the needle. Some patients complain of a shooting pain in their legs.

After

- Apply digital pressure and an adhesive dressing to the puncture site.

- Place the patient in the prone position with a pillow under the abdomen to increase the intraabdominal pressure, which will indirectly increase the pressure in the tissues surrounding the spinal cord. This retards continued CSF flow from the spinal canal.

PT Encourage the patient to drink increased amounts of fluid with a straw to replace the CSF removed during the lumbar puncture. Drinking with a straw will enable the patient to keep the head flat.

PT Usually keep the patient in a reclining position for 1 hour or up to several hours to avoid the discomfort of potential postpuncture spinal headache. Instruct the patient to turn from side to side as long as the head is not raised.

- Label and number the specimen jars appropriately and deliver them immediately to the laboratory after the test. Refrigeration will alter test results. A delay between collection time and testing can invalidate results, especially cell counts.

- Assess the patient for numbness, tingling, and movement of the extremities; pain at the injection site; drainage of blood or CSF at the injection site; and the ability to void. Notify the physician of any unusual findings.

🏠 **Home care responsibilities**

- The patient should be kept flat in bed for a designated time period (1 hour–several hours) to avoid a postprocedure spinal headache.
- Encourage the patient to drink increased amounts of fluid to replace CSF removed during the LP.
- Instruct the patient to report any abnormalities, such as numbness and tingling in the legs, to the physician.

Abnormal findings

Brain neoplasm
Spinal cord neoplasm
Cerebral hemorrhage
Encephalitis
Myelitis
Tumor
Neurosyphilis
Degenerative brain disease
Autoimmune disorder
Hepatic encephalopathy
Coma
Meningitis
Encephalitis
Viral or tubercular meningitis
Cerebral abscess
Degenerative cord or brain disease
Multiple sclerosis
Acute demyelinating polyneuropathy
Subarachnoid bleeding
Reye's syndrome
Metastatic tumor

notes

lung biopsy

Type of test Microscopic examination of tissue

Normal findings No evidence of pathology

Test explanation and related physiology

This invasive procedure is used to obtain a specimen of pulmonary tissue for a histologic examination by using either an open or a closed technique. The *open method* involves a limited thoracotomy. The *closed technique* includes methods such as transbronchial lung biopsy, transbronchial needle aspiration biopsy, transcatheter bronchial brushing, percutaneous needle biopsy, and video-assisted thoracotomy (VAT)(see p. 903).

Lung biopsy is indicated to determine the pathology of pulmonary parenchymal disease. Carcinomas, granulomas, infections, and sarcoidosis can be diagnosed with this procedure. The procedure is also useful in detecting environmental exposures, infections, or familial disease, which may lead to better prevention and treatment.

Contraindications

- Patients with bullae or cysts of the lung
- Patients with suspected vascular anomalies of the lung
- Patients with bleeding abnormalities
- Patients with pulmonary hypertension
- Patients with respiratory insufficiency

Potential complications

- Pneumothorax
- Pulmonary hemorrhage
- Empyema

Procedure and patient care

Before

- **PT** Explain the procedure to the patient.
- Ensure that informed and signed consent is obtained.
- **PT** Instruct the patient that fasting is usually ordered. The patient may be kept NPO after midnight on the day of the test.
- Administer the preprocedural medications 30 to 60 minutes before the test as ordered.

PT Instruct the patient to remain still during the lung biopsy. Any movement or coughing could cause laceration of the lung by the biopsy needle.

During

- Note that the patient's position depends on the method used and that the histologic lung specimen may be obtained by several different methods:

Transbronchial lung biopsy
1. This technique is performed via flexible fiberoptic bronchoscopy, using cutting forceps.
2. Fluoroscopy is used to ensure proper opening and positioning of the forceps on the lesions.
3. Fluoroscopy also permits visualization of the "tug" of the lung as the specimen is removed.

Transbronchial needle aspiration
1. The needle is inserted through the bronchoscope and into the tumor or desired area, where aspiration is performed with the attached syringe (Figure 27).
2. The needle is retracted within its sheath, and the entire catheter is withdrawn from the fiberoptic scope.

Transbronchial brushing
1. A small brush is moved back and forth over the suspicious area in the bronchus or its branches.
2. The cells adhere to the brush, which is then removed and used to make microscopic slides.

Percutaneous needle biopsy
1. In this method for obtaining a closed specimen, the biopsy is obtained after using fluoroscopic x-ray or CT scan determination of the desired site.
2. The procedure is carried out by using a cutting needle or by aspiration with a spinal-type needle to obtain a specimen.

Open lung biopsy
1. The patient is taken to the operating room, and general anesthesia is provided.
2. The patient is placed in the supine or lateral position, and an incision is made into the chest wall.
3. After a piece of lung tissue is removed, the lung is sutured.
4. Chest tube drainage is used for approximately 24 hours after an open lung biopsy.

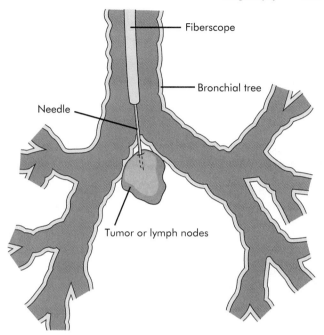

Figure 27 Transbronchial needle biopsy. The diagram shows a transbronchial needle penetrating the bronchial wall and entering a mass of subcarinal lymph nodes or tumor.

Thorascopic lung biopsy

1. The lung is collapsed with a double lumen endotracheal tube placed during induction of general anesthesia.
2. With the use of a thoracoscope (similar to a laparoscope [p. 579]), the lung is grasped, and a piece is cut off with the use of a cutting/stapling device. Large wedge lung resections can be obtained.
3. The scope and trocars are removed, and a small chest tube is left in place.
4. The tiny incisions are closed, and the procedure is completed.

- Note that this procedure is performed by a surgeon in 30 to 60 minutes.
- During the lung biopsy procedure, assess the patient carefully for signs of respiratory distress (e.g., shortness of breath, rapid pulse, cyanosis).

PT Tell the patient that most patients describe this procedure as painful.

After

- Place biopsy specimens in appropriate containers for histologic and microbiologic examination.
- Observe the patient's vital signs frequently for signs of bleeding (increased pulse, decreased blood pressure) and shortness of breath.
- Assess the patient's breath sounds and report any decrease on the biopsy side.
- Obtain a chest x-ray film to check for complications (e.g., pneumothorax).
- Observe the patient for signs of pneumothorax (e.g., dyspnea, tachypnea, decrease in breath sounds, anxiety, restlessness).

Abnormal findings

Carcinoma
Granuloma
Exposure lung diseases (e.g., black lung, asbestosis)
Sarcoidosis
Infection

notes

lung scan (Ventilation/perfusion scanning [VPS], Pulmonary scintiphotography, V̇/Q̇ scan)

Type of test Nuclear scan

Normal findings Diffuse and homogeneous uptake of nuclear material by the lungs

Test explanation and related physiology

This nuclear medicine procedure is used to identify defects in blood *perfusion* of the lung in patients with suspected pulmonary embolism. Blood flow to the lungs is evaluated using a macroaggregated albumin (MAA) tagged with technetium (Tc), which is injected into the patient's peripheral vein. Because the diameter of the radionuclide aggregates is larger than that of the pulmonary capillaries, the aggregates become temporarily lodged in the pulmonary vasculature. A scintillator (gamma camera) detects the gamma rays from within the lung microvasculature. With the use of light conversion, a realistic image of the lung is obtained on film.

A homogeneous uptake of particles that fills the entire pulmonary vasculature conclusively rules out pulmonary embolism. If a defect in an otherwise smooth and diffusely homogeneous pattern is seen, a perfusion abnormality exists. This can indicate pulmonary embolism. Unfortunately, many other serious pulmonary parenchymal lesions (e.g., pneumonia, pleural fluid, emphysematous bullae) also cause a defect in pulmonary blood perfusion. Therefore, although the scan may be sensitive, it is not specific, because many different pathologic conditions can cause the same abnormal results.

The chest x-ray film aids in assessing the perfusion scan, because a defect on the perfusion scan seen in the same area as an abnormality on the chest x-ray film does not indicate pulmonary embolism. Rather, the defect may represent pneumonia, atelectasis, effusion, and so on. However, when a perfusion defect occurs in an area of the lung that is normal on a chest x-ray study, pulmonary embolus is likely.

Specificity of a perfusion scan also can be enhanced by performance of a *ventilation scan,* which detects parenchymal abnormalities in ventilation (e.g., pneumonia, pleural fluid, emphysematous bullae). The ventilation scan reflects the patency of the pulmonary airways, using krypton gas or Tc-diethylenetriamine-pentaacetic acid (DTPA) as an aerosol. When vascular obstruction (embolism) is present by perfusion scan, ventilation scans demonstrate a normal wash-in and wash-out of radioactivity from the embolized lung area. If parenchymal disease (e.g., pneumonia) is responsible for the perfusion abnormality, however, wash-in or wash-out will be abnormal. Therefore, the "mismatch" of perfusion and ventilation findings is characteristic of embolic disorders, whereas the "match" is indicative of parenchymal disease. When ventilation and perfusion scan are performed synchronously, this is called a *ventilation/perfusion ($\dot{V}/\dot{Q}$) scan.* Most nuclear physicians read the lung scan as one of several categories: negative for PE, low probability of PE, high probability of PE, or positive for PE.

Contraindications

- Patients who are pregnant, unless the benefits outweigh the risks

Interfering factors

- Pulmonary parenchymal problems (e.g., pneumonia, emphysema, pleural effusion, tumors) will give the picture of a perfusion defect and simulate pulmonary embolism.

Procedure and patient care

Before

PT Explain the procedure to the patient.
- Obtain informed consent if required by the institution.
PT Assure the patient that he or she will not be exposed to large amounts of radioactivity, because only tracer doses of isotopes are used.
- Although rarely done, if iodine-131 will be administered, give the patient 10 drops of Lugol's solution several hours before the test as a blocking agent for the thyroid gland. This will prevent iodine uptake by the thyroid gland.
PT Tell the patient that no fasting is required.
- Note that a recent chest x-ray film should be available.
PT Instruct the patient to remove jewelry around the chest area.

During

- Note the following procedural steps:
  1. The unsedated, nonfasting patient suspected of having a pulmonary embolism is taken to the nuclear medicine department.

Perfusion scan

2. The patient is given a peripheral IV injection of radionuclide-tagged MAA.

3. While the patient lies in the appropriate position, a gamma ray detector is passed over the patient and records radionuclide uptake on Polaroid or x-ray film.

4. The patient is placed in the supine, prone, and various lateral positions, which allows for anterior, posterior, lateral, and oblique views, respectively.

5. The results are interpreted by a physician trained in diagnostic nuclear medicine.

Ventilation scan

6. The patient breathes the tracer through a face mask with a mouthpiece.

7. Less patient cooperation is needed with a krypton tracer. Ventilation scans can even be performed on comatose patients using krypton. Krypton images can be obtained before, during, or after perfusion images.

8. In contrast, Tc-DTPA images are usually done before perfusion images and require patient cooperation with deep breathing and appropriate use of breathing equipment to prevent contamination.

- Note that this test is usually performed by a physician in approximately 30 minutes.

PT Tell the patient that no discomfort is associated with this test other than the peripheral venipuncture.

After

- Apply pressure to the venipuncture site.

PT Inform the patient that no radiation precautions are necessary.

Abnormal findings

Pulmonary embolism
Pneumonia
Tuberculosis
Emphysema
Tumor
Asthma
Atelectasis
Bronchitis
Chronic obstructive pulmonary disease

luteinizing hormone (LH assay, Lutropin) and follicle-stimulating hormone (FSH) assay

Type of test Blood
Normal findings

	LH (IU/L)	FSH (IU/L)
Adult		
Male	1.24-7.8	1.42-15.4
Female		
Follicular phase	1.68-15	1.37-9.9
Ovulatory peak	21.9-56.6	6.17-17.2
Luteal phase	0.61-16.3	1.09-9.2
Postmenopause	14.2-52.3	19.3-100.6
Child (age 1-10 years)		
Male	0.04-3.6	0.3-4.6
Female	0.03-3.9	0.68-6.7

(Values may vary, depending on laboratory method.)

Test explanation and related physiology

LH and FSH are glycoproteins that are produced in the anterior pituitary gland. These two hormones then act on the ovary or testes. In the female, FSH stimulates the development of follicles in the ovary. In the male, FSH stimulates Sertoli cell development. In the female, LH stimulates follicular production of estrogen, ovulation, and formation of a corpus luteum. In the male, LH stimulates testosterone production from the Leydig cells. In females, the midcycle peak of FSH is necessary for follicle/ovum formation. LH also must peak at about that same time to stimulate corpus luteal formation that could potentially support an embryo if fertilization were to occur.

Spot urine tests for LH have become very useful in the evaluation and treatment of infertility. Because LH is rapidly excreted into the urine, the plasma LH surge that precedes ovulation by 24 hours can be recognized quickly and easily. This is used to indicate the period when a woman is most fertile. The best time to obtain a urine specimen is between 11 AM and 3 PM. Usually the woman begins to test her urine on the day following her menses and continues to do so daily. Home kits using a color change as an endpoint are now marketed to make this process even more convenient.

These hormones are used in the evaluation of infertility. Performing an LH assay is an easy way to determine if ovulation has occurred. An LH surge in blood levels indicates that ovulation has taken place. Daily samples of serum LH around the woman's midcycle can detect the LH surge, which is believed to occur on the day of maximal fertility.

These assays also determine whether a gonadal insufficiency is primary (problem with the ovary/testicle) or secondary (caused by pituitary insufficiency resulting in reduced levels of FSH and LH). Elevated levels of FSH and LH in patients with gonadal insufficiency indicate primary gonadal failure, as may be seen in women with polycystic ovaries or menopause. In secondary gonadal failure, LH and FSH levels are low as a result of pituitary failure or some other pituitary-hypothalamic pathology.

Interfering factors

- Recent use of radioisotopes may affect test results if the testing method is performed by radioimmunoassay.
- Human chorionic gonadotropin (HCG) and thyroid-stimulating hormone may interfere with some immunoassay methods. Therefore patients with HCG-producing tumors and hypothyroid patients should be expected to have falsely high LH levels.
- Drugs that may *increase* LH levels include anticonvulsants, clomiphene, naloxone, and spironolactone.
- Drugs that may *decrease* LH levels include estrogens, progesterones, testosterone, digoxin, oral contraceptives, and phenothiazines.

Procedure and patient care

Before
PT Explain the procedure to the patient.
PT Tell the patient that no food or fluid restrictions are needed.

During
- Collect approximately 7 to 10 ml of venous blood in a red-top tube.
- Note that the patient may also perform LH assays at home using a home urine test or a 24-hour urine test.
- Indicate the date of the last menstrual period on the laboratory slip. Note if the woman is postmenopausal.

After
- Apply pressure to the venipuncture site.

Abnormal findings

▲ **Increased levels**

Menopause
Ovarian dysgenesis
  (Turner's syndrome)
Testicular dysgenesis
  (Klinefelter's syndrome)
Castration
Anorchia
Hypogonadism
Polycystic ovaries
Complete testicular
  feminization syndrome
Precocious puberty
Pituitary adenoma

▼ **Decreased levels**

Pituitary failure
Hypothalamic failure
Stress
Anorexia nervosa
Malnutrition

notes

Lyme disease test

Type of test Blood

Normal findings Negative (low titers of IgM and IgG antibodies)

Test explanation and related physiology

Lyme disease was first recognized in Lyme, Connecticut, in 1975. It is caused by a spirochete called *Borrelia burgdorferi.* The disease usually begins in the summer with a skin lesion called erythema chronicum migrans (ECM), which occurs at the site of a bite by a deer tick, usually *Ixodes dammini* or *pacificus.* Ticks are the best-documented vectors of this spirochete, which is the causative agent for Lyme disease.

Cultures of ECM can isolate the spirochete in half the cases. However, it is hard to culture and takes a long time to grow. Cultures of the blood or cerebrospinal fluid are even less helpful. Currently, serologic studies are the most sensitive and specific tests for the detection of Lyme disease. These tests determine titers of specific immunoglobulin M (IgM) and specific IgG antibodies to the *B. burgdorferi* spirochete. Levels of specific IgM antibody peak during the third to sixth week after disease onset and then gradually decline.

Titers of specific IgG antibodies are generally low during the first several weeks of illness, reach maximal levels 4 to 6 months later, usually after the patient has developed arthritis, and often remain elevated for years. A single titer of specific IgM antibody may suggest the diagnosis. Acute and convalescent sera can be tested to verify the diagnosis.

The Centers for Disease Control and Prevention (CDC) require the following for the diagnosis to be made with certainty:

Isolation of *B. burgdorferi* from an infected tissue or specimen

Identification of IgM and IgG antibodies to *B. burgdorferi* in the blood or CSF

Acute and convalescent blood samples with significant positive antibody titers

Interfering factors

- Previous infection with *B. burgdorferi* can cause positive serologic testing. These patients no longer have Lyme disease.

- Other spirochete diseases (syphilis or leptospirosis) can cause false-positive results.

Procedure and patient care

Before
PT Explain the procedure to the patient.
PT Tell the patient that no fasting or special preparation is required.

During
- Collect approximately 7 to 10 ml of venous blood in a red-top tube.

After
- Apply pressure to the venipuncture site.

Abnormal findings
Lyme disease

notes

lymphangiography (Lymphangiogram, Lymphography)

Type of test X-ray with contrast dye

Normal findings Normal-sized lymph nodes containing no filling defects

Test explanation and related physiology

The lymphatic system consists of lymph vessels and lymph nodes. Assessment of this system is important, because cancer lymphomas and Hodgkin's disease often spread via the lymphatic system. With the help of lymphangiography, pathologic lymph nodes can be localized for surgical removal or for inclusion in radiation therapy ports.

Lymphangiography is especially useful in patients suspected of having lymphatic pathology (lymphoma or metastatic tumor). The test allows one to demonstrate the extent and level of lymphatic metastasis. The lymphangiogram is also useful in staging lymphoma patients and in evaluating the results of chemotherapy or radiation therapy. Because the contrast medium remains in the lymph nodes for 6 months to 1 year, repeat plain x-ray films may be done for continued follow-up of disease progression or response to treatment.

This test is also useful in the evaluation of patients with chronic leg swelling. Lack of flow of the dye into the pelvic lymphatic vessels indicates lymphatic vessel obstruction as the cause of the leg edema.

Contraindications

- Patients with an allergy to iodine dye or shellfish
- Patients with severe chronic lung diseases, cardiac disease, or advanced kidney or liver disease

Potential complications

- Lipoid (lipid) pneumonia
  This occurs if the contrast medium flows into the thoracic duct and causes micropulmonary emboli. These small emboli usually disappear after several weeks or months.
- Allergic reaction or allergy to iodine dye

Procedure and patient care

Before

PT Explain the procedure to the patient.

■ Obtain informed consent if required by the institution.

PT Tell the patient that no fasting or sedation is required.

PT Inform the patient that if a blue dye is used, he or she may note a bluish tinge in the urine. Excessive infiltration or IV administration of the lymphatic stain may create a transient bluish tint to a part of or the entire skin surface.

During

■ Note the following procedural steps:

1. In the radiology department the patient is placed on an x-ray table in the supine position.

2. A lymphatic stain is injected into the subcutaneous tissue between each of the first three toes in each foot to outline the lymphatic vessels. See Figure 28. (The stain can also be injected into the web of the skin between the fingers.)

3. After the stain is taken up by the lymphatic vessels, they can be easily seen.

4. A local anesthetic is injected.

5. A small incision is made on the top of the foot (or hand).

6. The lymphatic vessel is identified and cannulated to infuse the iodine contrast agent.

7. The dye is slowly infused into the vessel. Usually a low-rate infusion pump is used. The patient must lie very still during the injection.

8. The flow of iodine dye is followed by fluoroscopy.

9. When the dye reaches the upper lumbar level, the flow of dye is discontinued.

10. X-ray films are taken of the chest, abdomen, and pelvis to demonstrate the filling of the lymph nodes. Often the patient is asked to return in 24 hours to have additional x-ray studies done.

11. On completion of the injection, the cannula is removed and the incision is sutured closed.

■ See p. xix for appropriate interventions concerning the care of patients with iodine allergy.

■ Note that this procedure is performed by a radiologist in approximately 3 hours. Additional x-ray films are usually taken 24 to 48 hours later.

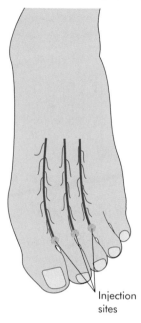

Injection
sites

Figure 28 Lymphangiography. Note the small lymphatic vessels that become apparent after the injection of a lymphatic stain into the web space of the feet.

PT Inform the patient that discomfort may be felt when the blue stain is injected subcutaneously and the feet are locally anesthetized.

After

PT Observe the injection and incision sites for evidence of cellulitis. If the patient will be returning home, instruct him or her to evaluate the site for redness, pain, and swelling.

PT Inform the patient that the sutures should be removed 7 to 10 days after the test.

Abnormal findings

Hodgkin's disease
Metastatic tumor involving the lymph glands
Lymphoma

lymphocyte immunophenotyping (AIDS T-lymphocyte cell markers, CD4 marker, CD4/CD8 ratio, CD4 percentage)

Type of test Blood

Normal findings

Cells	Percent	No. of cells/μl
T-cells	60-95	800-2500
T-helper (CD4) cells	60-75	600-1500
T-suppressor (CD8) cells	25-30	300-1000
B-cells	4-25	100-450
Natural killer cells	4-30	75-500

CD4/CD8 ratio: >1

Test explanation and related physiology

This test is used to detect the progressive depletion of CD4 T-lymphocytes, which is associated with an increased likelihood of clinical complications from acquired immunodeficiency syndrome (AIDS). Test results can also indicate if an AIDS patient is at risk for developing opportunistic infections.

T-lymphocytes, and especially CD4 counts, when combined with HIV RNA viral load testing (p. 529), are used to determine the time to initiate antiviral therapy. They also can be used to monitor antiviral therapy. Successful antiviral therapy is associated with an increase in CD4 counts. Worsening of disease or unsuccessful therapy is associated with decreasing T-lymphocyte counts.

T-lymphocytes are responsible for cellular immunity. CD4 helper cells and CD8 suppressor cells are examples of T-lymphocytes. There are three related measurements of CD4 T-lymphocytes. The first measurement is the *total CD4 cell count*. This is measured in whole blood and is the product of the white blood cell count, the lymphocyte differential count, and the percentage of lymphocytes that are CD4 T-cells. The second measurement, the *CD4 percentage*, is a more accurate prognostic marker. It measures the percentage of CD4 lymphocytes in the whole blood sample by using immunophenotyping with flow cytometry. This procedure relies on detecting specific antigenic determinants on the surface of the CD4 lymphocyte by antigen-specific monoclonal antibodies labeled with a fluorescent dye. The third prognostic marker, which is also more reliable than the total CD4 count, is the *ratio of CD4 cells to CD8 (T-suppressor) cells.*

Of the three T-cell measurements, the total CD4 count is the most variable. The Multicenter AIDS Cohort Study suggests that the last two measurements are more accurate than the total CD4 count.

The pathogenesis of AIDS is largely attributed to a decrease in the T-lymphocyte that bears the CD4 receptor. Progressive depletion of CD4 T-lymphocytes is associated with an increased likelihood of clinical complications from AIDS. Therefore CD4 measurement is a prognostic marker that can indicate whether a patient infected with HIV is at risk for developing opportunistic infections. The measurement of CD4 cell levels is used for deciding the initiation of *Pneumocystis carinii* pneumonia pro-phylaxis and the use of antiviral therapy and for determining the prognosis of patients with human immunodeficiency virus (HIV) infection.

The dosage of immunosuppressive medications used after organ transplant is also monitored with the use of lymphocyte phenotyping. Lymphomas and other lymphoproliferative dis-eases are now classified and treated according to the predomi-nant lymphocyte type identified. In some instances, prognosis of these diseases depends on lymphocyte phenotyping.

As the CD4 cell measurements decrease, the percentage of persons developing AIDS increases. Forty-eight percent of patients can be expected to develop AIDS within 6 months when their CD4 count is 100 cells/mm^3. It is recommended that antiviral therapy be started in patients whose CD4 count is less than 500 to 600 cells/mm^3. *Pneumocystis carinii* pneumo-nia prophylaxis should start when the CD4 count is less than 200 to 300 cells/mm^3.

CD4 prognostic markers also can be useful in guiding the approach to the patient's symptoms. Complaints such as cough and headache are common in most people; however, in patients infected with HIV, these symptoms often raise concerns about opportunistic infections. If the CD4 cell count exceeded 500 cells/mm^3 in the past 6 months, there is a very low proba-bility that these symptoms result from opportunistic infections. Knowing this, the patient and physician can feel comfortable with routine care.

Contraindications

- Patients who are not emotionally prepared for the prognosis that the results may indicate

Interfering factors

- Diurnal variation occurs.
- A recent viral illness can decrease total T-lymphocyte counts.
- Nicotine and very strenuous exercise have been shown to decrease lymphocyte counts.
- ✗ Steroids can *increase* lymphocyte counts.
- ✗ Immunosuppressive drugs will *decrease* lymphocyte counts.

Procedure and patient care

Before

- **PT** Explain the procedure to the patient.
- **PT** Tell the patient that no fasting or preparation is required.
- **PT** Maintain a nonjudgmental attitude toward the patient's sexual practices. Allow the patient ample time to express his or her concerns regarding the results.

During

- Record the time of day when the blood specimen is being obtained.
- Observe universal body and blood precautions. Wear gloves when handling blood products from all patients.
- Obtain 10 ml of blood in a large green-top tube (containing sodium heparin).
- Obtain 5 ml of blood in a small purple-top tube (containing ethylenediaminetetraacetic acid).
- Never recap needles. Dispose of needles and syringes required for obtaining the blood specimen in a puncture-proof container designed for this purpose.

After

- Keep the specimen at room temperature. Do not refrigerate.
- The specimen must be evaluated within 24 hours.
- Most specimens are sent to a central laboratory. Be sure to draw the blood immediately before the courier's departure to the central laboratory.
- Apply pressure to the venipuncture site.
- **PT** Instruct the patient to observe the venipuncture site for infection. Patients with AIDS are immunocompromised and susceptible to infection.

PT Encourage the patient to discuss his or her concerns regarding the prognostic information that may be obtained by these results.

🏠 Home care responsibilities

- Do not give test results over the phone. Decreasing CD4 counts can have devastating consequences.
- Decreasing CD4 counts are associated with worsening of disease or unsuccessful therapy.
- CD4 counts and HIV viral loads are used to determine the initiation of antiviral therapy.

Abnormal findings

▲ **Increased counts**

Chronic lymphocytic
  leukemia
B-cell lymphoma
T-cell lymphoma

▼ **Decreased counts**

Organ transplant
  patients
HIV-positive patients
Congenital
  immunodeficiency

notes

magnesium

Type of test Blood

Normal findings

Adult: 1.3-2.1 mEq/L or 0.65-1.05 mmol/L (SI units)
Child: 1.4-1.7 mEq/L
Newborn: 1.4-2 mEq/L

Possible critical values <0.5 mEq/L or >3 mEq/L

Test explanation and related physiology

Most of the magnesium found within the body exists intracellularly. About half is in the bone. Most of the magnesium is bound to an adenosine triphosphate (ATP) molecule and is important in phosphorylation of ATP (important as the main source of energy for the body). Therefore, this electrolyte is critical in nearly all metabolic processes.

Most organ functions, including neuromuscular tissue, also depend on magnesium. It is especially important to monitor magnesium levels in cardiac patients. Low magnesium may increase cardiac irritability and aggravate cardiac arrhythmias. Hypermagnesemia retards neuromuscular conduction and is demonstrated as cardiac conduction slowing (widened PR and Q-T intervals with wide QRS).

As intracellular elements, potassium, magnesium, and calcium (in order of quantity) are intimately tied together in maintaining a neutral intracellular electrical charge. That is why it is hard to maintain a normal potassium level when a patient has low magnesium blood levels.

Magnesium deficiency occurs in patients who are malnourished. Toxemia of pregnancy is also believed to be associated with reduced magnesium levels. Symptoms of magnesium depletion are mostly neuromuscular (i.e., weakness, irritability, tetany, electrocardiographic changes, delirium, and convulsions).

Increased magnesium levels most commonly are associated with ingestion of magnesium-containing antacids. Because most of the serum magnesium is excreted by the kidney, chronic renal diseases cause elevated magnesium levels. Symptoms of increased magnesium include lethargy, nausea and vomiting, and slurred speech.

Interfering factors

- Hemolysis should be avoided when collecting this specimen.
- Drugs that *increase* magnesium levels include thyroid medication, antacids, laxatives, calcium-containing medication, lithium, loop diuretics, and aminoglycoside antibiotics.
- Drugs that *decrease* magnesium levels include diuretics, some antibiotics, and insulin.

Procedure and patient care

Before

PT Explain the procedure to the patient.

PT Tell the patient that no special diet or fasting is required.

During

- Collect approximately 5 to 7 ml of venous blood in a red- or green-top tube.
- Avoid hemolysis.
- Indicate on the laboratory slip any drugs that may affect test results.

After

- Apply pressure to the venipuncture site.

Abnormal findings

▲ **Increased levels**

Renal insufficiency
Uncontrolled diabetes
Addison's disease
Hypothyroidism
Ingestion of magnesium-
    containing antacids
    or salts

▼ **Decreased levels**

Malnutrition
Malabsorption
Hypoparathyroidism
Alcoholism
Chronic renal disease
Diabetic acidosis

notes

magnetic resonance imaging (MRI, Nuclear magnetic resonance imaging [NMRI])

Type of test   Magnetic field study

Normal findings   No evidence of pathology

Test explanation and related physiology

MRI is a noninvasive diagnostic scanning technique that provides valuable information about the body's anatomy by placing the patient in a magnetic field. MRI is based on how hydrogen atoms behave when they are placed in a magnetic field and then disturbed by radiofrequency signals. The unique feature about MRI is that is does not require exposure to ionizing radiation. MRI has several advantages over computed tomography (CT) scanning, including the following:

1. MRI provides better contrast between normal tissue and pathologic tissue.
2. Obscuring bone artifacts that occur in CT scanning do not occur in MRI scanning.
3. Because rapidly flowing blood appears dark, which results from its quick motion, many blood vessels appear as dark lumens. This provides a natural contrast from other tissues to the blood vessels when using MRI.
4. Because spatial information depends only on how the magnetic fields are varied in space, it is possible to image the transverse, sagittal, and coronal planes directly with MRI.

Although the full usefulness of MRI is yet to be determined, it shows promise in the evaluation of the following areas:

1. Head and surrounding structures
2. Spinal cord and surrounding structures
3. Face and surrounding structures
4. Neck
5. Mediastinum
6. Heart and great vessels
7. Liver
8. Kidney
9. Prostate
10. Bone and joints
11. Breast
12. Extremities and soft tissues

An important advantage of MRI is that serial studies can be performed on the patient without any risk. This is useful in assessing the response of cancer to radiotherapy and chemotherapy. A major disadvantage of MRI is that patient eligibility is reduced as compared with CT scanning. For example, examination of patients requiring cardiac monitoring or having metal implants, metal joint replacements, pins for open reduction of fractures, pacemakers, or cerebral aneurysm clips will result in image degradation and may endanger the patient.

The uses and indications for MRI continue to expand as new technologies emerge. For example, *magnetic resonance angiography (MRA)* is a noninvasive procedure for viewing possible blockages in arteries. MRA uses radio waves and magnetic fields to visualize blood flow through the arteries. MRA has been useful in evaluation of the cervical carotid artery and large-caliber intracranial arterial and venous structures. Cardiac abnormalities, aortic aneurysm, and anatomic variants can be identified. This procedure also has proved useful in the noninvasive detection of intracranial aneurysms and vascular malformations, and especially in renal artery stenosis.

Imaging of the blood vessels with MRI is obtained by visualizing incoming blood as a bright signal while at the same time suppressing the surrounding tissue. This is the "time of flight" technique. A second method to visualize the blood vessels is to compare two contrasting pictures (phases) of the same sequence. In one sequence, the moving parts (blood) are highlighted and in the other, the motion effect is not recognized. When compared, only the blood vessels are obvious. This is called the "phase contrast" method. Either method is extremely reliable, except when there is turbulence in blood flow (area immediately distal to vascular stenosis). The vascular image is distorted in areas where blood flow is multidirectional.

MRI of the breast has expanded significantly over the past few years. With examiner experience, this procedure is more sensitive and specific than mammography or ultrasonography of the breast. Furthermore, lesions that previously were difficult to visualize (e.g., those close to the chest wall) are easily seen with this technique. MRI is fast becoming the most reliable technique for breast imaging.

Magnetic resonance spectroscopy (MRS) is a noninvasive procedure that generates high-resolution clinical images based on the distribution of chemicals in the body. For example, this technique has been used to investigate myocardial metabolism without exposing the patient to ionizing radiation. MR spectroscopy has also been used to assess chemical abnormalities in the brain associated with HIV infection without having to perform a brain biopsy. This procedure has been used in a wide variety of disorders including stroke, head injury, coma, Alzheimer's disease, multiple sclerosis, tumors, and heart disease.

Contraindications

- Patients who are extremely obese (more than 300 lb)
- Patients who are pregnant, because the long-term effects of MRI are not known at this time
- Patients who are confused or agitated
- Patients who are claustrophobic if using an enclosed scanner
- Patients who are unstable and require continuous life-support equipment, because monitoring equipment cannot be used inside the scanner room
- Patients with implantable metal objects such as pacemakers, infusion pumps, aneurysm clips, inner ear implants, and metal fragments in one or both eyes, because the magnet may move the object within the body and injure the patient

Interfering factors

- Movement during the scan may cause artifacts on MRI.

Procedure and patient care

Before

PT Explain the procedure to the patient.

PT Inform the patient that there is no exposure to radiation.

- Obtain informed consent if required by the institution.

PT Tell the patient that he or she can drive without assistance after the procedure.

PT Tell parents of young patients that they may read or talk to a child in the scanning room during the procedure, because no risk of radiation from the procedure exists.

- Assess the patient for any contraindications for testing (e.g., aneurysm clips).

PT If available, show the patient a picture of the scanning machine and encourage verbalization of anxieties. Some patients may experience claustrophobia. Antianxiety medications may be helpful for those with mild claustrophobia. If possible, an open MRI system can be used for these patients.

PT Instruct the patient to remove all metal objects (e.g., dental bridges, jewelry, hair clips, belts, credit cards), because they will create artifacts on the scan. The magnetic field can damage watches and credit cards. Also, movement of metal objects within the magnetic field can be detrimental to anyone within the field.

PT Inform the patient that he or she will be required to remain motionless during this study. Any movement can cause artifacts on the scan.

PT Tell the patient that during the procedure he or she may hear a thumping sound. Earplugs are available if the patient wishes to use them.

PT Inform the patient that no fluid or food restrictions are necessary before MRI.

PT For comfort, instruct the patient to empty the bladder before the test.

During

- Note the following:
  1. The patient lies on a platform that slides into a tube containing the doughnut-shaped magnet.
  2. The patient is instructed to lie very still during the procedure.
  3. During the scan, the patient can talk to and hear the staff via microphone or earphones placed in the scanner.
  4. A contrast medium called gadolinium (Magnevist) has been approved by the U.S. Food and Drug Administration. This is a paramagnetic enhancement agent that crosses the blood-brain barrier. It is especially useful for distinguishing edema from tumors. If this is to be administered, approximately 10 to 15 ml is injected in the vein. Imaging can begin shortly after the injection. No dietary restrictions are necessary before using this agent.

- Note that this procedure is performed by a qualified radiologic technologist in approximately 30 to 90 minutes.

PT Tell the patient that the only discomfort associated with this procedure may be lying still on a hard surface and a possible tingling sensation in teeth containing metal fillings. Also, an injection may be needed for administration of Magnevist.

After

PT Inform the patient that no special postprocedural care is needed.

Abnormal findings

Brain

Cerebral tumor
Cerebral infarction
Aneurysm
Arteriovenous malformation
Hemorrhage
Subdural hematoma
Multiple sclerosis
Dementia

Other

Tumor (primary or metastatic)
Myocardial infarction
Atherosclerotic plaques
Aortic dissection
Aortic occlusion and stenosis
Abscess
Edema
Congenital heart disease
Bone destructive lesion
Joint disorder
Degenerative vertebral disks

notes

mammography (Mammogram)

Type of test   X-ray

Normal findings

Class I: negative
Class II: benign
Class III: benign—short-term follow-up suggested
Class IV: suspicious—further evaluation suggested
Class V: cancer highly suspected

Test explanation and related physiology

Mammography is an x-ray examination of the breast used to identify cancers. In many cases these cancers can be detected before they become palpable lesions.

Although mammography is not a substitute for breast biopsy, it is reliable and accurate when interpreted by a skilled radiologist. The accuracy of detection of breast cancer with mammography has been approximately 85%. Usually cancers that are not detected by mammography are in areas of the breast not well imaged by an x-ray machine (the high axillary tail of the breast). Almost 35% of breast cancers are not palpable and are detected only by mammography. The combination of mammography and close physical examination provides the best approach to detect breast cancer at its earliest stage.

The American Cancer Society suggests that every woman older than age 40 should have a mammogram yearly. The National Cancer Institute (NCI) suggests that women in their 40s should have mammography every other year and annually after 50. However, the NCI suggests that women who are at increased risk for breast cancer should have them annually after 40.

Mammography also can detect other diseases of the breast. These include acute suppurative mastitis, abscess, fibrocystic changes, gross cysts, benign tumors (e.g., fibroadenoma), and intraglandular lymph nodes.

A woman receives minimal radiation exposure during this mammography (about 0.5 rad per view). Most mammograms include two views of each breast. Females younger than age 25 are most susceptible to the neoplastic effects of ionizing radiation. Therefore mammography is rarely performed in these women.

Mammography can also be used to locate a nonpalpable mammographically identifiable lesion for biopsy. The most common method is called *preoperative mammogram localization* of the mammogram abnormality, followed by open biopsy. Before surgery, a wire is placed to lead the surgeon to the abnormality. Nonoperative *stereotactic biopsy* with needle or *mammotomy* probes is the newest and least invasive manner of obtaining tissue from a nonpalpable mammographic abnormality. With the use of stereotaxis, a computer guides a core biopsy needle or mammotome probe into the abnormality. When fired, the biopsy equipment is in the center of the lesion, and specimens are obtained for biopsy. No surgery or sutures are required.

Contraindications

- Patients who are pregnant, unless the benefits outweigh the risk of fetal damage.
- Women younger than age 25

Interfering factors

- Talc powder can give the impression of calcification within the breast.
- Jewelry worn around the neck can preclude total visualization of the breast.
- Breast augmentation implants prevent total visualization of the breast.
- Previous breast surgery can alter or distort the mammogram findings.

Procedure and patient care

Before

PT Explain the procedure to the patient.

PT Inform the patient that some discomfort may be experienced during breast compression. This compression allows better visualization of the breast tissue. Assure the patient that the breast will not be harmed by the compression.

PT Tell the patient that no fasting is required.

PT Explain to the patient that a minimal radiation dose will be used during the test.

PT Instruct the patient to disrobe above the waist and put on an x-ray gown.

During

- Note the following procedural steps:
  1. The patient is taken to the radiology department and seated in front of a mammogram machine.

2. One breast is placed on the x-ray plate.
3. The x-ray cone is brought down on top of the breast to compress it gently between the broadened cone and the x-ray plate.
4. The x-ray film is exposed. This is the craniocaudal view.
5. The x-ray plate is turned about 45 degrees medially and placed on the inner aspect of the breast.
6. The broadened cone is brought in medially and again gently compresses the breast. This creates the mediolateral view.
7. Occasionally other views such as *direct lateral* (90 degree) or *magnified spot views* are obtained to visualize more clearly an area of suspicion.

- Note that mammography is performed by a radiologic technologist in approximately 10 minutes. The x-ray films are interpreted by a radiologist. Tell the patient that some discomfort may be caused by the pressure required to compress the breast tissue while the x-ray films are being taken. If the patient has very tender breasts, this may be painful.

M

After

PT Take this opportunity to instruct the patient in breast self-examination.

Abnormal findings

Breast cancer
Benign tumor (e.g., fibroadenoma)
Breast cyst
Fibrocystic changes
Breast abscess
Suppurative mastitis

notes

Meckel's diverticulum nuclear scan

Type of test Nuclear medicine

Normal findings No increased uptake of radionuclide in the right lower quadrant of the abdomen

Test explanation and related physiology

Meckel's diverticulum is the most common congenital abnormality of the intestinal tract. It is a persistent remnant of the omphalomesenteric tract. The diverticulum usually occurs in the ileum, approximately 2 feet proximal to the ileocecal valve. Approximately 20% to 25% of Meckel's diverticulum is lined internally by ectopic gastric mucosa. This gastric mucosa can secrete acid and cause ulceration of the intestinal mucosa nearby. Bleeding, inflammation, and intussusception are other potential complications of this congenital abnormality. The majority of these complications occur by 2 years of age.

Both normal gastric mucosa within the stomach and ectopic gastric mucosa in Meckel's diverticulum concentrate ^{99m}Tc pertechnetate. When this radionuclide is injected intravenously, it is concentrated in the ectopic gastric mucosa of Meckel's diverticulum. One can then expect to see a hot spot in the right lower quadrant of the abdomen at about the same time as the normal stomach mucosa is visualized. This is a very sensitive and specific test for this congenital abnormality.

It is possible that Meckel's diverticulum is present but contains no ectopic gastric mucosa within. Usually these are not symptomatic. No concentration of radionuclide will occur within the diverticulum. This test is not helpful in these cases.

Other conditions can simulate a hot spot compatible with Meckel's diverticulum containing ectopic gastric mucosa. Usually these are associated with inflammatory processes within the abdomen (e.g., appendicitis or ectopic pregnancy).

Procedure and patient care

Before

PT Explain the procedure to the patient.

PT Advise the patient to refrain from eating or drinking anything for 6 to 12 hours before the examination.

■ A histamine H_2-receptor antagonist is usually given for 1 to 2 days before the scan. This blocks secretion of the radionuclide from the ectopic gastric mucosa and improves visualization of Meckel's diverticulum.

During

- The patient lies in a supine position, and a large-view nuclear detector camera is placed over the patient's abdomen to identify concentration of nuclear material after intravenous injection.
- Images are taken at 5-minute intervals for 1 hour.
- Patients may be asked to lie on their left side to minimize the excretion of the radionuclide from the normal stomach, flooding the intestine with radionuclide and precluding visualization of Meckel's diverticulum.
- Occasionally glucagon is provided to prolong intestinal transit time and avoid downstream contamination with the radionuclide.
- Occasionally gastrin is given to increase the uptake of the radionuclide by the ectopic gastric mucosa.
- There is no pain associated with this test.

After

- The patient is asked to void, and a repeat image is obtained. This is to ensure that Meckel's diverticulum has not been hidden by a distended bladder.
- **PT** Because only tracer doses of radioisotopes are used, inform the patient that no precautions need to be taken by others against radiation.

Abnormal findings

Meckel's diverticula

notes

mediastinoscopy

Type of test Endoscopy

Normal findings No abnormal mediastinal lymph node tissue

Test explanation and related physiology

Mediastinoscopy is a surgical procedure in which a mediastinoscope (a lighted instrument scope) is inserted through a small incision made at the suprasternal notch. The scope is passed into the superior mediastinum to inspect the mediastinal lymph nodes and to remove biopsy specimens. Because these lymph nodes receive lymphatic drainage from the lungs, their assessment can provide information on intrathoracic diseases such as carcinoma, granulomatous infections, and sarcoidosis. Therefore mediastinoscopy is used in establishing the diagnosis of various intrathoracic diseases.

This procedure is also used to "stage" patients with lung cancer and to assess whether they are surgical candidates. Evidence of metastasis is usually a contraindication to thoracotomy because the tumor is considered inoperable. Tumors occurring in the mediastinum (e.g., thymoma or lymphoma) can also be biopsied through the mediastinoscope.

Potential complications

- Puncture of the esophagus, trachea, or blood vessels

Procedure and patient care

Before

PT Explain the procedure to the patient.
- Ensure that the physician has obtained the informed consent for this procedure.
- Check whether the patient's blood needs to be typed and crossmatched.
- Provide preoperative care as with any other surgical procedure.
- Keep the patient NPO after midnight on the day of the test.
- Administer preprocedure medication approximately 1 hour before the test as ordered.

During

- Note the following procedure steps:
  1. The patient is taken to the operating room for this surgical procedure.
  2. The patient is placed under general anesthesia.
  3. An incision is made in the suprasternal notch.
  4. The mediastinoscope is passed through this neck incision and into the superior mediastinum.
  5. The lymph nodes are biopsied.
  6. The scope is withdrawn, and the incision is sutured closed.
- Note that this procedure is performed by a surgeon in approximately 1 hour.

PT Inform the patient that he or she is asleep during the procedure.

After

- Provide postoperative care as with any other surgical procedure.
- Assess for mediastinal crepitus on auscultation, which may indicate mediastinal air from pneumothorax or the bronchus or esophagus.
- Note that distended neck veins and pulsus paradoxus may indicate lack of cardiac filling due to a large mediastinal hematoma.

🏠 Home care responsibilities

- Assess for cough or shortness of breath, which may indicate a pneumothorax.
- Note that subcutaneous emphysema may indicate a pneumothorax.
- Observe for hypotension and tachycardia, which may indicate bleeding from the biopsy site or the great vessels.
- Evaluate for hoarseness, which may indicate injury to the recurrent laryngeal nerve.
- Assess for fever, chills, and sepsis, which may indicate mediastinitis from infection.

Abnormal findings

Lung cancer
Metastasis
Sarcoidosis
Thymoma
Tuberculosis
Hodgkin's disease
Lymphoma
Infection

notes

methemoglobin (Hemoglobin M)

Type of test Blood

Normal findings
0.06-0.24 g/dl or 9.3-37.2 μmol/L (SI units)
0.4%-1.5% of total hemoglobin

Possible critical values >40% of total hemoglobin

Test explanation and related physiology
Methemoglobin is formed during the production of normal adult hemoglobin. If oxygenation of the iron component in the protohemoglobin occurs without subsequent reduction to normal hemoglobin, excess methemoglobin accumulates. The iron form in methemoglobin is unable to combine with oxygen to carry the oxygen to the peripheral tissues. Therefore, the oxyhemoglobin dissociation curve is "shifted to the left," resulting in cyanosis and hypoxia.

Methemoglobinemia can be congenital or acquired. Hemoglobin M disease is a genetic defect that results in a group of abnormal hemoglobins that are methemoglobins. Another genetic mutation can cause a deficiency in reduced nicotinamide adenine dinucleotide (NADH) methemoglobin reductase enzyme that is required to deoxygenate methemoglobin to normal adult hemoglobin. These forms of methemoglobinemia occur in infants, are usually severe, are not amenable to treatment, and are often fatal.

Acquired methemoglobinemia is a result of ingestion of nitrates (e.g., from well water) or drugs such as phenacetin, sulfonamides, isoniazid, local anesthetics, and some antibiotics. This form of the disease commonly occurs in older individuals and results in an acute crisis that is treated effectively with ascorbic acid or methylene blue.

Interfering factors
- Tobacco use and carbon monoxide poisoning are associated with increased methemoglobin levels.
- Drugs that may cause *increased* levels include, sulfonamides, isoniazid, local anesthetics, and some antibiotics.

M

Procedure and patient care

Before
PT Explain the procedure to the patient.
PT Tell the patient that no fasting is required.

During
- Collect approximately 5 to 7 ml of venous blood in a green-top (heparin) tube.
- Methemoglobin is very unstable. Place the specimen in an ice slush immediately after collection.
- Avoid hemolysis.
- List on the laboratory slip any drugs that the patient has taken over the last 7 to 14 days.

After
- Apply pressure to the venipuncture site.
- Be prepared to provide oxygen support and close monitoring in the event the patient becomes increasingly hypoxic.

Abnormal findings

Methemoglobinemia (hereditary or acquired)

notes

microalbumin (MA)

Type of test Urine

Normal findings

MA: 0.2-1.9 mg/dl
MA/creatinine ratio: 0-30 mg/g

Test explanation and related physiology

Microalbuminuria refers to an albumin concentration in the urine that is greater than normal, but not detectable with routine protein testing. Normally only small amounts of albumin are filtered through the renal glomeruli, and that small quantity can be reabsorbed by the renal tubules. However, when the increased glomerular permeability of albumin overcomes tubular reabsorption capability, albumin is spilled in the urine. Preceding this stage of disease is a period of microalbuminuria that would normally go undetected. Therefore MA is an early indication of renal disease.

For the diabetic patient, the amount of albumin in the urine is related to duration of the disease, and the degree of glycemic control. MA is the earliest indicator for the development of diabetic complications (nephropathy, cardiovascular disease [CVD], and hypertension). MA can identify diabetic nephropathy 5 years before routine protein urine tests. Diabetics with elevated MA have a 5- to 10-fold increase in the occurrence of CVD mortality, retinopathy, and end-stage kidney disease.

It is recommended that all diabetics older than the age of 12 be screened annually for MA. This can be done through a spot urine specimen using a semiquantitative Micral Urine Test Strip. If MA is present, the test should be repeated two more times. If two of three MA urine tests are positive, a quantitative measurement using a 24-hour urine specimen should be performed.

The presence of MA in nondiabetics is an early indicator of lower life expectancy due to CVD and hypertension. Nondiabetic nephropathies also may be associated with microalbuminuria. Life insurance underwriters are increasingly using MA testing to indicate life expectancy.

Interfering factors

- Urinary tract infection, blood, or acid-base abnormalities can cause elevated MA levels and falsely indicate more serious prognosis.
- Oxytetracycline may interfere with test results.

Procedure and patient care

Before

PT Explain the procedure to the patient.

- Ensure that the patient does not have any acute infection or urinary bleeding that could cause a false-positive result.

During

- Collect a fresh urine specimen in a urine container.
- If the urine specimen contains vaginal discharge or bleeding, a clean-catch or midstream specimen will be needed (see p. xvi).
- Ensure that the urine sample is at room temperature for testing.
- If using a Micral Urine Test Strip:
  1. Dip the test strip into the urine for 5 seconds.
  2. Allow the strip to dry for 1 minute.
  3. Compare the strip with the color scale on the label.

After

- Transport the urine specimen to the laboratory promptly.
- If a 24-hour urine collection is requested, the specimen should be refrigerated. However, it will be warmed to room temperature prior to testing.

PT If the results are positive, inform the patient that the test should be repeated in 1 week.

Abnormal findings

▲   **Increased levels**

Diabetes mellitus
Hypertension
Cardiovascular disease
Nephropathy
Urinary bleeding
Hemoglobinuria
Myoglobinuria

notes

mononucleosis spot test (Mononuclear heterophil test, Heterophil antibody test, Monospot test)

Type of test Blood

Normal findings Negative (<1:28 titer)

Test explanation and related physiology

The mononucleosis test is performed to aid in the diagnosis of infectious mononucleosis (IM), a disease caused by the Epstein-Barr virus (EBV). Usually young adults are affected by mononucleosis. The clinical presentation is fever, pharyngitis, lymphadenopathy, and splenomegaly. Approximately 2 weeks after the onset of the disease, many patients are found to have immunoglobulin M (IgM) heterophil antibodies in their serum that react against warm red blood cells (RBCs). When these antibodies are present in serial dilutions of greater than 1:56, infectious mononucleosis can be strongly considered. However, false-positive results can occur in patients who have other diseases that cause elevation of heterophil antibodies. Examples include patients with lymphoma, systemic lupus erythematosus, Burkitt's lymphoma, leukemia, and some gastrointestinal cancers. Burkitt's lymphoma is strongly associated with EBV.

Several heterophil agglutination tests are available, but the most frequently performed is the rapid slide test for infectious mononucleosis (Monospot test). Heterophil antibodies normally present in most individuals are produced in increased quantities in patients with IM. These antibodies strongly and readily agglutinate horse RBCs. The rapid slide test is performed by adding the patient's serum to horse RBCs on a slide. If agglutination occurs, heterophil antibodies are present in the patient's serum, indicating an EBV virus infection. About 30% of the cases of IM are "heterophil antibody negative." When a diagnosis of IM is still suspected, a repeat Monospot test or EBV serology is done (see p. 399).

Procedure and patient care

Before

PT Explain the procedure to the patient.

PT Tell the patient that no fasting or special preparation is required.

During
- Collect approximately 7 to 10 ml of venous blood in a red-top tube.

After
- Apply pressure to the venipuncture site.

Abnormal findings

Infectious mononucleosis
Chronic EBV infection
Chronic fatigue syndrome
Burkitt's lymphoma
Some forms of chronic hepatitis

notes

myelography (Myelogram)

Type of test X-ray with contrast dye

Normal findings Normal spinal canal

Test explanation and related physiology

By placing radiopaque dye (or air) into the subarachnoid space of the spinal canal, the contents of the canal can be radiographically outlined. Cord tumors, meningeal tumors, metastatic spinal tumors, herniated intravertebral disks, and arthritic bone spurs can be readily detected by this study. These lesions appear as canal narrowing or as varying degrees of obstruction to the flow of the dye column within the canal. The entire canal (from lumbar to cervical areas) can be examined. This test is indicated in patients with severe back pain or localized neurologic signs that suggest the canal as the location of these injuries. Because this test is usually performed by lumbar puncture (LP, see p. 602), all the potential complications of that procedure exist.

Different types of contrast material can be used for myelography. Pantopaque is most often used as the *oil-based medium*. An oil-based dye can cause meningeal irritation.

A *water-soluble* contrast material, metrizamide (Amipaque), is now frequently used for myelography. Metrizamide has two advantages over the oil-based medium. First, metrizamide does not need to be removed at the end of the procedure, because it is water soluble and will be completely resorbed. Second, metrizamide is less viscous than an iodinated, oil-based dye and therefore permits better visualization of small areas (e.g., nerves, nerve roots, nerve sheaths). Metrizamide may precipitate seizure activity after the procedure. To prevent this, the patient should be well hydrated and should avoid medications that could decrease the seizure threshold. A water-soluble contrast agent, Omnipaque, has a significantly lower risk of central nervous system (CNS) toxicity than does metrizamide and is now more routinely used.

To avoid the side effects associated with radiopaque dyes, some neurosurgeons prefer to use *air-contrast* myelography. After air myelography, the patient is positioned with the head lower than the trunk to prevent air from gravitating to the cerebral space and causing headaches.

M

Contraindications

- Patients with multiple sclerosis, because exacerbation may be precipitated by myelography
- Patients with increased intracranial pressure, because LP may cause herniation of the brain
- Patients with infection near the LP site, because this may precipitate a bacterial meningitis
- Patients who are allergic to shellfish or iodinated dye

Potential complications

- Headache
- Meningitis
- Herniation of the brain
- Seizures
- Allergic reaction to iodinated dye
- Hypoglycemia or acidosis may occur in patients who are taking metformin (Glucophage) and receive iodinated dye.

Procedure and patient care

Before

PT Explain the procedure to the patient.

- Ensure that the physician has obtained written and informed consent for this procedure.
- Assess the patient for allergies to iodinated contrast dye or shellfish.
- Ascertain whether the patient has recently taken phenothiazines, tricyclic antidepressants, CNS stimulants, or amphetamines if a water-soluble contrast (metrizamide) will be used. These medications should be avoided, because they could decrease the seizure threshold.
- Have the patient empty the bladder and bowel before myelography if possible.

PT Explain to the patient that he or she must lie very still during the procedure.

- Note that food and fluid restrictions vary according to the type of dye used. Check with the radiology department for specific restrictions.

PT Inform the patient that he or she will be tilted into an up-and-down position on the table so that the dye can properly fill the spinal canal and provide adequate visualization in the desired area.

During

- Note the following procedural steps:
  1. A lumbar puncture (see p. 602) is performed.
  2. Fifteen milliliters of cerebrospinal fluid (CSF) is withdrawn, and 15 ml or more of radiopaque dye or air is injected into the spinal canal. Because the specific gravity of the dye is greater than that of the CSF, the direction of dye flow will depend on the tilt of the table and the patient's position.
  3. With the needle in place, the patient is placed in the prone position on the tilt table with the head tilted down. A foot support and shoulder brace or harness will keep the patient from sliding.
  4. The lights are turned off, and the column of dye is followed in a cephalad direction with fluoroscopy.
  5. Representative x-ray films are taken.
  6. Obstructions to the flow of the dye are evident, and the level of the lesion is easily detected.
  7. After myelography is performed, the needle is removed and a dressing is applied.
  8. The patient is returned to the unit on a stretcher and is kept on bed rest.
- Note that this procedure is done by a radiologist in approximately 45 minutes.
- Keep in mind that patient response varies from mild discomfort to severe pain.

M

After

- Note that nursing interventions after the procedure depend on the type of contrast used.
- **PT** Usually place the patient on bed rest for several hours afterward, as indicated. Position the patient as specifically ordered by the physician in consultation with the radiologist. The head position varies with the dye used. For example, the head is usually elevated after using oil-based and water-soluble contrast agents. After an air-contrast study, the head is positioned lower than the trunk.
- Observe the patient for signs and symptoms of meningeal irritation (e.g., fever, stiff neck, occipital headache, photophobia).
- Observe the patient for seizure activity if metrizamide dye was used.
- If metrizamide was used, do *not* administer medications (e.g., phenothiazines) that may precipitate seizure activity.

- Monitor the patient's vital signs and ability to void.
PT Encourage the patient to drink fluids to enhance excretion of the dye and to hasten replacement of CSF.
- See p. xix for appropriate interventions concerning the care of patients with iodine allergy.

🏠 Home care responsibilities

- After this test, safe positioning of the patient's head will be determined by the type of dye used in the procedure.
- Encourage the patient to drink fluids to enhance excretion of the dye and to replace CSF.
- Tell the patient to report any signs of meningeal irritation such as fever, stiff neck, occipital headache, and photophobia.

Abnormal findings

Cord tumor
Meningeal tumor
Metastatic spinal tumor
Meningioma
Cervical ankylosing spondylosis
Arthritic lumbar stenosis
Herniated intravertebral disks
Arthritic bone spurs
Neurofibroma
Avulsion of nerve roots
Cysts
Astrocytoma

notes

myoglobin

Type of test Blood

Normal findings <90 mcg/L or <90 mcg/L (SI units)

Test explanation and related physiology

Myoglobin is an oxygen-binding protein found in cardiac and skeletal muscle. Measurement of myoglobin provides an early index of damage to the myocardium in myocardial infarction (MI) or reinfarction. Increased levels, which indicate cardiac muscle injury or death, occur in about 3 hours. Although this test is more sensitive than creatine phosphokinase (CPK) isoenzymes (see p. 322), it is not as specific. Trauma, inflammation, or ischemic changes to the noncardiac skeletal muscles also can cause elevated levels of myoglobin. The benefit of myoglobin over CPK-MB (see p. 322) is that it may become elevated earlier in some patients. This may prove beneficial, as revascularization is to be started within the first 6 hours after an MI.

As already indicated, disease or trauma of the skeletal muscle also causes elevations in myoglobin. With sudden and severe muscle injury, myoglobin levels can get very high. Myoglobin can also be measured in the urine. Because myoglobin is excreted in the urine and is nephrotoxic, urine levels must be monitored in these patients. The routine urine dipstick for hemoglobin will also react to screen for myoglobin.

Interfering factors

- Recent administration of radioactive substances may affect test results.
- Increased myoglobin levels can occur after IM injections.

Procedure and patient care

Before

PT Explain the procedure to the patient.

PT Tell the patient that no fasting is required.

During

- Collect approximately 5 ml of venous blood in a red-top tube.

After

- Apply pressure to the venipuncture site.

Abnormal findings

▲   **Increased levels**

Myocardial infarction
Skeletal muscle inflammation (myositis)
Malignant hyperthermia
Muscular dystrophy
Skeletal muscle ischemia
Skeletal muscle trauma
Rhabdomyolysis

notes

natriuretic peptides (Atrial natriuretic peptide [ANP], Brain natriuretic peptide [BNP], C-type natriuretic peptide [CNP])

Type of test Blood

Normal findings

ANP 22-77 pg/ml or 22-77 ng/L (SI units)

BNP <100 pg/ml

BNP levels are generally higher in healthy women than healthy men. BNP levels are higher in older patients.

CNP—yet to be determined

Test explanation and related physiology

Natriuretic peptides are a group of substances that oppose the activity of the renin–angiotensin system. There are three major natriuretic peptides: ANP is synthesized in the cardiac atrial muscle; BNP is actually a misnomer because its highest level does not exist in the brain, but rather in the cardiac ventricular muscle; CNP is synthesized in the brain. Both ANP and BNP are released in response to atrial and ventricular stretch, respectively, and will cause vasorelaxation, inhibition of aldostereone from the adrenal gland and renin from the kidney, thereby increasing natriuresis and reduction in blood volume. CNP has a vasorelaxation effect, but does not stimulate natriuresis.

ANP and BNP are secreted when there is stretch in the atrial or ventricular muscles, respectively. BNP, in particular, corresponds well to left ventricular pressures. As a result, BNP is a good marker for congestive heart failure (CHF). The higher the levels of BNP, the more severe the CHF. This test is becoming increasingly used in urgent care settings to aid in the diagnosis of "shortness of breath [SOB]." If BNP is elevated, the SOB is caused by CHF. If BNP levels are normal, the SOB is pulmonary and not cardiac. This is particularly helpful in evaluating SOB in patients with cardiac and chronic lung disease.

Furthermore, BNP is a helpful prognosticator and is used in CHF risk stratification. CHF patients whose BNP levels do not rapidly return to normal with treatment experience a significantly higher risk of mortality in the ensuing months than do those whose BNP levels rapidly normalize with treatment. BNP is elevated in early rejection of heart transplants. BNP also is elevated in patients with prolonged systemic hypertension and in those with acute myocardial infarction.

N

Procedure and patient care

Before

PT Explain the procedure to the patient.

PT Tell the patient that no fasting is required.

During

- Obtain 5 to 7 ml of venous blood in an EDTA (usually lavender)-containing tube.

After

- Apply pressure to the venipuncture site.
- Assess the venipuncture site for bleeding.
- Continue with aggressive medical care for suspected CHF.

Abnormal findings

Congestive heart failure
Myocardial infarction
Systemic hypertension
Cor pulmonale

notes

5′-nucleotidase

Type of test Blood

Normal findings 0-1.6 units at 37° C or 0-1.6 units at 37° C (SI units)

Test explanation and related physiology

5′-Nucleotidase is an enzyme specific to the liver. The 5′-nucleotidase level is elevated in patients with liver diseases, especially those associated with cholestasis. It provides information similar to alkaline phosphatase (ALP). However, ALP is not specific to the liver. Diseases of the bone, sepsis, pregnancy, and other diseases can cause ALP to be elevated. When doubt as to the cause of an elevated ALP exists, 5′-nucleotidase is recommended. If that enzyme is elevated along with the ALP, the source of the pathology is certainly in the liver. If the 5′-nucleotidase is normal in the face of an elevated ALP, the source of pathology is outside the liver (bone, kidney, or spleen). Gamma-glutamyl transpeptidase (GGTP) (p. 463) is used similarly because it is also specific to the liver.

Interfering factors

- Drugs that may cause *increased* 5′-nucleotidase levels include hepatotoxic agents.

Procedure and patient care

Before

PT Explain the procedure to the patient.

PT Tell the patient that no fasting is required.

During

- Collect approximately 7 to 10 ml of venous blood in a red-top tube.
- Indicate on the laboratory slip any medication the patient may be taking to aid in the interpretation of test results.

After

- Apply pressure to the venipuncture site. Patients with liver dysfunction often have prolonged clotting times.

Abnormal findings

▲ **Increased levels**

Bile duct obstruction
Cholestasis
Hepatitis
Cirrhosis
Hepatic necrosis
Hepatic ischemia
Hepatic tumor
Hepatotoxic drugs

notes

obstruction series

Type of test X-ray

Normal findings

No evidence of bowel obstruction
No abnormal calcifications
No free air

Test explanation and related physiology

The obstruction series is a group of x-ray films performed on the abdomen of patients with suspected bowel obstruction, paralytic ileus, perforated viscus, abdominal abscess, kidney stones, appendicitis, or foreign body ingestion. This series of films usually consists of at least two x-ray studies. The first is an *erect abdominal* film that should include visualization of both diaphragms. The film is examined for evidence of free air under either diaphragm, which is pathognomonic for a perforated viscus. This view is also used to detect air-fluid levels within the intestine; the presence of an air-fluid level is compatible with bowel obstruction or paralytic ileus. Occasionally patients are too ill to stand erect. In this case, an x-ray film can be taken with the patient in the left lateral decubitus position. If free air is present, it will be seen between the liver and the right side of the abdominal wall. As with the erect-position film, air-fluid levels also can be detected.

The second view in the obstruction series is usually a *supine abdominal* x-ray study. This x-ray is also called a *KUB* (kidney, ureter, and bladder) film. A calcification within the course of the ureter could indicate a kidney or ureteral stone. An abdominal abscess may be seen as a cluster of tiny bubbles within one localized area. A small calcification in the right lower quadrant on the film of a patient complaining of pain in this quadrant may be an appendicolith. A gas-filled distended bowel is compatible with bowel obstruction or paralytic ileus. The obstruction series can also be used to monitor the clinical course of patients with gastrointestinal (GI) disease. For example, repeated obstruction series on patients who have a partial small bowel obstruction or paralytic ileus can indicate worsening or improvement of the clinical situation.

Frequently a *cross-table lateral* view of the abdomen is included in an obstruction series to detect abdominal aorta calcification,

O

which often occurs in older patients. The calcification represents the anterior wall of the aorta. If an aortic aneurysm exists, this calcification will be seen to protrude from the spine.

Finally, the *supine abdominal* x-ray study can be used as a "scout film" before performing GI or abdominal x-ray studies that use contrast, such as a barium enema (see p. 146) or intravenous pyelogram (see p. 560).

Contraindications

- Patients who are pregnant, unless the benefits outweigh the risk to the fetus

Interfering factors

- Previous GI barium contrast study
  Although at times barium within the GI tract can preclude the identification of other important calcifications (e.g., kidney stones), it can be helpful in outlining the GI anatomy.

Procedure and patient care

Before

PT Explain the procedure to the patient.
- Ensure that all radiopaque clothing has been removed.
PT Remind the patient that no GI contrast will be used.

During

- Although the procedure varies from facility to facility, note that usually a supine abdominal x-ray film, erect abdominal film, and perhaps a lower erect chest film are taken. Often a cross-table lateral x-ray film is also included.
- Note that the obstruction series is performed in minutes in the radiology department by a radiologic technologist; however, it can be performed at the bedside with a portable x-ray machine. A radiologist interprets the films.
PT Tell the patient that no discomfort is associated with this study.

After

- Note that no special aftercare is needed.

Abnormal findings

Kidney stone
Bowel obstruction
Organomegaly
Presence of a foreign body
Bladder distention
Abdominal abscess
Perforated viscus
Abdominal aortic calcification
Appendicolithiasis
Paralytic ileus
Abdominal aortic aneurysm
Peritoneal effusion/ascites
Abnormal position of the kidneys
Soft tissue masses

notes

O

octreotide scan (Carcinoid nuclear scan, Neuroendocrine nuclear scan)

Type of test Nuclear scan

Normal findings No evidence of increased uptake throughout the body

Test explanation and related physiology

Octreotide scans are used to identify and localize neuroendocrine primary and metastatic tumors. These scans are indicated on patients with known neuroendocrine tumors.

Most neuroendocrine tumors have a somatostatin receptor on the cellular membrane. Octreotide is an analogue of somatostatin. When combined with a radiopharmaceutical (such as I^{123} or indium-111 DTPA), the radiolabeled octreotide will attach to the somatostatin receptors of the neuroendocrine tumor cells. With the use of a scintillator camera, the uptake can be identified. This test is used to identify primary and metastatic neuroendocrine tumors. It is also used to monitor the course of the disease.

The use of single-photon emission computed tomography (SPECT) imaging improves the sensitivity of this test. Many different types of hormone-producing tumors can be detected by this scan, most notably carcinoid, gastrinoma, insulinoma, glucagonoma, pheochromocytoma, and small-cell lung cancer. Other abnormalities can pick up octreotide, including granulomatous infections such as sarcoidosis or tuberculosis, rheumatoid arthritis, and nonhormonal cancers (breast, lymphoma, and non-small cell lung cancers).

Contraindications

- Patients who are pregnant or lactating, because of risk of damage to the fetus or infant

Interfering factors

- Barium in the gastrointestinal (GI) tract overlying the liver or spleen will produce defects on the scan that may be mistaken for masses.

Procedure and patient care

Before

PT Explain the procedure to the patient.

PT Tell the patient that no fasting or premedication is required.

PT Assure the patient that he or she will not be exposed to large amounts of radiation, because only tracer doses of isotopes are used.

- If an iodinated radionuclide is to be used, ensure that the patient does not have an allergy to iodine.

- If an iodinated dye is to be used, administer 5 drops of Lugol's solution (iodine) daily for 3 days. This will avoid uptake of the radionuclide by the thyroid gland.

PT If the patient has been receiving octreotide as a form of anti-neoplastic treatment, this must be discontinued for 2 weeks before scanning.

During

- Note the following procedural steps:
  1. The patient is taken to the nuclear medicine department, where the radionuclide is administered intravenously.
  2. One hour after injection, a gamma ray detector/camera is successively placed over the entire body.
  3. The patient is placed in supine, lateral, and prone positions so that all surfaces can be visualized.
  4. The radionuclide image is recorded on film. SPECT images may also be performed.
  5. Usually the patient is given a fatty meal 2 hours after octreotide injection to clear the radiopharmaceutical from the gallbladder.
  6. After 4 hours the patient is given a strong laxative to clear the octreotide from the bowel.
  7. Repeat scanning is performed at 2, 4, 24, and 48 hours after administration of the octreotide.

- Note that the imaging procedure is performed by a trained technologist in approximately ½ hour. A physician trained in nuclear medicine interprets the results.

PT Inform the patient that the only discomfort associated with this procedure is the IV injection of the radionuclide.

After

PT Because only tracer doses of radioisotopes are used, inform the patient that no precautions need to be taken by others against radiation exposure.

Abnormal findings

Carcinoid tumors

Neuroendocrine tumors

Granulomatous infections, such as sarcoidosis and tuberculosis

oncoscint scan (Immunoscintigraphy)

Type of test Nuclear medicine

Normal findings No increased uptake of radionuclide in the body

Test explanation and related physiology

Immunoscintigraphy is a new procedure. At present it is used to detect recurrent metastatic colorectal or ovarian cancer. The radionuclide indium-111 chloride is attached to a monoclonal antibody that is commonly on the cell surface of colorectal and ovarian cancer cells. When injected, this radionuclide-antibody conjugate attaches to the cancer cells. With the use of a gamma camera, whole-body images are obtained. Areas of increased uptake may represent tumor.

This scan is not 100% accurate and can be incorrectly negative up to 30% of the time. When positive, however, its accuracy meets or exceeds the accuracy of a computed tomography (CT) scan. It is very helpful in determining the source of a rising tumor marker (see CEA, p. 230, or CA-125, p. 215) in patients with an otherwise normal diagnostic evaluation. Also, it is very helpful in differentiating CT-recognized postsurgical or post-radiation anatomic changes from recurrent cancer. The first two do not take up tracer; recurrent cancer does. One must be aware that uptake of the radionuclide normally occurs in the liver, spleen, and bowel.

Contraindications

- Patients who are lactating

Procedure and patient care

Before
PT Explain the procedure to the patient.
PT Explain that no fasting is required before the test.
- Because the radionuclide can be concentrated in areas of degenerative joint disease, abdominal aortic aneurysms, abdominal inflammatory processes, or inflammatory bowel disease, a careful history should be obtained before scanning.

During
- The patient is injected with the radiolabeled monoclonal antibody.

- Initial images are obtained 48 to 72 hours after IV infusion.
- The patient is asked to lie on a padded table.
- A nuclear counter camera is placed over the anterior or posterior surface of the chest, abdomen, and pelvis. Approximately 10 minutes is required for each view.
- The patient may be asked to return the following day or the day after that for repeated images.
- Little or no discomfort is associated with this procedure.
- The procedure takes approximately 1 hour each day over 1 to 4 days.
- This procedure is performed in the nuclear medicine department.

After

PT Because only tracer doses of radioisotopes are used, inform the patient that no precautions need to be taken by others against radiation exposure.

Abnormal findings

▲ **Increased uptake**
Colorectal cancer
Ovarian cancer

O

notes

osmolality, blood (Serum osmolality)

Type of test Blood

Normal findings

Adult/elderly: 285-295 mOsm/kg H_2O or 285-295 mmol/kg (SI units)

Child: 275-290 mOsm/kg H_2O

Possible critical values

<265 mOsm/kg H_2O
>320 mOsm/kg H_2O

Test explanation and related physiology

Osmolality measures the concentration of dissolved particles in blood. As the amount of free water in the blood increases or the amount of particles decreases, osmolality decreases. As the amount of water in the blood decreases or the amount of particles increases, osmolality increases. Osmolality increases with dehydration and decreases with overhydration.

The serum osmolality test is useful in evaluating fluid and electrolyte imbalance. The test is very helpful in the evaluation of seizures, ascites, hydration status, acid-base balance, and suspected antidiuretic hormone (ADH) abnormalities. Osmolality is also helpful in identifying the presence of organic acids, sugars, or ethanol. In these cases there is an "osmolar gap." This gap represents the difference between what the osmolality should be (based on calculations of serum sodium, glucose, and BUN—the three most important solutes in the blood) and the osmolality as truly measured. If the "gap" is large, the presence of solutes such as organic acids (ketones), unusually high levels of glucose, or ethanol by-products is suspected.

Finally, osmolality also has an important role in evaluation of coma patients. Values of 385 mOsm/kg H_2O are associated with stupor in patients with hyperglycemia. When values of 400 to 420 are detected, grand mal seizures can occur. Values greater than 420 can be lethal. The simultaneous use of urine osmolality (p. 670) helps in the interpretation and evaluation of problems with osmolality.

Interfering factors

- Diseases such as cerebrovascular accident (stroke) or brain tumors may interfere with test results through inappropriate secretion of ADH.

Procedure and patient care

Before

PT Explain the procedure to the patient.

PT Tell the patient that no fasting is required.

During

- Collect approximately 5 to 10 ml of venous blood in a red-top tube.
- For pediatric patients, draw blood from a heel stick.

After

- Apply pressure to the venipuncture site.

Abnormal findings

▲ **Increased levels**

Hypernatremia
Dehydration
Hyperglycemia
Mannitol therapy
Azotemia
Uremia
Ingestion of ethanol, methanol, or ethylene glycol
Hyperosmolar nonketotic hyperglycemia
Diabetes insipidus
Hypercalcemia
Renal tubular necrosis
Severe pyelonephritis
Ketosis
Shock

▼ **Decreased levels**

Hyponatremia
Overhydration
Syndrome of inappropriate antidiuretic hormone (SIADH) secretion
Paraneoplastic syndromes associated with lung carcinoma

O

notes

osmolality, urine (Urine osmolality)

Type of test Urine

Normal findings

12- to 14-hour fluid restriction: >850 mOsm/kg H_2O
(SI units)

Random specimen: 50-1200 mOsm/kg H_2O, depending on
fluid intake or 50-1200 mmol/kg (SI units)

Test explanation and related physiology

Osmolality is the measurement of the number of dissolved
particles in a solution. It is a more exact measurement of urine
concentration than specific gravity, because specific gravity
depends on the number and precise nature of the particles in the
urine. Specific gravity also requires correction for the presence of
glucose or protein, as well as for temperature; in contrast, osmolality depends only on the number of particles of solute in a unit
of solution. Osmolality also can be measured over a wider range
than specific gravity and with greater accuracy.

Osmolality is used in the precise evaluation of the concentrating ability of the kidney. This test is also used to monitor fluid
and electrolyte balance. Osmolality is valuable in the workup of
patients with renal disease, the syndrome of inappropriate antidiuretic hormone (SIADH) secretion, and diabetes insipidus.
Osmolality may be used as part of the urinalysis when the patient
has glycosuria or proteinuria or has had tests that use radiopaque
substances. In these situations, the urine "osmolar gap" is
increased because of other organic osmolal particles. The osmolar gap is the sum of all the particles expected to be in the urine
(electrolytes, urea, and glucose) compared with the actual measurement of the osmolality. Normally, the osmolar gap is 80 to
100 mOsm/kg of H_2O. The urine osmolality is more easily
interpreted when the serum osmolality (p. 668) is simultaneously performed. The normal ratio between the urine and serum
osmolality is 1:3.

Procedure and patient care

Before

PT Explain the procedure to the patient.

PT Tell the patient that no special preparation is necessary for a
random urine specimen.

PT Inform the patient that preparation for a fasting urine specimen may require a high-protein diet for 3 days before the test. Instruct the patient to eat a dry supper the evening before the test and to drink no fluids until the test is completed the next morning.

During

- Collect a first-voided urine specimen for a random sample.
- For a fasting specimen, instruct the patient to empty the bladder at approximately 6 AM and to discard the urine. Collect the test urine at 8 AM.
- Indicate on the laboratory slip the patient's fasting status.

After

- Send the specimen to the laboratory.
- Provide food and fluids for the patient.

Abnormal findings

▲ **Increased levels**

SIADH secretion
Acidosis
Shock
Hypernatremia
Hepatic cirrhosis
Congestive heart failure
Addison's disease

▼ **Decreased levels**

Diabetes insipidus
Hypercalcemia
Excess fluid intake
Renal tubular necrosis
Aldosteronism
Hypokalemia
Severe pyelonephritis

O

notes

oximetry (Pulse oximetry, Ear oximetry, Oxygen saturation)

Type of test Photodiagnostic

Normal findings ≥95%

Possible critical values ≤75%

Test explanation and related physiology

Oximetry is a noninvasive method of monitoring arterial blood oxygen saturation (SaO_2). The SaO_2 is the ratio of oxygenated hemoglobin to the total amount of hemoglobin. The SaO_2 is expressed as a percentage; for example, a saturation of 95% indicates that 95% of the total hemoglobin attachments for oxygen have oxygen attached to them. The SaO_2 is an accurate approximation of oxygen saturation obtained from arterial blood gas study (see p. 117). By correlating the SaO_2 and the patient's physiologic status, a close estimate of the partial oxygen pressure (PO_2) can be obtained.

Oximetry is typically used for monitoring the patient's oxygenation status during the perioperative period (or any time of heavy sedation) and for patients receiving mechanical ventilation. This test is also frequently used in many clinical situations, such as pulmonary rehabilitation programs, stress testing, and sleep laboratories. Oximetry can be used to assess the body's response to various drugs such as theophylline, which causes bronchodilation, and methacholine, which evokes bronchospasm in people with asthma. This test is commonly used to titrate levels of oxygen on hospitalized patients.

Procedure and patient care

Before
PT Explain the procedure to the patient.
PT Tell the patient that no fasting is required.

During
- Rub the patient's earlobe, pinna (upper part of the ear), or fingertip to increase blood flow.
- Clip the monitoring probe or sensor to the ear or finger. The sensor warms and increases blood flow to the tissue. A beam of light passes through the tissue, and the sensor measures the amount of light the tissue absorbs (Figure 29).

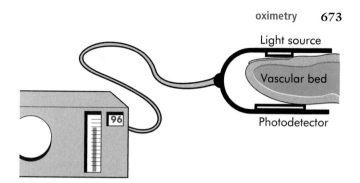

Figure 29 Oximetry. The pulse oximeter passes a beam of light through the tissue. The amount of light absorbed by the oxygen-saturated hemoglobin is measured by the sensor.

- Note that this study is usually performed by a respiratory therapist or nurse at the patient's bedside in a few minutes.
- **PT** Tell the patient that no discomfort is associated with this study.

After

- Note that no special aftercare is needed.

Abnormal findings

▲ **Increased levels**

Increased inspired O_2
Hyperventilation

▼ **Decreased levels**

Inadequate O_2 in inspired air
Hypoxic lung diseases
Hypoxic cardiac diseases
Severe hypoventilation states

notes

Papanicolaou smear (Pap smear, Pap test, Cytologic test for cancer)

Type of test Microscopic examination

Normal findings No abnormal or atypical cells

Test explanation and related physiology

A Pap smear is taken to detect neoplastic cells in cervical and vaginal secretions. This test is based on the fact that normal cells and abnormal cervical and endometrial neoplastic cells are shed into the cervical and vaginal secretions. By examining these secretions microscopically, one can detect early cellular changes compatible with premalignant conditions or an existing malignant condition. The Pap smear is 95% accurate in detecting cervical carcinoma; however, its accuracy in detection of endometrial carcinoma is only approximately 40%. In the past, the cells were classified as Class 1 (indicating absence of atypical or abnormal cells) through Class 5 (cytologic findings conclusive of malignancy).

Later, Pap smears were reported in terms of cervical intraepithelial neoplasia (CIN). This is a simple designation of the spectrum of intraepithelial dysplasia, which usually occurs before invasive cervical cancer. The subclasses of CIN are defined as follows.

CIN 1: mild and mild-to-moderate dysplasia
CIN 2: moderate and moderate-to-severe dysplasia
CIN 3: severe dysplasia and carcinoma in situ

Most recently, the Bethesda System for reporting cervical and vaginal cytologic diagnoses was developed and revised by the National Cancer Institute. This system was updated in 2001 and includes evaluation of the following five components:

1. Adequacy of specimen
2. General categorization (optional)
3. Interpretation/result
   Negative for Intraepithelial Lesion or Malignancy (includes infection or reactive changes)
   Epithelial Cell Abnormalities from atypical to cancer for both the squamous and glandular cancer lines.
4. Automated Review and Ancillary Testing (where appropriate)
5. Educational notes (optional)

A Pap smear also may be performed to follow some abnormalities (e.g., infertility). An abnormal maturation index (MI) is characteristic of an estrogen-progesterone imbalance. The MI is calculated by determining the ratio of parabasal cervical cells to intermediate cells to superficial cells. The normal ovulating adult MI is 0/70/30. The MI is used more frequently for determination of menstrual status and ovarian function.

Pap smears should be part of the routine pelvic examination, which is usually performed once a year in women older than age 18 (or even earlier when the patient is sexually active). Opinions differ regarding the necessity for annual Pap smears. The American Cancer Society recommends that a Pap smear be taken annually for two negative examinations, then repeated once every 3 years until age 65 in asymptomatic women. More frequent testing may be indicated for patients with venereal infections, those with a family history of cervical cancer, and those whose mothers had ingested diethylstilbestrol during their pregnancies.

A new method of Pap smear collection has been the *"thin prep" Pap smear* or *liquid-based cervical cytology*. With this newer technique, the specimen that is obtained from the cervix is placed into a preservative solution instead of smearing it onto a slide. Any blood cells and debris are then isolated, leaving only a thin film of cervical cells to be evaluated and tested. Furthermore, if cytologic abnormalities of undetermined significance are found that could be better elucidated with further testing, cells are still available in the fluid solution for that testing (rather than having to obtain another cervical sample). In particular, it is very easy (and, therefore, more often done) to identify evidence of human papillomavirus (HPV) infection with further testing. HPV has been incriminated in more than 95% of cervical cancers. HPV testing is now routinely performed by the *hybrid capture DNA test*. With an RNA probe, a semiquantitative estimate of HPV load can be provied. The more that HPV infections are recognized, the more women can address their increased risk for cervical cancer.

Contraindications

- Patients currently having routine, normal menses, because this can alter test interpretation
- Patients with vaginal infections
  Cellular changes that may be misinterpreted as dysplastic may transiently occur during these infections.

Interfering factors

- A delay in fixing a specimen allows the cells to dry, destroys effectiveness of the stain, and makes cytologic interpretation difficult.
- Using lubricating jelly on the speculum can alter the specimen.
- Douching and tub bathing may wash away cellular deposits and interfere with the test results.
- Menstrual flow may alter test results.
- Infections may interfere with hormonal cytology.
- Drugs such as digitalis and tetracycline may alter the test results by affecting the squamous epithelium.

Procedure and patient care

Before

PT Explain the procedure to the patient.

PT Instruct the patient not to douche or tub bathe during the 24 hours before the Pap smear. (Some physicians prefer that patients refrain from sexual intercourse for 24 to 48 hours before the test.)

PT Instruct the patient to empty her bladder before the examination.

PT Tell the patient that no fasting or sedation is required.

During

- Note the following procedural steps:
  1. The patient is placed in the lithotomy position.
  2. A vaginal speculum is inserted to expose the cervix.
  3. Material is collected from the cervical canal by rotating a moist saline cotton swab or spatula within the cervical canal and in the squamocolumnar junction (Figure 30).
  4. The cells are immediately wiped across a clean glass slide and fixed either by immersing the slide in equal parts of 95% alcohol and ether or by using a commercial spray (e.g., Aqua Net hair spray). The secretions must be fixed before drying because drying will distort the cells and make interpretation difficult.
  5. If a liquid-based cytology is performed, the cervical specimen is placed in the fixative preservative solution. Once placed in this solution, cells can be evaluated anytime within the next 3 weeks (if kept frozen).
  6. The slide is labeled with the patient's name, age, and parity and with the date of her last menstrual period.

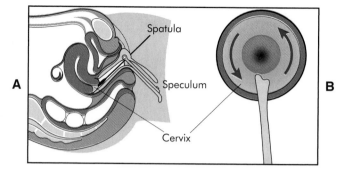

Figure 30 Papanicolaou (Pap) smear. **A,** The vaginal speculum is shown in position to allow direct visualization of the cervix. **B,** The cervix is scraped with the bifid end of a wooden spatula.

7. The patient's medication history (e.g., oral contraceptives) and the reason for the examination should be written on the laboratory request form.

- Note that a Pap smear is obtained by a nurse or a physician in approximately 10 minutes
PT Tell the patient that no discomfort, except for insertion of the speculum, is associated with this procedure.

After

PT Inform the patient that usually she will not be notified unless further evaluation is necessary.

Abnormal findings

Cancer
Infertility
Venereal disease
HPV infection
Reactive inflammatory changes
Fungal infection
Parasitic infection
Herpes infection

notes

paracentesis (Peritoneal fluid analysis, Abdominal paracentesis, Ascitic fluid cytology, Peritoneal tap)

Type of test Fluid analysis

Normal findings

Gross appearance: clear, serous, light yellow, <50 ml
Red blood cells (RBCs): none
White blood cells (WBCs): <300/μl
Protein: <4.1 g/dl
Glucose: 70-100 mg/dl
Amylase: 138-404 units/L
Ammonia: <50 mcg/dl
Alkaline phosphatase
    Adult male: 90-240 units/L
    Female <45 years: 76-196 units/L
    Female >45 years: 87-250 units/L
Lactate dehydrogenase (LDH): similar to serum lactate
    dehydrogenase
Cytology: no malignant cells
Bacteria: none
Fungi: none
Carcinoembryonic antigen (CEA): negative

Test explanation and related physiology

Paracentesis is an invasive procedure entailing the insertion of a needle or catheter into the peritoneal cavity (Figure 31) for removal of ascitic fluid for diagnostic and therapeutic purposes.

Diagnostically, paracentesis is performed to obtain and analyze fluid to determine the etiology of the peritoneal effusion. Peritoneal fluid is classified as to whether it is a transudate or exudate. This is an important differentiation and is very helpful in determining the etiology of the effusion. *Transudates* are most frequently caused by congestive heart failure, cirrhosis, nephrotic syndrome, myxedema, peritoneal dialysis, and hypoproteinemia. *Exudates* are most often found in infectious or neoplastic conditions. However, collagen vascular disease, gastrointestinal diseases, trauma, and drug hypersensitivity also may cause an exudative effusion.

Therapeutically, this procedure is done to remove large amounts of fluid from the abdominal cavity. Usually these patients experience transient relief of symptoms (shortness of

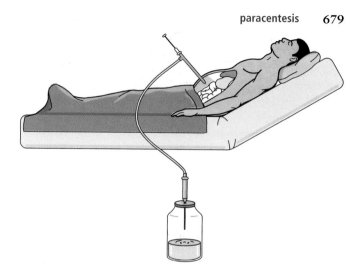

Figure 31 Paracentesis. A catheter is placed through the skin and abdominal muscle wall, into the peritoneal cavity containing free fluid.

breath, distention, and early satiety) because of the fluid within the abdominal cavity.

The peritoneal fluid is usually evaluated for gross appearance, RBCs, WBCs, protein, glucose, amylase, ammonia, alkaline phosphatase, LDH, cytology, bacteria, fungi, and other tests, such as CEA levels. Each is discussed separately. Urea and creatinine may be measured if there is a question that the fluid may represent urine from a perforated bladder.

Gross appearance

Transudative peritoneal fluid may be clear, serous, and light yellow, especially in patients with hepatic cirrhosis. Milk-colored peritoneal fluid may result from the escape of chyle from blocked abdominal or thoracic lymphatic ducts. Conditions that may cause lymphatic blockage include lymphoma, carcinoma, and tuberculosis involving the abdominal or thoracic lymph nodes. The triglyceride value in a chylous effusion exceeds 110 mg/dl.

Exudative fluid is cloudy or turbid. Bloody fluid may be the result of a traumatic tap (the aspirating needle penetrates a blood vessel), intra-abdominal bleeding, tumor, or hemorrhagic pancreatitis. Bile-stained green fluid may result from a ruptured gallbladder, acute pancreatitis, or perforated intestines.

Cell counts

Normally, no RBCs should be present. The presence of RBCs may indicate neoplasms, tuberculosis, or intra-abdominal bleeding. Increased WBC counts may be seen with peritonitis, cirrhosis, and tuberculosis.

Protein count

Total protein levels greater than 3 g/dl are characteristic of exudates, whereas transudates usually have a protein content of less than 3 g/dl. It is now thought that the *albumin gradient* between serum and ascitic fluid can differentiate better between the transudate and exudate nature of ascites than can the total protein content. This gradient is obtained by subtracting the ascitic albumin value from the serum albumin value. Values of 1.1 g/dl or more suggest a transudate, and values less than 1.1 g/dl suggest an exudate. The total protein ratio (fluid/serum) has been used to differentiate exudate from transudate. A total protein ratio of fluid to serum of greater than 0.5 is considered to be an exudate.

Glucose

Usually peritoneal glucose levels approximate serum glucose levels. Decreased levels may indicate tuberculous/bacterial peritonitis or peritoneal carcinomatosis.

Amylase

Increased amylase levels may be seen in patients with pancreatic trauma; pancreatic pseudocyst; acute pancreatitis; and intestinal necrosis, perforation, or strangulation. In these diseases the amylase level is usually greater than 1.5 times higher than serum levels.

Ammonia

High ammonia levels occur in ruptured or strangulated intestines and also with a ruptured appendix or ulcer.

Alkaline phosphatase

Levels of alkaline phosphatase are greatly increased in infarcted or strangulated intestines.

Lactate dehydrogenase

A peritoneal fluid/serum LDH ratio of greater than 0.6 is typical of an exudate. An exudate is identified with a higher degree of accuracy if the peritoneal fluid/serum protein ratio is greater than 0.5 and the peritoneal fluid/serum LDH ratio is greater than 0.6.

Cytology

A cytologic study is performed to detect tumors. It can be difficult to differentiate malignancy from severe inflammatory mesothelial cells. Cytology examination of the fluid is improved by spinning down a large volume of fluid and examining the sediment. Large numbers of cells can be seen and compared with each other.

Bacteria

Usually the fluid is cultured, and the antibiotic sensitivities are determined. Gram stains are often performed.

Gram stain and bacteriologic culture

The presence of bacteria may indicate intra-abdominal infection. Culture and Gram stains identify the organisms involved in the infection (see p. 872).

Fungi

Fungi may indicate infections with histoplasmosis, candidiasis, or coccidioidomycosis.

Carcinoembryonic antigen

Peritoneal fluid levels for CEA are associated with abdominal malignancy, usually arising from the gastrointestinal tract.

Contraindications

- Patients with coagulation abnormalities or bleeding tendencies
- Patients with only a small amount of fluid and extensive previous abdominal surgery

Potential complications

- Hypovolemia if a large volume of peritoneal fluid is removed
- Peritonitis

Procedure and patient care

Before

PT Explain the procedure to the patient.
- Obtain informed consent for this procedure.
PT Tell the patient that no fasting or sedation is necessary.
PT Have the patient urinate or empty the bladder before the test. This will help to prevent accidental bladder trauma.
- Measure abdominal girth.
- Obtain the patient's weight.
- Obtain baseline vital signs.

During

- Note the following procedural steps:
  1. Position the person in a high Fowler's position in bed.
  2. Paracentesis is performed under strict sterile technique. A paracentesis tray usually contains all necessary supplies.
  3. The needle insertion site is aseptically cleansed and anesthetized locally.
  4. A scalpel may be used to make a stab wound in the skin to allow the cannula or needle to enter.
  5. A trocar, cannula, or needle is threaded through the incision.
  6. Tubing is attached to the cannula. The other end of the tubing is placed in the collection receptacle (usually a container with a pressurized vacuum).
- Note that this procedure is performed by a physician at the patient's bedside, in a procedure room, or in the physician's office in less than 30 minutes. Usually the volume removed is limited to about 4 L at any one time to avoid hypovolemia if the ascites is rapidly reaccumulated.
- **PT** Although local anesthetics eliminate pain at the insertion site, tell the patient that he or she will feel a pressurelike pain as the needle is inserted.

After

- All tests performed on peritoneal fluid should be performed immediately to avoid false results due to chemical or cellular deterioration.
- Place a small bandage over the needle site.
- Label the specimen with the patient's name, date, source of fluid, and diagnosis.
- Send the specimen promptly to the laboratory.
- Observe the puncture site for bleeding, continued drainage, or signs of inflammation.
- Measure the abdominal girth and weight of the patient; compare with baseline values.
- Monitor vital signs for evidence of hemodynamic changes. Watch for signs of hypotension if a large volume of fluid was removed.
- Write any recent antibiotic therapy on the laboratory requisition slip.
- Because of the high protein content of ascitic fluid, albumin infusions may be ordered after paracentesis to compensate for

protein loss. Monitor serum protein and electrolyte (especially sodium) levels.

- Occasionally ascitic fluid continues to leak out of the needle tract after removal of the needle. A suture can stop that. If unsuccessful, a collection bag should be applied to the skin to allow for measurement of the volume of fluid loss.

Abnormal findings

Exudate

Lymphoma
Carcinoma
Tuberculosis
Peritonitis
Pancreatitis
Ruptured viscus

Transudate

Hepatic cirrhosis
Portal hypertension
Nephrotic syndrome
Hypoproteinemia
Congestive heart failure
Abdominal trauma
Peritoneal bleeding

P

notes

parathyroid hormone (PTH, Parathormone)

Type of test Blood

Normal findings

Intact (whole): 10-65 pg/ml or 10-65 ng/L (SI units)
N terminal: 8-24 pg/ml
C terminal: 50-330 pg/ml

Test explanation and related physiology

PTH is secreted by the parathyroid gland in response to hypocalcemia. This test is useful in establishing a diagnosis of hyperparathyroidism and distinguishing nonparathyroid from parathyroid causes of hypercalcemia. Increased PTH levels are seen in patients with hyperparathyroidism (primary, secondary or tertiary); in patients with nonparathyroid, ectopic PTH-producing tumors (pseudohyperparathyroidism); or as a normal compensatory response to hypocalcemia in patients with malabsorption or vitamin D deficiency.

It is important to measure serum calcium simultaneously with the measurement of PTH. Most laboratories have a PTH/calcium nomogram already made up, indicating what PTH level is considered normal for each calcium level.

Decreased PTH levels are seen in patients with hypoparathyroidism or as a compensatory response to hypercalcemia in patients with metastatic bone tumors, sarcoidosis, vitamin D intoxication, or milk-alkali syndrome. Of course, surgical ablation of the parathyroids is another cause of hypoparathyroidism.

Whole (intact) PTH is metabolized to several different fragments, including an N terminal, a midregion or midmolecule, and a C terminal. Intact PTH and all fragments generally provide accurate information concerning the level of PTH in the blood. Intact PTH is probably most often tested since it is most reliable.

Interfering factors

- Recent injection of radioisotopes may interfere with this test.
- Drugs that *increase* PTH include anticonvulsants, steroids, isoniazid, lithium, and rifampin.
- Drugs that *decrease* PTH include cimetidine and propranolol.

Procedure and patient care

Before

PT Explain the procedure to the patient.

- Keep the patient NPO except for water after midnight on the day of the test.

During

- Obtain a morning blood specimen, because diurnal rhythm affects PTH levels. (Check with the laboratory if the patient works at night.)
- Collect 5 to 10 ml of venous blood in a red-top tube. Note that some laboratories require 15 ml of blood in an iced plastic syringe.
- Obtain a serum calcium level determination at the same time if ordered. Serum PTH and serum calcium levels are important in the differential diagnosis.

After

- Indicate the time the blood was drawn on the laboratory slip, because a diurnal rhythm affects test results.
- Apply pressure to the venipuncture site.

Abnormal findings

▲ Increased levels

Hyperparathyroidism secondary to adenoma or carcinoma of the parathyroid gland
Non–PTH-producing tumors (paraneoplastic syndrome)
Lung carcinoma
Kidney carcinoma
Hypocalcemia
Chronic renal failure
Malabsorption syndrome
Vitamin D deficiency
Rickets
Osteomalacia
Congenital renal defect

▼ Decreased levels

Hypoparathyroidism
Hypercalcemia
Metastatic bone tumor
Sarcoidosis
Autoimmune destruction of the parathyroid glands
Vitamin D intoxication
Milk-alkali syndrome
Graves' disease
Hypomagnesemia
DiGeorge's syndrome

P

parathyroid scan (Parathyroid scintigraphy)

Type of test Nuclear medicine

Normal findings No increased parathyroid uptake

Test explanation and related physiology

Hypercalcemia can be caused by hyperparathyroidism. Parathyroid hyperplasia, adenoma, or cancer can cause hyperparathyroidism. It is important for the surgeon planning resection of the parathyroid abnormality to know how many parathyroid glands are involved and their location. Preoperative parathyroid scanning is the most accurate method of providing this information. Parathyroid hyperplasia causes enlargement of all four parathyroid glands. A parathyroid adenoma or cancer, however, causes enlargement of only one parathyroid gland and suppression of the other three glands. Based on the parathyroid scan, the surgeon will know whether he or she is dealing with hyperplasia or adenoma/cancer.

Parathyroids are located most commonly on the lateral borders of the thyroid lobes—two on each side. However, parathyroid anatomic location varies considerably, and they may be located anywhere from the upper neck to the lower mediastinum. They can even be located in the center of the thyroid lobe. Parathyroid scanning demonstrates the location of the pathologic parathyroids to the surgeon with high degree of resolution and accuracy. Single photon emission computed tomography (SPECT) scanning is even more accurate than routine nuclear imaging.

Scanning is now done more frequently in newly diagnosed patients. In some centers, scanning is reserved for those patients in whom an initial neck exploration failed to identify all four parathyroid glands and the hypercalcemia persisted after the operation.

There are two methods of parathyroid scanning. The first is the *single tracer double phase (STDP)* test using technetium-99m Sestamibi. With this method, the patient is injected with the Sestamibi tracer. Images are obtained at 15 minutes and 3 hours. The tracer initially lights up both the thyroid and the parathyroid glands. At 3 hours, however, the tracer is washed out of all normal endocrine tissue and remains only in the pathologic parathyroid tissue.

The second method is the *double tracer subtraction test (DTST)* in which technetium-99m pertechnetate or iodine-123 is administered. Only the thyroid gland takes up either of these two later tracers. Scanning is performed. Technetium-99m sestamibi is then administered and is taken up by both the thyroid and the parathyroid glands. Scanning is repeated and that first image is then "subtracted" from the second image leaving an image of only the parathyroid glands.

Contraindications

- Patients who are allergic to iodine if radioactive iodine is to be used
- Patients who are pregnant, unless the benefits outweigh the risks

Interfering factors

- Patient movement can inhibit the quality of imaging, especially when subtraction scanning is performed.
- Iodine-containing foods or drugs (including cough medicines) can affect test results.
- Recent administration of x-ray contrast agents can alter test results.

Procedure and patient care

Before

- PT Explain the procedure to the patient.
- PT Tell the patient that fasting is usually not required. Check with the laboratory.
- Check the patient for allergies to iodine.
- PT Instruct the patient about medications and food that need to be restricted for weeks before the test (e.g., thyroid drugs, medications or food containing iodine).
- Obtain a history concerning recent contrast x-ray studies, nuclear scanning, or intake of any thyroid-suppressive or antithyroid drugs.

During

- Note the following procedural steps:

STDP method

1. Technetium sestamibi is injected intravenously.
2. At 15 minutes and 3 hours, the patient is placed in a supine position and a detector is passed over the neck and upper chest area and the radioactive counts are recorded and displayed.

DTST method

1. Technetium-99m pertechnetate or iodine-123 is injected intravenously
2. At 15 minutes the patient is placed in a supine position and a detector is passed over the neck and upper chest area and the radioactive counts are recorded and displayed.
3. Technetium sestamibi is then injected intravenously and imaging is repeated.
4. With the computer, subtraction images are obtained leaving only the parathyroid gland images.

- Note that this study is performed by a radiologic technologist.

PT Tell the patient that no discomfort is associated with this study.

After

PT Assure the patient that the dose of radioactive technetium used in this test is minute and therefore harmless. No isolation and no special urine precautions are needed.

Abnormal findings

Parathyroid adenoma, carcinoma, or hyperplasia
Aberrantly placed parathyroid tissue in the upper neck, thyroid gland, or mediastinum

notes

partial thromboplastin time, activated (APTT, Partial thromboplastin time [PTT])

Type of test Blood

Normal findings

APTT: 30-40 seconds
PTT: 60-70 seconds
Patients receiving anticoagulant therapy: 1.5-2.5 times control value in seconds

Possible critical values

APTT: >70 seconds
PTT: >100 seconds

Test explanation and related physiology

The PTT test is used to assess the intrinsic system and the common pathway of clot formation. PTT evaluates factors I (fibrinogen), II (prothrombin), V, VIII, IX, X, XI, and XII. When any of these factors exists in inadequate quantities, as in hemophilia A and B or consumptive coagulopathy, PTT is prolonged. Because factors II, IX, and X are vitamin K-dependent factors, biliary obstruction, which precludes gastrointestinal absorption of fat and fat-soluble vitamins (e.g., vitamin K), can reduce their concentration and thus prolong PTT. Because coagulation factors are made in the liver, hepatocellular diseases will also prolong PTT.

Heparin has been found to inactivate prothrombin (factor II) and prevent the formation of thromboplastin. These actions prolong the intrinsic clotting pathway for approximately 4 to 6 hours after each dose of heparin. Thus heparin is capable of providing therapeutic anticoagulation. The appropriate dose of heparin can be monitored by PTT. PTT test results are given in seconds, along with a control value. The control value may vary slightly from day to day because of the reagents used.

Recently activators have been added to PTT test reagents to shorten normal clotting time and provide a narrow normal range. This shortened time is called the *activated* PTT (APTT). Normal APTT is 30 to 40 seconds. Desired ranges for therapeutic anticoagulation are 1.5 to 2.5 times normal (e.g., 70 seconds). The APTT specimen should be drawn 30 to 60 minutes before the patient's next heparin dose is given. If the APTT is less than 50 seconds, the patient may not be receiving therapeutic

P

anticoagulation and needs more heparin. An APTT greater than 100 seconds indicates that too much heparin is being given; the risk of serious spontaneous bleeding exists when the APTT is this high. The effects of heparin can be reversed immediately by the administration of 1 mg of protamine sulfate for every 100 units of the heparin dose.

Heparin's effect, unlike that of warfarin, is immediate and short-lived. When a thromboembolic episode (e.g., pulmonary embolism, arterial embolism, thrombophlebitis) occurs, immediate and complete anticoagulation is most rapidly and safely achieved by heparin administration. This drug is often given during cardiac and vascular surgery to prevent intravascular clotting during clamping of the vessels. Often, small doses of heparin (5000 units subcutaneously every 12 hours) are given to prevent thromboembolism in high-risk patients. This dose alters the PTT very little, and the risk of spontaneous bleeding is minimal.

Interfering factors

- ✖ Drugs that may prolong PTT test values include antihistamines, ascorbic acid, chlorpromazine, heparin, and salicylates.

Procedure and patient care

Before

PT Explain the procedure to the patient.
- If the patient is receiving heparin by intermittent injection, plan to draw the blood specimen for the APTT 30 minutes to 1 hour before the next dose of heparin.
- If the patient is receiving continuous heparin, draw the blood at any time.

During

- Collect 5 to 14 ml of venous blood in one or two blue-top tubes.

After

- Apply pressure to the venipuncture site. Remember, if the patient is receiving anticoagulants or has coagulopathies, the bleeding time will be increased.
- Assess the patient to detect possible bleeding. Check for blood in the urine and all other excretions and assess the patient for bruises, petechiae, and low back pain.

- If severe bleeding occurs, note that the anticoagulant effect of heparin can be reversed by parenteral administration of protamine sulfate.

Abnormal findings

▲ **Increased levels**

Acquired or congenital clotting factor deficiencies
Cirrhosis of the liver
Vitamin K deficiency
Leukemia
Disseminated intravascular coagulation
Heparin administration
Hypofibrinogenemia
von Willebrand's disease
Hemophilia

▼ **Decreased levels**

Early stages of disseminated intravascular coagulation
Extensive cancer

notes

parvovirus B19 antibody

Type of test Blood

Normal findings Negative for immunoglobulin M (IgM)- and IgG-specific antibodies to parvovirus B19

Test explanation and related physiology

The parvovirus group includes several species-specific viruses of animals. The parvovirus B19 is known to be a human pathogen. Many of the severe manifestations of B19 viremia relate to the ability of the virus to infect and lyse red blood cell precursors in the bone marrow. The name B19 was derived from the code number of the human serum in which the virus was discovered.

Erythema infectiosum is the most common manifestation of B19 infection and occurs predominantly in children. This pathogen is also referred to as fifth disease because it was classified in the late nineteenth century as the fifth in a series of six exanthems of childhood. This infection is also sometimes referred to as "academy rash." Recently, parvovirus B19 has been associated with a number of other clinical problems, including joint inflammation, purpura, hydrops fetalis, and aplastic anemia.

Because of the recently discovered spectrum of disease caused by parvovirus B19, laboratory diagnosis has come into great demand. Serologic testing for parvovirus B19-specific IgM and IgG antibodies can be detected. Acute infections can be determined by B19-compatible symptoms and the presence of IgM antibodies that remain detectable up to a few months. Past infection or immunity is documented by IgG antibodies that persist indefinitely. Fetal infection may be recognized by hydrops fetalis and the presence of B19 DNA in amniotic fluid or fetal blood.

Procedure and patient care

Before

PT Explain the procedure to the patient.

PT Tell the patient that no fasting or special preparation is necessary.

During

- Collect a venous blood sample according to the laboratory protocol.

After

- Apply pressure to the venipuncture site.
- **PT** Inform the patient that it normally requires approximately 2 to 3 days to get test results.

Abnormal findings

▲ **Increased levels**

Erythema infectiosum (fifth disease)
Joint arthralgia and arthritis
Hydrops fetalis
Fetal loss
Transient aplastic anemia
Chronic anemia in immunodeficient patients
Bone marrow failure

notes

P

pelvic ultrasonography (Obstetric echography, Pregnant uterus ultrasonography, Pelvic ultrasonography in pregnancy, Obstetric ultrasonography, Vaginal ultrasound, Fetal nuchal translucency [FNT])

Type of test Ultrasound

Normal findings Normal fetal and placental size and position

Test explanation and related physiology

Ultrasound examination of the female patient is a harmless, noninvasive method of evaluating the female genital tract and fetus. In real-time ultrasound, high-frequency sound waves are emitted from the transducer and penetrate the structure (uterus, ovaries, parametria, placenta, fetus) to be studied. These sound waves are bounced back to a sensor within the transducer and by electronic conversion are arranged into a pictorial image of the desired organ.

It should be noted that pelvic ultrasonography can be performed with the transducer placed on the anterior abdomen (see Figure 1, p. 2) or in the vagina with a specially designed vaginal probe. The view obtained from both transducers complements the information gained from either one alone. Vaginal ultrasound adds significant accuracy in identifying paracervical, endometrial, and ovarian pathology that otherwise may not be detected with the anterior abdominal probe.

Pelvic ultrasonography may be useful in the *obstetric patient* in the following circumstances:

1. Making an early diagnosis of normal pregnancy and abnormal pregnancy (e.g., tubal pregnancy)
2. Identifying multiple pregnancies
3. Differentiating a tumor (e.g., hydatidiform mole) from a normal pregnancy
4. Determining the age of the fetus by the diameter of the head. This is often combined with computed tomography scan of the pelvis to compare measurements of the fetal head to the maternal pelvis. This is helpful in identifying cephalopelvic disproportion.
5. Measuring the rate of fetal growth
6. Identifying placental abnormalities such as abruptio placentae and placenta previa
7. Determining the position of the placenta (Ultrasound localization of the placenta is done before amniocentesis.)

8. Making differential diagnoses of various uterine and ovarian enlargements (e.g., polyhydramnios, neoplasms, cysts, abscesses)
9. Determining fetal position
10. Diagnosing ectopic pregnancy

Ultrasound is quickly becoming a very accurate and easily performed screening test to recognize risks of fetal abnormalities (see *Amniotic Fluid Index*, p. 435). *Fetal nuchal translucency (FNT)* is an ultrasound measurement of subcutaneous edema in the neck region of the fetus. It is performed at 10 to 14 weeks of gestation. Major heart defects, trisomy 21, and other genetic defects are associated with increased edema in this location at this age of gestation. Screening for chromosomal defects by measurement of FNT identifies 80% of fetuses with trisomy 21 for a false-positive rate of 5%. This is especially helpful for older pregnant women. With FNT, these abnormalities can be identified earlier in the pregnancy when abortion is still possible. Although there may be advantages in early detection of fetal anomalies, a disadvantage should be considered. Many pregnancies complicated by fetal abnormality, both aneuploidy and other anomalies, will end in an early miscarriage. If these pregnancies are identified early, parents may be asked to make difficult decisions regarding termination of pregnancy. This imposes a potential burden and long-term consequence that may have been avoided had the pregnancy been lost spontaneously.

Pelvic ultrasound is used in the *nonpregnant woman* to monitor the endometrium in patients who take tamoxifen and to aid in the diagnosis of:

1. Ovarian cyst
2. Ovarian tumor
3. Tubo-ovarian abscess
4. Uterine fibroids
5. Uterine cancer
6. Pelvic inflammatory disease (PID)
7. Thickened uterine endometrium (stripe) (caused by cancer, hyperplasia, etc.)

When a woman is unable to visualize or palpate the string of an intrauterine device (IUD), ultrasound is indicated to determine whether the IUD has perforated the uterus, been expulsed, or been incorporated with an intrauterine pregnancy. IUDs have a particular type-specific morphology and can be easily recognized with ultrasound. If an IUD can be seen on the abdominal x-ray film but cannot be shown to be in the endometrial cavity by ultrasound, one must strongly suspect that the IUD has perforated the uterus.

Contraindications

- Patients with latex allergy
  Vaginal ultrasound requires placement of the probe in a latex condomlike sac. Patients with a latex allergy may react significantly to that contact.

Interfering factors

- Patients who have had recent gastrointestinal (GI) contrast studies, because barium creates severe distortion of reflective sound waves
- Patients with air-filled bowels, because gas does not transmit the sound waves well
- Failure to fill the bladder may make the image uninterpretable.

Procedure and patient care

Before

- **PT** Explain the procedure to the patient.
- **PT** Assure the patient that this study has no known deleterious effect on maternal or fetal tissues, even when it is repeated several times.
- **PT** Give the patient three to four glasses (200 to 350 ml) of water or other liquid 1 hour before the examination, and instruct her *not* to void until after the procedure is completed. This will permit visualization of the bladder, which is used as a reference point in pelvic anatomy.
- No water is required if the ultrasound is to be done vaginally only.
- If a transabdominal ultrasound is required urgently and there is not time to fill the bladder by ingestion or administration of fluids, a bladder catheter is inserted, and the bladder is filled with water.
- **PT** Tell the patient that no fasting or sedation is required.

During

- Note the following procedural steps:
  1. The patient is taken to the ultrasound room and placed in the supine position on the examining table.
  2. The ultrasonographer, usually a radiologist, applies a greasy conductive paste to the abdomen to enhance sound transmission and reception.

3. A transducer is passed vertically and horizontally over the skin.
4. If a vaginal probe is used, it is inserted via the vagina and angled to identify the various parts of the pelvis.
5. Pictures are taken of the reflections.
6. During the examination, fetal structures are pointed out to the mother.

- Note that this procedure is performed in approximately 20 minutes.

PT Inform the patient that no discomfort is associated with this study, other than having a full bladder and the urge to void. Some patients may be uncomfortable lying on a hard x-ray table.

After

- Remove the lubricant from the patient's skin.
- Provide an opportunity for the patient to void.

Abnormal findings

Tubal pregnancy
Abdominal pregnancy
Hydatidiform mole
Intrauterine growth retardation
Multiple fetuses
Fetal death
Abruptio placentae
Abnormal fetal position (e.g., breech, transverse)
Fetal anomalies
Placenta previa
Polyhydramnios
Neoplasm of the ovaries, uterus, or fallopian tubes
Cysts
Abscesses
Hydrocephalus of the fetus
Intrauterine device localization

P

notes

pericardiocentesis

Type of test Fluid analysis

Normal findings Minimal amount of clear, straw-colored fluid without evidence of any bacteria, blood, or malignant cells

Test explanation and related physiology

Pericardiocentesis, which involves the aspiration of fluid from the pericardial sac with a needle, may be performed for therapeutic and diagnostic purposes. Therapeutically, the test is performed to relieve cardiac tamponade by removing fluid and improving diastolic filling. Diagnostically, pericardiocentesis is performed to remove a sample of pericardial fluid for laboratory examination to determine the cause of the fluid. This is similar to the evaluation described for peritoneal and pleural fluid on p. 678 and p. 723, respectively.

Contraindications

- Patients who are uncooperative, because of the risk of lacerations to the epicardium or coronary artery
- Patients with a bleeding disorder
  Inadvertent puncture of the myocardium may create uncontrollable bleeding into the pericardial sac, leading to tamponade.

Potential complications

- Laceration of the coronary artery or myocardium
- Needle-induced ventricular arrhythmias (dysrhythmias)
- Myocardial infarction
- Pneumothorax caused by inadvertent puncture of the lung
- Liver laceration caused by inadvertent puncture
- Pleural infection
- Vasovagal arrest

Procedure and patient care

Before

PT Explain the procedure to the patient.
- Obtain informed consent for this procedure.
- Restrict fluid and food intake for at least 4 to 6 hours (if this is an elective procedure).
- Obtain IV access for infusion of fluids and cardiac medications if required.

- Administer pretest medication. Atropine is frequently given to prevent the vasovagal reflex of bradycardia and hypotension.

During

- Note the following procedural steps:
  1. The patient is placed in the supine position.
  2. An area in the fifth to sixth intercostal space at the left sternal margin (or subxyphoid) is prepared and draped.
  3. After skin anesthesia is performed, a large-bore pericardiocentesis needle is placed on a 50-ml syringe and introduced into the pericardial sac (Figure 32).

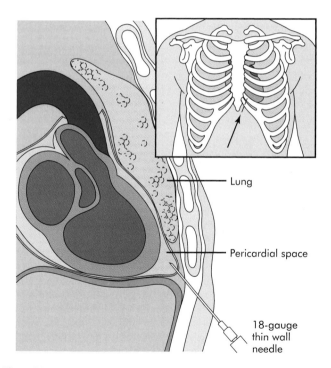

Lung

Pericardial space

18-gauge thin wall needle

Figure 32 Pericardiocentesis using subxiphoid route for aspiration of pericardial fluid. The 18-gauge needle is introduced at a 30- to 40-degree angle.

4. An electrocardiographic lead is often attached by a clip to the needle to identify any ST-segment elevations, which may indicate penetration into the epicardium.

5. Pericardial fluid is aspirated and placed in multiple specimen containers.

6. Some patients who have recurring cardiac tamponade may require placement of an indwelling pericardial catheter for continuous draining for 1 to 3 days.

7. With certain types of pericarditis, medications (e.g., antibiotics, antineoplastic drugs, corticosteroids) may be instilled during pericardiocentesis.

- Note that a physician usually performs this procedure in the cardiac catheterization laboratory, operating room, or emergency room in approximately 10 to 20 minutes.

PT Tell the patient that this procedure is associated with very little discomfort. Most patients feel pressure as the needle is inserted into the pericardial sac.

After

- Closely monitor the patient's vital signs. An increased temperature may indicate infection. Pericardial bleeding would be marked by hypotension or pulsus paradoxus (abnormal decrease in systolic blood pressure during inspiration).

- Label and number the specimen tubes that contain the pericardial fluid and deliver them to the appropriate laboratories for examination. Note the following possibilities:

1. Usually the fluid is taken to the chemistry laboratory, where the color, turbidity, glucose, albumin, protein, and lactic dehydrogenase levels are obtained (see discussion of thoracentesis, p. 897).

2. A tube of blood often goes to the hematology laboratory, where the quantities of red and white blood cells are recorded.

3. The bacteriology laboratory performs routine cultures, Gram stains, fungal studies, acid-fast bacilli smears, and cultures.

4. When malignancy is suspected, the fluid should be sent for cytology.

- Apply a sterile dressing to the catheter if one has been left for continuing pericardial drainage.

- Establish a closed system if continued pericardial drainage is required. This is usually performed via the straight drainage method.

- Note that to minimize infection, pericardial catheters, if used, are usually removed after 2 days, although there are exceptions. After the sutures are cut and the catheter is removed, apply a sterile dressing to the puncture site.

🏠 Home care responsibilities

- Check the dressing frequently for drainage.
- Note than an increased temperature may indicate infection.
- Instruct the patient to report any drop in BP. Hypotension may be a sign of pericardial bleeding.

Abnormal findings

Pericarditis
Uremia
Hypoproteinemia
Congestive heart failure
Metastatic cancer
Blunt or penetrating cardiac trauma
Rupture of ventricular aneurysm

notes

P

phenylketonuria test (PKU test, Guthrie test, Phenylalanine screening)

Type of test   Blood; urine

Normal findings

Blood: negative ≤2 mg/dl (Guthrie technique) or
  ≤121 μmol/L (SI units)

Urine: no green coloration

Possible critical values   ≥4 mg/dl (Guthrie technique)

Test explanation and related physiology

An inherited disease, PKU is characterized by deficiency of the enzyme phenylalanine hydroxylase, which converts phenylalanine to tyrosine. Phenylalanine is an essential amino acid necessary for growth; however, any excess must be degraded by conversion to tyrosine. An infant with PKU lacks the ability to make this necessary conversion. Thus phenylalanine accumulates in the body and spills over into the urine. If the amount of phenylalanine is not restricted in infants with PKU, progressive mental retardation results. Dietary control must begin early to avoid brain damage; therefore, diagnosis must be made early.

Routine screening of newborn infants for PKU is now mandatory in most of the United States. It is important to note that this test is not valid until the newborn has ingested an ample amount (for 2 or 3 days) of the amino acid phenylalanine, which is a constituent of both human and cow's milk. If the child is not eating well or does not weigh at least 5 lb, the test should not be done because results may be invalid. The urine PKU test is normally done after 6 weeks of age if, for some reason, a blood test was not done in the hospital. If the tests are positive, a blood phenylalanine test should be performed.

Interfering factors

- Premature infants may have false-positive results because of delayed development of liver enzymes.
- Ketonuria can produce an altered urine color reaction.
- Infants tested before 24 hours of age may have false-negative results.
- Feeding problems (e.g., vomiting) may cause false-negative results.

☀ Drugs that may influence screening results include antibiotics, aspirin, and salicylates.

Procedure and patient care

Before

PT Inform the parents about the purpose of the test and the method of performance.

- Assess the infant's feeding patterns before performing the PKU test. An inadequate amount of protein ingested before performing the test can cause false-negative results.

During

- Place a few drops of blood from a heel stick on filter paper for the Guthrie test. This test is performed after the newborn has ingested an ample amount (for 2 to 3 days) of the amino acid phenylalanine.
- Indicate on the laboratory slip the present date and time, date and time of birth, and time of first milk feeding.
- Note that urine tests also may be used to detect PKU in infants who are at least 6 weeks of age. These tests are usually done at the infant's first checkup:
  1. For the *diaper test,* drop 10% ferric chloride on a diaper that contains fresh urine. A green spot indicates probable PKU.
  2. For the *Phenistix* test, press a test stick against a diaper containing urine or dip the stick in the urine. A green color reaction indicates probable PKU.

After

PT If test results are positive, inform the mother that dietary control must begin immediately to prevent brain damage in the infant. This is done by substituting Lofenalac for milk. Later, strained foods low in protein are added to the infant's diet. The dietary treatment is monitored by blood and urine testing.

PT Instruct women with PKU who wish to have children to begin a low-phenylalanine diet before conception and continue throughout the pregnancy. The risk of producing a mentally retarded infant is very high if the mother remains on a general diet.

Abnormal findings

PKU
Low-birthweight infants
Galactosemia
Hepatic encephalopathy

pheochromocytoma suppression and provocative testing (Clonidine suppression test [CST], Glucagon stimulation test)

Type of test   Blood

Normal findings

Glucagon stimulation
Norepinephrine <3 times basal levels

Clonidine suppression
Norepinephrine >50% reduction in basal levels or <500 pg/ml
Epinephrine <275 pg/ml

Test explanation and related physiology

In patients with significantly high blood pressure, refractory to treatment, the diagnosis of pheochromocytoma is often considered. When catecholamine levels are excessive (norepinephrine >2000 pg/ml), the diagnosis is easily made. However, when basal levels are not significantly elevated, it is difficult to differentiate essential hypertension from a functioning pheochromocytoma. Suppression and provocative tests may be necessary. Normally, glucagon, metoclopramide, and naloxone are commonly used as provocative agents. In patients with pheochromocytoma, however, the response is accentuated. Clonidine is normally a potent suppressor of catecholamine production, yet it has little to no effect on patients with pheochromocytoma.

Potential complications

- Drowsiness during CST
- Hypotension during CST, especially in patients treated aggressively for hypertension
- Extremely high blood pressure during provocative testing

Interfering factors

- False suppression with CST may occur in patients with low basal catecholamine levels.

Procedure and patient care

Before
PT Explain the procedure to the patient.
- Identify the medications being administered prior to testing

- The patient must be reclining calmly for 30 minutes prior to testing

During

- Collect 3 to 9 ml of blood from an antecubital vein in a heparinized tube for determination of basal catecholamine levels.
- Monitor vital signs closely throughout the testing period.

Glucagon provocative test

- Administer 1 mg of glucagon intravenously.
- Two minutes later, obtain a blood specimen as described above.

Clonidine suppression test

- Administer 300 mcg of clonidine orally.
- Three hours later, obtain a blood specimen as described above.

After

- Monitor vital signs for at least 1 hour after conclusion of the procedure.

Abnormal findings

Pheochromocytoma

notes

P

phosphate (PO$_4$, Phosphorus [P])

Type of test Blood

Normal findings

Adult: 3-4.5 mg/dl or 0.97-1.45 mmol/L (SI units)
Elderly: values slightly lower than adult
Child: 4.5-6.5 mg/dl or 1.45-2.1 mmol/L (SI units)
Newborn: 4.3-9.3 mg/dl or 1.4-3 mmol/L (SI units)

Possible critical values <1 mg/dl

Test explanation and related physiology

Phosphorus in the body is in the form of a phosphate. Phosphorus and phosphate will be used interchangeably throughout this and other discussions. Most of the phosphate in the body is a part of organic compounds. Only a small part of total body phosphate is inorganic phosphate (i.e., not part of another organic compound). It is the *inorganic* phosphate that is measured when one requests a "phosphate," "phosphorus," "inorganic phosphorus," or "inorganic phosphate." Most of the body's inorganic phosphorus is combined with calcium within the skeleton; however, approximately 15% of the phosphorus exists in the blood as a phosphate salt.

Dietary phosphorus is absorbed in the small bowel. The absorption is very efficient, and only rarely is hypophosphatemia caused by gastrointestinal malabsorption. Phosphorus levels are determined by calcium metabolism, parathormone (parathyroid hormone [PTH]), renal excretion, and, to a lesser degree, intestinal absorption. Because an inverse relationship exists between calcium and phosphorus, a decrease of one mineral results in an increase in the other. The regulation of phosphate by PTH is such that PTH tends to decrease phosphate resorption in the kidney. PTH and vitamin D, however, tend to stimulate phosphate absorption weakly within the gut.

Interfering factors

- Laxatives or enemas containing sodium phosphate can increase phosphorus levels.
- Recent carbohydrate ingestion, including IV glucose administration, causes decreased phosphorus levels because phosphorus enters the cell with glucose.

✶ Drugs that may cause *increased* levels include methicillin and vitamin D (excessive).

✶ Drugs that may cause *decreased* levels include antacids and mannitol.

Procedure and patient care

Before

PT Explain the procedure to the patient.
- Keep the patient NPO after midnight on the day of the test.
- If indicated, discontinue IV fluids with glucose for several hours before the test.

During

- Collect approximately 5 to 10 ml of venous blood in a red-top tube.
- Avoid hemolysis. Handle the tube carefully.
- Use a heel stick to draw blood from infants.

After

- Take the specimen to the laboratory immediately.
- Indicate on the laboratory slip the time the blood was obtained. Apply pressure to the venipuncture site.

Abnormal findings

▲ **Increased levels (hyperphosphatemia)**

Renal failure
Increased dietary or IV intake of phosphorus
Acromegaly
Hypoparathyroidism
Bone metastasis
Sarcoidosis
Hypocalcemia
Liver disease
Renal failure
Acidosis
Rhabdomyolysis
Advanced lymphoma or myeloma
Hemolytic anemia

▼ **Decreased levels (hypophosphatemia)**

Inadequate dietary ingestion of phosphorus
Chronic antacid ingestion
Hyperparathyroidism
Hypercalcemia
Chronic alcoholism
Vitamin D deficiency
Diabetic acidosis
Hyperinsulinism
Rickets (childhood)
Osteomalacia (adult)
Malnutrition
Alkalosis
Sepsis

P

plasminogen (Fibrinolysin)

Type of test Blood

Normal findings 2.4-4.4 Committee on Thrombolytic Agents (CTA) units/ml

Test explanation and related physiology

This test is used to diagnose suspected plasminogen deficiency in patients who have multiple thromboembolic episodes. Plasminogen is a protein involved in the fibrinolytic process of intravascular blood clot dissolution (see Figure 11, p. 282). Plasminogen is converted to plasmin by proteolytic cleavage. This reaction can be catalyzed by urokinase, streptokinase, or tissue plasminogen activator (t-PA). Plasmin can destroy fibrin and dissolve clots. This fibrinolytic system is a normal part of the balance between coagulation and fibrinolysis.

Plasminogen levels are occasionally measured during fibrinolytic therapy (for coronary and peripheral arterial occlusion) and are diminished with full fibrinolysis. Decreased levels of plasminogen are also found in hyperfibrinolytic states (e.g., disseminated intravascular coagulation [DIC], primary fibrinolysis). Because plasminogen is made in the liver, patients with cirrhosis or other severe liver diseases can be expected to have decreased levels. There are rare cases of hereditary deficiencies of this protein. Pregnancy and, especially, eclampsia are associated with increased levels of plasminogen. Inflammatory conditions may have mild elevations of plasminogens, which are "acute phase reactant" proteins.

Procedure and patient care

Before

PT Explain the procedure to the patient.

PT Tell the patient that no fasting is required.

During

- Collect a venous blood sample in a blue-top tube containing sodium citrate.
- Avoid excessive agitation of the blood sample.

After

- Apply pressure to the venipuncture site, especially if the patient is suspected of having a hyperfibrinolytic process (e.g., DIC).

Abnormal findings

▲ **Increased levels**
Pregnancy

▼ **Decreased levels**
Hyperfibrinolytic state
(e.g., DIC,
fibrinolysis)
Primary liver disease
Syndrome associated
with hypercoagulation
(e.g., venous and
arterial clotting)
Rare congenital
deficiencies
Malnutrition

notes

P

platelet aggregation test

Type of test Blood

Normal findings Depends on the platelet agonist used

Test explanation and related physiology

Platelet aggregation is an important part of hemostasis. Surrounding an area of acute blood vessel endothelial injury is a clump of platelets. Normal platelets adhere to this area of injury, and through a series of chemical reactions, they attract other platelets to the area. This is platelet aggregation, the first step of hemostasis. After this step, the normal coagulation factor waterfall occurs (see Figure 11, p. 282). Certain diseases that affect either platelet number or function can inhibit platelet aggregation and thereby prolong bleeding times. Congenital syndromes, uremia, myeloproliferative disorders, and certain drugs are associated with abnormal platelet aggregation. If blood is passed through a heart-lung or dialysis pump, platelet injury can occur and aggregation can be reduced.

Platelet aggregation is measured by determining the turbidity of platelet-rich plasma in which platelet aggregation has been stimulated in vitro. Turbidity is then measured within an aggregometer, and a curve indicating light transmission per unit of time is plotted. Normal curves have been identified for each platelet aggregation stimulant that is used.

Interfering factors

- Factors that may cause increased levels include blood storage temperature, hyperbilirubinemia, hemoglobinemia, hyperlipidemia, and platelet count.
- Drugs that may cause *decreased* levels include aspirin, antibiotics, sodium warfarin (Coumadin), and heparin.

Procedure and patient care

Before

PT Explain the procedure to the patient.

PT Tell the patient that no fasting is required.

During

- Collect 5 to 7 ml of venous blood in a blue-top tube.
- If the patient is receiving any drugs that may interfere with platelet aggregation or has any diseases such as jaundice,

hyperlipidemia, or hemolysis, this should be listed on the laboratory request slip.

After

- Apply pressure to the venipuncture site.
- Remember that abnormalities in platelet aggregation can prolong bleeding time, and a significant hematoma at the venipuncture site may occur.

Abnormal findings

Prolonged platelet aggregation

Various congenital disorders (e.g., Wiskott-Aldrich syndrome, Bernard-Soulier syndrome, glycogen storage)

Connective tissue disorder (e.g., lupus erythematosus)

Recent cardiopulmonary or dialysis bypass

Various myeloproliferative diseases

Primary protein disease

von Willebrand's disease

Uremia

notes

P

platelet antibody detection (Antiplatelet antibody detection)

Type of test Blood

Normal findings No antiplatelet antibodies identified

Test explanation and related physiology

Immune-mediated destruction of platelets may be caused either by autoantibodies directed against antigens located on the same person's platelets or by alloantibodies that develop after exposure to transfused platelets received from a donor. These antibodies are usually directed to an antigen on the platelet membrane such as human lymphocyte antigen (HLA) (see p. 538) or platelet-specific antigens such as PLA1, PLA2.

Antibodies directed to platelets cause early destruction of the platelets and subsequent thrombocytopenia. Immunologic thrombocytopenia includes the following:

Idiopathic thrombocytopenia purpura (ITP)
Platelet-associated IgG antibodies are detected in 90% of these patients.

Posttransfusion purpura
This is a rare syndrome characterized by the sudden onset of severe thrombocytopenia a few hours to a few days after transfusion of red blood cells or platelets. This is usually associated with an antibody to ABO, HLA, or PLA antigens on the RBC.

Maternal-fetal platelet antigen incompatibility (neonatal thrombocytopenia)
This occurs when the fetal platelet contains a PLA1 antigen that is absent in the mother. Neonatal thrombocytopenia can also occur if the mother has ITP autoantibodies that are passed through the placenta and destroy the fetal platelets.

Drug-induced thrombocytopenia
This is usually caused by platelet-associated IgG antibodies. These antibodies are the result of a hypersensitivity to certain drugs. A host of drugs is known to induce autoimmune-mediated thrombocytopenia. They are *cimetidine,* analgesics (salicylates, acetaminophen), antibiotics (cephalosporins, penicillin, *sulfonamides*), *quinidine*-like drugs, hypnotics (phenobarbital), oral hypoglycemic agents

(e.g., chlorpropamide), heavy metals (e.g., gold, organic arsenicals), diuretics (e.g., chlorothiazide), and others (e.g., digoxin, propylthiouracil, disulfiram [Antabuse], *heparin*). **Note:** The medications in italics are the most common offenders.

Interfering factors

- Blood transfusion may cause the development of isoantibodies to HLA antigens on the platelets or red blood cells.

Procedure and patient care

Before

PT Explain the procedure to the patient.
PT Tell the patient that no fasting is required.

During

- Collect 10 to 30 ml of blood in a red-top tube. The amount of blood required depends on the initial platelet count.

After

- Apply pressure to the venipuncture site.
- Ensure adequate hemostasis in all patients who are suspected to have thrombocytopenia.

Abnormal findings

Idiopathic thrombocytopenia purpura
Neonatal thrombocytopenia
Posttransfusion purpura
Drug-induced thrombocytopenia
Paroxysmal hemoglobinuria

notes

platelet count (Thrombocyte count)

Type of test Blood

Normal findings

Adult/elderly: 150,000-400,000/mm^3 or 150-400 × 10^9/L (SI units)
Premature infant: 100,000-300,000/mm^3
Newborn: 150,000-300,000/mm^3
Infant: 200,000-475,000/mm^3
Child: 150,000-400,000/mm^3

Possible critical values <50,000 or >1 million/mm^3

Test explanation and related physiology

The platelet count is a count of the number of platelets (thrombocytes) per cubic milliliter of blood. It is performed on all patients who develop petechiae (small hemorrhages in the skin), spontaneous bleeding, or increasingly heavy menses. It is also used to monitor the course of the disease or therapy for thrombocytopenia or bone marrow failure.

Platelet activity is essential to blood clotting. Counts of 150,000 to 400,000/mm^3 are considered normal. Counts less than 100,000/mm^3 are considered to indicate *thrombocytopenia*; *thrombocytosis* is said to exist when counts are greater than 400,000/mm^3. *Thrombocythemia* is a term used to indicate a platelet count in excess of 1 million/mm^3. The most common associative disease with spontaneous thrombocytosis is malignancy (leukemia, lymphoma, or solid tumors, such as colon). Thrombocytosis may also occur with polycythemia vera and postsplenectomy syndromes.

Spontaneous hemorrhage may occur with thrombocytopenia. If thrombocytopenia is severe, the platelets are often hand counted. Spontaneous bleeding is a serious danger when platelet counts fall below 20,000/mm^3. Petechiae and ecchymosis also occur at that level of thrombocytopenia. With counts above 40,000/mm^3, spontaneous bleeding rarely occurs, but prolonged bleeding from trauma or surgery may occur at this level. Causes of thrombocytopenia (decreased number of platelets) include the following:

1. Reduced production of platelets (secondary to bone marrow failure or infiltration of fibrosis, tumor, etc.)

2. Sequestration of platelets (secondary to hypersplenism)
3. Accelerated destruction of platelets (secondary to antibodies [see antiplatelet antibodies p. 712], infections, drugs, prosthetic heart valves)
4. Consumption of platelets (secondary to disseminated intravascular coagulation)
5. Platelet loss from hemorrhage
6. Dilution with large volumes of blood transfusions that contain very few, if any, platelets

Interfering factors

- Living at high altitudes may cause increased platelet levels.
- Because platelets can clump together, automated counting is subject to at least a 10% to 15% error.
- Strenuous exercise may cause increased levels.
- Decreased levels may be seen before menstruation.
- ♥ Drugs that may cause *increased* levels include oral contraceptives.
- ♥ Drugs that may cause *decreased* levels include acetaminophen, aspirin, chemotherapeutic agents, chloramphenicol, colchicine, H_2-blocking agents (cimetidine, ranitidine [Zantac]), hydralazine, indomethacin, isoniazid (INH), Levaquin, quinidine, streptomycin, sulfonamides, thiazide diuretics, and tolbutamide (Orinase).

Procedure and patient care

Before

PT Explain the procedure to the patient.
PT Tell the patient that no fasting is required.

During

- Collect approximately 5 to 7 ml of peripheral venous blood in a lavender-top tube.
- List on the laboratory slip any drugs or other factors that may affect test results.

After

- Apply pressure to the venipuncture site.
- If the results indicate that the patient has a serious platelet deficiency:
    1. Observe the patient for signs and symptoms of bleeding.
    2. Check for blood in the urine and all excretions.
    3. Assess the patient for bruises, petechiae, bleeding from the gums, epistaxis, and low back pain.

4. Reassess all venipuncture sites for signs of hematoma formation.

Abnormal findings

▲ **Increased levels (thrombocytosis)**

Malignant disorder
Polycythemia vera
Postsplenectomy syndrome
Rheumatoid arthritis
Iron deficiency anemia

▼ **Decreased levels (thrombocytopenia)**

Hypersplenism
Hemorrhage
Immune thrombocytopenia
Leukemia and other myelofibrosis disorders
Thrombotic thrombocytopenia
Inherited thrombocytopenia disorders (e.g., Wiskott-Aldrich, Bernard-Soulier, or Zieve syndromes)
Disseminated intravascular coagulation
Systemic lupus erythematosus
Pernicious anemia
Hemolytic anemia
Cancer chemotherapy
Infection

notes

platelet volume, mean (Mean platelet volume [MPV])

Type of test Blood

Normal findings 7.4-10.4 fL

Test explanation and related physiology

The MPV is a measure of the volume of a large number of platelets determined by an automated analyzer. MPV is to platelets as mean corpuscular volume (see p. 785) is to the red blood cell.

The MPV varies with total platelet production. In cases of thrombocytopenia, despite a normal reactive bone marrow (e.g., hypersplenism), the normal bone marrow releases immature platelets to attempt to maintain a normal platelet count. These immature platelets are larger, and the MPV is elevated. When bone marrow production of platelets is inadequate, the platelets that are released are small. This will be reflected as a low MPV; in this way, the MPV is very useful in the differential diagnosis of thrombocytopenic disorders.

Procedure and patient care

Before

PT Explain the procedure to the patient.

PT Tell the patient that no fasting is required.

During

- Collect 5 to 7 ml of venous blood in a lavender-top tube.

After

- Apply pressure to the venipuncture site.
- If the patient is known to have a low platelet count:
    1. Observe the patient for signs and symptoms of bleeding.
    2. Check for blood in the urine and all excretions.
    3. Assess the patient for bruises, petechiae, bleeding of the gums, epistaxis, and low back pain.

P

Abnormal findings

▲ **Increased levels**

Valvular heart disease
Immune thrombocytopenia
Massive hemorrhage
B_{12} or folate deficiency
Myelogenous leukemia

▼ **Decreased levels**

Aplastic anemia
Chemotherapy-induced
  myelosuppression
Wiskott-Aldrich
  syndrome

notes

plethysmography, arterial

Type of test Manometric

Normal findings

<20 mm Hg difference in systolic blood pressure of the lower extremity compared with the upper extremity

Normal pulse wave amplitude showing a steep upswing, an acute narrow peak, and a more gentle downslope containing a dicrotic notch (normal arterial pulse wave)

Test explanation and related physiology

Plethysmography is usually performed to rule out occlusive disease of the lower extremities; however, it also can identify arteriosclerotic disease in the upper extremities. This test does require one normal extremity against which the other extremities may be compared.

Arterial plethysmography is performed by applying three blood pressure cuffs to the proximal, middle, and distal parts of an extremity. These are then attached to a pulse volume recorder (plethysmograph), and each pulse wave can be displayed. A reduction in amplitude of a pulse wave in any of the three cuffs indicates arterial occlusion immediately proximal to the area where the decreased amplitude is noted. Also, measurements of arterial pressures are performed at each cuff site. A difference in pressure greater than 20 mm Hg indicates a degree of arterial occlusion in the extremity. A positive result is reliable evidence of arteriosclerotic peripheral vascular occlusion. However, a negative result does not definitely exclude this diagnosis, because extensive vascular collateralization can compensate for even a complete arterial occlusion.

Although it is not as accurate as arteriography (see p. 126), plethysmography is performed without serious complications and can be done for extremely ill patients who cannot be transported to the arteriography laboratory.

Interfering factors

- Arterial occlusion proximal to the extremity
- Nicotine from cigarette smoking can cause transient arterial constriction.

Procedure and patient care

Before

PT Explain the procedure to the patient.

PT Tell the patient that no fasting is required.

PT Inform the patient that this test is painless.

PT Tell the patient that he or she must lie still during the testing procedure.

■ Remove all clothing from the patient's extremities.

PT Instruct the patient to avoid smoking for at least 30 minutes before the test. Nicotine creates constriction of the peripheral arteries and alters the test results.

During

■ Note the following procedural steps:
   1. The patient is placed in the semirecumbent position.
   2. The cuffs are applied to the extremities and then inflated to 65 mm Hg to increase their sensitivity to pulse waves.
   3. The pulse waves are recorded on plethysmographic paper.
   4. The amplitudes and form of the pulse wave of each cuff are measured and compared. A marked reduction in wave amplitude indicates arterial occlusive disease.

■ Note that this noninvasive test usually is performed in the vascular laboratory or at the patient's bedside by a vascular technologist in approximately 30 minutes.

PT Inform the patient that results are usually interpreted by a physician and are available in a few hours.

PT Remind the patient that no discomfort is associated with this test.

After

■ Encourage the patient to verbalize any concerns regarding the test results.

Abnormal findings

Arterial occlusive disease
Arterial trauma
Small vessel diabetic changes
Vascular diseases (e.g., Raynaud's phenomenon)
Arterial embolization

plethysmography, venous (Cuff pressure test)

Type of test Manometric

Normal findings Patent venous system without evidence of thrombosis or occlusion

Test explanation and related physiology

Plethysmography measures changes in the volume of an extremity. Usually this test is performed on a leg to exclude deep-vein thrombosis. During this test, blood pressure cuffs are placed on the proximal, middle, and distal parts of the extremity and attached to a pulse volume recorder. The leg volume can then be recorded as a baseline value. The venous system is occluded by inflating the most proximal cuff *(occlusion cuff)*; the most distal cuff *(recording cuff)* should record a sudden increase in venous volume. When the occlusion cuff is released, the venous volume of the leg should return to preocclusion baseline levels. In patients with venous obstruction, no initial increase in leg volume is recorded. Because venous outflow is obstructed, the venous volume of the leg will not dissipate quickly.

The results of venous plethysmography are less accurate than those of venography (see p. 985); however, no complications are associated with this noninvasive study. Plethysmography can be performed easily and quickly on any patient with suspected venous disease. Furthermore, with the use of portable plethysmography, this test can be performed at the bedside for extremely ill patients.

Doppler flow studies are now being performed to identify deep-vein thrombosis, but they are less accurate in evaluating the venous system below the knee.

Interfering factors

- Venous occlusion more proximal to the site of the occlusion cuff

Procedure and patient care

Before

PT Explain the procedure to the patient.
PT Tell the patient that no fasting is required.
PT Assure the patient that no discomfort is associated with the study.

PT Instruct the patient to lie still during the testing.

- Remove all clothing from the patient's extremity to be tested.

During

- Note the following procedural steps:
    1. A large, inflatable occlusion cuff is placed on the proximal part of the extremity, usually a leg.
    2. A second, smaller plethysmographic monitor or recording cuff is placed more distal on the leg. A third cuff may be placed in between the proximal and distal cuffs.
    3. The second cuff is inflated to 10 mm Hg to facilitate recognition of small changes in the leg's venous volume.
    4. The effects of respiration on the leg's venous volume are evaluated. If no significant changes occur with respiration, venous occlusion can be suspected.
    5. The occlusion cuff is inflated to 50 mm Hg. The monitor cuff should demonstrate a rise in venous volume, displayed on the pulse-monitor recorder.
    6. After the highest volume is recorded in the monitor cuff, the occlusion cuff is rapidly deflated. The leg should return to its preocclusion volume within 1 second. If return to preocclusion baseline values is delayed for a long period, venous thrombosis is suspected.
    7. Often this test is performed concomitantly with Doppler ultrasound of the venous system (see p. 982).
- Note that this noninvasive test is usually performed in the vascular laboratory or at the patient's bedside by a vascular technologist in approximately 30 minutes.

PT Remind the patient that no discomfort is associated with this test.

After

- Note that no special aftercare is needed.

Abnormal findings

Partial venous obstruction
Total venous obstruction

notes

pleural biopsy

Type of test Microscopic examination of tissue

Normal findings No evidence of pathology

Test explanation and related physiology

This test is indicated when the pleural fluid obtained by thoracentesis (see p. 897) is exudative fluid, which suggests infection, neoplasm, or tuberculosis. The pleural biopsy is indicated to distinguish among these disease processes. It is also performed when a plain chest x-ray indicates a pleural-based tumor, reaction, or thickening.

Pleural biopsy is the removal of pleural tissue for histologic examination. It is usually performed by a percutaneous needle biopsy. It also can be performed via thoracoscopy, which is done by inserting a laparoscope into the pleural space for inspection and biopsy of the pleura. Pleural tissue also may be obtained by an *open pleural biopsy,* which involves a limited thoracotomy and requires general anesthesia. For this procedure, a small intercostal incision is made, and the biopsy of the pleura is done under direct observation. The advantage of these open procedures is that a larger piece of pleura can be obtained.

Contraindications

- Patients with prolonged bleeding or clotting times

Potential complications

- Bleeding or injury to the lung
- Pneumothorax

Procedure and patient care

Before

PT Explain the procedure to the patient.
- Obtain informed consent for this procedure.
PT Tell the patient that no fasting or sedation is required.
PT Instruct the patient to remain very still during the procedure. Any movement may cause inadvertent needle damage.

During

- Note the following procedural steps for percutaneous needle biopsy:
  1. This procedure is usually performed with the patient in a sitting position with his or her shoulders and arms elevated and supported by a padded overbed table.
  2. After the presence of fluid has been determined by the thoracentesis technique, the skin overlying the biopsy site is anesthetized and pierced with a scalpel blade.
  3. A needle is inserted with a cannula until fluid is removed (some fluid is left in the pleural space after the thoracentesis to make the biopsy easier).
  4. The inner needle is removed, and a blunt-tipped, hooked biopsy trocar attached to a three-way stopcock is inserted into the cannula.
  5. The patient is instructed to expire all air and then perform the Valsalva maneuver to prevent air from entering the pleural space.
  6. The cannula and biopsy trocar are withdrawn while the hook catches the parietal wall and takes a specimen with its cutting edge.
  7. Usually three biopsy specimens are taken from different sites at the same session.
  8. The specimens are placed in a fixative solution and sent to the laboratory immediately.
  9. After the specimens are taken, additional parietal fluid can be removed.
- Note that this procedure is performed by a physician at the patient's bedside, in a special procedure room, or in the physician's office in approximately 30 minutes.
- **PT** Because of the local anesthetic, tell the patient that little discomfort is associated with this procedure.

After

- Apply an adhesive bandage to the biopsy site.
- Note that a chest x-ray film is usually taken to detect the potential complication of pneumothorax.
- Observe the patient for signs of respiratory distress (e.g., shortness of breath, diminished breath sounds) on the side of the biopsy.
- Observe the patient's vital signs frequently for evidence of bleeding (increased pulse, decreased blood pressure).
- Ensure that the biopsy specimen is sent immediately to the laboratory.

🏠 **Home care responsibilities**

- Instruct the patient to report any signs of shortness of breath.
- Note any signs of bleeding, such as decreasing blood pressure or increasing pulse.

Abnormal findings

Neoplasm
Tuberculosis

notes

P

porphyrins and porphobilinogens

Type of test   Urine (fresh and 24-hour)

Normal findings

	Male (mcg/24 hr)	*Female (mcg/24 hr)*
Total porphyrins	8-149	3-78
Uroporphyrin	4-46	3-22
Coproporphyrin	<96	<60

Porphobilinogens: 0-2 mg/24 hr or 0-8.8 μmol/day (SI units)

Test explanation and related physiology

This test is a quantitative measurement of porphyrins and porphobilinogen. Along with measurement of aminolevulinic acid, the various forms of porphyria can be identified.

Porphyria is a group of genetic disorders associated with enzyme deficiencies involved with porphyrin synthesis. Porphyrins (e.g., uroporphyrin and coproporphyrin) and porphobilinogens are important building blocks in the synthesis of heme. Heme is incorporated into hemoglobin within the erythroid cells. Porphyrias are classified according to the location of the accumulation of the porphyrin precursors. In most forms of porphyria, increased levels of porphyrins and porphobilinogen are found in the urine. Heavy metal (lead) intoxication is also associated with increased porphyrins in the urine.

This test is a quantitative analysis of urinary porphyrins and porphobilinogens. If porphyrins are present, the urine may be amber-red or burgundy and may turn even darker after standing in the light. Urine tests for porphyrins are not as accurate as plasma measurements and pattern identification for the various forms of porphyria. However, urine tests are an accurate screening for porphyria, especially the intermittent variety. Although the test can also be done on a fresh stool specimen, random and 24-hour urine collections are more accurate.

Interfering factors

✘ Drugs that may alter test results include aminosalicylic acid, barbiturates, chloral hydrate, chlorpropamide (Diabinese), ethyl alcohol, griseofulvin, morphine, oral contraceptives, phenazopyridine (Pyridium), procaine, and sulfonamides.

Procedure and patient care

Before
PT Explain the procedure to the patient.
PT Tell the patient that no fasting is required.

During

Porphobilinogens
- Collect a freshly voided urine specimen.
- Protect the specimen from light.
- For both porphobilinogens and porphyrins, indicate on the laboratory slip any drugs that may affect test results.

Porphyrins
PT Instruct the patient to begin a 24-hour urine collection after voiding. Discard the initial specimen and start the 24-hour timing at that point.
- Collect all the urine passed during the next 24 hours.
PT Instruct the patient to avoid alcohol during the collection period.
PT Show the patient where to store the urine container.
- Keep the specimen on ice or refrigerated during the 24 hours.
- Keep the urine in a light-resistant specimen bottle with a preservative to prevent degradation of the light-sensitive porphyrin.
- Indicate the starting time on the urine container and the laboratory slip.
- Post the times for urine collection in a prominent place to prevent accidental discarding of the specimen.
PT Instruct the patient to void before defecating so that urine is not contaminated by feces.
PT Remind the patient not to put toilet paper in the collection container.
PT Encourage the patient to drink fluids during the 24 hours unless contraindicated for medical purposes.
PT Instruct the patient to collect the last specimen as close as possible to the end of the 24-hour period. Add this urine to the collection.

After
- Transport the urine specimens promptly to the laboratory.

P

Abnormal findings

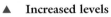 **Increased levels**

Porphyrias
Liver disease
Lead poisoning
Pellagra

notes

positron emission tomography (PET scan of the brain, PET scan of the heart, Oncologic PET scan)

Type of test Nuclear scan, x-ray

Normal findings Normal patterns of tissue metabolism

Test explanation and related physiology

PET scanning is used in many areas of medicine, most commonly for evaluation of the heart and brain. It is also commonly used in many aspects of oncology. In PET scanning, radioactive chemicals are administered to the patient. These chemicals are used in the normal metabolic process of the particular organ being imaged. Positrons emitted from the radioactive chemicals in the organ are sensed by a series of detectors positioned around the patient. These detectors receive positron counts and—with the combination of computed tomography—the positron emissions are recorded into a high-resolution two- or three-dimensional image indicating a particular metabolic process in a specific anatomic site. Therefore PET provides images representing not only anatomy but also physiology. Depending on the particular radionuclide used, PET can demonstrate the glucose metabolism, oxygenation, blood flow, and tissue perfusion of any specific area. Pathologic conditions are recognized and diagnosed by alterations in the normal metabolic process.

Certain radioactive chemical compounds provide specific information depending on the information required and the organ being evaluated. A cyclotron is used to create the radioactive chemical. Radioactive oxygen is used to make radioactive water $(H_2^{15}O)$. This is used to evaluate blood flow and tissue perfusion of an organ. Radioactive fluorine is applied to a glucose analogue and called fluorodeoxyglucose (FDG). Because most cells use glucose as an energy source, FDG is particularly useful in concentrating in regions of high metabolic activity of a particular organ. Radioactive carbon–labeled glucose is also useful for this purpose. PET scanning is becoming more widely applied and commonly used as research continues. Its greatest use thus far has been in the fields of neurology, cardiology, and oncology.

Brain

Most brain imaging is performed with FDG. The brain uses glucose as its sole metabolic fuel. The areas of the brain that are

P

more metabolically active (e.g., cancer) would take up more of the FDG than normal areas of the brain would. Alzheimer's disease is classically recognized as hypometabolism in multiple areas of the brain (temporal and parietal lobe) as scanning is performed during cognitive exercises. Epilepsy, Parkinson's disease, and Huntington's disease are identified as localized areas of increased metabolic activity, indicating rapid nerve firing. Brain trauma resulting in a hematoma or bleeding is evident as decreased metabolic activity in the area of trauma. With the use of radioactive water ($H_2{}^{15}O$), brain blood flow can be determined. Areas of decreased blood flow will take up less $H_2{}^{15}O$ than normal areas and represent areas at risk for stroke.

Heart

Flow studies (e.g., thallium scan) matched with PET metabolism FDG studies allow visualization of areas of decreased blood flow where cardiac muscle metabolism persists. This would indicate that the myocardium is viable despite decreased blood flow; infarction has not yet occurred and surgical revascularization has a good chance of completely returning the function of that area of the heart to normal. Muscle dysfunction and dyskinesia secondary to infarction will be associated with hypometabolism and lack of FDG concentration in that specific area.

Oncology

FDG is an accurate contrast agent for use in oncology. Rapidly growing tumors are associated with a high metabolic rate and will therefore concentrate FDG more than normal tissue would. PET can be used to visualize rapidly growing tumors and indicate their anatomic location. It is used to determine tumor response to therapy, identify recurrence of tumor after surgical removal, and differentiate tumor from other pathologic conditions (e.g., infection).

PET is particularly helpful in identifying regional and metastatic spread for a particular tumor. PET is more accurate in oncologic staging than CT scan. PET is also helpful in determining the site for biopsy of a suspected tumor. PET has been particularly useful for lung, melanoma, breast, pancreas, colon, lymphoma, and brain cancers.

Interfering factors

- High glucose levels in diabetics may confound PET scans using FDG as the radionuclide.

- Recent use (within 24 hours) of caffeine, alcohol, or tobacco may affect test results.
- Excessive anxiety may affect brain function evaluation.
- Excessive exercise within the preceding 3 days can cause factitious update of the contrast material in the musculature.
- Drugs that may influence results include tranquilizers and sedatives.

Procedure and patient care

Before

PT Explain the procedure to the patient. Because many patients have not heard of this study, they are often anxious and require emotional support.

- Obtain informed consent if required by the institution.

PT Inform the patient that he or she may have two IV lines inserted.

PT Inform the patient that he or she may need to restrict food or fluids for 4 hours on the day of the test. The patient should refrain from alcohol, caffeine, and tobacco for 24 hours before the test.

PT Instruct patients with diabetes to take their pretest dose of insulin at a meal 3 to 4 hours before the test.

PT Tell the patient that no sedatives or tranquilizers should be taken because he or she may need to perform certain mental activities during the test.

PT Tell the patient to empty the bladder before the test for comfort.

P

During

- Note the following procedural steps:
  1. The patient is positioned in a comfortable, reclining chair.
  2. The radioactive material can be infused through an IV line or inhaled as a radioactive gas.
  3. The gamma rays that penetrate the tissues are recorded outside the body by a circular array of detectors and are displayed by a computer.
  4. If the brain is being scanned, the patient may be asked to perform different cognitive activities (e.g., reciting the Pledge of Allegiance) to measure changes in brain activity during reasoning or remembering.
  5. Extraneous auditory and visual stimuli are minimized by a blindfold and ear plugs.
- Note that this procedure is performed by a physician or trained technologist in approximately 40 to 90 minutes.

PT Tell the patient that the only discomfort associated with this study is insertion of the two IV lines.

After

PT Instruct the patient to change position slowly from lying to standing to avoid postural hypotension.

PT Encourage the patient to drink fluids and urinate frequently to aid removal of the radioisotope from the bladder.

Abnormal findings

Myocardial infarction
Cerebrovascular accident (stroke)
Epilepsy
Parkinson's disease
Dementia
Alzheimer's disease
Coronary artery disease
Brain tumor
Breast tumor
Huntington's disease

notes

potassium, blood (K)

Type of test Blood

Normal findings

Adults/elderly: 3.5-5 mEq/L or 3.5-5 mmol/L (SI units)
Child: 3.4-4.7 mEq/L
Infant: 4.1-5.3 mEq/L
Newborn: 3.9-5.9 mEq/L

Possible critical values

Adult: <2.5 or >6.5 mEq/L
Newborn: <2.5 or >8 mEq/L

Test explanation and related physiology

Potassium is the major cation within the cell. Intracellular potassium concentration is approximately 150 mEq/L, whereas normal serum potassium concentration is approximately 4 mEq/L. Because the serum concentration of potassium is so small, minor changes in concentration have significant consequences. K is excreted by the kidneys. There is no resorption of K from the kidneys. Therefore if K is not adequately supplied in the diet (or by IV administration in patients who are unable to eat), serum K levels can drop rapidly.

Serum potassium concentration depends on many factors, including the following:

1. *Aldosterone* (and, to a lesser extent, the glucocorticosteroids). This hormone tends to increase renal losses of potassium.
2. *Sodium resorption.* As sodium is resorbed, potassium is lost.
3. *Acid-base balance.* Alkalotic states tend to lower serum potassium levels by causing a shift of potassium into the cell. Acidotic states tend to raise serum potassium levels by reversing that shift.

Symptoms of *hyperkalemia* include irritability, nausea, vomiting, intestinal colic, and diarrhea. An electrocardiogram may demonstrate peaked T waves, a widened QRS complex, and depressed ST segment. Signs of *hypokalemia* are related to a decrease in contractility of smooth, skeletal, and cardiac muscles, which results in weakness, paralysis, hyporeflexia, ileus, increased cardiac sensitivity to digoxin, cardiac arrhythmias, flattened T waves, and prominent U waves. This electrolyte has profound

P

effects on the heart rate and contractility. The potassium level should be carefully followed in patients with uremia, Addison's disease, vomiting and diarrhea, and steroid therapy, and in patients taking potassium-depleting diuretics. K must be closely monitored in patients taking digitalis-like drugs because cardiac arrhythmias may be induced by hypokalemia and digoxin.

Interfering factors

- Movement of the forearm with a tourniquet in place may increase potassium levels.
- Hemolysis of blood during venipuncture causes increased levels.
- ✗ Drugs that may cause *increased* potassium levels include aminocaproic acid, antibiotics, antineoplastic drugs, captopril, epinephrine, heparin, histamine, isoniazid (INH), lithium, mannitol, potassium-sparing diuretics, potassium supplements, and succinylcholine.
- ✗ Drugs that may cause *decreased* levels include acetazolamide, aminosalicylic acid, amphotericin B, carbenicillin, cisplatin, diuretics (potassium wasting), glucose infusions, insulin, laxatives, lithium carbonate, penicillin G sodium (high doses), phenothiazines, salicylates (aspirin), and sodium polystyrene sulfonate (Kayexalate).

Procedure and patient care

Before

PT Explain the procedure to the patient.
PT Tell the patient that no special diet or fasting is required.

During

PT Instruct the patient to avoid opening and closing the hand after a tourniquet is applied.
- Collect approximately 5 to 7 ml of venous blood in a red- or green-top tube.
- Avoid hemolysis.
- Indicate on the laboratory slip any drugs that may affect test results.

After

- Apply pressure to the venipuncture site.
- Evaluate patients with increased or decreased potassium levels for cardiac arrhythmias.
- Monitor for hypokalemia in patients taking digoxin and diuretics.

■ If indicated, administer resin exchanges (e.g., Kayexalate enema) to correct hyperkalemia.

Abnormal findings

▲ **Increased levels (hyperkalemia)**

Excessive dietary intake
Excessive IV intake
Acute or chronic renal failure
Hypoaldosteronism
Aldosterone-inhibiting
  diuretics
Crush injury to tissues
Hemolysis
Transfusion of hemolyzed
  blood
Infection
Acidosis
Dehydration

▼ **Decreased levels (hypokalemia)**

Deficient dietary intake
Deficient IV intake
Burns
Gastrointestinal
  disorders
  (e.g., diarrhea,
  vomiting)
Diuretics
Hyperaldosteronism
Cushing's syndrome
Renal tubular acidosis
Licorice ingestion
Insulin administration
Glucose administration
Ascites
Renal artery stenosis
Cystic fibrosis
Trauma
Surgery

P

notes

potassium, urine (K)

Type of test Urine (24-hour)

Normal findings

25-100 mEq/L/day or 25-100 mmol/day (SI units)
(Values vary greatly with diet.)

Test explanation and related physiology

Potassium is the major cation within the cell (see p. 733). Potassium can be measured in both a spot collection and a 24-hour urine collection.

Potassium concentration in the urine depends on many factors. Aldosterone and, to a lesser extent, glucocorticosteroids tend to increase the renal losses of potassium. Acid-base balance is dependent on potassium excretion to a small degree. In alkalotic states, hydrogen can be resorbed in exchange for potassium. The kidneys cannot resorb potassium. Therefore, the intake of potassium is balanced by kidney excretion through the urine.

Interfering factors

- Dietary intake affects potassium levels.
- Excessive intake of licorice may cause increased levels of potassium in the urine.
- ✶ Drugs that may cause *increased* levels include diuretics, glucocorticoids, and salicylates.

Procedure and patient care

Before
PT Explain the procedure to the patient.
PT Tell the patient that no special diet is required.

During
PT Instruct the patient to begin the 24-hour urine collection after voiding.
- Discard the initial specimen and start the 24-hour timing at that point.
- Collect all urine passed during the next 24 hours.
PT Show the patient where to store the urine container.
- Keep the specimen on ice or refrigerated during the entire 24 hours.
- Indicate the starting time on the urine container and the laboratory slip.

- Post the hours for urine collection in a noticeable place to prevent accidental discarding of the specimen.
PT Instruct the patient to void before defecating so that the urine is not contaminated by feces.
PT Remind the patient not to put toilet paper in the collection container.
PT Encourage the patient to drink fluids during the 24 hours.
PT Instruct the patient to collect the last specimen as close as possible to the end of the 24-hour collection. Add this urine to the container.

After
- Transport the urine specimen promptly to the laboratory.

Abnormal findings

▲ **Increased levels**

Chronic renal failure
Renal tubular acidosis
Cushing's syndrome
Hyperaldosteronism
Excessive intake of licorice
Alkalosis
Diuretic therapy

▼ **Decreased levels**

Dehydration
Addison's disease
Malnutrition
Vomiting
Diarrhea
Malabsorption
Acute renal failure

notes

P

prealbumin (PAB, Thyroxine-binding prealbumin [TBPA], Thyretin, Transthyretin)

Type of test Blood; urine (24-hour); cerebrospinal fluid (CSF) analysis

Normal findings

Serum
Adult/elderly: 15-36 mg/dl or 150-360 mg/L (SI units)
Child
    <5 days: 6-21 mg/dl
    1-5 years: 14-30 mg/dl
    6-9 years: 15-33 mg/dl
    10-13 years: 22-36 mg/dl
    14-19 years: 22-45 mg/dl

Urine (24-hour)
0.017-0.047 mg/day

Cerebrospinal fluid
Approximately 2% of total CSF protein

Possible critical values Serum prealbumin levels <10.7 mg/dl indicate severe nutritional deficiency.

Test explanation and related physiology

Prealbumin is one of the major plasma proteins. Because prealbumin can bind thyroxine, it is also called *thyroxine-binding prealbumin (TBA)*. However, prealbumin is secondary to thyroxine-binding globulin in the transportation of triiodothyronine (T_3) and thyroxine (T_4). Prealbumin also plays a role in the transport and metabolism of vitamin A.

Since prealbumin levels in serum fluctuate more rapidly in response to alterations in synthetic rate than do those of other serum proteins, clinical interest in the quantification of serum prealbumin has centered on its usefulness as a marker of nutritional status. Its half-life of 1.9 days is much less than the 21-day half-life of albumin (see p. 758). Because prealbumin has a short half-life, it is a sensitive indicator of any change affecting protein synthesis and catabolism. For this reason, prealbumin is frequently ordered to monitor the effectiveness of total parenteral nutrition (TPN).

Prealbumin is significantly reduced in hepatobiliary disease because of impaired synthesis. Prealbumin is also a negative acute-phase reactant protein; serum levels decrease in inflammation, malignancy, and protein-wasting diseases of the intestines or kidneys. Since zinc is required for synthesis of prealbumin, low levels occur with a zinc deficiency. Increased levels of prealbumin occur in Hodgkin's disease and during chronic kidney disease.

Interfering factors

- Coexistent inflammation may make test result interpretation impossible.
- ✘ Drugs that may cause *increased* levels include anabolic steroids, androgens, and prednisolone.
- ✘ Drugs that may cause *decreased* levels include amiodarone, estrogens, and oral contraceptives.

Procedure and patient care

Before

PT Explain the procedure to the patient.
PT Tell the patient that no food or fluid restrictions are needed.
- If the patient is going to collect a 24-hour urine specimen, provide a collection bottle. (See p. 416 for guidelines.)

During

- Collect a venous blood sample in a red-top tube.

After

- Apply pressure to the venipuncture site.
- Transport the 24-hour urine specimen promptly to the laboratory.
PT Inform the patient how and when to obtain the results of this study.

Abnormal findings

▲ **Increased levels**

Some cases of nephrotic syndrome
Hodgkin's disease
Chronic kidney disease
Pregnancy

▼ **Decreased levels**

Malnutrition
Liver damage
Burns
Salicylate poisoning
Inflammation

notes

pregnancy tests (Human chorionic gonadotropin [HCG])

Type of test Blood; urine

Normal findings

Qualitative: negative; *positive* in pregnancy

Quantitative

Whole HCG *Gestation (wk)*	*Whole HCG (milli-international units/ml)*
<1	5-50
2	50-500
3	100-10,000
4	1000-30,000
5	3500-115,000
6-8	12,000-270,000
12	15,000-220,000
Males and nonpregnant females	<5

B subunit: normal values depend on the method and test used.

Test explanation and related physiology

All pregnancy tests are based on the detection of HCG, which is secreted by the placental trophoblast after the ovum is fertilized. HCG will appear in the blood and urine of pregnant women as early as 10 days after conception. In the first few weeks of pregnancy, HCG rises markedly, and serum levels are higher than urine levels. After about a month, HCG is about the same in either specimen.

HCG is made up of alpha and beta subunits. The alpha subunit is the same for all the glycoprotein hormones. The beta subunit is specific for HCG.

It is important to know that all these pregnancy studies demonstrate the presence of HCG. Methods of pregnancy testing fall into three categories: immunologic, radioimmunologic, and radioreceptor assays. Biologic (animal) tests have been used since the 1920s. They are primarily of historical interest today and are not discussed here.

Immunologic tests (agglutination inhibition test [AIT]) (blood and urine)

Immunologic tests are performed using commercially prepared antibodies against the whole HCG molecule and can be completed within 2 minutes or 2 hours, depending on the method used. Previous immunologic tests had a high false-positive rate and were usually not positive until about 28 days after the last menses. However, immunologic testing for the beta subunit of HCG greatly improved accuracy and shortened the time for positive testing (18 days). Now, with the development of monoclonal antibodies, immunoassays can identify very small levels of HCG, and pregnancy can be detected 3 to 7 days after conception. Several immunologic tests are now commercially available for testing by the public. In these tests, the patient's urine is examined, and its color is compared to a standard containing a known small amount of HCG. If the color matches that standard, pregnancy is present. These tests take from 5 to 120 minutes to perform.

Radioimmunoassay (RIA) (serum)

The RIA is a highly sensitive and reliable blood test for the detection of the beta unit of HCG. This study requires a blood sample; however, RIA also may be performed with a urine test. The test can be done in 1 to 5 hours. This test is so sensitive that pregnancy can be diagnosed before the first missed menstrual period.

Radioreceptor assay (RRA) (serum)

The RRA for serum HCG is highly sensitive and accurate. This test can be performed in 1 hour. The major advantage of this study is its reliable diagnosis of early gestation in patients requesting an early termination of pregnancy and in cases in which infertile couples are anxious to confirm pregnancy. This study is 90% to 95% accurate 6 to 8 days after conception. Even the minute amounts of HCG secreted in an ectopic pregnancy can be measured. This test is also used in looking for early spontaneous abortion in patients who have difficulties maintaining early pregnancy.

● ● ●

Normally HCG is not present in nonpregnant women. In a very small number of women (<5%), HCG exists in minute levels. The presence of HCG does not necessarily indicate a normal pregnancy. Ectopic pregnancy, hydatidiform mole of the uterus, and choriocarcinoma of the uterus can all produce HCG. However, HCG levels in ectopic pregnancy fail to double appropriately and decreased levels eventually result relative to the values expected in normal pregnancies of similar gestational age. Germ cell tumors (choriocarcinoma and embryonal cell cancers) of the testes or ovaries can produce HCG in men and nonpregnant women, respectively. Primary liver cell cancers (hepatoma) can also make HCG. In tumors, HCG is a valuable marker that can be used to monitor and identify tumor activity.

Interfering factors

- Tests performed too early in the pregnancy, before a significant HCG level exists, may cause false-negative results.
- Hematuria and proteinuria in the urine may cause false-positive results.
- Hemolysis of blood may interfere with test results.
- Urine pregnancy tests can vary according to the dilution of the urine. HCH levels may not be detectable on a dilute urine but may be quite detectable on a concentrated urine.
- ⚕ Drugs that may cause false-negative urine results include diuretics (by causing diluted urine) and promethazine.
- ⚕ Drugs that may cause false-positive results include anticonvulsants, antiparkinsonian drugs, hypnotics, and tranquilizers (especially promazine and its derivatives).

Procedure and patient care

Before

PT Explain the procedure to the patient.

- If a urine specimen will be collected, give the patient a urine container the evening before so that she can provide a first-voided morning specimen. This specimen generally contains the greatest concentration of HCG.

During

- Collect the first-voided urine specimen for urine testing.
- Collect approximately 7 to 10 ml of venous blood in a red-top tube for serum testing. Avoid hemolysis.

After

- Apply pressure to the venipuncture site.
- PT Emphasize to the patient the importance of antepartal health care.

Abnormal findings

▲ **Increased levels**

Pregnancy
Ectopic pregnancy
Hydatidiform mole of the
    uterus
Choriocarcinoma of the
    uterus, testes, or ovaries
Tumor

▼ **Decreased levels**

Threatened abortion
Incomplete abortion
Dead fetus

pregnanediol

Type of test Urine (24-hour)

Normal findings

<2 years: <0.1 mg/day
<9 years: <0.5 mg/day
10-15 years: 0.1-1.2 mg/day
Adult male: 0-1.9 mg/day
Adult female
   Follicular phase: <2.6 mg/day
   Luteal: 2.6-10.6 mg/day
Pregnancy
   First trimester: 10-35 mg/day
   Second trimester: 35-70 mg/day
   Third trimester: 70-100 mg/day

Test explanation and related physiology

Urinary pregnanediol is measured to evaluate progesterone production by the ovaries and placenta. The main effect of progesterone is on the endometrium. It initiates the endometrial secretory phase in anticipation of implantation of a fertilized ovum. Normally, progesterone is secreted by the ovarian corpus luteum after ovulation. Both serum progesterone levels and the urine concentration of progesterone metabolites (pregnanediol and others) are significantly increased during the later half of an ovulatory cycle. Pregnanediol is the most easily measured metabolite of progesterone.

Because pregnanediol levels rise rapidly after ovulation, this study is useful in documenting whether ovulation has occurred and, if so, its exact time. During pregnancy, pregnanediol levels normally rise because of the placental production of progesterone. Repeated assays can be used to monitor the status of the placenta in women who are having difficulty becoming pregnant or maintaining a pregnancy. It is also used to monitor "high-risk" pregnancies.

Hormone assays for urinary pregnanediol are primarily used today to monitor progesterone supplementation in patients with an inadequate luteal phase. Urinary assays may be supplemented by plasma assays (progesterone assay, see p. 746), which are quicker and more accurate.

P

Interfering factors

- ✘ Drugs that may cause *increased* levels include adrenocorticotropic hormone.
- ✘ Drugs that may cause *decreased* levels include oral contraceptives and progesterones.

Procedure and patient care

Before

PT Explain the procedure to the patient.

PT Tell the patient that usually no special diet is required.

PT Inform the patient that no sedation or fasting is necessary.

During

PT Instruct the patient to begin the 24-hour urine collection. Discard the initial specimen and start the 24-hour timing at that point.

- ■ Collect all urine passed for the next 24 hours.

PT Show the patient where to store the urine collection.

- ■ Keep the specimen on ice or refrigerated during the 24 hours. Check with the laboratory to see if a preservative is needed.
- ■ Indicate the starting time on the urine container and the laboratory slip.
- ■ Post the hours for urine collection in a noticeable place to prevent accidental discarding of the specimen.

PT Instruct the patient to void before defecating so that the urine is not contaminated by feces.

PT Remind the patient not to put toilet paper in the collection container.

PT Encourage the patient to drink fluids during the 24 hours.

PT Instruct the patient to collect the last specimen as close as possible to the end of the 24-hour collection. Add this urine to the container.

After

- ■ Record on the laboratory slip the date of the last menstrual period or the week of gestation during pregnancy.

Abnormal findings

▲ **Increased levels**

Ovulation
Pregnancy
Luteal cysts of ovary
Arrhenoblastoma of ovary
Hyperadrenocorticalism
Choriocarcinoma of ovary
Adrenocortical hyperplasia

▼ **Decreased levels**

Threatened abortion
Fetal death
Toxemia of pregnancy
Amenorrhea
Ovarian hypofunction
Placental failure
Preeclampsia
Ovarian neoplasm
Breast neoplasm

notes

P

progesterone assay

Type of test Blood

Normal findings (extraction/radioimmunoassay)

<9 years: <20 ng/dl
10-15 years: <20 ng/dl
Adult male: 10-50 ng/dl
Adult female
    Follicular phase: <50 ng/dl
    Luteal: 300-2500 ng/dl
    Postmenopausal: <40 ng/dl
Pregnancy
    First trimester: 725-4400 ng/dl
    Second trimester: 1950-8250 ng/dl
    Third trimester: 6500-22,900 ng/dl

Test explanation and related physiology

The major effect of progesterone is to induce the development of the secretory phase of the endometrium in anticipation of implantation of a fertilized ovum. Normally, progesterone is secreted by the ovarian corpus luteum following ovulation. Serum progesterone level is significantly increased during the second half of the ovulatory cycle. Normally, blood samples drawn at days 8 and 21 of the menstrual cycle show a large increase in progesterone levels in the latter specimen, indicating that ovulation has occurred. Therefore, this study is useful in documenting whether ovulation has occurred and, if so, its exact time. This is very useful information for a woman who has difficulty becoming pregnant. A series of measurements can help define the day of ovulation.

In pregnancy, progesterone is produced by the corpus luteum for the first few weeks. After that, the placenta begins to make progesterone. Progesterone levels should progressively rise during pregnancy because of placental production. Repeated assays can be used to monitor the status of the placenta in cases of "high-risk" pregnancy. Progesterone assay is also used today to monitor progesterone supplementation in patients with an inadequate luteal phase to maintain an early pregnancy.

Interfering factors

- Recent use of radioisotopes may affect test results.
- Hemolysis caused by rough handling of the sample may affect test results.
- Drugs that may interfere with test results include estrogen and progesterone.

Procedure and patient care

Before

PT Explain the procedure to the patient.
PT Tell the patient that no fasting is required.

During

- Collect approximately 5 to 7 ml of venous blood in a red-top tube.
- Indicate the date of the last menstrual period on the laboratory slip.

After

- Apply pressure to the venipuncture site.

Abnormal findings

▲ **Increased levels**

Ovulation
Pregnancy
Luteal cysts of ovary
Hyperadrenocorticalism
Adrenocortical hyperplasia
Choriocarcinoma of ovary
Molar pregnancy

▼ **Decreased levels**

Preeclampsia
Toxemia of pregnancy
Threatened abortion
Placental failure
Fetal death
Ovarian neoplasm
Amenorrhea
Ovarian hypofunction

notes

progesterone receptor assay (PR assay, PRA, PgR)

Type of test Tumor-specimen analysis

Normal findings

Negative: <5% of the cells stain for receptors
Positive: >5% of the cells stain for receptors

Test explanation and related physiology

The PR assay is used in determining the prognosis and treatment of breast cancer and, to a lesser degree, other cancers. These assays help determine whether a tumor is likely to respond to endocrine medical or surgical therapy. The test is done on breast cancer specimens when a primary or recurrent cancer is identified; it is usually done in conjunction with estrogen receptor (ER) assay (see p. 418) to increase the predictability of a tumor response to hormone therapy. Breast tumors in postmenopausal women tend to be PR positive more often than in premenopausal women. PR-positive tumors are suspected to be associated with a better prognosis than PR-negative tumors. Tumor response rates to medical or surgical hormonal manipulation are potentiated if the ER assay is positive. Response rates are as follows:

ER positive, PR positive: 75%
ER negative, PR positive: 60%
ER positive, PR negative: 35%
ER negative, PR negative: 25%

In the past, 1 g of the breast cancer specimen has been sent to a centralized laboratory, where the PR protein is biochemically quantified in the cytoplasm or nucleus of breast cancer cells. A newer method, however, provides more accurate information on paraffin-embedded tissue using immunohistochemical staining for PR proteins. Positive reactivity by immunohistochemistry is observed in the nuclei of the tumor cells. Routinely positive and negative controls are performed with the specimen testing in order to avoid false-positive and false-negative results. This method of measuring ER receptors is considered very accurate. The testing is usually performed in a reference laboratory. Only a small portion of the paraffin-embedded tissue is required for testing. Results are usually available in about 1 week. Only the cancerous tissue is evaluated for PR receptors. Normal tissue usually contains PR receptors.

Other tumors (such as ovarian, melanoma, uterine, or pancreatic) are occasionally studied for ER and PR assay. This is done mostly within clinical trials. To date, hormonal therapy has not been very successful with these tumors.

Interfering factors

✠ Use of hormones such as progesterone or estrogen may cause false-negative results.

Procedure and patient care

Before

PT Explain the procedure to the patient.
- Prepare the patient for breast biopsy per routine protocol.
- Record the menstrual status of the patient.
- Record any exogenous hormone the patient may have used during the last 2 months.

PT Instruct the patient to discontinue exogenous hormones before breast biopsy. This is done in consultation with the physician.

During

- The surgeon obtains tissue.
- This tissue should be placed on ice or placed in formalin.
- Part of the tissue is used for routine histology. A portion of the paraffin block is sent to a reference laboratory.
- Results are usually available in 1 week.

After

- Provide routine postoperative care.

Abnormal findings

▲ **Increased levels**
Hormonally dependent cancer

notes

prolactin levels (PRLs)

Type of test Blood

Normal findings

Adult male: 0-20 ng/ml or <20 mcg/L (SI units)
Adult female: 0-25 ng/ml or <25 mcg/L (SI units)
Pregnant female: 20-400 ng/ml or 20-400 mcg/L (SI units)

Test explanation and related physiology

Prolactin is a hormone secreted by the anterior pituitary gland (adenohypophysis). In females, prolactin promotes lactation. Its role in males is not clear. During sleep, prolactin levels increase twofold to threefold, to circulating levels equaling those of pregnant women. With breast stimulation, pregnancy, nursing, stress, or exercise, a surge of this hormone occurs. It is elevated in patients with prolactin-secreting pituitary acidophilic or chromophobic adenomas. To a lesser extent, moderately high prolactin levels have been observed in women with secondary amenorrhea (i.e., postpubertal) and galactorrhea. Paraneoplastic tumors (e.g., lung cancer) may cause ectopic secretion of prolactin as well. In general, very high prolactin levels are more likely to be caused by pituitary adenoma than other causes.

The prolactin level is helpful for monitoring the disease activity of pituitary adenomas. Several *prolactin stimulation tests* (with TRH or chlorpromazine) and *prolactin suppression tests* (with levodopa) have been designed to help differentiate pituitary adenoma from some of the other causes of prolactin overproduction.

Interfering factors

- Stress from illness, trauma, surgery or even the fear of a blood test can elevate prolactin levels. In cases in which the patient is fearful of venipuncture, it is best to place a heparin lock and withdraw the blood specimen 2 hours later.
- Drugs that may cause *increased* values include phenothiazines, oral contraceptives, reserpine, opiates, verapamil, histamine antagonists, monoamine oxidase inhibitors, estrogens, and antihistamines.
- Drugs that may cause *decreased* values are ergot alkaloid derivatives, clonidine, levodopa, and dopamine.

Procedure and patient care

Before

PT Explain the procedure to the patient.

PT Tell the patient no fasting or special preparation is required.

PT Inform the patient that this blood sample should be drawn in the morning.

- Record the use of any medication that may affect results.

During

- Obtain 5 to 7 ml of venous blood in a red-top tube.
- Transfer the specimen to the laboratory as soon as possible. If a delay occurs, the specimen should be placed on ice.

After

- Apply pressure to the venipuncture site.

Abnormal findings

▲ **Increased levels**

Galactorrhea

Amenorrhea

Prolactin-secreting pituitary tumor

Infiltrative diseases of the hypothalamus and pituitary stalk (e.g., granuloma, sarcoidosis)

Hypothyroidism

Renal failure

Anorexia nervosa

Perineoplastic ectopic production of prolactin

Metastatic cancer to the pituitary gland

Polycystic ovary syndrome

Stress such as anorexia nervosa, surgery, strenuous exercise, trauma, or severe illness

Empty sella syndrome

▼ **Decreased levels**

Pituitary apoplexy

Pituitary destruction from tumor (craniopharyngioma)

P

prostate/rectal sonogram (Ultrasound prostate)

Type of test Ultrasound

Normal findings Normal size, contour, and consistency of the prostate gland

Test explanation and related physiology

Rectal ultrasound of the prostate is a very valuable tool in the early diagnosis of prostate cancer. When combined with rectal digital examination and prostate-specific antigen (see p. 755), very small prostate cancers can be identified. Prostate/rectal sonography is also helpful in evaluating the seminal vessels and other perirectal tissue. Ultrasound is very helpful in guiding the direction of a prostate biopsy (Figure 33) and can be extremely helpful in quantitating the volume of prostate cancer. When radiation therapy implantation is required for treatment, ultrasound is used to map the exact location of the prostate cancer. Rectal ultrasound is very helpful in staging rectal cancers as well. The depth of transmural involvement and presence of extrarectal extension can be accurately assessed.

Real-time ultrasonography requires the emission of high-frequency sound waves from a special transducer placed in the rectum. The sound waves are bounced back to the transducer and electronically converted into a pictorial image.

Contraindications

- Patients with latex allergy
  Rectal ultrasound requires placement of the probe in a latex condom-like sac. Patients with a latex allergy may react significantly to that contact.

Interfering factors

- Stool within the rectum

Procedure and patient care

Before

PT Explain the procedure to the patient.

PT Instruct the patient that a small-volume rectal enema is required approximately 1 hour before the ultrasound examination.

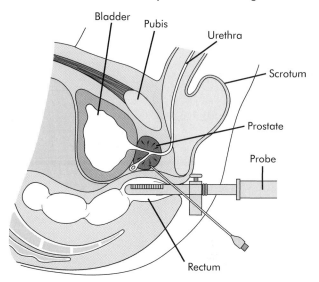

Figure 33 Rectal ultrasonography. Diagram demonstrating transrectal biopsy of the prostate.

P

During
- The patient is placed in the left lateral decubitus position.
- A digital rectal examination may be performed to assess the prostate gland or rectal tumor.
- A draped and lubricated ultrasound probe is placed within the rectum.
- Scans are performed in various spatial planes.

After
- Provide the patient with tissue material to cleanse the perianal area.

Abnormal findings

Prostate cancer
Benign prostatic hypertrophy
Prostatitis
Seminal vesicle tumor
Prostate abscess
Perirectal abscess
Intrarectal or perirectal tumor

notes

prostate-specific antigen (PSA)

Type of test Blood

Normal findings <4 ng/ml or <4 mcg/L (SI units)

Test explanation and related physiology

PSA is a glycoprotein (part carbohydrate, part protein) normally found in the cytoplasm of prostatic epithelial cells. This antigen can be detected in all males; however, its level is greatly increased in patients with prostatic cancer. The higher the levels, the greater the tumor burden. Furthermore, the PSA assay is a sensitive test for monitoring response to therapy. Successful surgery, radiation, or hormone therapy is associated with a marked reduction in the PSA blood level. Subsequent significant elevation in PSA indicates the recurrence of prostatic cancer.

Prostate-specific antigen is more sensitive and specific than other prostatic tumor markers such as prostatic acid phosphatase (PAP, see p. 7). Also, PSA is more accurate than PAP in monitoring response and recurrence of tumor after therapy.

The American Urological Association and the American Cancer Society have recommended annual PSA screening for men older than age 50. For men with a family history of prostate cancer or men of African-American descent, PSA testing should begin at age 40. It is important to be aware that some patients with early prostate cancer will not have elevated levels of PSA. It is equally important to recognize that PSA levels above 4 are not always associated with cancer. The PSA is limited by a lack of specificity within the "diagnostic gray zone" of 4.0 to 10.0 ng/ml. PSA levels also may be minimally elevated in patients with benign prostatic hypertrophy (BPH) and prostatitis. PSA levels greater than 10.0 ng/ml indicate a high probability of prostate cancer. Lower values may be compatible with BPH or early prostate cancer.

Several factors affect the predictability and specificity of PSA. Gland volume affects PSA levels (i.e., patients with large benign glands have a higher PSA). Several formulas have been created to partially correct for gland volume. One such *volume adjusted* formula is:

Predicted PSA = 0.12 × Gland volume (in cubic centimeters) as determined by ultrasound

PSA density is an adjustment that divides the PSA measurement by the gland volume. A number of other modalities have been proposed to enhance the accuracy of PSA. PSA levels have been *age adjusted* by some investigators. Older men have a higher PSA than younger men. Levels above those predicted by age would be compatible with cancer. *PSA velocity* monitors the change in PSA with time, allowing for longitudinal measurements of PSA levels. PSA velocity can improve the ability to detect prostate cancer when at least three serial PSA values are measured during a 2-year period. A PSA velocity of greater than 0.75 ng/ml per year is suggestive of cancer.

Percent free PSA (%FPSA) is also helpful in differentiating between cancer and benign prostate disorders in men with total PSA levels within this diagnostic gray zone. It has been noted that when the %FPSA is less than 25%, there is a high likelihood of cancer. If prostate digital examination and ultrasound exams are normal, blind biopsy should be performed. Levels of %FPSA greater than 25% are associated with a low probability of cancer. Some research reports have used lower cutoff points.

Prostatic-specific membrane antigen may, with further study, represent an excellent marker for prostate cancer. It is more frequently present than PSA in more advanced cancer.

Although PSA was originally measured by histochemical techniques, radioimmunoassay techniques have recently provided increased accuracy.

Interfering factors

- Rectal examinations, known to falsely elevate PAP levels, may also minimally elevate PSA levels. To avoid this problem, the PSA specimen should be drawn before rectal examination of the prostate or several hours afterward.
- Prostatic manipulation by biopsy or transurethral resection of the prostate (TURP) may elevate PSA levels. The blood test should be done before the surgery or 6 weeks afterward.
- Ejaculation within 24 hours of blood testing will be associated with elevated PSA levels.
- Recent urinary tract infection or prostatitis can cause elevations of PSA as much as five times baseline for as long as 6 weeks.
- Finasteride (Propecia, Proscar) may cause *increased* levels of PSA.

Procedure and patient care

Before

PT Explain the procedure to the patient.

PT Tell the patient that no fasting is required.

During

- Collect approximately 5 ml of blood in a red-top tube.
- The use of the percent-free PSA demands strict sample handling not required with the total PSA. Appropriate sample handling is necessary for accurate and consistent assay performance. Check with your laboratory for specific guidelines.

After

- Apply pressure to the venipuncture site.

Abnormal findings

▲ **Increased levels**

Prostate cancer

Benign prostatic hypertrophy

Prostatitis

notes

P

protein, blood (Albumin, blood; Serum albumin; Serum globulin; Total protein; Protein electrophoresis)

Type of test   Blood

Normal findings

Adult/elderly
   Total protein: 6.4-8.3 g/dl or 64-83 g/L (SI units)
   Albumin: 3.5-5 g/dl or 35-50 g/L (SI units)
   Globulin: 2.3-3.4 g/dl
      Alpha$_1$ globulin: 0.1-0.3 g/dl or 1-3 g/L (SI units)
      Alpha$_2$ globulin: 0.6-1 g/dl or 6-10 g/L (SI units)
      Beta globulin: 0.7-1.1 g/dl or 7-11 g/L (SI units)
Children
   Total protein
      Premature infant: 4.2-7.6 g/dl
      Newborn: 4.6-7.4 g/dl
      Infant: 6-6.7 g/dl
      Child: 6.2-8 g/dl
   Albumin
      Premature infant: 3-4.2 g/dl
      Newborn: 3.5-5.4 g/dl
      Infant: 4.4-5.4 g/dl
      Child: 4-5.9 g/dl

Test explanation and related physiology

   Proteins are constituents of muscle, enzymes, hormones, transport vehicles, hemoglobin, and several other key functional and structural entities within the body. They are the most significant component contributing to the osmotic pressure within the vascular space. This osmotic pressure keeps fluid within the vascular space, minimizing extravasation of fluid.

   Albumin and globulin constitute most of the protein within the body and are measured in the total protein. *Albumin* is a protein that is formed within the liver. It makes up approximately 60% of the total protein. The major effect of albumin within the blood is to maintain colloidal osmotic pressure. Furthermore, albumin transports important blood constituents such as drugs, hormones, and enzymes. Albumin is synthesized within the liver and is therefore a measure of hepatic function. When disease affects the liver cell, the hepatocyte loses its ability to synthesize albumin. The serum albumin level is greatly decreased. Because the half-life of albumin is 12 to 18 days, however, severe impairment of hepatic albumin synthesis may not be recognized until after that period.

Globulins are the key building block of antibodies. Their role in maintaining osmotic pressure is far less than that of albumin. Alpha$_1$ globulins are mostly alpha$_1$ antitrypsin. Some transporting proteins such as thyroid and cortisol-binding globulin also contribute to this electrophoretic zone. Alpha$_2$ globulins include serum haptoglobins (bind hemoglobin during hemolysis), ceruloplasmin (carrier for copper), prothrombin, and cholinesterase (an enzyme used in the catabolism of acetylcholine). Beta$_1$ globulins include lipoproteins, transferrin, plasminogen, and complement proteins; beta$_2$ globulins include fibrinogen. Gamma globulins are the immune globulins (antibodies) (see p. 555). To a lesser degree, globulins also act as transport vehicles.

Serum albumin and globulin are measures of nutrition. Malnourished patients, especially after surgery, have a greatly decreased level of serum proteins. Burn patients and patients who have protein-losing enteropathies and uropathies have low levels of protein, despite normal synthesis. Pregnancy, especially the third trimester, is usually associated with reduced total proteins.

In some diseases, albumin is selectively diminished, and globulins are normal or increased to maintain a normal total protein level. For example, in collagen vascular diseases (e.g., lupus erythematosus), capillary permeability is increased. Albumin, a molecule much smaller than globulin, is selectively lost into the extravascular space. Another group of diseases similarly associated with low albumin, high globulin, and normal total protein levels is chronic liver diseases. In these diseases the liver cannot produce albumin, but globulin is adequately made in the reticuloendothelial system. In both these types of diseases, the albumin level is low, but the total protein level is normal because of increased globulin levels. These changes, however, can be detected if one measures the albumin/globulin ratio. Normally this ratio exceeds 1.0. The diseases just described that selectively affect albumin levels are associated with lesser ratios. Increased total protein levels, particularly the globulin fraction, occur with multiple myeloma and other gammopathies. It is important to note that the albumin fraction of the total protein can be factitiously elevated in dehydrated patients.

Serum protein electrophoresis can separate the various components of blood protein into bands or zones according to their electrical charge. Several well-established electrophoretic patterns have been identified and can be associated with specific diseases (Table 18).

TABLE 18 Protein electrophoresis patterns in specific diseases

Pattern	Electrophoresis	Disease
Acute reaction	↓ Albumin ↑ Alpha$_2$ globulin	Acute infections, tissue necrosis, burns, surgery, stress, myocardial infarction
Chronic inflammatory	sl. ↓ Albumin sl. ↑ Gamma globulin N Alpha$_2$ globulin	Chronic infection, granulomatous diseases, cirrhosis, rheumatoid-collagen diseases
Nephrotic syndrome	↓↓ Albumin ↑↑ Alpha$_2$ globulin N ↑ Beta globulin	Nephrotic syndrome
Far-advanced cirrhosis	↓ Albumin ↑ Gamma globulin Incorporation of beta and gamma peaks	Far-advanced cirrhosis
Polyclonal gamma globulin elevation	↑↑ Gamma globulin with a broad peak	Cirrhosis, chronic infection, sarcoidosis, tuberculosis, endocarditis, rheumatoid-collagen diseases
Hypogamma-globulinemia	↓ Gamma globulin with normal other globulin levels	Light-chain multiple myeloma
Monoclonal gammopathy	Thin spikes in gamma globulin	Myeloma, macroglobulinemia, gammopathies

↓, Decreased; ↑, increased; sl. ↓, slightly decreased; sl. ↑, slightly increased; N, normal; ↓↓, greatly decreased; ↑↑, greatly increased.

In most centers, when the protein electrophoresis is abnormal, *immunofixation electrophoresis (IFE)* is performed. This is described on p. 553. IFE has become particularly useful for the identification of various monoclonal gammopathies such as multiple myeloma or Waldenström's macroglobulinemia (see p. 557).

Interfering factors

- Prolonged application of a tourniquet can increase both fractions of total proteins.
- Sampling of peripheral venous blood proximal to an IV administration site can result in an inaccurately low protein level. Likewise, massive IV infusion of crystalloid fluid can result in acute hypoproteinemia.
- ☤ Drugs that may cause *increased* protein levels include anabolic steroids, androgens, corticosteroids, dextran, growth hormone, insulin, phenazopyridine, and progesterone.
- ☤ Drugs that may cause *decreased* protein levels include ammonium ions, estrogens, hepatotoxic drugs, and oral contraceptives.

Procedure and patient care

Before
PT Explain the procedure to the patient.
PT Tell the patient that no fasting is usually required.

During
- Collect approximately 5 to 7 ml of blood in a red-top tube.

After
- Apply pressure to the venipuncture site. Patients with liver dysfunction often have prolonged clotting times.

Abnormal findings

▲ **Increased albumin levels**
Dehydration

▼ **Decreased albumin levels**
Malnutrition
Pregnancy
Liver disease
Protein-losing
  enteropathies
Protein-losing
  nephropathies
Third-space losses
Overhydration
Increased capillary
  permeability
Inflammatory disease
Familial idiopathic
  dysproteinemia

▲ **Increased alpha$_1$ globulin levels**
Inflammatory disease

▼ **Decreased alpha$_1$ globulin levels**
Juvenile pulmonary
  emphysema

▲ **Increased alpha$_2$ globulin levels**
Nephrotic syndrome
Inflammatory disease

▼ **Decreased alpha$_2$ globulin levels**
Hemolysis
Wilson's disease
Hyperthyroidism
Severe liver dysfunction

▲ **Increased beta globulin levels**
Hypercholesterolemia
Iron deficiency anemia

▼ **Decreased beta globulin levels**
Malnutrition

▲ **Increased gamma globulin levels**
(see p. 557 for specific gamma immunoglobulin specifics)
Multiple myeloma
Waldenström's macroglobulinemia
Chronic inflammatory disease
Malignancy
Hyperimmunization
Acute and chronic infection

▼ **Decreased gamma globulin levels**
Genetic immune disorders
Secondary immune deficiency

notes

P

protein C, protein S

Type of test Blood

Normal findings
Protein S: 60%-130% of normal activity
Protein C: 70%-150% of normal activity
(Protein C decreases with age and in females.)

Test explanation and related physiology
The plasma coagulation system is tightly regulated between thrombosis and fibrinolysis. This precise regulation is important. The "protein C–protein S" system is an important inhibitor of coagulation. Protein C inhibits the activation of factor VIII and factor V (see Figure 11, p. 282). This inhibitory function of protein C is enhanced by protein S. Inherited or acquired deficiencies of these vitamin K–dependent proteins will cause spontaneous intravascular thrombosis. Furthermore, dysfunctional forms of the proteins will result in a hypercoagulable state. In addition, nearly 50% of hypercoagulable states are caused by the presence of a factor V (factor V Leiden) that is resistant to protein C inhibition.

When protein C is tested, protein S activity also should be tested, because the decreased activity of protein C may be the result of decreased protein S. When decreased protein C activity is noted, protein C resistance (presence of factor V Leiden) should be tested.

These proteins are vitamin K-dependent and are decreased in liver diseases and severe malnutrition. Complement 4 (C4) binding protein can inactivate protein S. Therefore, diseases that increase C4 binding proteins (such as autoimmune diseases and other inflammatory diseases) are associated with an acquired protein S deficiency.

Interfering factors
- Decreased protein C may occur in the postoperative states.
- Pregnancy or the use of exogenous sex hormones is associated with decreases in proteins C and S.
- The concentration of citrate in the collection tube varies and can affect activity results.
- Heparin *decreases* proteins C and S levels.

Procedure and patient care

Before

PT Explain the procedure to the patient.

PT Tell the patient that fasting is usually not required.

During

- Collect 5 ml of venous blood in a blue-top tube. If more than one blood test is to be obtained, draw the blood for protein C or S second to avoid contamination with tissue thromboplastin that may occur in the first tube. If only blood for protein C or S is being drawn, draw a red-top tube first (and throw it away), and then draw the blood for this study in a blue-top tube (two-tube method of blood draw).
- Place the tube in an ice bath.

After

- Apply pressure to the venipuncture site.

PT If the patient is found to be deficient in either protein, encourage the patient's family to be tested, as they may be similarly affected.

Abnormal findings

Congenital deficiency of protein C or protein S
Disseminated intravascular coagulation (DIC)
Hypercoagulable states
Pulmonary emboli
Arterial or venous thrombosis
Vitamin K deficiency
Malignancy
Autoimmune diseases
Inflammation
Warfarin (Coumadin)-induced skin necrosis

P

notes

prothrombin time (PT, Pro-time, International normalized ratio [INR])

Type of test Blood

Normal findings

11.0-12.5 seconds; 85%-100%
Full anticoagulant therapy: 1.5-2 times control value;
    20% to 30%

Possible critical values

>20 seconds
Full anticoagulant therapy: >3 times control value

Test explanation and related physiology

The PT is used to evaluate the adequacy of the extrinsic system and common pathway in the clotting mechanism. The PT measures the clotting ability of factors I (fibrinogen), II (prothrombin), V, VII, and X. When these clotting factors exist in deficient quantities, PT is prolonged. Many diseases and drugs are associated with decreased levels of these factors. These include the following:

1. *Hepatocellular liver disease* (e.g., cirrhosis, hepatitis, and neoplastic invasive processes)

    Factors I, II, V, VII, IX, and X are produced in the liver. With severe hepatocellular dysfunction, synthesis of these factors will not occur, and serum concentration of these factors will be decreased. Even a small decrease in factor VII will result in marked prolongation of PT.

2. *Obstructive biliary disease* (e.g., bile duct obstruction secondary to tumor or gallstones, or intrahepatic cholestasis secondary to sepsis or drugs)

    As a result of the biliary obstruction, the bile necessary for fat absorption fails to enter the gut, and fat malabsorption results. Vitamins A, D, E, and K are fat soluble and also are not absorbed. Because the synthesis of factors II, VII, IX, and X depends on vitamin K, these factors will not be adequately produced, and serum concentrations will fall. Factor VII is the first to decrease and will result in prolongation of PT.

    Parenchymal (hepatocellular) liver disease can be differentiated from obstructive biliary disease by determination of the patient's response to parenteral vitamin K administration. If PT returns to normal after 1 to 3 days of vitamin K administration (10 mg IM twice a day), one can safely assume that the patient has obstructive biliary disease that is causing vitamin K malabsorption. If, on the other hand, PT does not return to normal with the vitamin K injections, one can assume that severe hepatocellular disease exists and that the liver cells are incapable of synthesizing the clotting factors, no matter how much vitamin K is available.

3. *Coumarin ingestion*

The coumarin derivatives dicumarol and warfarin (Coumadin, Panwarfin) are used to prevent coagulation in patients with thromboembolic disease (e.g., pulmonary embolism, thrombophlebitis, arterial embolism). These drugs interfere with the production of vitamin K–dependent clotting factors, which results in a prolongation of PT, as already described. The adequacy of coumarin therapy can be monitored by following the patient's PT. Appropriate coumarin therapy for full anticoagulation should prolong PT by 1.5 to 2 times the control value (or 20% to 30% of the normal value if percentages are used).

• • •

PT test results are usually given in seconds, along with a control value. The control value usually varies somewhat from day to day because the reagents used may vary. The patient's PT should be approximately equal to the control value. Some laboratories report PT values as percentages of normal activity, because the patient's results are compared with a curve representing normal clotting time. Normally, the patient's PT is 85% to 100%.

To have uniform PT results for physicians in different parts of the country and the world, the World Health Organization has recommended that PT results now include the use of the *international normalized ratio (INR)* value. The reported INR results are independent of the reagents or methods used because the standard method of obtaining therapeutic anticoagulation by keeping PT ratios of 1.5 to 2 times the control value in certain clinical indications would be converted to a figure that takes the sensitivity of the thromboplastin used as reagent and the

TABLE 19 Preferred INR according to indication for anticoagulation

Indication	Preferred INR
Deep-vein thrombosis prophylaxis	1.5-2.0
Orthopedic surgery	2.0-3.0
Deep-vein thrombosis	2.0-3.0
Prevention of embolus in patients in atrial fibrillation*	2.0-3.0
Pulmonary embolism	3.0-4.0
Prosthetic valve prophylaxis	2.5-3.5

*Often not recommended.

type of instrument into account. These international sensitivity indices are different for various thromboplastins and according to whether mechanical or photo-optical methods and instruments are used. Many hospitals are now reporting PT times in both absolute and INR numbers. Therapeutic INR is usually considered to be 2 to 3.5 in most institutions, depending on the clinical situation (Table 19).

Interfering factors

- Alcohol intake can increase PT levels.
- A high-fat diet may decrease PT levels.
- Drugs that may cause *increased* levels include allopurinol, aminosalicylic acid, barbiturates, beta-lactam antibiotics, chloral hydrate, cephalothins, chloramphenicol, chlorpromazine (Thorazine), cholestyramine, cimetidine, clofibrate, colestipol, ethyl alcohol, glucagon, heparin, methyldopa (Aldomet), neomycin, oral anticoagulants, propylthiouracil, quinidine, quinine, salicylates, and sulfonamides.
- Drugs that may cause *decreased* levels include anabolic steroids, barbiturates, chloral hydrate, digitalis, diphenhydramine (Benadryl), estrogens, griseofulvin, oral contraceptives, and vitamin K.

Procedure and patient care

Before

PT Explain the procedure to the patient.
PT Tell the patient that no fasting is required.

- If the patient is receiving warfarin, obtain the blood specimen before the patient is given the daily dose of warfarin. The daily dose may be increased, decreased, or kept the same, depending on the PT test results for that day.

During

- Collect approximately 5 to 7 ml of venous blood in a blue-top tube.
- List on the laboratory slip any drugs that may affect test results.

After

- Apply pressure to the venipuncture site. Remember, hemostasis will be delayed if the patient is taking warfarin or if the patient has any coagulopathies.
- If the PT is greatly prolonged, evaluate the patient for bleeding tendencies (i.e., check for blood in the urine and all excretions and assess the patient for bruises, petechiae, and low back pain.
- If severe bleeding occurs, the anticoagulant effect of warfarin can be reversed by the slow parenteral administration of vitamin K (phytonadione).
- **PT** Because of drug interactions, instruct the patient not to take any medication unless specifically ordered by the physician.

P

🏠 **Home care responsibilities**

- Patients taking warfarin will be regulated by PT and INR values.
- Teach these patients to evaluate themselves for bleeding tendencies. Patients should assess themselves for bruises, petechiae, low back pain, and bleeding gums. Blood may be detected in the urine and stool.
- Because of many drug interactions, instruct patients on warfarin therapy not to take any other medications unless approved by their physician.

Abnormal findings

▲   **Increased levels**

Cirrhosis
Hepatitis
Vitamin K deficiency
Salicylate intoxication
Bile duct obstruction
Coumarin ingestion
Disseminated intravascular coagulation
Massive blood transfusion
Hereditary factor deficiency

notes

pulmonary angiography (Pulmonary arteriography, Bronchial angiography)

Type of test X-ray with contrast dye

Normal findings Normal pulmonary vasculature

Test explanation and related physiology

Through an injection of a radiographic contrast material into the pulmonary arteries, pulmonary angiography permits visualization of the pulmonary vasculature. Angiography is used to detect pulmonary embolism and a variety of congenital and acquired lesions of the pulmonary vessels.

When pulmonary embolism is suspected, lung scanning should be performed first. If the lung scan is normal, pulmonary embolism is ruled out. If the scan is equivocal, however, the diagnosis of pulmonary embolism is questionable, because pathologic parenchymal processes (e.g., emphysema, pneumonia) also may cause abnormalities on the lung scan. Definitive diagnosis for pulmonary embolism may require pulmonary angiography. This may be especially important in patients with peptic ulcers for whom anticoagulant treatment for pulmonary embolism may be associated with significant risks. Also, in rare instances, pulmonary embolectomy rather than anticoagulation is considered critical for patient survival. In these cases, the angiographic location of the clot is important.

Bronchial angiography is now being done in some facilities to identify bleeding sites in the lungs. For this procedure, catheters are placed transarterially into the orifice of bronchial arteries. Radiopaque material is then injected, and the arteries are visualized. If a bleeding site is identified, the site can be injected with a sclerosing agent to prevent further bleeding.

Contraindications

- Patients with allergies to shellfish or iodinated dye
- Patients who are pregnant, unless the benefits outweigh the risks
- Patients with bleeding disorders

Potential complications

- Allergic reaction to iodinated dye
- Hypoglycemia or acidosis may occur in patients who are taking metformin (Glucophage) and receive iodine dye.

P

- Cardiac arrhythmia
  Premature ventricular contractions during right-sided heart catheterization may lead to ventricular tachycardia and ventricular fibrillation.

Procedure and patient care

Before

PT Explain the procedure to the patient.

- Ensure that written and informed consent for this procedure is obtained.

PT Inform the patient that a warm flush will be felt when the dye is injected.

- Check the patient for allergies to iodinated dyes and shellfish.
- Determine if the patient has ventricular arrhythmias (dysrhythmias).
- Keep the patient NPO after midnight on the day of the test.
- Administer preprocedural medications as ordered. Atropine may be given to decrease secretions. Meperidine may be used for sedation and relaxation.

During

- Note the following procedural steps:
  1. The patient is placed on an x-ray table in the supine position.
  2. Electrocardiographic electrodes are attached for cardiac monitoring.
  3. The catheter is placed into the femoral vein and passed into the inferior vena cava.
  4. With fluoroscopic visualization, the catheter is advanced to the right atrium and the right ventricle.
  5. The catheter is manipulated into the main pulmonary artery, where the dye is injected.
  6. X-ray films of the chest are immediately taken in timed sequence. This allows all vessels visualized by the injection to be photographed. If filling defects are seen in the contrast-filled vessels, pulmonary emboli are present.
  7. If *bronchial angiography* is performed, the femoral artery is cannulated instead of the vein. The rest of the procedure is similar to that in preceding paragraphs.
- Note that this test is performed by a physician in approximately 1 hour.

PT During injection of dye, inform the patient that he or she will feel a burning sensation and flush throughout the body.

After

- Observe the catheter insertion site for inflammation, hemorrhage, and hematoma.
- Assess the patient's vital signs for evidence of bleeding (decreased blood pressure, increased pulse).
- Apply cold compresses to the puncture site if needed to reduce swelling or discomfort.
- **PT** Inform the patient that coughing may occur after this study.
- **PT** Educate the patient regarding the need for bed rest for 12 to 24 hours after the test.

Abnormal findings

Pulmonary embolism
Congenital and acquired lesions of the pulmonary vessels
(e.g., pulmonary hypertension)
Tumor

notes

P

pulmonary function tests (PFTs)

Type of test   Airflow assessment

Normal findings   Vary with the patient's age, sex, height, and weight

Test explanation and related physiology

PFTs are performed to detect abnormalities in respiratory function and to determine the extent of any pulmonary abnormality. The main reasons for pulmonary function tests include the following:

1. Preoperative evaluation of the lungs and pulmonary reserve. When planned thoracic surgery will result in loss of functional pulmonary tissue, as in lobectomy (removal of part of a lung) or pneumonectomy (removal of an entire lung), a significant risk of pulmonary failure exists if preoperative pulmonary function is already severely compromised by other diseases such as chronic obstructive pulmonary disease (COPD).

2. Evaluation of response to bronchodilator therapy. Some patients with COPD have a spastic component to their obstructive disease that may respond to long-term use of bronchodilators. Pulmonary function studies performed before and after the use of bronchodilators will identify that group of patients.

3. Differentiation between restrictive and obstructive forms of chronic pulmonary disease. *Restrictive* defects (e.g., pulmonary fibrosis, tumors, chest-wall trauma) occur when ventilation is disturbed by a limitation in chest expansion. Inspiration is primarily affected. *Obstructive* defects (e.g., emphysema, bronchitis, asthma) occur when ventilation is disturbed by an increase in airway resistance. Expiration is primarily affected.

4. Determination of the diffusing capacity of the lungs (D_L). Rates are based on the difference in concentration of gases in inspired and expired air.

5. Performance of inhalation tests in patients with inhalation allergies.

PFTs routinely include spirometry, measurement of airflow rates, and calculation of lung volumes and capacities. Exercise pulmonary stress testing can also be performed to provide data concerning the patient's pulmonary reserve.

Spirometry is performed first. On the basis of age, height, weight, race, and sex, normal values for the volumes and flow rates can be predicted. If the actual values are greater than 80% of predicted values, the person is considered normal. Spirometry provides information about obstruction or restriction of airflow. If airflow rates are significantly diminished (<60% of normal), spirometry can be repeated after bronchodilators are administered by nebulizer. If airflow rates are improved by 20%, the chronic use of bronchodilators may be recommended to the patient. Measurement of lung capacities (combination of two or more lung volumes) can be performed.

Gas exchange studies measure the diffusing capacity of the lung (D_L) (i.e., the amount of gas exchanged across the alveolar-capillary membrane per minute). Arterial blood gases (see p. 117) are also a part of pulmonary function studies; the information obtained is used in calculations of lung function data.

PFTs routinely include determination of the following:

Forced vital capacity. FVC is the amount of air that can be forcefully expelled from a maximally inflated lung position. This volume is decreased below the expected value in obstructive and restrictive pulmonary diseases.

Forced expiratory volume in 1 second. FEV_1 is the volume of air expelled during the first second of the FVC. In patients with obstructive disease, airways are narrowed and resistance to flow is high. Therefore not as much air can be expelled in 1 second, and FEV_1 will be reduced below the predicted value. In restrictive lung disease, FEV_1 is decreased not because of airway resistance but because the amount of air originally inhaled is less. One should therefore measure the FEV_1/FVC ratio. A normal value of 80% is found in patients with restrictive lung disease. In obstructive lung disease this ratio is considerably less than 80%. The FEV_1 measurement will reliably improve with bronchodilator therapy if a spastic component to an obstructive disease exists.

Maximal midexpiratory flow. MMEF is the maximal rate of airflow through the pulmonary tree during forced expiration. This is also called *forced midexpiratory flow*. This test is independent of the patient's effort or cooperation. MMEF is reduced below expected values in obstructive diseases and normal in restrictive diseases.

Maximal volume ventilation. MVV, formerly called *maximal breathing capacity*, is the maximal volume of air that the patient can breathe in and out during 1 minute. MVV is

P

decreased below the expected value in both restrictive and obstructive pulmonary disease.

A comprehensive pulmonary function study also may include evaluation of the following lung volumes and lung capacities, many of which are illustrated in Figure 34:

Tidal volume. TV or V_T is the volume of air inspired and expired with each normal respiration.

Inspiratory reserve volume. IRV is the maximal volume of air that can be inspired from the end of a normal inspiration. It represents forced inspiration over and beyond the tidal volume.

Expiratory reserve volume. ERV is the maximal volume of air that can be exhaled after a normal expiration.

Residual volume. RV is the volume of air remaining in the lungs following forced expiration.

Inspiratory capacity. IC is the maximal amount of air that can be inspired after a normal expiration (IC = TV + IRV).

Functional residual capacity. FRC is the amount of air left in the lungs after a normal expiration (FRC = ERV + RV).

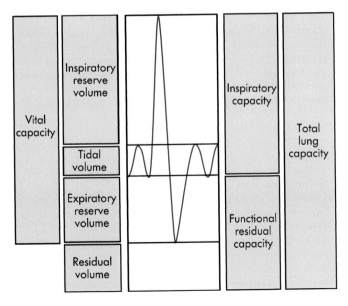

Figure 34 Relationship of lung volumes and capacities.

Vital capacity. VC is the maximal amount of air that can be expired after a maximal inspiration (VC = TV + IRV + ERV).

Total lung capacity. TLC is the volume to which the lungs can be expanded with the greatest inspiratory effort (TLC = TV + IRV + ERV + RV).

Minute volume. MV, sometimes called *minute ventilation,* is the volume of air inhaled and exhaled per minute.

Dead space. Dead space is the part of the tidal volume that does not participate in alveolar gas exchange. This would include the air within the trachea.

Forced expiratory flow$_{200-1200}$. FEF$_{200-1200}$ is the airflow rate of expired air between 200 ml and 1200 ml during the FVC. This is the portion of the airflow curve that is most affected by airway obstruction.

Forced expiratory flow$_{25-75}$. FEF$_{25-75}$ is the airflow rate of expired air between 25% and 75% of the flow during the FVC. This is the part of the airflow curve that is most affected by airway obstruction.

Peak inspiratory flow rate. PIFR is the flow rate of inspired air during maximum inspiration. This is used to indicate large (trachea and bronchi) airway disease.

Peak expiratory flow rate. PEFR is the maximum airflow rate during forced expiration.

Spirometry is the standard method for measuring most relative lung volumes; however, it is incapable of providing information about absolute volumes of air in the lung. Thus a different approach is required to measure residual volume, functional residual capacity, and total lung capacity. Two of the most common methods of obtaining information about these volumes are *body plethysmography* and *gas dilution tests.*

In body plethysmography, the patient sits inside an airtight box, inhales or exhales to a particular volume (usually functional residual capacity [FRC]), and then a shutter drops across the breathing tube. The subject makes respiratory efforts against the closed shutter. Changes in total lung volumes can be easily measured instead of calculated. From those values, assuming pressures in the box are stable, airway resistance and lung compliance can be measured. Body plethysmography is particularly appropriate for patients who have air spaces within the lung that do not communicate with the bronchial tree.

Gas dilution or gas exchange studies measure the D_L (i.e., the amount of gas exchanged across the alveolar-capillary membrane per minute). Gases, like helium, have densities lower than air.

These gases are not affected by turbulent airflow. As a result, the use of helium provides an extremely accurate method of measuring even the most minimal airway resistance existing in the small airways. This is used to test *volume of isoflow (VisoV)*, which is helpful in identifying early obstructive changes.

Contraindications

- Patients who are in pain because of the inability to cooperate by deep inspiration and expiration
- Patients who are unable to cooperate because of age or mental incapability

Procedure and patient care

Before

PT Explain the test to the patient.

PT Inform the patient that cooperation is necessary to obtain accurate results.

PT Instruct the patient not to use bronchodilators or smoke for 6 hours before this test (if requested by physician).

PT Tell the patient to withhold the use of small-dose meter inhalers and aerosol therapy before this study.

- Measure and record the patient's height and weight before this study to determine the predicted values.
- List on the laboratory slip any medications the patient is taking.

During

- Note the following procedural steps:

Spirometry and airflow rates

  1. The unsedated patient is taken to the pulmonary function laboratory.
  2. The patient breathes through a sterile mouthpiece and into a spirometer to measure and record the desired values.
  3. The patient is asked to inhale as deeply as possible and then forcibly exhale as much air as possible. This is repeated several times (usually two to three times). The two best are used for calculations. This test may be repeated with bronchodilators if the patient's values are deficient.
  4. From this, the machine computes FVC, FEV_1, FEV_1/FVC, PIFR, PEFR, and MMEF.

5. The patient is asked to breathe in and out as deeply and frequently as possible for 15 seconds. The total volume breathed is recorded and multiplied by 4 to obtain the MVV.

6. The patient is asked to breathe in and out normally into the spirometer and then exhale forcibly from the end tidal volume expiration point. This provides measurement of ERV.

7. The patient is asked to breathe in and out normally into the spirometer and then inhale forcibly from the end tidal volume expiration point. This provides measurement of IC.

8. The patient is asked to breathe in and out maximally (but not forced). This is a measure of VC and the calculated TLC.

Gas exchange/diffusing capacity of the lung (D_L)

1. The D_L of CO is usually measured by having the patient inhale a CO mixture.

2. $D_L CO$ is calculated with an analysis of the amount of CO exhaled compared with the amount inhaled. Some procedures require arterial blood gases to be performed at the same time as the gas exchange maneuvers.

Inhalation tests (bronchial provocation studies)

1. These tests also may be performed during pulmonary function studies to establish a cause-and-effect relationship in some patients with inhalant allergies.

2. The *methacholine* or *histamine challenge* test is typically used to detect the presence of hyperactive airway diseases. This test would not be indicated for a patient known to have asthma. A positive methacholine challenge is a greater than 20% reduction in the patient's FEV_1.

3. Care is taken during this challenge test to reverse any severe bronchospasm with prompt administration of an inhalant bronchodilator (e.g., isoproterenol).

After

- Note that patients with severe respiratory problems are occasionally exhausted after the testing and will need rest.

Abnormal findings

Pulmonary fibrosis
Interstitial lung diseases
Tumor
Chest wall trauma
Emphysema
Chronic bronchitis
Asthma
Inhalant pneumonitis
Postpneumonectomy
Bronchiectasis
Airway infection
Pneumonia
Neuromuscular disease
Hypersensitivity bronchospasm

notes

rabies-neutralizing antibody test

Type of test Blood

Normal findings <1:16

Test explanation and related physiology

Identification and documentation of the presence of rabies-neutralizing antibody is important for veterinary health care workers and others who may be or may have been exposed to the rabies virus. This test is performed on patients who are at great risk for animal bites and have received the human diploid cell rabies vaccine (HDCV). A low rabies titer of greater than 1:16 is considered to be protective.

The rabies antibody test is also used in making the diagnosis of rabies in a patient suspected of having been exposed to the virus. A fourfold rise in antibody titer over several weeks in a person not previously exposed to the HDCV indicates rabies exposure.

Procedure and patient care

Before

PT Explain the procedure to the patient.

PT Tell the patient that no fasting or special preparation is required.

During

- Collect 7 to 10 ml of venous blood in a red-top tube.

After

- Apply pressure to the venipuncture site.

Abnormal findings

Exposure to rabies vaccine
Recent bite exposure to rabies virus
Active rabies in patient or animal

notes

red blood cell count (RBC count, Erythrocyte count)

Type of test Blood

Normal findings (RBC $\times 10^6$/µl or RBC $\times 10^{12}$/L [SI units])

Adult/elderly
    Male: 4.7-6.1
    Female: 4.2-5.4
Children
    Newborn: 4.8-7.1
    2-8 weeks: 4-6
    2-6 months: 3.5-5.5
    6 months-1 year: 3.5-5.2
    1-6 years: 4-5.5
    6-18 years: 4-5.5

Test explanation and related physiology

This test is a count of the number of circulating red blood cells (RBCs) in 1 mm^3 of peripheral venous blood. The RBC count is routinely performed as part of a complete blood count. Within each RBC are molecules of hemoglobin that permit the transport and exchange of oxygen to the tissues and carbon dioxide from the tissues. RBCs are produced by the erythroid elements in the bone marrow. Under the stimulation of erythropoietin, RBC production is increased.

Normally, RBCs survive in the peripheral blood for approximately 120 days. During that time, RBCs are transported through the bloodstream. In the smallest of capillaries, the RBCs must fold and bend to conform to the size of these tiny vessels. Toward the end of the life of an RBC, the cell membrane becomes less pliable; the aged RBC is then lysed and extracted from the circulation by the spleen. Abnormal RBCs have a shorter life span and are extracted earlier (see RBC survival study p. 789). Intravascular RBC trauma, such as that caused by artificial heart valves or peripheral vascular atherosclerotic plaques, also shorten the life of the RBC. An enlarged spleen, such as that caused by portal hypertension or leukemia, may inappropriately destroy and remove normal RBCs from the circulation.

Normal RBC values vary according to gender and age. Women tend to have lower values than do men, and RBC counts tend to decrease with age. When the value is decreased by more than 10% of the expected normal value, the patient is said to be anemic. Low RBC values are caused by many factors, including the following:

1. Hemorrhage, as in gastrointestinal bleeding or trauma
2. Hemolysis, as in glucose-6-phosphate dehydrogenase deficiency, spherocytosis, or secondary splenomegaly
3. Dietary deficiency, as of iron or vitamin B_{12}
4. Genetic aberrations, as in sickle cell anemia or thalassemia
5. Drug ingestion, as of chloramphenicol, hydantoins, or quinidine
6. Marrow failure, as in fibrosis, leukemia, or antineoplastic chemotherapy
7. Chronic illness, as in tumor or sepsis
8. Other organ failure, as in renal disease

RBC counts greater than normal can be physiologically induced as a result of the body's requirements for greater oxygen-carrying capacity (e.g., at high altitudes). Diseases that produce chronic hypoxia (e.g., congenital heart disease) also provoke this physiologic increase in RBCs. Polycythemia vera is a neoplastic condition involving uncontrolled production of RBCs.

Interfering factors

- Normal decreases are seen in RBCs during pregnancy because of normal body fluid increases and dilution of the RBCs.
- Persons living at high altitudes have increased RBCs.
- Hydration status: Dehydration factitiously increases the RBC count, and overhydration decreases the RBC count.
- Drugs that may cause *increased* RBC levels include gentamicin and methyldopa.
- Drugs that may cause *decreased* RBC levels include chloramphenicol, hydantoins, and quinidine.

Procedure and patient care

Before
PT Explain the procedure to the patient.
PT Tell the patient that no fasting is required.

During
- Collect approximately 5 to 7 ml of blood in a lavender-top tube.

- Thoroughly mix the blood with the anticoagulant by tilting the tube.
- Avoid hemolysis.
- List on the laboratory slip any drugs or other patient factors that may affect RBC levels.

After

- Apply pressure to the venipuncture site.

Abnormal findings

▲ **Increased levels**

High altitude
Congenital heart disease
Polycythemia vera
Dehydration/
    hemoconcentration
Cor pulmonale
Pulmonary fibrosis

▼ **Decreased levels**

Hemorrhage
Hemolysis
Anemia
Hemoglobinopathy
Advanced cancer
Bone marrow fibrosis
Leukemia
Antineoplastic
    chemotherapy
Chronic illness
Renal failure
Overhydration
Multiple myeloma
Pernicious anemia
Rheumatoid disease
Subacute endocarditis
Pregnancy
Dietary deficiency

notes

red blood cell indices (RBC indices, MCV, MCH, MCHC, Blood indices, Erythrocyte indices, Red cell distribution width [RDW])

Type of test Blood

Normal findings

Mean corpuscular volume (MCV)
Adult/elderly/child: 80-95 μm^3
Newborn: 96-108 μm^3

Mean corpuscular hemoglobin (MCH)
Adult/elderly/child: 27-31 pg
Newborn: 32-34 pg

Mean corpuscular hemoglobin concentration (MCHC)
Adult/elderly/child: 32-36 g/dl (or 32%-36%)
Newborn: 32-33 g/dl (or 32%-33%)

Red blood cell distribution width (RDW)
Adult: 11%-14.5%

Test explanation and related physiology

The RBC indices provide information about the size (MCV and RDW), weight (MCH), and hemoglobin concentration (MCHC) of RBCs. This test is routinely performed as part of a complete blood count (CBC). The results of the RBC, hematocrit, and hemoglobin tests are necessary to calculate the RBC indices. When investigating anemia, it is helpful to categorize the anemia according to the RBC indices, as shown in Table 20. Cell size is indicated by the terms *normocytic, microcytic,* and *macrocytic.* Hemoglobin content is indicated by the terms *normochromic, hypochromic,* and *hyperchromic.* Additional information about RBC size, shape, color, and intracellular structure is described in the blood smear study (see p. 174).

Mean corpuscular volume

The MCV is a measure of the average volume, or size, of a single RBC and is therefore used in classifying anemias. MCV is calculated as follows:

$$MCV = \frac{Hematocrit\ (\%) \times 10}{RBC\ (million/mm^3)}$$

TABLE 20 Categorization of anemia according to RBC indices

Normocytic,[1] normochromic[2] anemia
Iron deficiency (detected early)
Chronic illness (e.g., sepsis, tumor)
Acute blood loss
Aplastic anemia (e.g., chloramphenicol toxicosis)
Acquired hemolytic anemias (e.g., from a prosthetic cardiac valve)

Microcytic,[3] hypochromic[4] anemia
Iron deficiency (detected late)
Thalassemia
Lead poisoning

Microcytic, normochromic anemia
Renal disease (because of the loss of erythropoietin)

Macrocytic,[5] normochromic anemia
Vitamin B_{12} or folic acid deficiency
Hydantoin ingestion
Chemotherapy

---

[1]Normocytic—normal RBC size.
[2]Normochromic—normal color (normal hemoglobin content).
[3]Microcytic—smaller than normal RBC size.
[4]Hypochromic—less than normal color (decreased hemoglobin content).
[5]Macrocytic—larger than normal RBC size.

When the MCV value is increased, the RBC is said to be abnormally large, or *macrocytic*. This is most frequently seen in megaloblastic anemias (e.g., vitamin B_{12} or folic acid deficiency). When the MCV value is decreased, the RBC is said to be abnormally small, or *microcytic*. This is associated with iron deficiency anemia or thalassemia.

Mean corpuscular hemoglobin

The MCH is a measure of the average amount (weight) of hemoglobin within an RBC. MCH is calculated as follows:

$$MCH = \frac{\text{Hemoglobin (g/dl)} \times 10}{\text{RBC (million/mm}^3)}$$

Because macrocytic cells generally have more hemoglobin and microcytic cells have less hemoglobin, the causes for these values closely resemble those for the MCV value.

Mean corpuscular hemoglobin concentration

The MCHC is a measure of the average concentration or percentage of hemoglobin within a single RBC. MCHC is calculated as follows:

$$MCHC = \frac{Hemoglobin\ (g/dl) \times 100}{Hematocrit\ (\%)}$$

When values are decreased, the cell has a deficiency of hemoglobin and is said to be *hypochromic* (frequently seen in iron deficiency anemia and thalassemia). When values are normal, the anemia is said be *normochromic* (e.g., hemolytic anemia). RBCs cannot be considered *hyperchromic*. Only 37 g/dl of hemoglobin can fit into the RBC.

Red blood cell distribution width

The RDW is an indication of the variation in RBC size. It is calculated by a machine using the MCV and RBC values. Variations in the width of RBCs may be helpful when classifying certain types of anemia. The RDW is essentially an indicator of the degree of *anisocytosis,* a blood condition characterized by RBCs of variable and abnormal size.

Interfering factors

- Abnormal RBC size may affect indices.
- Extremely elevated white blood cell counts may affect RBC indices.
- Large red blood cell precursors (e.g., reticulocytes [see p. 805]) cause an abnormally high MCV.
- The presence of cold agglutinins also falsely elevates MCHC, MCH, and MCV.

Procedure and patient care

Before

PT Explain the procedure to the patient.

PT Tell the patient that no fasting is required.

During

- Collect approximately 5 to 7 ml of venous blood in a lavender-top tube.
- Avoid hemolysis.

- Transport the specimen to the hematology laboratory, where the blood is passed through automated machines that calculate the RBC indices.

After
- Apply pressure to the venipuncture site.

Abnormal findings

▲ **Increased MCV**

Liver disease
Antimetabolite therapy
Alcoholism
Pernicious anemia
  (vitamin B_{12} deficiency)
Folic acid deficiency

▼ **Decreased MCV**

Iron deficiency anemia
Thalassemia

▲ **Increased MCH**

Macrocytic anemia

▼ **Decreased MCH**

Microcytic anemia
Hypochromic anemia

▲ **Increased MCHC**

Spherocytosis
Intravascular hemolysis
Cold agglutinins

▼ **Decreased MCHC**

Iron deficiency anemia
Thalassemia

▲ **Increased RDW**

Iron deficiency anemia
B_{12} or folate deficiency
  anemia
Hemoglobinopathies
  (e.g., sickle cell disease)
Hemolytic anemias
Posthemorrhagic anemias

notes

red blood cell survival study (RBC survival study, Splenic sequestration study)

Type of test Nuclear scan

Normal findings

Half-life of RBC: 26-30 days
Spleen/liver ratio: 1:1
Spleen/pericardium ratio: <2:1

Test explanation and related physiology

In patients with hemolytic anemia, the RBCs are destroyed and normally sequestered in the spleen. As a result of this ongoing RBC destruction, RBC life span will be significantly reduced. This reduction in RBC survival indicates that active hemolysis is occurring and is the cause of the patient's anemia.

The nuclear medicine determination of RBC life span can provide a semiquantitative measurement of the degree of hemolysis. This quantitation can be performed best by determining the half-life of RBCs within the circulation. This part of the test is performed by extracting some of the patient's RBCs, labeling them with chromium-51 (^{51}Cr), and reinjecting them into the patient. Subsequent blood levels of ^{51}Cr indicate the half-life of the labeled RBCs. As RBC survival decreases, more labeled RBCs are sequestered by the spleen. As a result, the amount of ^{51}Cr activity in the blood decreases.

The second part of the test is the imaging of the spleen, liver, and pericardium. In patients with hemolytic anemia associated with abnormal splenic sequestration, the spleen/liver ratio is in excess of 1:1. However, this abnormally high ratio can occur in patients who have splenomegaly caused by a disease other than hemolytic anemia. Therefore spleen/pericardium ratios are performed; those greater than 2:1 indicate abnormal splenic sequestration of hemolyzed RBCs. A normal spleen/pericardium ratio with an increased spleen/liver ratio indicates splenomegaly.

This splenic sequestration part of the study is also helpful in determining which patients with hemolytic anemia will benefit from splenectomy. Patients with increased splenic sequestration can be expected to improve greatly as a result of splenectomy.

R

Contraindications

- Patients who are pregnant, unless the benefits outweigh the risks

Interfering factors

- Factors that can decrease RBC survival include recent RBC transfusion, increased RBC production, active bleeding, high white blood cell (WBC) counts in excess of 25,000, and high platelet counts greater than 500,000.
- Splenomegaly can increase spleen/pericardium ratios.
- Splenic infarctions can decrease spleen/pericardium ratios.

Procedure and patient care

Before

- **PT** Explain the procedure to the patient.
- **PT** Assure the patient that he or she will not be exposed to large amounts of radioactivity, because only tracer doses of the isotope are used.
- **PT** Tell the patient that no preparation or sedation is required.
- Notify the nuclear medicine technologist or physician if blood transfusion or hemorrhage has occurred shortly before or during the study.
- Note that usually a hematocrit, WBC count, platelet count, and reticulocyte count are performed before testing.

During

- Note the following procedural steps:
  1. Approximately 20 ml of blood is withdrawn from the patient, and the RBCs are labeled with ^{51}Cr.
  2. The RBCs are immediately reinjected into the patient.
  3. On the first day of testing, 10 ml of blood is withdrawn by a peripheral venipuncture into a red-top tube.
  4. The RBCs are quantitated for ^{51}Cr counts per minute.
  5. Nuclear imaging of the spleen, liver, and pericardium is carried out.
  6. This process is repeated three times a week for 3 weeks.
  7. The peripheral venous blood ^{51}Cr counts are plotted on a graph, and the half-life is determined.
  8. The spleen/liver and spleen/pericardium ratios and nuclear counts are determined.
- Note that this test takes place over 2 to 3 weeks. The results are available on the day after the study is completed. The study is performed by a nuclear medicine technologist or physician.

PT Tell the patient that no pain or discomfort is associated with this procedure. The patient must lie still during the nuclear imaging part of the test.

After

PT Inform the patient that because only tracer doses of radioisotopes are used, no precautions need to be taken against radioactive exposure.

Abnormal findings

▲ **Increased splenic sequestration**

  Hemolysis
  Splenomegaly

▼ **Decreased RBC survival**

  Hemolysis
  Hemorrhage
  Abnormally increased erythropoiesis
  Recent transfusion

notes

R

renal biopsy (Kidney biopsy)

Type of test Microscopic examination of tissue

Normal findings No pathologic conditions

Test explanation and related physiology

Biopsy of the kidney affords microscopic examination of renal tissue. Renal biopsy is performed for the following purposes:

1. To diagnose the cause of renal disease (e.g., poststreptococcal glomerulonephritis, Goodpasture's syndrome, lupus nephritis)
2. To detect primary and metastatic malignancy of the kidney in patients who may not be candidates for surgery
3. To evaluate the degree of rejection that occurs after kidney transplantation, which enables the physician to determine the appropriate dose of immunosuppressive agents

Renal biopsy is most often obtained percutaneously (Figure 35). During this procedure, a needle is inserted through the skin and into the kidney to obtain a sample of kidney tissue. The biopsy needle is more accurately placed when guided by ultrasonography or fluoroscopy. These techniques allow more precise localization of the desired kidney tissue.

Occasionally open renal biopsy is performed. This involves an incision through the flank and dissection to expose the kidney surgically. A renal biopsy can also be obtained by the *transurethral* approach. This is an alternative to percutaneous needle biopsy that avoids the need for an open operation in some patients. It can be readily used in patients who require cystoscopic evaluation.

Contraindications

- Patients with coagulation disorders, because of the risk of excessive bleeding
- Patients with operable kidney tumors, because tumor cells may be disseminated during the procedure
- Patients with hydronephrosis, because the enlarged renal pelvis can be easily entered and cause a persistent urine leak requiring surgical repair
- Patients with urinary tract infections, because the needle insertion may disseminate the active infection throughout the retroperitoneum

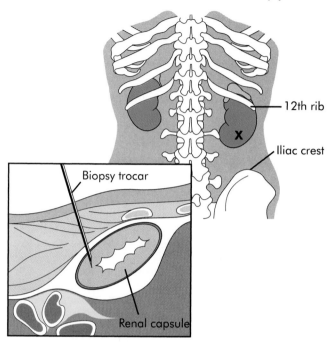

Figure 35 Renal biopsy. A biopsy needle is placed through the posterior lower chest wall and into the renal parenchyma from which tissue is extracted.

R

Potential complications

- Hemorrhage from the highly vascular renal tissue
- Inadvertent puncture of the liver, lung, bowel, aorta, and inferior vena cava
- Infection when an open biopsy is performed

Procedure and patient care

Before

PT Explain the procedure to the patient.

- Ensure that written and informed consent for this procedure is obtained by the physician.
- Keep the patient NPO after midnight on the day of the test in the event that bleeding or inadvertent puncture of an abdominal organ may necessitate surgical intervention.

- Assess the patient's coagulation studies (prothrombin time, partial thromboplastin time).
- Check the patient's hemoglobin and hematocrit values.
- Note that the patient may need to be typed and cross-matched for blood in the event of severe hemorrhage requiring transfusions.
- **PT** Tell the patient that no sedative is required.
- Note that the needle stick may be done at the bedside.
- If fluoroscopic or ultrasound guidance is to be used, note that the needle stick is performed in the radiology or ultrasonography department.

During
- Note the following procedural steps:
  1. The patient is placed in a prone position with a sandbag or pillow under the abdomen to straighten the spine.
  2. Under sterile conditions the skin overlying the kidneys is infiltrated with a local anesthetic (lidocaine).
  3. While the patient holds his or her breath to stop kidney motion, the physician inserts the biopsy needle into the kidney and takes a specimen.
  4. After this procedure is completed, the needle is removed, and pressure is applied to the site for approximately 20 minutes.
- Note that this procedure is performed by a physician in approximately 10 minutes.
- **PT** Tell the patient that this procedure is uncomfortable, but only minimally if enough lidocaine is used.

After
- After the test, apply a pressure dressing.
- Turn the patient on his or her back and keep on bed rest for approximately 24 hours.
- Check the patient's vital signs, puncture site, and hematocrit values frequently during the 24-hour period.
- **PT** Instruct the patient to avoid any activity that increases abdominal venous pressure (e.g., coughing).
- Assess the patient for signs and symptoms of hemorrhage (e.g., decrease in blood pressure, increase in pulse, pallor, backache, flank pain, shoulder pain, lightheadedness).
- Evaluate the patient's abdomen for signs of bowel or liver penetration (e.g., abdominal pain and tenderness, abdominal muscle guarding and rigidity, decreased bowel sounds).

- Inspect all urine specimens for gross hematuria. Usually the patient's urine will contain blood initially, but this generally will not continue after the first 24 hours. Urine samples may be placed in consecutive chronologic order to facilitate comparison for evaluation of hematuria. This is referred to as *rack* or *serial* urine samples.
- **PT** Encourage the patient to drink large amounts of fluid to prevent clot formation and urine retention.
- Frequently obtain blood for hemoglobin and hematocrit determination after the biopsy specimen to assess for active bleeding. One purple-top tube of blood is needed.

🏠 Home care responsibilities

- Instruct the patient to avoid strenuous exercise (e.g., heavy lifting, contact sports, horseback riding) or any activity that could cause jolting of the kidney for at least 2 weeks.
- Teach the patient the signs and symptoms of renal hemorrhage, and instruct him or her to call the physician if any of these symptoms occur.
- Instruct the patient to report burning during urination or any temperature elevations. These could indicate a urinary tract infection.

Abnormal findings

Renal disease (e.g., poststreptococcal conditions, glomerulonephritis, lupus nephritis)
Primary and metastatic malignancy of the kidney
Rejection of kidney transplant

R

notes

renal scanning (Kidney scan, Radiorenography, Renography, Radionuclide renal imaging, Nuclear imaging of the kidney, DSMA renal scan, DTPA renal scan, Captopril renal scan)

Type of test Nuclear scan

Normal findings Normal size, shape, and function of the kidney

Test explanation and related physiology

Renal scans are used to indicate the perfusion, function, and structure of the kidneys. They are also used to indicate the presence of ureteral obstruction or renovascular hypertension. Because this study uses no iodinated dyes (except when iodohippurate is used), it is safe to perform on patients who have iodine allergies or compromised renal function. Renal scans are used to monitor renal function in patients with known renal disease. This scan also plays a large part of the diagnosis of renal transplant rejection.

This nuclear procedure provides visualization of the urinary tract after IV administration of a radioisotope. The radioactive material is detected by a scintillator camera, which can detect the gamma rays emitted by the radionuclide in the kidney. Scans do not interfere with the normal physiologic process of the kidney. The resultant image (scan) indicates distribution of the radionuclide within the kidney and ureters.

There are several different kinds of renal scans, depending on what information is needed to be obtained. Different isotopes may be more suitable for different scans, based on the manner in which the kidney handles the radioisotope.

Renal blood flow (perfusion) scan

This type of renal scan is used to evaluate the blood flow to each kidney. It is used to identify renal artery stenosis, renovascular hypertension, and rejection of renal transplant. Also, it is used to demonstrate hypervascular lesions (renal cell carcinoma) in the kidney.

Decreased gamma activity is noted in a kidney with arterial stenosis or renovascular hypertension. Decreased activity relative to the aorta is noted in a transplanted kidney that is experiencing rejection. Localized increased gamma activity is noted in a kidney that contains a hypervascular tumor (cancer).

Renal structural scan

This type of renal scan is performed to outline the structure of the kidney to identify pathology that may alter normal anatomic structure (e.g., tumor, cyst, abscess). Congenital disorders (e.g., hypoplasia or aplasia of the kidney, malposition of the kidney) can also be detected. A filling defect in the renal parenchyma may indicate a tumor, cyst, abscess, or infarction. Horseshoe-shaped kidney, pelvic kidney, or absence of a kidney may be evident. Also, information concerning postrenal transplants can be obtained with this scan. Anatomic alterations in the parenchymal distribution of tracer may indicate transplant rejection. Tc-DTPA or DSMA can be used for this scan.

Renal function scan (renogram)

Renal function can be determined by documenting the capability of the kidney to take up and excrete a particular radioisotope. A well-functioning kidney can be expected to rapidly assimilate the isotope and then excrete it. A poorly functioning kidney will not be able to take up the isotope rapidly or excrete it in a timely manner. Renal function can be monitored by serially repeating this test and comparing results. Each radioactive tracer is handled by the kidney in a different manner. Different renal functions can be tested according to which isotope is used:

Technetium-99m diethylenetriamine pentaacetic acid (^{99m}Tc DTPA) measures glomerular filtration.

Tc disodium monomethane arsonate (DSMA) measures tubular cell secretion.

Iodine-131 (^{131}I) or ^{133}I hippurate measures both glomerular filtration and tubular cell secretion.

Renal hypertension scan

This scan is used to identify the presence and location of renovascular hypertension. It usually uses angiotensin-converting enzyme (ACE) inhibitors such as captopril. The *captopril scan* (captopril renography/scintigraphy) determines the functional significance of a renal artery or arteriole stenosis. These scans may predict the response of the blood pressure to medical treatment, angioplasty, or surgery.

Renal obstruction scan

This scan is performed to identify obstruction of the outflow tract of the kidney caused by obstruction of the renal pelvis, ureter, or bladder outlet.

Often several of these scans are combined to obtain the maximum possible information about the renal system. A *triple renal study* may use all of these techniques to evaluate renal blood perfusion, structure, and excretion. Radionuclear scans are also helpful in the evaluation of arterial trauma.

Contraindications

- Patients who are pregnant, unless the benefits outweigh the risk of fetal damage

Procedure and patient care

Before

PT Explain the procedure to the patient.

- Do not schedule a renal scan within 24 hours after an intravenous pyelogram.

PT Assure the patient that he or she will not be exposed to large amounts of radioactivity because only tracer doses of isotopes are used.

- Note that Lugol's solution (10 drops) may be ordered if ^{131}I orthoiodohippurate is used. This minimizes thyroid uptake of the radioisotope.

PT Remind the patient to void before the scan.

PT Tell the patient that no sedation or fasting is required but that good hydration is essential.

PT Instruct the patient to drink two to three glasses of water before the scan.

During

- Note the following procedural steps:
  1. The unsedated, nonfasting patient is taken to the nuclear medicine department.
  2. A peripheral IV injection of radionuclide is given. It takes only minutes for the radioisotopes to be concentrated in the kidneys.
  3. While the patient assumes a prone or sitting position, a gamma ray scintography camera is passed over the kidney area and records the radioactive uptake on film.
  4. Scans may be repeated at different intervals after the initial isotope injection.
  5. Unique features of the various scans:
     a. For a furosemide *(Lasix) renal scan* or a *diuretic renal scan,* images are obtained for 10 to 20 minutes; then 40 mg of furosemide is administered through an IV, and another 20 minutes of images are obtained.

b. For the *captopril renal scan,* the patient is scanned after the administration of captopril.

c. For the *renal blood flow* and the *renal function scans,* scanning is started immediately after the injection.

d. For *structural renal scans,* the patient is asked to lie still for the entire time of the scan (30 minutes).

- Note that the duration of this test varies from 1 to 4 hours, depending on the specific information required. Perfusion scans are done in approximately 20 minutes, and functional scans in less than 1 hour. Static structure scans require 20 minutes to 4 hours for completion.

- Note that this study is performed by a nuclear medicine technologist or physician.

PT Tell the patient that no pain or discomfort is associated with this procedure.

PT Inform the patient that he or she must lie still during this study.

After

PT Because only tracer doses of radioisotopes are used, inform the patient that no precautions need to be taken against radioactive exposure.

PT Tell the patient that the radioactive substance is usually excreted from the body within 6 to 24 hours. Encourage the patient to drink fluids.

Abnormal findings

Urinary obstruction
Pyelonephritis
Renovascular hypertension
Absence of kidney function
Renal infarction
Renal arterial atherosclerosis
Glomerulonephritis
Renal tumor
Congenital abnormalities
Renal trauma
Transplant rejection
Acute tubular necrosis
Renal abscess
Renal cyst

R

renin assay, plasma (Plasma renin activity [PRA], Plasma renin concentration [PRC])

Type of test   Blood

Normal findings

Plasma renin assay

Adult/elderly

Upright position, *sodium-depleted* (sodium-restricted diet)

Ages 20-39 years: 2.9-24.0 ng/ml/hr

>40 years: 2.9-10.8 ng/ml/hr

Upright position, *sodium-repleted* (normal sodium diet)

Ages 20-39 years: 0.1-4.3 ng/ml/hr

>40 years: 0.1-3.0 ng/ml/hr

Child

0-3 years: <16.6 ng/ml/hr

3-6 years: <6.7 ng/ml/hr

6-9 years: <4.4 ng/ml/hr

9-12 years: <5.9 ng/ml/hr

12-15 years: <4.2 ng/ml/hr

15-18 years: <4.3 ng/ml/hr

Renal vein

Renin ratio of involved kidney to uninvolved kidney <1.4

Test explanation and related physiology

Renin is an enzyme released by the juxtaglomerular apparatus of the kidney into the renal veins in response to hyperkalemia, sodium depletion, decreased renal blood perfusion, or hypovolemia. Renin activates the renin-angiotensin system, which results in angiotensin II, a powerful vasoconstrictor that also stimulates aldosterone production from the adrenal cortex. Angiotensin and aldosterone increase the blood volume, blood pressure, and serum sodium (Figure 36).

Renin is not actually measured in this test. The PRA test actually measures the rate of generation of angiotensin. This is the most commonly used renin assay. The *plasma renin concentration (PRC)* is used to measure the maximum renin effect.

The PRA is a screening procedure for the detection of essential, renal, or renovascular hypertension. A determination of the PRA and a measurement of the plasma aldosterone level (see p. 32) are used in the differential diagnosis of primary versus

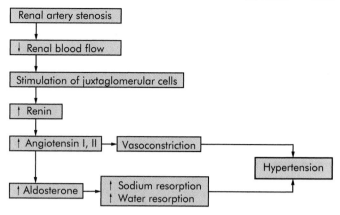

Figure 36 Physiology of renovascular hypertension.

secondary hyperaldosteronism. Patients with primary hyperaldosteronism (adrenal adenoma overproducing aldosterone—Conn's syndrome) have increased aldosterone production associated with decreased renin activity. Patients with secondary hyperaldosteronism (caused by renovascular occlusive disease or primary renal disease) have increased levels of plasma renin.

Renal vein assays for renin are used to diagnose and lateralize renovascular hypertension, that is, hypertension that is due to inappropriately high renin levels from a diseased kidney or hypoperfused kidney. The renal veins can be identified using injection of a radiopaque dye into the inferior vena cava. A catheter is placed into each renal vein, and blood is withdrawn from each vein. PRA is determined in each sample. If hypertension is caused by renal artery stenosis or renal pathology, the renal vein renin level of the affected kidney should be 1.4 or more times greater than that of the unaffected kidney. If the levels are the same, the hypertension is not caused by a renovascular source. This is very helpful in determining whether a stenosis seen on a renal angiogram is significantly contributing to hypertension.

The *renin stimulation test* can be performed to more clearly diagnose and separate primary from secondary hyperaldosteronism. In this test, PRA is obtained while the patient is in the recumbent and standing positions. In primary hyperaldosteronism, a change in position will not result in increased renin levels. In secondary hyperaldosteronism (or normal persons with essential hypertension), renin levels increase due to decreased renal perfusion while in the upright position.

The PRA is assessed as part of the *captopril test,* a screening test for renovascular hypertension (RVH). Patients with RVH have greater falls in blood pressure and increases in PRA after administration of angiotensin-converting enzyme (ACE) inhibitors than do those with essential hypertension.

Contraindications

- Patients who are allergic to shellfish or iodinated dye, because of potential allergic reaction to the radiopaque dye used during renal vein renin assay

Potential complications

- Allergic reaction to iodinated dye during renal vein renin assay

Interfering factors

- Renin levels are affected by pregnancy, salt intake, and licorice ingestion.
- Values are higher in patients on low-salt diets, and when the patient is in an upright position.
- Posture: renin is increased in the erect position and decreased in the recumbent position.
- Values are higher early in the day. There is a diurnal variation in renin production.
- ✗ Drugs that *increase* levels of renin include antihypertensives, ACE inhibitors, diuretics, estrogens, oral contraceptives, and vasodilators.
- ✗ Drugs that *decrease* renin levels include beta-blockers, clonidine, potassium, licorice, and reserpine.

Procedure and patient care

Before
- PT Explain the procedure to the patient.
- PT Instruct the patient to maintain a normal diet with a restricted amount of sodium (approximately 3 g/day) for 3 days before the test. A high-sodium diet causes a decrease in renin.
- PT Instruct the patient to discontinue medications (e.g., diuretics, steroids, antihypertensives, vasodilators, oral contraceptives) and licorice for 2 to 4 weeks before the test as ordered by the physican.

- Usually draw a fasting blood sample because renin values are higher in the morning.
PT For stimulation tests, instruct the patient to significantly reduce sodium intake (supplemented with potassium) for 3 days before testing.
- Ensure that the patient stands or sits upright for 2 hours before the blood is drawn.
- If a recumbent sample is ordered, have the patient remain in bed in the morning until the blood sample has been obtained.

During
- The test is usually performed with the patient in an upright position.
- For the stimulation tests, the blood is drawn in the recumbent and upright positions.
- It is best to release the tourniquet immediately prior to obtaining the blood specimen because stasis can lower renin levels.
- Collect approximately 7 to 12 ml of venous blood and place it in a chilled lavender-top tube with ethylenediaminetetraacetic acid as an anticoagulant.
- Gently invert the blood tube to allow adequate mixing of the blood sample and the anticoagulant.
- Record the patient's position, dietary status, and time of day on the laboratory slip. Also note any medication that the patient is currently taking.
- Place the tube of blood on ice and immediately send it to the laboratory.

R

After
- Apply pressure to the venipuncture site.
PT Tell the patient that usually a normal diet may be resumed.
- Note that medications that were withheld may be reordered.

Abnormal findings

▲ **Increased levels**

Essential hypertension
Malignant hypertension
Renovascular hypertension
Chronic renal failure
Salt-losing gastrointestinal
  disease (vomiting or
  diarrhea)
Addison's disease
Renin-producing renal tumor
Bartter's syndrome
Cirrhosis
Hyperkalemia
Hemorrhage

▼ **Decreased levels**

Primary
  hyperaldosteronism
Steroid therapy
Congenital adrenal
  hyperplasia

notes

reticulocyte count (Retic count)

Type of test Blood

Normal findings

Reticulocyte count:
    Adult/elderly/child: 0.5%-2%
    Infant: 0.5%-3.1%
    Newborn: 2.5%-6.5%
Reticulocyte index: 1.0

Test explanation and related physiology

The reticulocyte count is a test for determining bone marrow function and evaluating erythropoietic activity. This test is also useful in classifying anemias. A reticulocyte is an immature red blood cell (RBC) that can be readily identified under a microscope. Normally there are a small number of reticulocytes in the bloodstream.

The reticulocyte count gives an indication of RBC production by the bone marrow. Increased reticulocyte counts indicate that the marrow is putting an increased number of RBCs into the bloodstream, usually in response to anemia. A normal or low reticulocyte count in a patient with anemia indicates that the marrow response to the anemia by way of production of RBCs is inadequate and perhaps contributing to or the cause of the anemia (as in aplastic anemia, iron deficiency, vitamin B_{12} deficiency, or depletion of iron stores). An elevated reticulocyte count found in patients with a normal hemogram indicates increased RBC production compensating for an ongoing loss of RBCs (hemolysis or hemorrhage).

Because the reticulocyte count is a percentage of the total number of RBCs, a normal to low number of reticulocytes can appear high in the anemic patient, because the total number of mature RBCs is low. To determine if a reticulocyte count indicates an appropriate erythropoietic (RBC marrow) response in patients with anemia and a decreased hematocrit, one should calculate the *reticulocyte index:*

Reticulocyte index =

$$\text{Reticulocyte count (in \%)} \times \frac{\text{Patient's hematocrit}}{\text{Normal hematocrit}}$$

R

The reticulocyte index in a patient with a good marrow response to the anemia should be 1.0. If it is below 1.0, even though the reticulocyte count is elevated, the bone marrow response is inadequate in its ability to compensate.

Interfering factors

- Pregnancy may cause an increased reticulocyte count.
- RBCs containing Howell-Jolly bodies look like reticulocytes and are miscounted by the automated counter machines to be reticulocytes and give a falsely high number of reticulocytes.

Procedure and patient care

Before

PT Explain the procedure to the patient.
PT Tell the patient that no fasting is required.

During

- Collect approximately 5 to 7 ml of venous blood in a lavender-top tube.

After

- Apply pressure to the venipuncture site.

Abnormal findings

▲ **Increased levels**

Hemolytic anemia
Sickle cell anemia
Hemorrhage (3 to 4 days later)
Postsplenectomy
Erythroblastosis fetalis
Pregnancy
Leukemias
Recovery from nutritional anemias

▼ **Decreased levels**

Pernicious anemia
Folic acid deficiency
Adrenocortical hypofunction
Aplastic anemia
Radiation therapy
Marrow failure
Anterior pituitary hypofunction
Chronic infection
Cirrhosis
Malignancy

notes

retrograde pyelography

Type of test X-ray with contrast dye

Normal findings Normal outline and size of the ureters and bladder

Test explanation and related physiology

Retrograde pyelography refers to radiographic visualization of the urinary tract through ureteral catheterization and the injection of contrast material. The ureters are catheterized during cystoscopy. A radiopaque material is injected into the ureters, and x-ray films are taken. This test can be performed even if the patient has an allergy to IV contrast dye, because none of the dye injected into the ureters is absorbed.

Retrograde pyelography is helpful in radiographically examining the ureters in patients when visualization with intravenous pyelography (IVP, see p. 560) is inadequate or contraindicated. When a ureter is obstructed, IVP will visualize only the ureter proximal to the obstruction, if at all. To visualize the distal part of the ureter, retrograde pyelography is necessary. Also, in patients with unilateral renal disease, the involved kidney and collecting system are not visualized because renal function is so poor. As a result, no dye will be filtered into the collecting system by the nonfunctioning kidney. To rule out ureteral obstruction as a cause of the unilateral kidney disease, retrograde pyelography must be done. Tumors, benign strictures, tortuous ureters, stones, scarring, and extrinsic compression may cause ureteral obstruction.

Potential complications

- Urinary tract infection
  Infections may be caused by the invasive nature of this procedure.
- Sepsis by seeding the bloodstream with bacteria from infected urine
- Perforation of the bladder or ureter
- Hematuria
- Temporary obstruction to ureteral urine flow
  Manipulation of the ureters may cause edema, which can result in temporary, partial obstruction to urine flow.
- Allergic reaction to iodinated dye
  This rarely occurs, because the dye is not administered intravenously.

R

Interfering factors

- Retained barium from previous x-ray studies can obscure visualization.

Procedure and patient care

Before

PT Explain the procedure to the patient.
- Ensure that informed consent for this procedure is obtained.
- If enemas are ordered to clear the bowel, assist the patient as needed and record the results.
- If the procedure will be performed with the patient under general anesthesia, follow routine general anesthesia precautions. Keep the patient NPO after midnight on the day of the test. Fluids may be given intravenously.
- Administer preprocedure medications as ordered 1 hour before the study. Sedatives decrease the spasm of the bladder sphincter, thus decreasing the patient's discomfort.

During

- Note the following procedural steps:
  1. The ureteral catheters are passed into the ureters by means of cystoscopy (see p. 341).
  2. Radiopaque contrast material (Hypaque or Renografin) is injected into the ureteral catheters, and x-ray films are taken.
  3. The entire ureter and renal pelvis are demonstrated.
  4. As the catheters are withdrawn, more dye is injected, and more x-ray films are taken to visualize the complete outline of the ureters.
  5. A delayed film is often performed to assess the emptying capabilities of the ureter. This is usually done about 5 minutes after the last injection.
  6. If obstruction is noted, a stent may be left in the ureter so that the ureter can drain.
- Note that retrograde pyelography is performed by a urologist in approximately 1 hour in a cystoscopy room or operating room.

PT Inform the patient that this study is uncomfortable. If awake, the patient will feel pressure and an urge to void.

After

- Check and record the patient's vital signs as ordered. Watch for a decrease in blood pressure and increase in pulse as an indication of bleeding.
- Observe the patient for signs and symptoms of sepsis (elevated temperature, flush, chills, decreased blood pressure, increased pulse).
- Assess the patient's ability to void for at least 24 hours. Urinary retention may be secondary to edema caused by instrumentation.
- Note the color of the urine; a pink tinge is typically present. Report bright red blood or clots to the physician.
- **PT** Encourage the patient to increase intake of fluids. A dilute urine decreases dysuria. Fluids also maintain a constant flow of urine to prevent stasis and the accumulation of bacteria in the bladder.
- Monitor the patient for bladder spasms. Often, belladonna-and-opium suppositories are given to relieve bladder spasms.
- Administer analgesics as needed.

🏠 Home care responsibilities

- Observe the vital signs for indications of bleeding (e.g., decreased blood pressure, increased pulse) and sepsis (e.g., temperature, flush, chills).
- Monitor the urine output over the first 24 hours to detect urinary retention.
- Encourage the patient to drink lots of fluids to prevent stasis and to prevent the accumulation of bacteria in the bladder.

R

Abnormal findings

Tumor
Strictures
Stones
Ureteral obstruction
Intrinsic or extrinsic tumor affecting the ureters
Congenital anomaly

rheumatoid factor (RF)

Type of test Blood

Normal findings

Negative (<60 units/ml by nephelometric testing)
(Elderly patients may have slightly increased values.)

Test explanation and related physiology

Rheumatoid arthritis (RA) is a chronic inflammatory disease that affects most joints, especially the metacarpal and phalangeal joints, the proximal interphalangeal joints, and the wrists; however, any synovial joint can be involved.

In this disease, abnormal immunoglobulin G (IgG) antibodies produced by lymphocytes in the synovial membranes act as "antigens." Other IgG and IgM antibodies in the patient's serum react with the "fc" component of the abnormal synovial antigenic IgG to produce immune complexes. These immune complexes activate the complement system and other inflammatory systems to cause joint damage. The reactive IgM is called RF. Tissues other than the joints, including blood vessels, lungs, nerves, and heart, may also be involved in the autoimmune inflammation.

Tests for RF are directed toward identification of the IgM antibodies. The exact role, if any, that RF plays in the pathophysiology of the disease is not well known. Approximately 80% of patients with rheumatoid arthritis have positive RF titers. To be considered positive, RF must be found in a dilution of greater than 1:80; when RF is found in titers less than 1:80, diseases such as systemic lupus erythematosus, scleroderma, and other autoimmune conditions should be considered. Although the normal value is "no rheumatoid factor identifiable at low titers," a small number of normal patients will have RF present at a very low titer. Furthermore, a negative RF does not exclude the diagnosis of RA. RF is not a useful disease marker because its presence does not disappear in patients who are experiencing a remission from the disease symptoms.

Other autoimmune diseases (see Table 2, p. 89), such as systemic lupus erythematosus or Sjögren's syndrome, also may cause a positive RF test. RF is occasionally seen in patients with tuberculosis, chronic hepatitis, infectious mononucleosis, and subacute bacterial endocarditis as well.

Interfering factors

- Elderly patients often have false-positive results.

Procedure and patient care

Before

PT Explain the procedure to the patient.

PT Tell the patient that no fasting or preparation is required.

During

- Collect approximately 7 ml of venous blood in a red-top tube.

After

- Apply pressure to the venipuncture site.

Abnormal findings

▲   **Increased levels**

Rheumatoid arthritis

Other autoimmune diseases (e.g., systemic lupus erythematosus)

Chronic viral infection

Subacute bacterial endocarditis

Tuberculosis

Chronic hepatitis

Dermatomyositis

Scleroderma

Infectious mononucleosis

Leukemia

Cirrhosis

Syphilis

Renal disease

notes

rubella antibody test (German measles test, Hemagglutination inhibition [HAI])

Type of test Blood

Normal findings

Method	Result	Interpretation
HAI titer	<1:8	No immunity to rubella
HAI titer	>1:20	Immune to rubella
LA	negative	No immunity to rubella
ELISA—IgM	<0.9 international units/ml	No infection
ELISA—IgM	>1.1 international units/ml	Active infection
ELISA—IgG	<7 international units/ml	No immunity to rubella
ELISA—IgG	>10 international units/ml	Immune to rubella

LA, Latex agglutination; *ELISA,* enzyme-linked immunosorbent assay.

Possible critical values Evidence of susceptibility in pregnant women with recent exposure to rubella

Test explanation and related physiology

Screening for rubella antibodies is done to detect immunity to rubella. These tests detect the presence of immunoglobulin G (IgG) and/or IgM antibodies to rubella (the causative agent for German measles). They become elevated a few days to a few weeks after the onset of the rash, depending on what method of testing is used. IgM tends to disappear after about 6 weeks. IgG, however, persists at low but detectable levels for years. These antibodies become elevated in patients with active rubella infection or with past infections. In the past decade, children have been vaccinated with rubella to prevent the effects of the disease and to minimize infection. Rubella testing documents immunity to rubella. Rubella immunity testing is suggested for all health care workers. Most importantly, however, it is done to verify the presence or absence of rubella immunity in pregnant women, because congenital rubella infection in the first trimester of pregnancy is associated with congenital abnormalities of the fetus (heart defects, brain damage, deafness), abortion, or stillbirth. The term TORCH (**t**oxoplasmosis, **o**ther, **r**ubella, **c**ytomegalovirus, **h**erpes) has been applied to infections with recognized detrimental effects on the fetus. The effects on the fetus may be direct or indirect (e.g., precipitating abortion or premature labor). All of these tests are discussed separately (see separate listings).

If the woman's titer is greater than 1:10 to 1:20, she is not susceptible to rubella. If the woman's titer is 1:8 or less, she has little or no immunity to rubella. A fourfold increase in HAI rubella titer from the acute to the convalescent titer indicates that the rash was caused by an active rubella infection. Alternatively, an IgM antibody titer could be done. If the titer is positive, recent infection has occurred. IgM titers appear 1 to 2 days after onset of the rash and disappear 5 to 6 weeks after infection.

Antirubella antibody testing is also used to diagnose rubella in infants (congenital rubella). IgM antirubella antibodies cannot pass through the placenta. If an infant has IgM antibodies, acute congenital or newborn rubella is suspected. Antibody testing is often used in children with congenital abnormalities that may have come from congenital rubella infection.

Procedure and patient care

Before

PT Explain the purpose of the test to the patient.

During

- Collect approximately 7 ml of venous blood in a red-top tube.

After

- Apply pressure to the venipuncture site.
PT Inform the patient when to return for a follow-up HAI titer if indicated.

Abnormal findings

Active rubella infection
Previous rubella infection leading to immunity

notes

rubeola antibody

Type of test Blood

Normal findings Negative

Test explanation and related physiology

Rubeola is an RNA paramyxovirus that is known to cause the measles (not German measles – see Rubella, p. 812). Upper respiratory symptoms, fever, conjunctivitis, a rash, and Koplik's spots on the buccal mucosa highlight the disease. Since the 1970s, children have been vaccinated to prevent this disease. Although it is most usually a self-limiting disease, the virus can easily be spread (by respiratory droplets) to nonimmune pregnant women and cause preterm delivery or spontaneous abortion.

Testing for rubeola includes indirect immunofluorescence serologic identification of immunoglobulin G (IgG) and IgM antibodies. The first represents a previous infection. The latter indicates an acute infection. A fourfold rise in IgM indicates a current infection.

This test is used to diagnose measles in patients with a rash or viral syndrome when the diagnosis cannot be made clinically. Even more important, however, this test is used to establish and document immunity (active—by previous measles infection, or passive—by previous vaccination). Populations commonly tested to document immunity include college students, health care workers, and pregnant women.

Procedure and patient care

Before

PT Explain the purpose of the test to the patient.

During

- Collect approximately 7 ml of venous blood in a red-top tube.

After

- Apply pressure to the venipuncture site.
PT Inform the patient when to return for a follow-up rubeola titer if indicated.
PT If the results are negative for immunity, recommend immunization. For women of childbearing age, vaccination should precede future pregnancy.

Abnormal findings

Active rubeola infection
Previous rubeola infection leading to immunity

notes

R

salivary gland nuclear imaging (Parotid gland nuclear imaging)

Type of test Nuclear medicine

Normal findings

Normal function of the salivary gland. No tumor or duct obstruction.

Test explanation and related physiology

The ability of the epithelial cells of the salivary glands to transport large pertechnetate ions from the blood and to secrete them into the saliva provides the principle for imaging the salivary glands. The functional capabilities, structural integrity, and location of the glands can be assessed. Most usually, the parotid gland alone is visualized. Occasionally, the submandibular glands can be seen.

Indications for salivary gland imaging include patients with the following:

1. Xerostomia (dry mouth)
2. Pain
3. Tumors
4. Possible parotid duct obstruction

By following the radionuclide immediately after injection, blood flow can be evaluated. In about 10 minutes after injection, gland function becomes obvious by uptake of the nuclide into the gland. Five to 10 minutes later, one should see secretion of nuclear material into the mouth. Washout demonstrates complete salivary gland excretion. Usually the patient is asked to suck on a lemon to encourage rapid washout. This test can indicate inflammation, hypofunction, location and character of tumors, and duct obstruction.

Contraindications

Patients who are pregnant, unless the benefits outweigh the risks

Interfering factors

Rinsing mouth prior to study may reduce excretion.

Procedure and patient care

Before

PT Explain the procedure to the patient.

PT Tell the patient that no specific preparation is necessary.

- Make certain that the patient does not receive any thyroid-blocking agents within 48 hours of testing.

During

- Tc-99m pertechnetate is injected into the antecubital vein.
- Dynamic images are obtained immediately.
- Repeat images are obtained every 3 to 5 minutes for a total of 15 to 20 minutes.
- Administer a salivary gland stimulant after completion of static images. Either lemon juice or a lemon slice should be swished in the mouth and then expectorated.
- "Washout" images are obtained 5 to 10 minutes after the salivary gland stimulant. The thyroid gland is included for reference/comparison.

After

PT Assure the patient that the dose of radioactive technetium used in this test is minute and therefore harmless. No isolation or special urine precautions are needed.

Abnormal findings

Sjögren's syndrome
Benign mixed tumors/pleomorphic adenomas
Malignant lesions (e.g., adenocarcinomas, squamous cell carcinomas, undifferentiated and mixed carcinomas)
Salivary duct obstruction

notes

S

SARS viral testing

Type of test Blood; fluid analysis

Normal findings No SARS virus

Test explanation and related physiology

Severe acute respiratory syndrome, or SARS, has now killed more than 100 people and infected some 2600 in 20 countries. A coronavirus (CoV) causes SARS. China's southern Guangdong province, which includes Hong Kong, is believed to be the source of the virus, which has about an 8- to 10-day incubation period. Symptoms are similar to any pneumonia (fever, chills, and cough). The diagnosis should be suspected in a symptomatic patient who lives in or has traveled to an area having documented transmission of the illness. Routine testing for the SARS virus is not conducted unless a cluster of cases develops and health officials are able to rule out all other infectious agents.

Three tests are currently available. They are:

Enzyme-linked immunosorbent assay (ELISA)—This test detects antibodies to CoV. The test identifies antibodies 20 days after the start of symptoms. That means it cannot be used to detect cases in the early stage of illness.

Immunofluorescence assay (IFA)—This method detects SARS antibodies as early as 10 days after infection, but is a complex and relatively slow test that requires growing the virus in the laboratory.

Reverse transcriptase-polymerase chain reaction (RT-PCR)—This molecular test detects the SARS virus by amplifying RNA genetic information from a cultured sample by a reverse transcriptase-polymerase chain reaction. It is good at detecting early stages of the infection, and results can be available in 2 days.

The diagnosis can only be made with positive test results in the following situations with:

One specimen tested on two occasions using the original clinical specimen on each occasion,

Two clinical specimens from different sources (e.g., nasopharyngeal and stool), and

Two clinical specimens collected from the same source on two different days (e.g., two nasopharyngeal aspirates).

Eight types of respiratory specimens may be collected for viral and/or bacterial diagnostics: (1) nasopharyngeal wash/ aspirates, (2) nasopharyngeal swabs, (3) oropharyngeal swabs, (4) bronchoalveolar lavage, (5) tracheal aspirate, (6) pleural fluid tap, (7) sputum, and (8) postmortem tissue. Nasopharyngeal wash/aspirates are the specimen of choice for detection of most respiratory viruses.

Serum and blood (plasma) should be collected early in the illness for RT-PCR testing. The reliability of RT-PCR testing performed on blood specimens decreases as the illness progresses. Both acute and convalescent serum specimens should be collected for antibody testing. To confirm or rule out SARS-CoV infection, it is important to collect convalescent serum specimens more than 28 days after the onset of illness.

Procedure and patient care

Before

- ☛ Explain the procedure to the patient.
- Observe all universal precautions in handling specimen.
- Observe strict isolation technique. This disease is contagious.

During

- To obtain a *nasopharyngeal wash/aspirate*, have the patient sit with the head tilted slightly backward. Instill 1 to 1.5 ml of nonbacteriostatic saline (pH 7.0) into one nostril. Flush a plastic catheter or tubing with 2 to 3 ml of saline. Insert the tubing into the nostril. Aspirate nasopharyngeal secretions. Repeat this procedure for the other nostril. Collect the specimens in sterile vials.
- To obtain a *nasopharyngeal or oropharyngeal swab*, use only sterile dacron or rayon swabs with plastic shafts. Do not use a cotton swab or swabs with wooden sticks, as they may contain substances that inactivate some viruses and inhibit PCR testing. Insert the swab into the nostril. Leave the swab in place for a few seconds to absorb secretions. Swab both nostrils. (For *oropharyngeal culture*, swab the posterior pharynx and tonsillar areas, avoiding the tongue.)
- To collect *sputum*, educate the patient about the difference between sputum and oral secretions. Have the patient rinse the mouth with water and then expectorate deep-cough sputum directly into a sterile screw-cap sputum collection cup or sterile dry container.

S

- To collect *blood*, collect 5 to 10 ml of whole blood in a serum separator tube for serum RT-PCR testing or for ELISA antibody testing. Collect 5 to 10 ml of blood in an EDTA (purple-top) tube for plasma testing.

After
- Provide acute care for respiratory illness.
- If shipping the specimen domestically, use cold packs to keep the sample at 4° C. If shipping internationally, pack in dry ice.

Abnormal findings
SARS

notes

Schilling test (Vitamin B$_{12}$ absorption test)

Type of test Urine (24- to 48-hour); nuclear

Normal findings Excretion of 8%-40% of radioactive vitamin B$_{12}$ within 24 hours

Test explanation and related physiology

The Schilling test is performed to evaluate vitamin B$_{12}$ absorption. Normally ingested vitamin B$_{12}$ combines with intrinsic factor (IF), which is produced by gastric mucosa, and is absorbed in the distal part of the ileum. Pernicious anemia results when absorption of vitamin B$_{12}$ is inadequate. This may be caused by a primary malabsorption problem of the intestinal tract or from lack of IF.

The two-stage Schilling test can detect a defect in vitamin B$_{12}$ absorption. With normal absorption, the ileum absorbs more vitamin B$_{12}$ than the body needs and excretes the excess into the urine. With impaired absorption, however, little or no vitamin B$_{12}$ is excreted into the urine.

In the Schilling test, urinary B$_{12}$ levels are measured after the ingestion of radioactive vitamin B$_{12}$. The test can be performed in one stage (without IF) or two stages (with IF). Patients with pernicious anemia from lack of IF will have an abnormal first-stage and a normal second-stage Schilling test. Patients with malabsorption from an intestinal source will have an abnormal first- and second-stage Schilling test. A combined one-stage and two-stage test is now commonly used.

In some clinical situations, the Schilling test is repeated after a course of antibiotic or anti-inflammatory drug therapy. Because vitamin B$_{12}$ is absorbed primarily in the distal ileum, an abnormal response to the Schilling test may also indicate a pathologic condition of the distal small bowel. For example, in regional enteritis and lymphomas, the first- and second-stage Schilling tests are frequently abnormal. However, the Schilling test response may normalize after treatment with prednisone or sulfasalazine. The Schilling test may also be helpful in establishing a diagnosis of intestinal bacteria overgrowth of the small bowel. Under these conditions, the first- and second-stage Schilling tests frequently give an abnormal result. However, after appropriate antibiotic treatment, the Schilling test response usually returns to normal.

S

All bone marrow and hematologic studies along with serum vitamin B_{12} levels must be done before the Schilling test. The vitamin B_{12} that is administered during this test can significantly alter the test results.

Contraindications

- Patients who are pregnant, unless the benefits outweigh the risks
- Patients who are lactating

Interfering factors

- Radioactive nuclear material received 10 days before testing may affect results.
- Renal insufficiency may cause reduced excretion of radioactive vitamin B_{12}.
- Patients who are elderly, have hypothyroidism, or have diabetes may have reduced excretion of vitamin B_{12}.
- ✗ Drugs that may affect test results include laxatives, because they could *decrease* the rate of vitamin B_{12} absorption.

Procedure and patient care

Before

- PT Explain the procedure to the patient.
- PT Instruct the patient to remain NPO except for water 8 to 12 hours before the test. Food should not be given until after the patient receives the injections.
- PT Instruct the patient not to take laxatives during the test period.

During

- Note the following procedural steps:

First-stage Schilling test (without intrinsic factor)
1. Radioactive vitamin B_{12} is administered orally to the patient.
2. Shortly thereafter, nonradioactive vitamin B_{12} is administered to the patient intramuscularly to saturate tissue-binding sites and to permit some excretion of radioactive vitamin B_{12} in the urine if it is absorbed.
3. A 24- to 48-hour urine collection for vitamin B_{12} is obtained.
4. The patient is encouraged to drink fluids.

Second-stage Schilling test (with intrinsic factor)
1. If indicated, the second stage is performed approximately 1 week after the first stage.
2. The fasting patient is provided radioactive vitamin B_{12} combined with human intrinsic factor.

3. As before, an IM injection of nonradioactive vitamin B_{12} is administered.

4. Again, 24- to 48-hour urine collections are begun.

Combined one-stage and two-stage Schilling test

1. The fasting patient receives a capsule of cobalt-57–labeled vitamin B_{12} plus intrinsic factor.

2. A second capsule of cobalt-58–labeled vitamin B_{12} is also given.

3. One hour later an IM injection of nonradioactive vitamin B_{12} is administered.

4. Again the urine for vitamin B_{12} is collected for 24 to 48 hours.

5. Percentages of cobalt-57 and cobalt-58 are calculated. Cobalt-57–labeled vitamin B_{12} will be present only in patients with pernicious anemia secondary to lack of intrinsic factor. No vitamin B_{12} will be present in the urine of patients whose pernicious anemia is caused by primary bowel malabsorption.

After

- Ensure that the urine specimens are promptly transported to the laboratory.

Abnormal findings

▼ **Decreased levels**

Pernicious anemia
Intestinal malabsorption
Hypothyroidism
Liver disease
Regional enteritis
Lymphomas
Blind loop syndrome
Scleroderma
Small bowel diverticula

S

notes

scrotal nuclear imaging (Scrotal scan, Testicular imaging)

Type of test Nuclear medicine

Normal findings Symmetric and prompt blood flow to both testicles

Test explanation and related physiology

Scrotal imaging is helpful in the diagnosis of patients with a sudden onset of unilateral testicular swelling and pain. Scrotal imaging can differentiate unilateral testicular torsion from other causes of testicular pain (e.g., acute epididymitis, torsion of the testicular appendage, orchitis, strangulated hernia, testicular hemorrhage). Testicular torsion is a surgical emergency requiring prompt surgical exploration to salvage the involved testicle. It must be differentiated from other causes of testicular pain to provide immediate surgical care if the testicle is to be salvaged. The other causes of painful testicular swelling do not require surgery. Use of radionuclide scrotal imaging enables the surgeon to diagnose testicular torsion. However, in nearly all circumstances today, scrotal ultrasound (see p. 826) has supplanted this test for the diagnosis of testicular tortion.

The patient is positioned under the gamma ray camera with the scrotum supported between the abducted thighs. Technetium-99m pertechnetate is administered, and a dynamic radionuclide angiogram is obtained. Static images are obtained immediately afterward. An area of decreased perfusion corresponding to the involved testis indicates a high probability of torsion of the testicle. If the clinically involved testis is normally perfused or hypervascular, a disease other than torsion of the testicle (as described earlier) exists. In 95% of all cases of testicular torsion, the scrotal image will make the diagnosis. This information can be obtained 10 to 15 minutes after injection of the nuclear material.

Procedure and patient care

Before

PT Explain the procedure to the patient.

PT Tell the patient that no fasting or premedication is required.

PT Assure the patient that he will not be exposed to large amounts of radiation, because only tracer doses of isotope are used.

■ If the patient is a child, encourage the parent(s) to be present.

During

- The patient is placed on a padded table in the supine position.
- The patient's legs are abducted, and the testicles are supported with tape or a lead shield. The penis is taped to the lower abdomen.
- A small IV injection of technetium-99m pertechnetate is administered.
- Radionuclide imaging is then immediately performed over both testicles. Both dynamic and static images are obtained.

After

PT Because only tracer doses of radioisotopes are used, inform the patient that no precautions need to be taken by others against radiation exposure.

- If the patient is identified as having torsion of the testicle, prepare him for surgery.

Abnormal findings

▲ **Increased testicular blood flow**

Epididymitis
Torsion of the testicular appendage
Orchitis
Trauma

▼ **Decreased testicular blood flow**

Testicular torsion of the spermatic cord

notes

S

scrotal ultrasound (Ultrasound of testes)

Type of test Ultrasound

Normal findings Normal size, shape, and configuration of the testicles

Test explanation and related physiology

With the advent of scrotal ultrasound, a noninvasive, nonionizing, rapid method for scrotal examination was developed. Through the use of reflected sound waves, ultrasonography provides accurate visualization of the scrotum and its contents. Ultrasonography requires the emission of high-frequency sound waves from the transducer to penetrate the organ being studied. The sound waves are bounced back to the transducer and electronically converted into a pictorial image.

Present uses for scrotal ultrasound include:

1. Evaluation of scrotal masses
2. Measurement of testicular size
3. Evaluation of scrotal trauma
4. Evaluation of scrotal pain
5. Evaluation of occult testicular neoplasm
6. Surveillance of patients with prior primary or metastatic testicular neoplasms
7. Follow-up for testicular infections
8. Location of undescended testicles
9. Ultrasound guided needle biopsy of a suspected testicle tumor

With the real-time ultrasound transducer, the scrotum is examined. The testicle and extratesticular intrascrotal tissues are examined. The accuracy of scrotal ultrasound is 90% to 95%. Both benign and malignant tumors (primary and metastatic) can be identified with ultrasound. Benign abnormalities such as testicular abscess, orchitis, testicular infarction, and testicular torsion also can be identified. Extratesticular lesions such as hydrocele, hematocele (blood in the scrotum), and pyocele (pus in the scrotum) can be identified as well. Scrotal and groin ultrasound has been very helpful in locating cryptorchid (undescended) testicles.

There is very little discomfort associated with testicular ultrasound. It is usually performed by an ultrasound technologist and interpreted by an ultrasound physician.

Procedure and patient care

Before
PT Explain the procedure to the patient.
PT Tell the patient that no fasting is required.

During
▪ Note the following procedural steps:
1. Careful examination of the scrotum is performed by the physician. Usually a short history is obtained.
2. The scrotum is supported by a towel or cradled by the examiner's gloved hand.
3. A greasy, conductive paste is applied to the scrotum before scanning. This paste enhances sound wave transmission and reception.
4. Thorough scanning in the sagittal, transverse, and oblique projections is performed.
▪ The test takes approximately 20 to 30 minutes.

After
▪ Remove the coupling agent (grease) from the patient's scrotum.

Abnormal findings

Benign testicular tumor
Malignant testicular tumor
Occult testicular tumor
Testicular infection (orchitis)
Hydrocele
Hematocele
Pyocele
Varicocele
Epididymitis
Spermatocele
Scrotal hernia
Cryptorchidism
Hematoma
Testicular torsion

S

secretin-pancreozymin (Pancreatic enzymes)

Type of test Fluid analysis

Normal findings

Volume: 2-4 ml/kg body weight
HCO_3 (bicarbonate): 90-130 mEq/L
Amylase: 6.6-35.2 units/kg

Test explanation and related physiology

Cystic fibrosis is an inherited disease characterized by abnormal secretion by exocrine glands within the bronchi, small intestines, pancreatic ducts, bile ducts, and skin (sweat glands). Because of this abnormal exocrine secretion, children with cystic fibrosis develop mucous plugs that obstruct their pancreatic ducts. The pancreatic enzymes (e.g., amylase, lipase, trypsin, chymotrypsin) cannot be expelled into the duodenum and therefore are either completely absent or present only in diminished quantities within the duodenal aspirate. For the same reasons, bicarbonate and other neutralizing fluids cannot be secreted from the pancreas.

In this test, secretin and pancreozymin are used to stimulate pancreatic secretion of these enzymes and bicarbonate into the duodenum. The duodenal contents are then aspirated and examined for pH, bicarbonate, and enzyme levels; amylase is the most frequently measured enzyme. Diminished values are suggestive of cystic fibrosis. This test is indicated in children with recurrent respiratory tract infections, malabsorption syndromes, or failure to thrive.

Procedure and patient care

Before
PT Explain the procedure to the patient and/or parents.
PT Instruct the adult patient to fast for 12 hours before testing.
- Determine pediatric fasting times according to the patient's age.

During
- Note the following procedural steps:
    1. With the use of fluoroscopy, a Dreiling tube is passed through the patient's nose and into the stomach.

2. The distal lumen of the tube is placed within the duodenum.
3. The proximal lumen of the tube is placed within the stomach.
4. Both lumens are aspirated. The gastric lumen is continually aspirated to avoid contamination of the gastric contents in the duodenum aspirate.
5. A control specimen of the duodenal juices is collected for 20 minutes.
6. The patient is tested for sensitivity to secretin and pancreozymin by low-dose intradermal injection.
7. If no sensitivity is present, these hormones are administered intravenously. Secretin can be expected to stimulate pancreatic water and bicarbonate secretion. Pancreozymin can be expected to stimulate pancreatic enzyme (lipase, amylase, trypsin, chymotrypsin) secretion.
8. Four duodenal aspirates are collected at 20-minute intervals and placed in the specimen container.
9. Each specimen is analyzed for pH, volume, bicarbonate, and amylase levels.

- Note that a physician performs this test in approximately 2 hours in the laboratory or at the patient's bedside.
- **PT** Tell the patient that he or she may have discomfort and gagging during placement of the Dreiling tube.

After

- Place the aspirated specimens on ice. Send them to the chemistry laboratory as soon as the test is completed.
- Remove the Dreiling tube after completion of the test. Give appropriate nose and mouth care.
- Allow the patient to resume a normal diet.

Abnormal findings

Cystic fibrosis
Sprue

notes

semen analysis (Sperm count, Sperm examination, Seminal cytology, Semen examination)

Type of test Fluid analysis

Normal findings

Volume: 2-5 ml
Liquefaction time: 20-30 minutes after collection
pH: 7.12-8.00
Sperm count (density): 50-200 million/ml
Sperm motility: 60%-80% actively motile
Sperm morphology: 70%-90% normally shaped

Test explanation and related physiology

Semen analysis is one of the most important aspects of the fertility workup because the cause of a woman's inability to conceive often lies with the man. After 2 to 3 days of sexual abstinence, sperm is collected and examined for volume, sperm count, motility, and morphology.

The freshly collected semen is first measured for volume. After liquefaction of the white, gelatinous ejaculate, a sperm count is done. Men with very low or very high counts likely are infertile. The motility of the sperm is then evaluated; at least 60% should show progressive motility. Morphology is studied by staining a semen preparation and calculating the number of normal versus abnormal sperm forms. A single sperm analysis, especially if it indicates infertility, is inconclusive, because sperm count varies from day to day. A semen analysis should be done at least twice, and possibly a third time, 3 weeks apart.

Semen production depends on the function of the testicles. Semen analysis is a measure of testicular function. Inadequate sperm production can be the result of primary gonadal failure (Klinefelter's syndrome, infection, radiation, or surgical orchidectomy) or secondary gonadal failure (caused by pituitary diseases). Men with *aspermia* (no sperm) or *oligospermia* (20 million/ml) should be evaluated endocrinologically for pituitary, thyroid, or testicular aberrations.

A normal semen analysis alone does not accurately assess the male factor unless the effect of the partner's cervical secretion on sperm survival is also determined (see Sims-Huhner test, p. 852). In addition to its value in infertility workups, semen analysis is also helpful in documenting adequate sterilization after a vasectomy. It is usually performed 6 weeks after the surgery. If any sperm are seen, the adequacy of the vasectomy must be questioned.

Interfering factors

✠ Drugs that may cause *decreased* semen levels include antineoplastic agents (e.g., nitrogen mustard, procarbazine, vincristine, methotrexate), cimetidine, estrogens, and methyltestosterone.

Procedure and patient care

Before

PT Explain the procedure to the patient.

PT Instruct the patient to abstain from sexual activity for 2 to 3 days before collecting the specimen. Prolonged abstinence before the collection should be discouraged because the quality of the sperm cells, and especially their motility, may diminish.

■ Give the patient the proper container for the sperm collection.

PT Instruct the patient to avoid alcoholic beverages for several days before the collection.

■ For evaluation of the adequacy of vasectomy, the patient should ejaculate once or twice before the day of examination.

During

■ Note that semen is best collected by ejaculation into a clean container. For best results, the specimen should be collected in the physician's office or laboratory by masturbation.

PT Note that less satisfactory specimens can be obtained in the patient's home by coitus interruptus or masturbation. Note the following procedural steps:

1. Instruct the patient to deliver these home specimens to the laboratory within 1 hour after collection.
2. Tell the patient to avoid excessive heat and cold during transportation of the specimen.

After

■ Record the date of the previous semen emission, along with the collection time and date of the fresh specimen.

PT Tell the patient when and how to obtain the test results. Remember that abnormal results may have a devastating effect on the patient's sexuality.

S

Abnormal findings

Infertility
Vasectomy (obstruction of vas deferens)
Orchitis
Testicular atrophy
Testicular failure
Hyperpyrexia

notes

sentinel lymph node biopsy (SLNB, Lymphoscintigraphy)

Type of test Nuclear scan

Normal findings Uptake is noted in one or more lymph nodes. No tumor is noted in sentinel node.

Test explanation and related physiology

With this procedure, the first (sentinel) lymph node in line to catch metastatic tumor cells from a primary tumor can be identified. In order to stage cancers such as breast, melanoma, and others, a lymph node dissection has been required. With the use of SLNB, the first lymph node in the chain of lymph nodes can be identified and biopsied. If results are negative, the rest of the lymph contents can be safely assumed to be free of tumor and are not removed. This saves the patient potential complications associated with a full lymph node dissection such as swelling, cellulitis, postoperative pain, and reduced range of motion of the affected extremity. Furthermore, this test can identify unusual locations for lymph node metastasis that would not normally be examined.

A tracer (isosulfan blue dye or technetium) is injected into the tissue surrounding the tumor. If *technetium* is used, a handheld gamma detector is used to identify the region of maximum radioactivity. If *isosulfan blue dye* is injected, a blue node is seen at surgery. The sentinel lymph node is the blue node or "hot" node. If the sentinel lymph node does not contain any tumor, the lymph node dissection procedure is aborted. If the sentinel lymph node contains tumor, a full lymph node dissection is carried out. In some instances, immunochemical stains are applied to the sentinel lymph node. Tumor can be more easily detected with these special stains.

This test is quickly becoming an important part of the standard treatment for breast and melanoma cancer surgery. A similar diagnostic procedure for colon cancer will soon be developed. It is important to note that uptake of dye or radionuclide does not indicate whether a lymph node contains metastatic tumor. It only locates the lymph node that is most likely to contain tumor, if metastasis occurred.

S

Contraindications

- Patients with prior surgery to the lymph node area to be studied

Potential complications

- Anaphylaxis has been reported with injection of isosulfan blue dye.

Interfering factors

- A poorly placed injection of dye or nuclide can interfere with identification of the sentinel lymph node.

Procedure and patient care

Before
PT Explain the procedure to the patient.
- Because this is an operative procedure, routine preoperative procedures should be carried out, including obtaining operative consent, keeping the patient on NPO status, and surgical site preparation as ordered.

During
- Note the following procedural steps:
Technetium
1. The patient is taken to the nuclear medicine department, where the radionuclide is injected around the tumor.
2. The site of lymph node drainage is then scanned immediately and 2 to 24 hours later.
3. Lymph node uptake is reported to the surgeon.
4. In the operating room, a handheld gamma detector locates "hot" areas of radionuclide uptake in the lymph node–bearing area.
Isosulfan blue
1. In the operating room, 4 to 5 ml of isosulfan blue dye is injected around the tumor.
2. After 5 to 9 minutes, a small incision is made overlying the lymph node–bearing area and the proximal blue lymph node is removed as the sentinel lymph node.
PT Inform the patient that the only discomfort associated with the test is the preoperative injections required around the tumor.

After

PT Inform the patient that no radiation precautions are required if technetium is used because the radionuclide dose is minimal.

PT If isosulfan blue dye is used, inform the patient that the skin may develop a transient blue hue (looking almost like severe cyanosis). This will dissipate over the next 6 to 12 hours.

PT Warn the patient that the urine will have a blue tinge as a result of the isosulfan blue dye injection.

■ Observe the patient for signs of allergy (rare) due to the blue dye injection.

Abnormal findings

Metastatic tumor to lymph node

notes

S

sexual assault testing

Type of test Blood; fluid analysis

Normal findings No physical evidence of sexual assault

Test explanation and related physiology

The sexual assault victim needs to have psycho-emotional support, treatment of any physical injuries, and accurate and reliable evidentiary testing. Nearly all acute care centers have protocols in place that provide care to victims of sexual assault. Furthermore, in most circumstances, there are nurses specifically trained in obtaining the appropriate specimens. This person knows the importance of following the chain of evidence protocols to ensure that evidence is admissible in court.

While being provided with emotional support and assistance, the patient is first interviewed in a nonjudgmental manner. A thorough gynecologic history is obtained. A brief summary of the assault (if there was vaginal, oral, or anal penetration during the assault) and timing of the assault is important. After 72 hours, very little evidence still exists. It is important to ascertain if the victim changed clothing, showered, or used a douche before coming to the hospital. These will affect the presence of evidence. The general demeanor of the patient, status of the clothing, and physical maturation assessment is documented.

The victim's clothes are removed and separately placed in a paper bag for possible DNA sources of the victim's or assailant's body parts. Plastic bags are not used because bacteria may grow in them and can destroy DNA. Photographs of all injuries should be obtained, if possible. The victim is then examined for signs of external and internal injuries. A pelvic exam is then performed. A "sexual assault evidence collection kit" is used to obtain all the needed specimens. The directions must be carefully followed to ensure that any and all evidence is obtained and is useful toward identification and conviction of the perpetrator.

Vaginal secretions are obtained for sperm (see p. 830), or other cells from the assailant. Acid phosphatase (see p. 7) or PSA (see p. 755) are also obtained using this specimen. Cervical secretions are obtained for sexually transmitted disease (STD) (see p. 840) testing. These anatomic areas, along with the anorectal area, are swabbed per directions in the kit. In the male victim, penile and anorectal areas are swabbed. Pubic hair is obtained by combing or plucking. STD testing would include syphilis (p. 888), trichomoniasis (p. 841), gonorrhea (p. 841), and chlamydia (p. 257). Later, blood testing for human immunodeficiency virus (HIV) (p. 529) and pregnancy (p. 740) is obtained.

Next blood specimens are obtained for DNA testing per the testing kit directions, usually an EDTA-containing tube (lavender topped). More blood or urine also may be collected for evidence of mind-altering drugs/alcohol or STDs. After this testing, a more detailed examination of the vagina, cervix, and rectum is performed using a Wood's lamp to identify more easily saliva or sperm from the assailant. These areas are examined for subtle injuries from forced penetration. Two methods used to identify these injuries are the toluidine blue dye test and a colposcope (see p. 289). The *toluidine blue dye test* also can be used to identify recent or healed genital or anorectal injuries. A 1% aqueous solution is applied to the area of concern and washed off with a lubricant (e.g., K-Y jelly) or a 1% acetic acid solution. Injured mucosa will retain the dye and become more apparent to the naked eye. Finally, the fingernails are scraped underneath, which may potentially contain tissue from the assailant. Upon completion of the exam, the victim is usually interviewed by the police for further investigation.

Unless medically contraindicated, all survivors should be offered antimicrobial therapy to prevent STDs. The following combination of drugs is used in public hospitals: ciprofloxacin 250 mg po stat dose; doxycycline 100 mg bid for 7 days; and metronidazole 2 g stat. The use of antiretroviral drugs in the prevention of HIV transmission may be recommended, and the current guideline for postexposure prophylaxis after needle stick injuries should be used. It may also be advisable to offer survivors a hepatitis B vaccination or Hepatitis B immunoglobulin, as the disease may be fatal. Survivors who are at risk for HIV infection should also be given counseling on HIV/acquired immunodeficiency syndrome (AIDS).

A pregnancy test should be done before any treatment or drugs are prescribed. If there is a risk of pregnancy, the survivor should be offered postcoital contraception if the rape occurred less than 72 hours before examination by the healthcare worker. If it occurred more than 72 hours but less than 7 days before the examination, an intrauterine contraceptive device may be used to prevent pregnancy. Pregnancy testing may be repeated in the week after the rape.

Contraindications

- The patient is emotionally unable to undergo the examination.

Interfering factors

- Delays in examination after the alleged attack diminish the possibility of identifying meaningful evidence.

Procedure and patient care

Before

PT Explain the procedure to the patient and provide emotional support.
- Obtain consent to treat the patient or family.
- Notify any family members the patient would like present during the exam.
- Assess the patient's emotional position and determine if the victim is able to undergo sexual assault testing.

During

- Obtain a thorough history as described above.
- Use the SAPS Sexual Assault Evidence Collection Kit (SAECK) or similar test kit exactly as described to maintain the chain of evidence.
- Properly handle the kit specimens to maintain the chain of custody.
- Refrigerate all samples containing biological evidentiary material such as DNA to prevent putrefaction (decomposition).
- It is important to examine carefully all areas of the body to help corroborate the survivor's version of the alleged events.

After

- Notify police of the alleged assault.
- Assess the patient's need for urgent counseling support and make arrangements, as needed.
- If additional or ongoing counseling is required, the patient should be referred to a trained counselor in a victim support.

| Box 1 | DNA evidence collection: special precautions |

To avoid contamination of evidence that may contain DNA, the special sexual assault kit should be used and the following precautions taken:
- Wear gloves and change them often.
- Use disposable instruments or clean them thoroughly before and after handling each sample.
- Avoid touching any area where you believe DNA may be present.
- Avoid talking, sneezing, or coughing over evidence.
- Avoid touching your face, nose, and mouth when collecting and packaging evidence.
- Keep evidence dry and transport it at room temperature.
- Ensure that the chain of custody is maintained at all times.

Abnormal findings

Rape
Sexual assault

notes

S

sexually transmitted disease cultures (STD cultures; Culture of cervix, urethra, and anus)

Type of test Microscopic examination; blood

Normal findings No evidence of sexually transmitted disease

Test explanation and related physiology

STDs can cause urethritis, vaginitis, endometritis, pelvic inflammatory disease, pharyngitis, proctitis, epididymitis, prostatitis, and salpingitis. Children born of infected mothers may develop conjunctivitis, pneumonia, neonatal blindness, neonatal neurologic injury, and even death.

Cultures for STD infections are performed on men and women with suggestive symptoms. If the culture is positive, sexual partners should be evaluated and treated. Cervical cultures are usually done for women; urethral cultures are done for men. Rectal and throat cultures are performed in persons who have engaged in anal and oral intercourse. Because rectal gonorrhea accompanies genital gonorrhea in a high percentage of women, rectal cultures are recommended in all women with suspected gonorrhea.

Other STDs are identified by culture or smear of a genital lesion, tissue biopsy, serologic testing, and observation of classic clinical lesion (Table 21).

Interfering factors

- *Neisseria gonorrhoeae* can be destroyed by the use of lubricants and disinfectants.
- Menses may alter test results.
- Female douching within 24 hours of a cervical culture makes fewer organisms available for culture.
- Male voiding within 1 hour of a urethral culture washes secretions out of the urethra.
- Fecal material may contaminate an anal culture.

Procedure and patient care

Before

PT Explain the purpose and procedure to the patient. Use a matter-of-fact, nonjudgmental approach.

PT Tell the patient that no fasting or sedation is required.

TABLE 21 Sexually transmitted diseases (STDs) and methods of diagnosis

Disease	Method of diagnosis
Gonorrhea	Cervical, urethral, anal, oropharyngeal cultures
Chlamydia Lymphogranuloma venereum *C. trachomatis*	Cervical, urethral culture, serology, DNA probe testing (see p. 257)
Herpes genitalis	Culture from lesion, serology (see p. 524)
Syphilis	Serology, fluid cultures (CNS), darkfield slide (see p. 888)
Hepatitis	Serology (see p. 519)
AIDS	Serology (see p. 23)
Trichomoniasis	Cervical, urethral, vaginal smear on a wet mount
Candida (Monilia)	Wet mount, Gram stain, fungal culture
Gardnerella vaginalis	Cervical, urethral, anal cultures

During

- Obtain cultures as follows:

Cervical culture

1. The female patient is told to refrain from douching and tub bathing before the cervical culture.
2. The patient is placed in the lithotomy position, and a moistened nonlubricated vaginal speculum is inserted to expose the cervix.
3. Cervical mucus is removed with a cotton ball held in a ring forceps.
4. A sterile cotton-tipped swab is inserted into the endocervical canal and moved from side to side to obtain the culture.
5. The swab is placed in sterile saline or a transporting fluid obtained from the laboratory. The specimen should be plated as soon as possible. The specimen should not be refrigerated.

Anal canal culture

1. An anal culture of the female or male patient is taken by inserting a sterile cotton-tipped swab approximately 1 inch into the anal canal (Figure 37).
2. If stool contaminates the swab, a repeat swab is taken.

Urethral culture

1. The urethral specimen should be obtained from the male patient before voiding. Voiding within 1 hour of collection washes secretions out of the urethra, making fewer organisms available for culture. The best time to obtain the specimen is before the first morning micturition.
2. A culture is taken by inserting a sterile swab gently into the anterior urethra (see Figure 38).
3. It is advisable to place the male patient in the supine position to prevent falling if vasovagal syncope occurs during introduction of the cotton swab or wire loop into the urethra.
4. The patient is observed for hypotension, bradycardia, pallor, sweating, nausea, and weakness.
5. Prostatic massage may increase the chances of obtaining positive cultures.

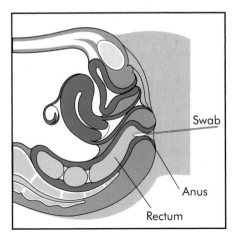

Figure 37 Rectal culture of the female. Method for obtaining an anorectal culture for sexually transmitted diseases on a female patient.

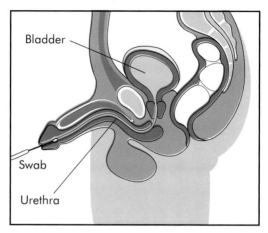

Figure 38 Urethral culture of the male. Method for obtaining a urethral culture for sexually transmitted diseases on a male patient.

Oropharyngeal culture
1. This culture should be obtained in male and female patients who have engaged in oral intercourse.
2. A throat culture is best obtained by depressing the patient's tongue with a wooden tongue blade and touching the posterior wall of the throat with a sterile cotton-tipped swab.

After
- Place the swabs for gonorrhea in a Thayer-Martin medium and roll them from side to side.
- Label and send the culture bottle to the microbiology laboratory.
- Transport the specimen to the laboratory as soon as possible.
- Handle all specimens as though they were capable of transmitting disease.
- Do not refrigerate the specimen.
- Mark the laboratory slip with the collection time, date, source of specimen, patient's age, current antibiotic therapy, and clinical diagnosis.
- **PT** Advise the patient to avoid intercourse and all sexual contact until test results are available.

PT If the culture results are positive, tell the patient to obtain treatment and to have sexual partners evaluated.

- Note that repeat cultures should be taken after completion of treatment to evaluate therapy.

Abnormal findings

STD

notes

sialography

Type of test X-ray

Normal findings No evidence of pathology in the salivary ducts and related structures

Test explanation and related physiology

Sialography is an x-ray procedure used to examine the salivary ducts (parotid, submaxillary, submandibular, sublingual) and related glandular structures after injection of a contrast medium into the desired duct. This procedure is used to detect calculi, strictures, tumors, or inflammatory disease in patients who complain of pain, tenderness, or swelling in these areas.

Contraindications

- Patients with mouth infections

Potential complications

- Allergic reaction to the iodinated dye
  This rarely occurs because the dye is not administered intravenously.

Procedure and patient care

Before

PT Explain the procedure to the patient. The thought of a dye injection in the mouth is frightening to many patients. Provide emotional support.

- Obtain informed consent if required by the institution.

PT Instruct the patient to remove jewelry, hairpins, and dentures, which could obscure x-ray visualization.

PT Instruct the patient to rinse his or her mouth with an antiseptic solution before the procedure to reduce the possibility of introducing bacteria into the ductal structures.

During

- Note the following procedural steps:
  1. X-ray studies are taken before the dye injection to ensure that stones are not present, which could prevent the contrast material from entering the ducts.
  2. The patient is placed in a supine position on an x-ray table.

3. The contrast medium is injected directly into the desired orifice via a cannula or a special catheter.
4. X-ray films are taken with the patient in various positions.
5. The patient is given a sour substance (e.g., lemon juice) orally to stimulate salivary excretion.
6. Another set of x-ray studies is taken to evaluate ductal drainage.

- Note that a radiologist performs this procedure in the radiology department in less than 30 minutes.

PT Tell the patient that he or she may feel a little pressure as the contrast medium is injected into the ducts.

After

PT Encourage the patient to drink fluids to eliminate the dye.

Abnormal findings

Calculi
Strictures
Tumor
Inflammatory disease

notes

sickle cell test (Sickle cell preparation, Sickledex, Hemoglobin [Hgb] S test)

Type of test Blood

Normal findings No sickle cells present

Test explanation and related physiology

Both sickle cell disease (homozygous for Hgb S) and sickle cell trait (heterozygous for Hgb S) can be detected by this study. Sickle cell anemia results from a genetic homozygous defect and is caused by the presence of Hgb S instead of Hgb A. When Hgb S becomes deoxygenated, it tends to bend in a way that causes the red blood cell (RBC) to assume a sickle shape. These sickled RBCs cannot freely pass through the capillaries, and thus they cause plugging of the microvascular tree. This may compromise the blood supply to various organs. Hgb S is found in varying quantities in 8% to 10% of the black population.

A routine peripheral blood smear of patients with sickle cell disease does not contain sickled RBCs unless hypoxemia is present. In the sickle cell test, a deoxygenating agent is added to the patient's blood. If 25% or more of the patient's hemoglobin is of the S variation, the cells will assume the crescent (sickle) shape, and the test is positive. If no sickling occurs, the test is negative. A negative test indicates that the patient has no or very little Hgb S. Other less common hemoglobin variants also may cause sickling.

This test is only a screening test, and its sensitivity varies according to the method used by the laboratory. The definitive diagnosis is made by hemoglobin electrophoresis (see p. 516), in which Hgb S can be identified and quantified.

Interfering factors

- Any blood transfusions within 3 to 4 months before the sickle cell test may cause false-negative results because the donor's normal hemoglobin may dilute the recipient's abnormal Hgb S.
- Polycythemia may cause false-negative results.
- Infants younger than age 3 months may have false-negative results.
- Drugs that may cause false-negative results include phenothiazines.

Procedure and patient care

Before

PT Explain the procedure to the patient.

PT Tell the patient that no fasting is required.

During

- Collect approximately 7 ml of venous blood in a lavender-top tube.

After

- Apply pressure to the venipuncture site.
- If the test is positive, offer the family genetic counseling. A patient with one recessive gene (heterozygous) is said to have sickle cell *trait*. A patient with two recessive genes (homozygous) has sickle cell *anemia*.

PT Inform patients with sickle cell anemia that they should avoid situations in which hypoxia may occur (e.g., strenuous exercise, air travel in unpressurized aircraft, travel to high-altitude regions).

Abnormal findings

Sickle cell trait

Sickle cell anemia

notes

sigmoidoscopy (Proctoscopy, Anoscopy)

Type of test   Endoscopy

Normal findings   Normal anus, rectum, and sigmoid colon

Test explanation and related physiology

Endoscopy of the lower gastrointestinal (GI) tract allows one to visualize and perform biopsies of tumors, polyps, hemorrhoids, or ulcers of the anus, rectum, and sigmoid colon. *Anoscopy* refers to examination of the anus; *proctoscopy* to examination of the anus and rectum; and *sigmoidoscopy* (the most frequent procedure) to examination of the anus, rectum, and sigmoid colon. This test can be performed with a rigid or flexible sigmoidoscope. Because the lower GI tract is difficult to visualize radiographically, direct visualization by sigmoidoscopy is helpful.

Furthermore, sigmoidoscopy, as with colonoscopy, can be therapeutic. Reduction of sigmoid volvulus, removal of polyps, and obliteration of hemorrhoids can be performed through the sigmoidoscope.

Contraindications

- Patients who are uncooperative
- Patients with diverticulitis
- Patients with painful anorectal conditions (e.g., fissures, fistulas)
- Patients with severe bleeding
  Blood clots obstruct the view of the scope.
- Patients suspected of having perforated colon lesions

Potential complications

- Perforation of the colon
- Bleeding from biopsy sites

Interfering factors

- Poor bowel preparation may obscure visualization of the bowel mucosa.
- Rectal bleeding may obstruct the lens system and preclude adequate visualization.

Procedure and patient care

Before

PT Explain the procedure to the patient.

- Obtain informed consent for this procedure.
- Assist the patient with bowel preparation. In most cases two Fleet enemas are sufficient.

PT Instruct the patient to ingest only a light breakfast on the morning of the endoscopy.

- Assure patients that they will be properly draped to avoid unnecessary embarrassment.

During

- Note the following procedural steps:
  1. The patient is placed on the endoscopy table or bed in the left lateral decubitus position. Physicians often prefer the knee-chest position; many operating and examining tables are easily converted to make the knee-chest position more comfortable. This procedure also can be performed with the patient in the lithotomy position.
  2. Usually no sedation is required.
  3. The anus is mildly dilated with a well-lubricated finger.
  4. The rigid or flexible sigmoidoscope is placed into the rectum and advanced to its point of maximal penetration.
  5. Air is insufflated during the procedure to distend more fully the lower intestinal tract.
  6. The sigmoid, rectum, and anus are visualized.
  7. Biopsies can be obtained, and polypectomy performed at the time of sigmoidoscopy.
- Note that a physician trained in GI endoscopy usually performs this procedure in the GI laboratory, operating room, patient's bedside, or outpatient clinic setting in approximately 15 to 20 minutes.

PT Tell the patient that he or she probably will feel discomfort and the urge to defecate as the sigmoidoscope is inserted.

After

PT Inform the patient that because air has been insufflated into the bowel during the procedure, he or she may have flatulence or gas pains. Ambulation may help.

- Observe the patient for signs of abdominal distention, increased tenderness, or rectal bleeding.

PT Tell the patient that slight rectal bleeding may occur if biopsies have been taken.

🏠 **Home care responsibilities**

- Observe for increasing abdominal pain, which may indicate bowel perforation.
- Note that fever and chills may indicate a bowel perforation.
- Inform the patient that frequent bloody bowel movements may indicate poor hemostasis if biopsy or polypectomy was performed.
- Observe for abdominal bloating and inability to pass flatus, which may indicate colon obstruction if a neoplasm was identified.

Abnormal findings

Tumor (benign or malignant)
Polyps
Ulcerative colitis
Pseudomembranous colitis
Crohn's disease (regional enteritis)
Intestinal ischemia
Irritable bowel syndrome

notes

S

Sims-Huhner test (Postcoital test, Postcoital cervical mucus test, Cervical mucus sperm penetration test)

Type of test Fluid analysis

Normal findings

Cervical mucus adequate for sperm transmission, survival, and penetration

6 to 20 active sperm per high-power field

Test explanation and related physiology

The Sims-Huhner test consists of a postcoital examination of the cervical mucus to measure the ability of the sperm to penetrate the mucus and maintain motility. This test is used in the evaluation of infertile couples. It evaluates interaction between the sperm and the cervical mucus. It also measures the quality of the cervical mucus. This test can determine the effect of vaginal and cervical secretions on the activity of the sperm. It is performed only after a previously performed semen analysis has been determined to be normal.

This test is performed during the middle of the ovulatory cycle, because at this time the secretions should be optimal for sperm penetration and survival. During ovulation, the quantity of cervical mucus is maximal, whereas the viscosity is minimal, thus facilitating sperm penetration. The *endocervical mucus sample* is examined for color, viscosity, and tenacity *(spinnbarkeit)*. The fresh specimen is then spread on a clean glass slide and examined for the presence of sperm. Estimates of the total number of sperm and of the number of motile sperm per high-power field are reported. Normally 6 to 20 active sperm cells should be seen in each microscopic high-power field; if sperm are present but not active, the cervical environment is unsuitable (e.g., abnormal pH) for their survival.

After the specimen has dried on the glass slide, the mucus can be examined for *ferning*. This pattern is correlated with estrogen activity and is therefore present in all ovulatory women at midcycle. When the cervical mucus is checked again immediately before menstruation, no ferning is found because of progesterone activity. The Sims-Huhner study is invaluable in fertility examinations; however, it is not a substitute for the semen analysis. If the results of the Sims-Huhner test are less than optimal, the test is usually repeated during the same or next ovulatory cycle.

This analysis is also helpful in documenting cases of suspected rape by testing vaginal and cervical secretions for sperm.

Procedure and patient care

Before

PT Explain the procedure to the patient.

PT Inform the patient that basal body temperature recordings should be used to indicate ovulation.

PT Tell the patient that no vaginal lubrication, douching, or bathing is permitted until after the vaginal cervical examination, because these factors will alter the cervical mucus.

PT Inform the patient that this study should be performed after 3 days of sexual abstinence.

PT Instruct the patient to remain in bed for 10 to 15 minutes after coitus to ensure cervical exposure to the semen. After resting, the patient should report to her physician for examination of her cervical mucus within 2 hours after coitus.

During

- Note that with the patient in the lithotomy position, the cervix is exposed by an unlubricated speculum. The specimen is aspirated from the endocervix and delivered to the laboratory for analysis.
- Note that this procedure is performed by a physician in approximately 5 minutes.

PT Tell the patient that the only discomfort associated with this study is insertion of the speculum.

After

PT Tell the patient how and when she may obtain the test results.

Abnormal findings

Infertility
Suspected rape

notes

skull x-ray

Type of test X-ray

Normal findings Normal skull and surrounding structures

Test explanation and related physiology

An x-ray film of the skull allows for visualization of the bones making up the skull, the nasal sinuses, and any cerebral calcification. Skull x-rays are rarely indicated today because of the availability of CT scanning of the brain (see p. 300).

Skull fractures are easily seen as abnormal radiolucent lines in an otherwise radiopaque skull bone. Metastatic tumors of the skull can easily be seen as radiolucent spots in an otherwise normal skull. Opacification of the nasal sinuses may indicate sinusitis, hemorrhage, or tumor.

Procedure and patient care

Before

PT Explain the procedure to the patient.

PT Instruct the patient to remove all objects above the neck because metal objects and dentures prevent x-ray visualization of the structures they cover.

■ Avoid hyperextension and manipulation of the head if surgical injuries are suspected.

PT Tell the patient that no sedation or fasting is required.

During

■ Note that the patient is taken to the radiology department and placed on an x-ray table. Axial (submentovertical), half-axial (Towne), posteroanterior, and lateral views of the skull are usually taken.

■ Note that a radiologic technologist takes skull films in a few minutes.

PT Tell the patient that this test is painless.

After

■ If a prosthetic eye is present, note this on the x-ray examination request, because it can present a confusing shadow on x-ray film.

Abnormal findings

Skull fracture
Metastatic tumor
Sinusitis
Hemorrhage
Tumor
Hematoma
Congenital anomaly
Paget's disease

notes

sleep studies (Polysomnography [PSG], Multiple sleep latency tests [MSLT], Multiple wake test [MWT])

Type of test Electrodiagnostic; various

Normal findings

Respiratory disturbance index (RDI): <5 episodes of apnea per hour

Normal progress through sleep stages

No interruption in nasal or oral airflow

End tidal CO_2: 30-45 mm Hg

Oximetry: ≥90%; no oxygen desaturation of >5%

Minimal snoring sounds

ECG: no disturbances in rate or rhythm

No evidence of restlessness

No apnea

MSLT: onset of sleep >9 minutes

Test explanation and related physiology

There are many types of sleep disorders. Most, however, are associated with impaired nighttime sleep and excessive daytime drowsiness. Sleep disorders can be caused by alterations in sleep times (e.g., nightshift workers), medications (stimulants), or psychiatric problems (e.g., depression, mania).

Sleep studies can identify the cause of the sleep disorders and indicate appropriate treatment. Sleep studies include polysomnography (PSG) and testing for wakefulness and sleepiness. A full PSG would include:

Electroencephalography: This is limited to two or more channels (see p. 373).

Electro-oculography: This documents eye movements (see Electronystagmography, p. 384).

Electromyography: This demonstrates muscle movement, usually of the chin and legs (see p. 376).

Electrocardiography: This determines heart rate and rhythm (see p. 368).

Chest impedance: This monitors chest wall movement and respirations.

Airflow monitors: This measures the amount of airflow in and out of the mouth and nose.

CO_2 monitor: This measures expiratory CO_2 levels.

Pulse oximetry: This monitors tissue oxygen levels (see p. 672).

Sound sensors: These are used to document snoring
  sounds.
Audiovisual recordings: These are used to document restless
  motion and fitfulness.
Esophageal pH probe: This is used only if gastroesophageal reflux
  is considered to be a cause of paroxysmal nocturnal dyspnea
  and coughing (see p. 406).

On occasions when sleep apnea alone is suspected, a four-channel PSG is performed. This more simplified test includes the ECG, chest impedance, airflow monitor, and O_2 oximetry. Audiovisual recordings are performed also.

Sleep apnea can be obstructive or central. Obstructive apnea is by far the most common and is caused by muscle relaxation of the posterior pharyngeal muscles. Breathing stops for 10 to 40 seconds. Central sleep apnea is highlighted by simple cessation of breathing not due to obstructed airway. Primary cardiac events that lead to significant and transient reduction in cardiac output can also cause apnea. Apnea from either cause is associated with increase in heart rate, decreased oxygen levels, change in brain waves, and increased expiratory CO_2. Obstructive apnea is also associated with progressively diminished airflow.

During a sleep study, electrodes for the ECG, EEG, electro-oculography, and electromyography are applied. The chest impedance belt monitors are also placed. Under audiovisual monitoring the patient is placed in a comfortable room, and sleeps. During sleep, information is synchronously gathered. The EEG determines the various stages of sleep, and the physiologic changes during each stage are documented.

Testing for obstructive sleep apnea is performed in a specially constructed sleep laboratory. This is a well-insulated room in which external sounds are blocked and room temperature is easily controlled. It is performed by a certified sleep technologist and interpreted by a physician trained in sleep disorders. The study is usually completed in one night, although occasionally two nights are required. A second day is often required to administer the *multiple sleep latency test (MSLT)* or the *multiple wake test (MWT)*. The MSLT is a measure of the patient's ability to sleep during a series of structured naps. The MSLT is typically done in the morning. The MWT is a measure of the patient's ability to not fall asleep during a period of what should be wakefulness. These tests are used to diagnose narcolepsy that follows a night of inadequate sleep. These tests can also be used to determine the success of therapy for sleep disorders.

S

Interfering factors

- Psychologic-induced insomnia associated with laboratory environmental changes compared to home may occur.
- Environmental noises, temperature changes, or other sensations may affect the sleep pattern.
- Times for sleep testing different from usual times may affect sleep patterns and should be avoided.

Procedure and patient care

Before

PT Explain the procedure to the patient.

PT Instruct the patient to avoid caffeine for several days before testing.

PT Reassure the patient that monitoring equipment will not interrupt the patient's sleeping pattern.

- Allow the patient to express concerns about videotaping and other forms of monitoring.
- Several sleep rating questionnaires are completed by both the patient and his or her sleeping partner.
- Age, weight, and medical history are recorded.

During

- Electrodes for ECG, EEG, and electromyography are applied to the patient. Excess hair may need to be shaved on male patients.
- Airflow, oximetry, and impedance monitors are also applied.
- Once the patient is comfortable, the patient is allowed to sleep per normal routine.
- The lights are turned off, and monitoring begins before sleeping.
- For PSG, the patient is asked to sleep per normal routine.

Multiple sleep latency testing

- The patient is asked to nap about every 2 hours throughout the testing period.
- The nap is terminated after 20 minutes.
- Between naps the patient must stay awake.

Multiple wake testing

- The patient is asked to stay awake and not nap.
- Monitoring is similar to that described for PSG except for impedance, sound, and airflow monitors.

After

- On completion of the sleep cycle, the monitors and electrodes are removed.
- Test results take several days to collate and interpret.

Abnormal findings

Obstructive sleep apnea
Central sleep apnea
Cardiac sleep apnea
Insomnia
Narcolepsy
Restless leg syndrome
Parasomnia
REM disorder

notes

small bowel follow-through (SBF, Small bowel enema)

Type of test X-ray with contrast dye

Normal findings

Normal positioning, motility, and patency of the small intestine
No evidence of intrinsic obstruction or extrinsic compression

Test explanation and related physiology

The SBF study is performed to identify abnormalities in the
small bowel. Usually the patient is asked to drink barium; in
patients who cannot drink, barium can be injected through a
nasogastric tube. X-ray films are then taken at timed intervals
(usually 30 minutes) to follow the progression of barium
through the small intestine. Significant delays in transit time of
the barium may occur with both benign and malignant forms of
obstruction or diminished intestinal motility (ileus). On the
other hand, the flow of barium is faster in patients who have
hypermotility states of the small bowel (malabsorption syndromes). Failure of the progression through the small bowel can
be seen in patients with partial mechanical small bowel obstruction or diminished intestinal motility, as seen in patients with
diabetes. Furthermore, SBF series are helpful in identifying and
defining the anatomy of small bowel fistulas (abnormal connections between the small bowel and other abdominal organs or
skin).

A more accurate radiographic evaluation of the small intestine
is provided by the *small bowel enema*. Unlike the SBF, in which
the barium is swallowed by the patient, during the small bowel
enema the barium is injected into a tube previously passed to the
small bowel. This small bowel enema provides better visualization of the entire small bowel, because the barium is not diluted
by gastric and duodenal juices, as occurs when the patient drinks
barium. This test is especially useful in the evaluation of patients
with partial small bowel obstruction of unknown etiology.
Tumors, ulcers, and small bowel fistulas are more easily identified and defined with the enema.

Contraindications

- Patients with a complete small bowel obstruction
  The introduction of barium into an obstructed bowel may
  create a stonelike impaction; however, this is extremely rare.

- Patients suspected of having a perforated viscus
  Barium should not be used in these patients because it may cause prolonged and recurrent abscesses if it leaks out of the bowel. Gastrografin, a water-soluble contrast medium, can be used if perforation is suspected. Unfortunately, Gastrografin becomes diluted very rapidly, minimizing the accuracy of the SBF with this contrast medium.
- Patients with unstable vital signs
  These patients should be closely supervised during the time required for this study.

Potential complications

- Barium-induced small bowel obstruction

Interfering factors

- Barium within the intestinal tract from a previous barium x-ray film may obstruct adequate visualization of the small bowel.
- Food or fluid within the gastrointestinal tract

Procedure and patient care

Before

PT Explain the procedure to the patient.

PT Instruct the patient not to eat anything for at least 8 hours before the test. Usually keep the patient NPO after midnight on the day of the test.

PT Inform the patient that the SBF series may take several hours. Suggest that the patient bring reading material or some paperwork to occupy his or her time.

- Accompany the patient to the radiology department if his or her vital signs are not stable.
- Arrange for transportation of the hospitalized patient back to the nursing unit between serial films.

During

- Note the following procedural steps:
  1. A specially prepared drink containing barium sulfate is mixed as a milkshake, which the patient drinks through a straw.
  2. Usually, an upper GI series is performed concomitantly (see p. 949).
  3. The barium flow is followed through the upper GI tract fluoroscopically.

S

4. At frequent intervals (15 to 60 minutes), repeat x-ray films are taken to follow the flow of barium through the small intestine. These films are repeated until barium is seen flowing into the right colon. This usually takes 60 to 120 minutes, but in patients with delayed progression of the barium, the test may take as much as 24 hours to complete.

Small bowel enema

1. This is usually performed by placing a long weighted tube transorally; however, a tube also can be placed into the upper small bowel endoscopically.
2. After the tube is in place, a thickened barium mixture is injected through the tube, and x-ray films are serially performed as described for the SBF.

- Note that this procedure is performed by a radiologist in the radiology department in approximately 30 minutes.

PT Tell the patient that this test is not uncomfortable.

After

PT Inform the patient of the need to evacuate adequately all the barium. Cathartics (e.g., magnesium citrate) are recommended. Initially stools will be white and should return to normal color with complete evacuation.

Abnormal findings

Small bowel tumor
Small bowel obstruction from intrinsic tumors
Small bowel obstruction from adhesions, extrinsic tumors, or hernia
Inflammatory small bowel disease (e.g., Crohn's disease)
Malabsorption syndromes (e.g., Whipple's disease, sprue)
Congenital anatomic anomaly (e.g., malrotation)
Congenital abnormalities (e.g., small bowel atresia, duplication, Meckel's diverticulum)
Small bowel intussusception
Small bowel perforation

notes

sodium (Na), blood

Type of test Blood

Normal findings

Adult/elderly: 136-145 mEq/L or 136-145 mmol/L
  (SI units)
Child: 136-145 mEq/L
Infant: 134-150 mEq/L
Newborn: 134-144 mEq/L

Possible critical values <120 or >160 mEq/L

Test explanation and related physiology

Sodium is the major cation in the extracellular space, where serum levels of approximately 140 mEq/L exist. The concentration of sodium intracellularly is only 5 mEq/L. Therefore, sodium salts are the major determinants of extracellular osmolality. The sodium content of the blood is a result of a balance between dietary sodium intake and renal excretion. Normally, individual nonrenal (e.g., sweat) sodium losses are minimal.

Many factors regulate homeostatic sodium balance. Aldosterone causes conservation of sodium by decreasing renal losses. Natriuretic hormone, or third factor, increases renal losses of sodium. Antidiuretic hormone (ADH), which controls the resorption of water at the distal tubules of the kidney, also affects sodium serum levels.

Physiologically, water and sodium are very closely interrelated. As free body water is increased, serum sodium is diluted, and the concentration may decrease. The kidney compensates by conserving sodium and excreting water. If free body water were to decrease, the serum sodium concentration would rise; the kidney would then respond by conserving free water. Aldosterone, adrenocorticotropic hormone (ADH), and natriuretic factor all assist in these compensatory actions of the kidney.

An average dietary intake of approximately 90 to 250 mEq/day is needed to maintain sodium balance in adults. Symptoms of hyponatremia may include weakness, confusion, lethargy, stupor, and coma. Symptoms of hypernatremia include dry mucous membranes, thirst, agitation, restlessness, hyperreflexia, mania, and convulsions.

S

Interfering factors

- Recent trauma, surgery, or shock may cause increased levels.
- Drugs that may cause *increased* levels include anabolic steroids, antibiotics, clonidine, corticosteroids, cough medicines, laxatives, methyldopa, carbenicillin, estrogens, and oral contraceptives.
- Drugs that may cause *decreased* levels include carbamazepine, diuretics, sodium-free IV fluids, sulfonylureas, triamterene, ACE inhibitors, captopril, haloperidol, heparin, nonsteroidal antiinflammatory drugs (NSAIDs), tricyclic antidepressants, and vasopressin.

Procedure and patient care

Before
- PT Explain the procedure to the patient.
- PT Tell the patient that no food or fluid is restricted.

During
- Collect 5 to 10 ml of venous blood in a red- or green-top tube.
- If the patient is receiving an IV infusion, obtain the blood from the opposite arm.
- List on the laboratory slip any drugs that may affect test results.

After
- Apply pressure to the venipuncture site.

Abnormal findings

▲ **Increased levels (hypernatremia)**

Increased sodium intake
Excessive dietary intake
Excessive sodium in
   IV fluids

Decreased sodium loss
Cushing's syndrome
Hyperaldosteronism

Excessive free body water loss
Excessive sweating
Extensive thermal burns
Diabetes insipidus
Osmotic diuresis

▼ **Decreased levels (hyponatremia)**

Decreased sodium intake
Deficient dietary intake
Deficient sodium in IV
   fluids

Increased sodium loss
Addison's disease
Diarrhea
Vomiting or nasogastric
aspiration
Diuretic administration
Chronic renal insufficiency

Increased free body water
Excessive oral water
   intake
Excessive IV water
   intake
Congestive heart failure
Syndrome of inappropriate ADH (SIADH)
secretion
Osmotic dilution

Third-space losses of sodium
Ascites
Peripheral edema
Pleural effusion
Intraluminal bowel loss
   (ileus or mechanical
   obstruction)

notes

sodium (Na), urine

Type of test Urine (24-hour)

Normal findings 40-220 mEq/day or 40-220 mmol/day (SI units)

(Values vary greatly with dietary intake.)

Test explanation and related physiology

This test evaluates sodium balance in the body by determining the amount of sodium excreted in urine over 24 hours. Sodium is the major cation in the extracellular space. Measuring the amount of sodium in the urine is useful for evaluating patients with volume depletion, acute renal failure, adrenal disturbances, and acid-base imbalances. This test is important, especially when the serum sodium concentration is low. For example, in patients with hyponatremia caused by inadequate sodium intake, urine sodium will be low. In patients with hyponatremia caused by chronic renal failure, however, urine sodium concentration will be high.

The sodium content in urine is the result of the balance between dietary sodium and the renal excretion of sodium. In a normal individual, nonrenal sodium losses are minimal. Many factors affect this delicate homeostatic sodium balance. For example, aldosterone tends to decrease urine sodium levels by stimulating conservation of sodium. Antidiuretic hormone, which increases the resorption of water in the distal tubules of the kidney, tends to increase urine sodium levels.

Interfering factors

- Dietary salt intake may increase sodium levels.
- Altered kidney function may affect levels.
- ℣ Drugs that may cause *increased* levels include antibiotics, cough medicines, laxatives, and steroids.
- ℣ Drugs that may cause *decreased* levels include diuretics (e.g., furosemide [Lasix]) and steroids.

Procedure and patient care

Before

PT Explain the procedure to the patient.

PT Tell the patient that no fasting is required.

During

PT Instruct the patient to begin the 24-hour urine collection after urinating. Discard the initial specimen and start the 24-hour timing at that point.

■ Collect all urine passed during the next 24 hours.

PT Show the patient where to store the urine specimen.

■ Keep the specimen on ice or refrigerated during the 24 hours.

■ Indicate the starting time on the urine container and on the laboratory slip.

■ Post the hours for urine collection in a noticeable place to prevent accidental discarding of the specimen.

PT Instruct the patient to void before defecating so that urine is not contaminated by feces.

PT Remind the patient not to put toilet paper in the collection container.

PT Encourage the patient to drink fluids during the 24 hours.

PT Instruct the patient to collect the last specimen as close as possible to the end of the 24-hour period. Add this urine to the container.

After

■ Transport the urine specimen promptly to the laboratory.

Abnormal findings

▲ **Increased levels**

Dehydration
Starvation
Adrenocortical insufficiency
Diuretic therapy
Hypothyroidism
Syndrome of inappropriate ADH (SIADH) secretion
Diabetic ketoacidosis
Toxemia of pregnancy

▼ **Decreased levels**

Congestive heart failure
Malabsorption
Diarrhea
Renal failure
Cushing's syndrome
Aldosteronism
Diaphoresis
Pulmonary emphysema
Inadequate sodium intake

S

notes

somatomedin C and insulin-like growth factor (IGF-1, insulin-like growth factor binding proteins [IGF BP])

Type of test Blood

Normal findings

Adults: 42-110 ng/ml
Children:

Age (yr)	Girls (ng/ml)	Boys (ng/ml)
0-8	5-128	2-118
9-10	24-158	15-148
11-13	65-226	55-216
14-15	124-242	114-232
16-17	94-231	84-211
18-19	66-186	56-177

Test explanation and related physiology

Growth hormone (GH) exerts its effects on many tissues through a group of peptides called somatomedins. The most commonly tested somatomedin is somatomedin C (also called insulin-like growth factor [IGF-1]).

Great variation in GH secretion occurs during the day. A random GH assay result may significantly overlap between normal and abnormal values. To diminish the common variations in GH secretion, screening for somatomedin C provides a more accurate reflection of the mean plasma concentration of growth hormone. Somatomedins are not affected by the time of day, food intake, or exercise as is GH because they circulate bound to proteins that are durable or long lasting. As a result, there is no overlap of results of somatomedin C among normal and abnormal values. Normally there is a large increase during the pubertal growth spurt.

Levels of somatomedin C depend on levels of GH. As a result, somatomedin levels are low when GH levels are deficient. See GH (p. 499) for a discussion of causes of and diseases associated with GH deficiency. Nonpituitary causes of reduced somatomedin C include malnutrition, severe chronic illnesses, severe liver disease, hypothyroidism, and Laron's dwarfism. Abnormally low test results require an abnormally reduced or absent GH during a GH stimulation test (see p. 502) to make the diagnosis of GH deficiency.

Pediatricians are now more commonly using *insulin-like growth factor binding proteins (IGF BP)* to even further diminish the impact of the variables affecting GH and somatomedin levels. Specifically, IGF BP 2 and IGF BP 3 are most commonly measured. These tests are expensive and not indicated for routine screening of children with short stature. However, if GH deficiency is strongly suspected, yet documentation using GH or somatomedins is questionable, IGF BP determinations are helpful. IGF BP 3 is less age dependent and is the most accurate (97% sensitivity and specificity). These proteins help to evaluate GH deficiencies and GH-resistant syndromes (e.g., Laron's dwarfism). Finally, these binding proteins are very useful to predict response to therapeutic exogenous GH administration.

Interfering factors

- A radioactive scan performed within the week before the test may affect test results.
- Drugs that may cause *decreased* levels include high doses of estrogens.

Procedure and patient care

Before
- PT Explain the procedure to the patient.
- PT Tell the patient that an overnight fast is preferred.

During
- Collect one lavender- or red-top tube of venous blood.

After
- Apply pressure to the venipuncture site.

Abnormal findings

▲ **Increased levels**

Acromegaly
Gigantism
Hyperpituitarism
Obesity
Pregnancy
Precocious puberty

▼ **Decreased levels**

GH deficiency
Laron's dwarfism
Inactive GH
Resistance to somatomedins
Nutritional deficiency
Delayed puberty
Pituitary tumor
Hypopituitarism
Cirrhosis of the liver

spinal x-rays (Cervical, thoracic, lumbar, sacral, or coccygeal x-ray studies)

Type of test X-ray

Normal findings Normal spinal vertebrae

Test explanation and related physiology

Spinal x-ray studies may be performed to evaluate any area of the spine. They usually include anteroposterior, lateral, and oblique views of these structures. These x-ray films are often done to assess back or neck pain, degenerative arthritic changes, traumatic fractures, tumor metastasis, spondylosis (stress fracture of the vertebrae), and spondylolisthesis (slipping of one vertebral disk on the other). Cervical spine x-ray studies are routinely performed in cases of multiple trauma to ensure no fracture before the patient is moved or the neck is manipulated. Spinal x-rays are very helpful in evaluating children and adults for spinal alignment abnormalities (e.g., kyphosis, scoliosis).

Contraindications

- Patients who are pregnant, unless the benefits outweigh the risks

Procedure and patient care

Before

PT Explain the procedure to the patient.

PT Instruct the patient to remove any metal objects covering the area to be visualized.

- Immobilize the patient if a spinal fracture is suspected. Apply a neck brace if a cervical spine fracture is suspected.

PT Tell the patient that no fasting or sedation is required; however, if a fracture is suspected, the patient may be kept NPO.

During

- Note that the patient is placed on an x-ray table. Anterior, posterior, lateral, and oblique x-ray films are taken of the desired area on the spinal cord.

- Note that a radiologic technologist takes spinal x-ray films in a few minutes.

PT Tell the patient that no discomfort is associated with this study.

After
- Note that positioning and patient activity depend on test results.

Abnormal findings

Degenerative arthritis changes
Traumatic or pathologic fracture
Spondylosis
Spondylolisthesis
Metastatic tumor invasion

notes

sputum culture and sensitivity (C&S, Culture and Gram stain)

Type of test   Sputum

Normal findings   Normal upper respiratory tract

Test explanation and related physiology

Sputum cultures are obtained to determine the presence of pathogenic bacteria in patients with respiratory infections, such as pneumonia. A *Gram stain* is the first step in the microbiologic analysis of sputum. Staining of sputum provides an opportunity to classify bacteria as gram positive or gram negative. This may be used to guide drug therapy until the C&S report is complete. The sputum sample is then applied to a series of bacterial culture plates. The bacteria that grow on those plates 1 to 3 days later are then identified. Determinations of bacterial sensitivity to various antibiotics are done to identify the most appropriate antimicrobial drug therapy. This is done by observing a ring of growth inhibition around an antibiotic plug in the culture medium. Sputum for C&S should be collected before antimicrobial therapy is initiated, unless the test is being performed to evaluate the effectiveness of medications already being given. Preliminary reports are usually available in 24 hours. Cultures require at least 48 hours for completion. Sputum cultures for fungus and *Mycobacterium tuberculosis* may take 6 to 8 weeks.

Procedure and patient care

Before

- PT Explain the procedure for sputum collection to the patient.
- PT Remind the patient that sputum must be coughed up from the lungs and that saliva is not sputum.
- Hold antibiotics until after the sputum has been collected.
- If an elective specimen is to be obtained, give the patient a sterile sputum container on the night before the sputum is to be collected so that the morning specimen may be obtained on arising.
- PT Instruct the patient to rinse out his or her mouth with water before the sputum collection to decrease contamination of the sputum by particles in the oropharynx.

During

- Note that sputum specimens are best when the patient first awakens in the morning and before eating or drinking.
- Collect at least 1 teaspoon of sputum in a sterile sputum container.
- Usually obtain sputum by having the patient cough after taking several deep breaths.
- If the patient is unable to produce a sputum specimen, stimulate coughing by lowering the head of the patient's bed or giving the patient an aerosol administration of a warm, hypertonic solution.
- Note that other methods to collect sputum include endotracheal aspiration, fiberoptic bronchoscopy, and transtracheal aspiration.

After

PT Inform the patient to notify the nurse as soon as the sputum is collected.

- Label the sputum and send it to the laboratory as soon as possible.
- Note any current antibiotic therapy on the laboratory slip.

Abnormal findings

Bacterial infection (e.g., pneumonia)
Viral infection
Atypical bacterial infection (e.g., tuberculosis)

notes

S

sputum cytology

Type of test Sputum

Normal findings Normal epithelial cells

Test explanation and related physiology

Tumors within the pulmonary system frequently slough cells into the sputum. When the sputum is gathered, the cells are examined. If the cytologic test is positive, malignant cells are seen, indicating a lung tumor. If only normal epithelial cells are seen, either no malignancy exists, or any existing tumor is not shedding cells. Therefore a positive test indicates malignancy; a negative test means nothing.

Bronchoscopy and percutaneous lung biopsy have supplanted the need for sputum cytology to a large degree. Now its greatest use is in patients who have an abnormal chest x-ray, productive cough, and nothing visible on bronchoscopy. It is also used to monitor smokers who have had some atypical changes on prior examination of the lower respiratory tract.

Procedure and patient care

Before

- **PT** Explain the procedure for sputum collection to the patient.
- **PT** Remind the patient that sputum must be coughed up from the lungs and that saliva is not sputum.
- ▪ Give the patient a sterile sputum container on the night before the sputum is to be collected so that the morning specimen may be obtained on arising.
- **PT** Instruct the patient to rinse out her or his mouth with water to decrease contamination of the sputum by particles in the oropharynx.

During

- ▪ Note that sputum specimens are best collected when the patient first awakens in the morning and before eating or drinking.
- ▪ Collect at least 1 teaspoon of sputum in the sterile sputum container.
- ▪ Usually obtain sputum by having the patient cough after taking several deep breaths.

- If the patient is unable to produce a sputum specimen, stimulate coughing by lowering the head of the patient's bed or giving the patient an aerosol administration of a warm hypertonic solution.
- Note that other methods to collect sputum include endotracheal aspiration, fiberoptic bronchoscopy, and transtracheal aspiration.
- Usually collect sputum for cytology on three separate occasions.

After

PT Instruct the patient to notify the nurse as soon as the sputum is collected.

- Label the specimen and send it to the laboratory as soon as possible.

Abnormal findings

Malignancies

notes

S

stool culture (Stool for culture and sensitivity [C&S], Stool for ova and parasites [O&P])

Type of test Stool

Normal findings Normal intestinal flora

Test explanation and related physiology

Normally, stool contains many bacteria and fungi. The more common bacteria include *Enterococcus, Escherichia coli, Proteus, Pseudomonas, Staphylococcus aureus, Candida albicans, Bacteroides,* and *Clostridium.* Bacteria are indigenous to the bowel. Sometimes normal stool flora can become pathogenic if overgrowth of the bacteria occurs as a result of antibiotics, immunosuppression, or overaggressive catharsis (e.g., *Clostridium difficile*). *Salmonella, Shigella, Campylobacter, Yersinia,* pathogenic *E. coli, Clostridium,* and *Staphylococcus* are acquired bacteria that can infect the bowel. Parasites also may affect the stool. Common parasites are *Ascaris* (hookworm), *Strongyloides* (tapeworm), and *Giardia* (protozoans). Identification of any of these pathogens in the stool incriminates that "bug" as the etiology of the infectious enteritis.

Infections of the bowel from bacteria, virus, or parasites usually present as acute diarrhea, excessive flatus, and abdominal discomfort. Patients who have been drinking well water, have been on prolonged antibiotics, or have traveled out of the United States are especially susceptible.

Interfering factors

- Urine may inhibit the growth of bacteria. Therefore urine should not be mixed with the feces during collection of a stool sample.
- Recent barium studies may obscure the detection of parasites.
- ♉ Drugs that may affect test results include antibiotics, bismuth, and mineral oil.

Procedure and patient care

Before

PT Explain the method of stool collection to the patient. Be matter-of-fact to avoid any embarrassment to the patient.

PT Instruct the patient not to mix urine or toilet paper with the stool specimen.

PT Instruct the patient to use an appropriate collection container.

During

PT Instruct the patient to defecate into a clean bedpan.
- Place a small amount of stool in a sterile collection container.
- Send mucus and blood streaks with the specimen.
- If a rectal swab is to be used, wear gloves and insert the cotton-tipped swab at least 1 inch into the anal canal. Then rotate the swab for 30 seconds and place it into the clean container.

Tape test
- Use this test when pinworms *(Enterobius)* are suspected.
- Place a clear tape in the patient's perianal region. (This is especially helpful in children.)
- Because the female worm lays her eggs at night around the perianal area, apply the tape before bedtime and remove it in the morning before the patient gets out of bed.
- Press the sticky surface of the tape directly to a glass slide and examine microscopically for pinworm ova.

After
- Handle the stool specimen carefully, as though it were capable of causing infection. Wear gloves when obtaining and handling the specimen.
- Indicate on the laboratory slip any antibiotics that the patient may be taking.
- Promptly send the stool specimen to the laboratory. Delays in transfer of the specimen may affect viability of the organism. If long delays are necessary, obtain a buffered glycerol-saline solution to be combined with the stool and used as a preservative.
- Note that some enteric pathogens occasionally take as long as 6 weeks to isolate.
- When pathogens are detected, maintain isolation of the patient's stool until therapy is completed.

S

Abnormal findings

Bacterial enterocolitis
Protozoan enterocolitis
Parasitic enterocolitis

stool for occult blood (Stool for OB)

Type of test Stool

Normal findings No occult blood within stool

Test explanation and related physiology

Normally only minimal quantities of blood are passed into the gastrointestinal (GI) tract. Usually this bleeding is not significant enough to cause a positive result in stool for OB testing. Tumors of the intestine grow into the lumen and are subjected to repeated trauma by the fecal stream. Eventually the friable tumor ulcerates, and bleeding occurs. Most often, bleeding is so slight that gross blood is not seen in the stool. The blood can be detected only by chemical assay through OB testing of the stool.

Benign and malignant GI tumors, ulcers, inflammatory bowel disease, arteriovenous malformations, diverticulosis, and hematobilia (hemobilia) can cause OB within the stool. Other more common abnormalities (e.g., hemorrhoids, swallowed blood from oral or nasal pharyngeal bleeding) may also cause OB within the stool. This test can detect occult blood when as little as 5 ml of blood is lost per day.

This test is a part of every routine physical examination. It is also a part of routine screening of asymptomatic individuals over the age of 50 years. It is important to note that many drugs and the ingestion of hemoglobin contained in red meats such as beef and pork may cause a false-positive OB stool test. The more sensitive the test method, the more false positives that will be obtained.

A positive result obtained on multiple specimens performed on successive days warrants a thorough GI evaluation. Most would agree that four positives out of six specimens would constitute criteria for a more thorough evaluation.

Interfering factors

- Vigorous exercise
- Bleeding gums following a dental procedure
- Ingestion of red meat within 3 days before testing
- Ingestion of fish, turnips, and horseradish
- Drugs that may cause GI bleeding include anticoagulants, aspirin, colchicine, iron preparations (large doses), nonsteroidal antiarthritics, and steroids.

✘ Drugs that may cause false-positive results include colchicine, iron, oxidizing drugs (e.g., iodine, bromides, boric acid), and rauwolfia derivatives.

✘ Drugs that may cause false-negative results include vitamin C.

Procedure and patient care

Before

PT Explain the procedure to the patient.

PT Instruct the patient to refrain from eating any red meat for at least 3 days before the test.

PT Instruct the patient to refrain from drugs known to interfere with OB testing.

PT Instruct the patient as to the method of obtaining appropriate stool specimens. Many procedures are available (e.g., specimen cards, tissue wipes, test paper). Tests may be done at home with specimen cards (Hemoccult) and mailed when collected.

PT Instruct the patient not to mix urine with the stool specimen.

PT Inform the patient as to the need for multiple specimens obtained on separate days to increase the test's accuracy.

■ Note that in some centers a high-residue diet is recommended to increase the abrasive effect of the stool.

■ Note on the laboratory slip any anticoagulant medications that the patient may be taking.

■ Be gentle in obtaining stool by digital rectal examination. Traumatic digital examination can cause a false-positive stool, especially in patients with prior anorectal disease such as hemorrhoids.

During

Hemoccult slide test

■ Place a stool sample on one side of guaiac paper.

■ Place two drops of developer on the other side.

■ Note that a bluish discoloration indicates OB in the stool.

Tablet test

■ Place a stool sample on the developer paper.

■ Place a tablet on top of the stool specimen.

■ Put two or three drops of tap water on the tablet and allow to flow onto the paper.

■ Note that a bluish discoloration indicates OB in the stool.

After

PT Inform the patient as to the results.

- If the tests are positive, inquire whether the patient violated any of the preparation recommendations.

Abnormal findings

GI tumor

Polyps

Ulcer

Varices

Inflammatory bowel disease

Diverticulosis

Ischemic bowel disease

GI trauma

Recent GI surgery

Hemorrhoids

Esophagitis

Gastritis

notes

substance abuse testing (Urine drug testing, Drug screening, Toxicology screening)

Type of test Urine; blood; various

Normal findings Negative

Test explanation and related physiology

Substance abuse testing is used mostly by employers and law enforcement agencies. Employers use drug testing to promote and protect the safety, health, and well-being of their employees. Because 40% of industrial fatalities are attributable to substance abuse, drug testing programs are becoming more common in the workplace. Furthermore, drug use is responsible for decreased productivity and increased absenteeism. Industrial testing is used at the time of preemployment, prepromotion, annual physical, postaccident, when there is reasonable suspicion, or for random testing or follow-up treatment surveillance.

Most commonly, a drug screen is performed to detect small amounts of any number of metabolites of commonly used drugs. If the screen result is positive, a more accurate and quantitative test is performed on the same specimen. Drug screens are available for a variety of substances. The most common are amphetamines, barbiturates, benzodiazepines, cocaine, methamphetamine, opiates (morphine and heroin), cannabinoids (marijuana [THC]), phencyclidine (PCP), and propoxyphene. Alcohol testing is most commonly used by law enforcement (see Ethanol, p. 420). Not only is drug testing helpful in identifying users, but it also acts as a deterrent. Athletes are tested for anabolic hormones that may unfairly improve their performance. Health and life insurance companies routinely test for illicit drugs.

Until recently, substance abuse testing has used urine exclusively as the sample of choice. Urine drug testing is generally inexpensive. Urine is easily obtained and plentiful, and it contains a large amount of drug and metabolites. More important, urine can identify drug usage for 7 to 14 days after the last usage, whereas blood testing reflects drug usage only during the past few hours. Saliva, breath, hair, and sweat are becoming increasingly important and accurate specimens for specific drug testing. These newer testing methods are very expensive, however. Hair samples detect the presence of drugs used during the past

S

3 months. In addition, hair and nail samples may be used to detect or document exposure to arsenic and mercury. Nevertheless, urine testing remains the mainstay for drug testing.

Several test kits are becoming increasingly available for "in-house" (i.e., on-site) drug screening. These kits can provide results in a few minutes. Results of more definitive urine or hair testing require approximately 2 to 4 days.

Because a positive result can have a profound effect on a person's life, job, and accountability, it is not uncommon for a drug abuser to attempt to alter the urine specimen. Therefore the urine sample is tested for odor, color, temperature, creatinine, pH, and specific gravity to ensure that it is a proper specimen. If the specimen does not meet these assessment standards, it is rejected and a second specimen is requested.

Toxicology screening tests for drug overdose (see Table 22 on p. 894) and poisoning (e.g., lead and carbon monoxide) are best performed on blood. Results indicate current drug levels, which are used to determine or alter therapy. Toxicology studies are used to incriminate drugs as a cause or factor in the death of a person. They are also used to assess patients when poisoning contributes to an illness.

Interfering factors

- Poppyseeds can cause false-positive opiate results.
- Secondhand marijuana smoke can cause false-positive THC results.
- Detergents, bicarbonates, salt tablets, or blood can all foil accurate drug testing in a urine specimen.
- ✗ Ibuprofen can cause a false-positive THC result.
- ✗ Cold remedies can cause false-positive amphetamine results.
- ✗ Antibiotics (e.g., amoxicillin) can cause false-positive results for heroin and/or cocaine.
- ✗ The aggressive use of diuretics can *decrease* drug levels in the urine.

Procedure and patient care

Before

PT Explain the procedure to the patient or significant others based on standard guidelines.

- If the specimen is obtained for medicolegal testing, ensure that the patient or family member has signed a consent form.
- Obtain a list of prescription medicines that the patient is taking that may alter or confuse screening results. Obtain as

much information as possible about the drug type, amount, and ingestion time.

- Carefully assess the patient for respiratory distress (a common adverse reaction of drug overdosage).

During

- Collect blood and urine samples as designated by the laboratory.
- Ensure that patients provide their own urine. Urine specimens for substance abuse testing are usually collected in the presence of the nurse.
- Be sure that the patient does not alter the urine specimen.
- For hair testing, cut 50 strands of hair from the scalp.
- At the laboratory, the specimen is usually divided for more definitive testing if the result is above the cutoff value.
- Collect gastric contents as indicated in the specific institution. An NG tube is required.

After

- Apply pressure to the venipuncture site.
- Refer the patient for appropriate drug and psychiatric counseling.
- Follow the chain of custody for the specimen as provided by standard guidelines of the institution.
- Place the specimen in the required container for delivery.
- Check the temperature of urine specimens within 3 minutes after voiding. Temperature should be between 97° and 99° F.
- The specimen is usually sent to a laboratory certified by the National Institute of Drug Abuse.

Abnormal findings

Positive drug level

notes

swallowing examination (Videofluoroscopy swallowing examination)

Type of test X-ray with contrast dye

Normal findings Normal swallowing function and complete clearing of radiographic material through the upper digestive tract

Test explanation and related physiology

This test is performed to identify the exact problems that exist in a patient who is unable to swallow. Problems in swallowing may result from local structural diseases such as tumors, upper esophageal diverticula, inflammation, extrinsic compression of the upper gastrointestinal (GI) tract, or surgery to the oropharyngeal tract. Motility disorders of the upper GI tract (such as Zenker's diverticulum) and neurologic disorders (such as stroke syndrome), Parkinson's disease, and neuropathies also may cause difficulty in swallowing. Videofluoroscopy of the swallowing function allows a speech pathologist to delineate more clearly the exact pathology in the swallowing mechanism. This videofluoroscopy then can be used to determine the most appropriate treatment and teach the patient proper swallowing technique.

This test is performed by asking the patient to swallow barium or a barium-containing meal. With the use of videofluoroscopy, the swallowing function is visualized and documented. Morphologic abnormalities and functional impairment can be identified easily using the slow-frame progression and reversal that is available with videofluoroscopy. Although this test is similar to the barium swallow (see p. 150), finer details of swallowing can be evaluated with the use of videofluoroscopy.

Contraindications

- Patients who obviously aspirate their saliva are not candidates for swallowing, because they will require nonswallowing methods of alimentation

Procedure and patient care

Before

PT Explain the procedure to the patient.

PT Explain to the patient that no preparation is required.

During

- In the radiology department the patient is asked to swallow a barium-containing meal. The consistency of the meal will be determined by the speech therapist and radiologist. The meal consistency simulates foods to which the patient is to be initially reintroduced. The food may be in the form of a liquid, semisoft (e.g., applesauce), or solids (e.g., a tea biscuit). While the patient is swallowing, videofluoroscopy is recorded in both the lateral and the anterior positions.
- The video is then repeatedly examined and reexamined by the radiologist and speech pathologist.

After

- No catharsis is required.

Abnormal findings

Oral pharyngeal inflammation
Cancer
Extrinsic compression
Neuromuscular disorder
Achalasia
Upper GI motility disorder (e.g., stroke syndrome, Parkinson's disease, peripheral neuropathy)
Diffuse esophageal spasms
Zenker's diverticulum

notes

S

sweat electrolytes test (Iontophoretic sweat test)

Type of test Fluid analysis

Normal findings

Sodium values in children
Normal: <70 mEq/L
Abnormal: >90 mEq/L
Equivocal: 70-90 mEq/L

Chloride values in children
Normal: <50 mEq/L
Abnormal: >60 mEq/L
Equivocal: 50-60 mEq/L

Test explanation and related physiology

Patients with cystic fibrosis have increased sodium and chloride contents in their sweat. This forms the basis of this test, which is both sensitive and specific for cystic fibrosis. Cystic fibrosis is an inherited disease characterized by abnormal secretion by exocrine glands within the bronchi, small intestines, pancreatic ducts, bile ducts, and skin (sweat glands). Sweat induced by electrical current *(pilocarpine iontophoresis)* is collected, and its sodium and chloride contents are measured. The degree of abnormality is no indication of the severity of cystic fibrosis; it merely indicates that the patient has the disease.

In children with recurrent respiratory tract infections, malabsorption syndromes, or failure to thrive, this test is indicated to diagnose cystic fibrosis. This test is also used to screen children or siblings of cystic fibrosis patients for the disease. Almost all patients with cystic fibrosis have sweat sodium and chloride contents 2 to 5 times greater than normal values. In patients with suspicious clinical manifestations, these levels are diagnostic of cystic fibrosis.

Procedure and patient care

Before
PT Explain the procedure to the patient and/or parents.
PT Tell the patient and/or parents that no fasting is required.

During

- Note the following procedural steps:
  1. For iontophoresis, a low-level electrical current is applied to the test area (the thigh in infants, the forearm in older children).
  2. The positive electrode is covered by gauze and saturated with pilocarpine hydrochloride, a stimulating drug that induces sweating.
  3. The negative electrode is covered by gauze saturated with a bicarbonate solution.
  4. The electrical current is allowed to flow for 5 to 12 minutes.
  5. The electrodes are removed, and the arm is washed with distilled water.
  6. Paper disks are placed over the test site with the use of clean, dry forceps.
  7. These disks are covered with paraffin to obtain an air-tight seal, preventing evaporation of sweat.
  8. After 1 hour the paraffin is removed. The paper disks are transferred immediately by forceps to a weighing jar and sent for sodium and chloride analysis.
  9. A *screening* test may be done to detect sweat chloride levels. For screening, a test paper containing silver nitrate is pressed against the child's hand for several seconds. The test is positive when the excess chloride combines with the silver nitrate to form white-silver chloride on the paper (i.e, the child with cystic fibrosis will leave a "heavy" handprint on the paper).
  10. A positive screening test is usually validated by iontophoresis.
- Note that an experienced technologist performs the sweat test in approximately 90 minutes in the laboratory or at the patient's bedside.
- PT Inform the patient that the electrical current is small and no discomfort or pain is generally associated with this test.

After

PT Initiate extensive education and counseling for the patient and/or parents if the results indicate cystic fibrosis.

Abnormal findings

Cystic fibrosis

---

syphilis detection test (Serologic test for syphilis [STS], Venereal Disease Research Laboratory [VDRL], Rapid plasma reagin [RPR], Fluorescent treponemal antibody test [FTA])

Type of test   Blood

Normal findings   Negative, or nonreactive

Test explanation and related physiology

These blood tests are used to diagnose and to document successful therapy of syphilis. Syphilis is caused by the spirochete *Treponema pallidum*. Two groups of antibodies form the basis for these tests. The first group detects the presence of a nontreponemal antibody, called *reagin*, which reacts to phospholipids in the patient's body (which are probably similar to lipids in the membrane of *T. pallidum*). The nontreponemal antibody tests are grouped as STS and are relatively nonspecific. These antibodies are most often detected by the *Wassermann test* or the *VDRL test*. A newer, more sensitive nontreponemal test is the RPR test. The VDRL and RPR tests, by virtue of their testing for a nonspecific antibody, have a high false-positive (or cross-reactive) rate. The VDRL test becomes positive approximately 2 weeks after the patient's inoculation with *Treponema* and returns to normal after adequate treatment is administered. The test is positive in nearly all primary and secondary stages of syphilis and in two thirds of patients with tertiary syphilis.

If the VDRL or RPR test is positive, the diagnosis may be confirmed by the *Treponema* test, such as the *FTA absorption test* (FTA-ABS). This second group of tests detects antibodies directed against the *Treponema* organism itself. The FTA test, which tests for a more specific antibody, is more accurate than the VDRL and RPR tests.

False-positive and false-negative results are rare in all stages of the disease. The FTA test is required before the diagnosis of syphilis can be made with certainty.

Screening for syphilis is usually done during the first prenatal checkup for pregnant women. Syphilis, if untreated, may cause abortion, stillbirth, and premature labor. The effect on the fetus can be central nervous system damage, hearing loss, and possible death.

Interfering factors

- Excessive hemolysis and gross lipemia may affect test results.
- Excess chyle in the blood may interfere with the test results.
- Many conditions cause false-positive results when VDRL and RPR tests are used. Some of these conditions include *Mycoplasma* pneumonia, malaria, acute bacterial and viral infections, autoimmune diseases, and pregnancy.
- Recent ingestion of alcohol may alter the test results.

Procedure and patient care

Before
PT Explain the procedure to the patient.
- Check with the laboratory regarding fasting requirements. Some prefer collecting the specimen before meals. Some laboratories request that the patient refrain from alcohol for 24 hours before the blood test.

During
- Collect approximately 7 ml of blood in a red-top tube.

After
- Apply pressure to the venipuncture site.
PT If the test is positive, instruct the patient to inform recent sexual contacts so they can be evaluated.
PT If the test is positive, be sure the patient receives the appropriate antibiotic therapy.

Abnormal findings

Syphilis

S

notes

testosterone (Total testosterone serum level)

Type of test Blood

Normal findings

Men: 3-10 ng/ml or 10-35 nmol/L (SI units)
Women: <1 ng/ml or <3.5 nmol/L (SI units)
Prepubertal boys and girls: 0.05-0.2 ng/ml or 0.17-0.7
  nmol/L (SI units)

Test explanation and related physiology

Testosterone is made in the male by the Leydig cells in the
testicle; this accounts for 95% of the circulating testosterone
in men. In women the ovary and adrenal glands secrete small
amounts of testosterone; the majority of the testosterone in
the female is made as a derivative of metabolism of androstenedione (see p. 65). Approximately 60% of circulating testosterone
binds strongly to sex hormone–binding globulin. Most of the
remaining testosterone is bound loosely to albumin, and approximately 2% is unbound.

Testosterone levels are used to evaluate ambiguous sex characteristics, precocious puberty, virilizing syndromes in the female,
and infertility in the male. This test can also be used as a tumor
marker for rare tumors of the ovary and testicle.

Physiologically, testosterone stimulates spermatogenesis and
influences the development of male secondary sexual characteristics. Overproduction of this hormone in the young male may
cause precocious puberty. This can be caused by testicular,
adrenal, or pituitary tumors or adrenal hyperplasia. Overproduction
of this hormone in females causes masculinization, which is
demonstrated by amenorrhea and excessive growth of body hair
(hirsutism). Ovarian and adrenal tumors/hyperplasia and medications (e.g., danazol) are all potential causes of masculinization
in the female. Reduced levels of testosterone in the male suggest
hypogonadism or Klinefelter's syndrome.

Several *testosterone stimulation tests* can be performed to more
accurately evaluate hypogonadism. Human chorionic gonadotropin,
clomiphene, and gonadotropin-releasing hormone (GnRH) can
be used to stimulate testosterone secretion.

Interfering factors

✔ Drugs that may cause *increased* testosterone levels include anticonvulsants, barbiturates, estrogens, and oral contraceptives.

✔ Drugs that may cause *decreased* testosterone levels include androgens, dexamethasone, diethylstilbestrol, digoxin, alcohol, steroids, ketoconazole, phenothiazine, and spironolactone.

Procedure and patient care

Before

PT Explain the procedure to the patient.

PT Tell the patient that no fasting is required.

▪ Because testosterone levels are highest in the early morning hours, blood should be drawn in the morning.

During

▪ Collect 7 ml of peripheral venous blood in a red-top tube.

After

▪ Apply pressure to the venipuncture site.

Abnormal findings

▲ **Increased levels (male)**

Idiopathic sexual precocity
Pinealoma
Encephalitis
Congenital adrenal
  hyperplasia
Adrenocortical tumor
Testicular or extragonadal
  tumor
Hyperthyroidism
Testosterone resistance
  syndromes

▼ **Decreased levels (male)**

Klinefelter's syndrome
Cryptorchidism
Primary and secondary
  hypogonadism
Down syndrome
Orchidectomy
Hepatic cirrhosis

T

▲ **Increased levels (female)**

Ovarian tumor
Adrenal tumor
Congenital adrenocortical hyperplasia
Trophoblastic tumor
Polycystic ovaries
Idiopathic hirsutism

notes

therapeutic drug monitoring (TDM)

Type of test Blood

Normal findings See Table 22.

Test explanation and related physiology

Therapeutic drug monitoring (TDM) entails taking measurements of blood drug levels to determine effective drug dosages and to prevent toxicity. It is also used to identify noncompliant patients. Patient age and size, extent and rate of drug absorption or excretion, and metabolic rate can all affect drug levels. Measurement of drug levels is very important in patients who are beyond the normal range in regard to variables that affect drug metabolism. TDM is helpful in patients who take other medicines that may affect drug levels or act in a synergistic or antagonistic manner with the drug to be tested. TDM is helpful in prescribing medicines (e.g., antiarrhythmics, bronchodilators, antibiotics, anticonvulsants, cardiotonics) that have a very narrow therapeutic margin (i.e., the difference between therapeutic and toxic drug levels is small).

Table 22 lists the therapeutic and toxic ranges for most patients. These ranges may not apply to all patients because clinical response is influenced by many factors (e.g., noncompliance, concurrent drug use, other clinical conditions, patient's age and size, extent and rate of drug absorption, metabolism). Also, note that different laboratories use different units for reporting test results and normal ranges. It is important that sufficient time pass between the administration of the medication and the collection of the blood sample to allow for therapeutic levels to occur.

Blood samples can be taken at the drug's *peak* level (the highest concentration) or at the *trough* level (the lowest concentration). Peak levels are useful when testing for toxicity, and trough levels are useful for demonstrating a satisfactory therapeutic level. Trough levels are often referred to as *residual* levels. The time when the sample should be drawn after the last dose of the medication varies according to whether a peak or trough level is requested and according to the half-life of the drug.

T

TABLE 22 Therapeutic drug monitoring data

Drug	Use	Therapeutic level*	Toxic level*
Acetaminophen	Analgesic, antipyretic	Depends on use	<250 mcg/ml
Amikacin	Antibiotic	15-25 mcg/ml	>25 mcg/ml
Aminophylline	Bronchodilator	10-20 mcg/ml	>20 mcg/ml
Amitriptyline	Antidepressant	120-150 ng/ml	>500 ng/ml
Amobarbital	Sedative, hypnotic	0.5-3.0 mcg/ml	>10 mcg/ml
Butabarbital	Sedative, hypnotic	0.5-3.0 mcg/ml	>10 mcg/ml
Carbamazepine	Anticonvulsant	5-12 mcg/ml	>12 mcg/ml
Chloramphenicol	Antiinfective	10-20 mcg/ml	>25 mcg/ml
Desipramine	Antidepressant	150-300 ng/ml	>500 ng/ml
Digitoxin	Cardiac glycoside	15-25 ng/ml	>25 ng/ml
Digoxin	Cardiac glycoside	0.8-2.0 ng/ml	>2.4 ng/ml
Disopyramide	Antiarrhythmic	2-5 mcg/ml	>5 mcg/ml
Ethosuximide	Anticonvulsant	40-100 mcg/ml	>100 mcg/ml
Gentamicin	Antibiotic	5-10 mcg/ml	>12 mcg/ml
Glutethimide	Sedative	0.5-3.0 mcg/ml	>10 mcg/ml
Imipramine	Antidepressant	150-300 ng/ml	>500 ng/ml
Kanamycin	Antibiotic	20-25 mcg/ml	>35 mcg/ml
Lidocaine	Antiarrhythmic	1.5-5.0 mcg/ml	>5 mcg/ml
Lithium	Manic episodes of bipolar psychosis	0.8-1.2 mEq/L	>2.0 mEq/L

Meprobamate	Antianxiety agent	0.5-3.0 mcg/ml	>10 mcg/ml
Methotrexate	Antitumor agent	>0.01 μmol/24 hr	>10 μmol/24 hr
Methyprylon	Hypnotic	0.5-3.0 mcg/ml	>10 mcg/ml
Nortriptyline	Antidepressant	50-150 ng/ml	>500 ng/ml
Phenobarbital	Anticonvulsant	10-30 mcg/ml	>40 mcg/ml
Phenytoin	Anticonvulsant	10-20 mcg/ml	>30 mcg/ml
Primidone	Anticonvulsant	5-12 mcg/ml	>15 mcg/ml
Procainamide	Antiarrhythmic	4-10 mcg/ml	>16 mcg/ml
Propranolol	Antiarrhythmic	50-100 ng/ml	>150 ng/ml
Quinidine	Antiarrhythmic	2-5 mcg/ml	>10 mcg/ml
Salicylate	Antipyretic, antiinflammatory, analgesic	100-250 mcg/ml	>300 mcg/ml
Theophylline	Bronchodilator	10-20 mcg/ml	>20 mcg/ml
Tobramycin	Antibiotic	5-10 mcg/ml	>12 mcg/ml
Valproic acid	Anticonvulsant	50-100 mcg/ml	>100 mcg/ml

*Levels vary according to the institution performing the test.

T

Procedure and patient care

Before
PT Explain the procedure to the patient.

PT Tell the patient that no food or fluid restrictions are needed.

During
- Collect approximately 7 to 10 ml of venous blood in a tube designated by the laboratory. *Peak* levels are usually obtained 1 to 2 hours after oral intake, approximately 1 hour after IM administration, and approximately 30 minutes after IV administration. *Residual* (trough) levels are usually obtained shortly before (0-15 minutes) the next scheduled dose. Consult with the pharmacy for specific times.

After
- Apply pressure to the venipuncture site.
- Clearly mark all blood samples with the following information: patient's name, diagnosis, name of drug, time of last drug ingestion, time of sample, and any other medications the patient is currently taking.
- Promptly send the specimen to the laboratory.

Abnormal findings

Nontherapeutic levels of drugs
Toxic levels of drugs

notes

thoracentesis and pleural fluid analysis (Pleural tap)

Type of test Fluid analysis

Normal findings

Gross appearance: Clear, serous, light yellow, 50 ml
Red blood cells (RBCs): None
White blood cells (WBCs): <300/ml
Protein: <4.1 g/dl
Glucose: 70-100 mg/dl
Amylase: 138-404 units/L
Alkaline phosphatase
   Adult male: 90-240 units/L
   Female: <45 years: 76-196 units/L
   Female: >45 years: 87-250 units/L
Lactate dehydrogenase (LDH): Similar to serum lactate
   dehydrogenase
Cytology: No malignant cells
Bacteria: None
Fungi: None
Carcinoembryonic antigen (CEA): <5 ng/ml

Test explanation and related physiology

Thoracentesis is an invasive procedure that entails insertion of a needle into the pleural space for removal of fluid (or, rarely, air) (Figure 39). Pleural fluid is removed for diagnostic and therapeutic purposes. *Therapeutically* it is done to relieve pain, dyspnea, and other symptoms of pleural pressure. Removal of this fluid also permits better radiographic visualization of the lung.

Diagnostically, thoracentesis is performed to obtain and analyze fluid to determine the etiology of the pleural effusion. Pleural fluid is classified according to transudate or exudate. This is an important differentiation and is very helpful in determining the etiology of the effusion. *Transudates* are most frequently caused by congestive heart failure, cirrhosis, nephrotic syndrome, and hypoproteinemia. *Exudates* are most often found in inflammatory, infectious, or neoplastic conditions. However, collagen vascular disease, pulmonary infarction, trauma, and drug hypersensitivity also may cause an exudative effusion.

Pleural fluid is usually evaluated for the following features.

T

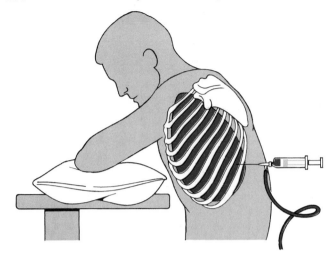

Figure 39 Thoracentesis. A needle is placed through the chest wall and into the fluid contained within the pleural cavity. A special one-way valve system is placed between the needle and the syringe to allow aspiration of fluid when the plunger of the syringe is pulled back and diversion of the fluid to a container when the plunger is pushed in.

Gross appearance

The color, optical density, and viscosity are noted as the pleural fluid appears in the aspirating syringe. Empyema is characterized by the presence of a foul odor and thick, puslike fluid. An opalescent, pearly fluid is characteristic of chylothorax (chyle in the pleural cavity).

Cell counts

The white blood cell (WBC) and differential counts are determined. A WBC count exceeding 1000/ml is suggestive of an exudate. The predominance of polymorphonuclear leukocytes usually is an indication of an acute inflammatory condition (e.g., pneumonia, pulmonary infarction, early tuberculosis effusion). When more than 50% of the WBCs are small lymphocytes, the effusion is usually caused by tuberculosis or tumor. Normally no RBCs should be present. The presence of RBCs may indicate neoplasms, tuberculosis, or intrathoracic bleeding.

Protein content

Total protein levels greater than 3 g/dl are characteristic of exudates, whereas transudates usually have a protein content of less than 3 g/dl. The *albumin gradient* between serum and pleural fluid can differentiate better between the transudate and exudate nature of pleural fluid than can the total protein content. This gradient is obtained by subtracting the pleural albumin value from the serum albumin value. Values of 1.1 g/dl or more suggest a transudate. Values less than 1.1 g/dl suggest an exudate but will not differentiate the potential cause of the exudate (malignancy from infection or inflammation). The total protein ratio (fluid/serum) has been considered to be another accurate criterion differentiating transudate from exudate. A total protein ratio of fluid to serum of greater than 0.5 is considered to be an exudate.

Lactic dehydrogenase

A pleural fluid/serum LDH ratio greater than 0.6 is typical of an exudate. An exudate is identified with a high degree of accuracy if the pleural fluid/serum protein ratio is greater than 0.5 and the pleural fluid/serum LDH ratio is greater than 0.6.

Glucose

Usually pleural glucose levels approximate serum levels. Low values appear to be a combination of glycolysis by the extra cells and impairment of glucose diffusion because of damage to the pleural membrane. Values less than 60 mg/dl are occasionally seen in tuberculosis or malignancy and typically occur in rheumatoid arthritis and empyema.

Amylase

In a malignant effusion the amylase concentration is slightly elevated. Amylase levels above the normal range for serum or two times the serum level are seen when the effusion is caused by pancreatitis or rupture of the esophagus associated with leakage of salivary amylase.

Triglyceride

Measurement of triglyceride levels is an important part of identifying chylous effusions. These effusions are usually produced by obstruction or transection of the lymphatic system caused by lymphoma, neoplasm, trauma, or recent surgery. The triglyceride value in a chylous effusion exceeds 110 mg/dl.

Gram stain and bacteriologic culture

These tests are routinely performed when bacterial pneumonia or empyema is a possible cause of the effusion. If possible, these should be done before initiation of antibiotic therapy.

Cultures for *Mycobacterium tuberculosis* and fungus

Tuberculosis is less often a cause for pleural effusion in the United States today than it was. Fungus may be a cause of pulmonary effusion in patients with compromised immunologic defenses.

Cytology

A cytologic study is performed to detect tumor cells in approximately 50% to 60% of patients with malignant effusions. Breast and lung are the two most common tumors; lymphoma is the third.

Carcinoembryonic antigen

Pleural fluid CEA levels are elevated in various malignant (gastrointestinal, breast) conditions. See p. 230.

Special tests

The pH of pleural fluid is usually 7.4 or greater. The pH is typically less than 7.2 when empyema is present. The pH may be 7.2 to 7.4 in tuberculosis or malignancy.

In some instances, the rheumatoid factor (see p. 810) and the complement levels (see p. 292) are also measured in pleural fluid.

Pleural fluid antinuclear antibody (ANA) levels and pleural fluid/serum ANA ratios are often used to evaluate pleural effusion secondary to systemic lupus erythematosus.

Contraindications

- Patients with significant thrombocytopenia

Potential complications

- Pneumothorax because of puncture of the visceral pleura or entry of air into the pleural space
- Interpleural bleeding because of puncture of tissue or a blood vessel
- Hemoptysis caused by needle puncture of a pulmonary vessel or by inflammation
- Reflex bradycardia and hypotension
- Pulmonary edema
- Seeding of the needle track with tumor when malignant pleural effusion exists

Procedure and patient care

Before

PT Explain the procedure to the patient.
- Obtain informed consent for this procedure.

PT Tell the patient that no fasting or sedation is necessary.

PT Inform the patient that movement or coughing should be minimized to avoid inadvertent needle damage to the lung or pleura during the procedure.
- Administer a cough suppressant before the procedure if the patient has a troublesome cough.
- Note that an x-ray film or ultrasound scan is often used to assist in location of the fluid. Fluoroscopy also may be used.

During

- Note the following procedural steps:
  1. The patient is usually placed in an upright position, with the arms and shoulders raised and supported on a padded overhead table. This position spreads the ribs and enlarges the intercostal space for insertion of the needle.
  2. Patients who cannot sit upright are placed in a side-lying position on the unaffected side with the side to be tapped uppermost.
  3. The thoracentesis is performed under strict sterile technique.
  4. The needle insertion site, which is determined by percussion, auscultation, and examination of a chest x-ray film, ultrasound scan, or fluoroscopy, is aseptically cleansed and anesthetized locally.
  5. The needle is positioned in the pleural space, and the fluid is withdrawn with a syringe and a three-way stopcock.
  6. Various mechanisms to stabilize the pleural needle are available to secure the needle depth during the fluid collection.
  7. A short polyethylene catheter may be inserted into the pleural space for fluid aspiration; this decreases the risk of puncturing the visceral pleura and inducing a pneumothorax.
  8. Also, large volumes of fluid may be collected by connecting the catheter to a gravity-drainage system.
- Note that this procedure is performed by a physician at the patient's bedside, in a procedure room, or in the physician's office in less than 30 minutes.
- Monitor the patient's pulse for reflex bradycardia and evaluate the patient for diaphoresis and the feeling of faintness during the procedure.

T

PT Although local anesthetics eliminate pain at the insertion site, tell the patient that he or she may feel a pressure-like pain when the pleura is entered and the fluid is removed.

After

- Place a small bandage over the needle site. Usually turn the patient on the unaffected side for 1 hour to allow the pleural puncture site to heal.
- Label the specimen with the patient's name, date, source of fluid, and diagnosis. Send the specimen promptly to the laboratory.
- Obtain a chest x-ray study as indicated to check for pneumothorax.
- Monitor the patient's vital signs.
- Observe the patient for coughing or expectoration of blood (hemoptysis), which may indicate trauma to the lung.
- Evaluate the patient for signs and symptoms of pneumothorax, tension pneumothorax, subcutaneous emphysema, and pyogenic infection (e.g., tachypnea, dyspnea, diminished breath sounds, anxiety, restlessness, fever).
- Assess the patient's lung sounds for diminished breath sounds, which could be a sign of pneumothorax.
- If the patient has no complaints of dyspnea, normal activity usually can be resumed 1 hour after the procedure.

Abnormal findings

Exudate
Empyema
Pneumonia
Tuberculosis effusion
Pancreatitis
Ruptured esophagus
Tumors
Lymphoma
Pulmonary infarction
Collagen vascular disease
Drug hypersensitivity

Transudate
Cirrhosis
Congestive heart failure
Nephrotic syndrome
Hypoproteinemia
Trauma

thoracoscopy

Type of test Endoscopy

Normal findings Normal pleura and lung

Test explanation and related physiology

This procedure is used to directly visualize the pleura, lung, and mediastinum. Tissue can be obtained for testing. It is also helpful in assisting in the staging and dissection of lung cancers.

With this technique, the parietal pleura, visceral pleura, and mediastinum can be directly visualized. Tumor involving the chest cavity can be staged by direct visualization. Any abnormality can be biopsied. Collections of fluid can be drained and aspirated for testing. Dissection for lung resection can be carried out with the thoracoscope *(video-assisted thoracotomy [VAT])*, thereby minimizing the extent of a thoracotomy incision.

Contraindications

- Patients with previous lung surgery, because it is difficult to obtain access to the free pleural space

Potential complications

- Bleeding
- Infection or empyema
- Prolonged pneumothorax

Procedure and patient care

Before

PT Explain the procedure to the patient.
- Ensure that an informed consent for this procedure is obtained.
- An open thoracotomy may be required because of the possibility of intrathoracic injury. Be sure the patient is aware of this.
- Because the procedure is usually performed with the patient under general anesthesia, follow routine general anesthesia precautions.
- Shave and prepare the patient's chest as ordered.
- Keep the patient NPO after midnight on the day of the test. IV fluids may be given.

T

During

- Note the following procedural steps:
  1. Thoracoscopy is performed in the operating room. The patient is initially placed in the lateral decubitus position.
  2. After the thorax is cleansed, a blunt-tipped (Verres) needle is inserted through a small incision, and the lung is collapsed.
  3. A thoracoscope is inserted through a trocar to examine the chest cavity. Other trocars can be placed as conduits for other instrumentation.
  4. After the desired procedure is completed, the scope and trocars are removed.
  5. Usually a small chest tube is placed to ensure full reexpansion of the lung.
  6. The incision(s) is closed with a few skin stitches and covered with an adhesive bandage.

After

- Assess the patient frequently for signs of bleeding (increased pulse rate, decreased blood pressure). Report any significant findings to the physician.
- Provide analgesics to relieve the minor to moderate pain that may be experienced.
- If a surgical procedure has been performed thoracoscopically, provide appropriate specific postsurgical care.
- A chest x-ray is performed after the procedure to ensure complete reexpansion of the lung.

Abnormal findings

Primary lung cancer
Metastatic cancer to the lung or pleura
Empyema
Pleural tumor
Pleural infection
Pleural inflammation
Pulmonary infection

notes

throat and nose cultures

Type of test Microscopic examination

Normal findings Negative

Test explanation and related physiology

Because the throat and nose are normally colonized by many organisms, cultures of these areas serve only to isolate and identify a few particular pathogens (e.g., streptococci, meningococci, gonococci, *Bordetella pertussis, Corynebacterium diphtheriae*). Identification of these bacterial pathogens indicates the need for treatment.

Streptococci are most often sought on a throat culture, because a beta-hemolytic streptococcal pharyngitis may be followed by rheumatic heart disease or glomerulonephritis. This type of streptococcal infection most frequently affects children between the ages of 3 and 15 years. Therefore all children with a sore throat and fever should have a throat culture done to attempt to identify streptococcal infections. In adults, however, fewer than 5% of patients with pharyngitis have a streptococcal infection. Therefore throat cultures in adults are indicated only when the patient has severe or recurrent sore throat, often associated with fever and palpable lymphadenopathy. These adults often have a history of streptococcal infections.

Rapid immunologic tests *(strept screen)* with antiserum against group A streptococcus antigen are now available and are very accurate. With these newer kits, the streptococcus organism can be identified directly from the swab specimen without culture. These tests can be performed in about 15 minutes. If the test is negative, no streptococcus infection exists.

Nasal and nasopharyngeal cultures are often done to screen for infections and carrier states caused by various other organisms such as *Staphylococcus aureus, Haemophilus influenzae, Neisseria meningitidis,* respiratory syncytial virus (RSV), and viruses causing rhinitis. Health care workers in the operating room and newborn nursery may have these cultures to screen potential sources of spread once an outbreak occurs in a hospital setting. These cultures are also used to detect infection in elderly and debilitated patients.

All cultures should be performed before antibiotic therapy is initiated. Otherwise, the antibiotic may interrupt the growth of the organism in the laboratory. Most organisms take approximately 24 hours to grow in the laboratory, and a preliminary report can be given at that time. Occasionally 48 to 72 hours is required for growth and identification of the organism. Cultures may be repeated on completion of appropriate antibiotic therapy to identify resolution of the infection.

Interfering factors

▼ Drugs that may affect test results include antibiotics and antiseptic mouthwashes.

Procedure and patient care

Before

PT Explain the procedure to the patient.

During

- Obtain a *throat culture* by depressing the tongue with a wooden tongue blade and touching the posterior wall of the throat and areas of inflammation, exudation, or ulceration with a sterile cotton swab. Two swabs are preferred. Growth of streptococcus from both swabs is more accurate, and the second swab can also be used in the strept screen. Avoid touching any other part of the mouth. Place the swabs in a sterile container.
- Obtain a *nasal culture* by gently raising the tip of the nose and inserting a flexible swab into the nares. Rotate the swab against the side of the nares. Remove the swab and place it in an appropriate culture tube.
- Obtain a *nasopharyngeal culture* by gently raising the tip of the nose and inserting a flexible swab along the bottom of the nares. Guide this swab until it reaches the posterior pharynx. Rotate the swab to obtain secretions and then remove it. Place the swab in an appropriate culture tube.
- Wear gloves and handle the specimen as if it were capable of transmitting disease.
- Indicate on the laboratory slip any medications that the patient may be taking that could affect test results.

After

- Label all specimens and send immediately to the microbiology lab.
- Notify the physician of any positive results so that appropriate antibiotic therapy can be initiated.

Abnormal findings

Bacterial pathogens (e.g., streptococci)
Respiratory syncytial virus
H. influenzae bacteria

notes

T

Thrombosis Indicators
fibrin monomers (Fibrin degradation products [FDPs], Fibrin split products [FSPs], Fibrin monomers)   **fibrinopeptide A** (FPA)   **prothrombin fragment** (F1+2)

Type of test Blood

Normal findings

FDP: <10 mcg/ml or <10 mg/L (SI units)

FPA:

  Male: 0.4-2.6 mg/ml

  Female: 0.7-3.1 mg/ml

F1+2:

7.4-103 mcg/L or 0.2-2.8 nmol/L

Possible critical values FDP >40 mcg/ml

Test explanation and related physiology

Identification of FDPs, FPA, and F1+2 is mostly used to document that fibrin clot formation and, therefore, thombosis is occurring in patients. These tests most commonly support the diagnosis of disseminated intravasular coagulation (DIC). They also provide an indication about the effectiveness of anticoagulation therapy. Finally, they are used to support the diagnosis and follow treatment for hypercoagulable states.

F1+2 is liberated when prothrombin is converted to thrombin in reaction 4 of secondary hemostasis (Figure 11). FPA is released into the bloodstream from alpha and beta chains of fibrinogen during its conversion to fibrin.

Measurement of FDPs provides a direct indication of the activity of the fibrinolytic system. Thrombin formation initiates fibrin formation, which stimulates the fibrinolytic system. This system degenerates fibrin polymer into fragment monomers called FDPs (X, D, E, and Y). These, therefore, are indirect evidence of thrombosis and DIC. FDPs also are increased with other secondary fibrinolytic disorders. Thrombolytic therapy used to treat vascular thrombsis is associated with increased FDPs. Streptokinase or urokinase stimulates the conversion of plasminogen to plasmin.

These tests are part of the DIC screening tests. These products of hemostasis and fibrinolysis also may be elevated in patients with extensive malignancy, tissue necrosis, and gram-negative sepsis.

Interfering factors

- Traumatic venipunctures may increase FPA levels.
- Surgery or massive trauma is associated with increased levels of these indicators.
- Menstruation may be associated with increased FDP levels.
- ⚹ Drugs that may cause *increased* levels include barbiturates, heparin, streptokinase, and urokinase.
- ⚹ Drugs that may cause *decreased* levels include warfarin (Coumadin) and other oral anticoagulants.

Procedure and patient care

Before

- **PT** Explain the procedure to the patient.
- **PT** Tell the patient that no fasting is required.
- Avoid prolonged used of a tourniquet.

During

- Draw the sample before initiating heparin therapy.
- Collect a venous blood sample (usually only 2 ml) in a small, blue-top tube or in the colored tube designated by the laboratory.
- Avoid excessive agitation of the blood sample.
- Note that it is best to place the blood on ice and take it immediately to the hematology laboratory.
- List on the laboratory slip any drugs that may cause elevated levels.

After

- Apply pressure to the venipuncture site.

Abnormal findings

▲ Increased levels

DIC
Heart or vascular surgery
Thromboembolism
Thrombosis
Advanced malignancy
Severe inflammation
Postoperative states
Massive trauma
Deficiency in protein S and C
Antithrombin III deficiency

▼ Decreased levels

Anticoagulation therapy

thyroid scanning (Thyroid scintiscan)

Type of test   Nuclear scan

Normal findings

Normal size, shape, position, and function of the thyroid gland
No areas of decreased or increased uptake

Test explanation and related physiology

Thyroid scanning allows the size, shape, position, and physiologic function of the thyroid gland to be determined with the use of radionuclear scanning. A radioactive substance such as technetium-99m is given to the patient to visualize the thyroid gland. A scanner is passed over the neck area, and an image is recorded.

Thyroid nodules are easily detected by this technique. Nodules are classified as functioning (warm/hot) or nonfunctioning (cold), depending on the amount of radionuclide taken up by the nodule. A functioning nodule could represent a benign adenoma or a localized toxic goiter. A nonfunctioning nodule may represent a cyst, carcinoma, nonfunctioning adenoma or goiter, lymphoma, or localized area of thyroiditis.

Scanning is useful in:

1. Patients with a neck or substernal mass
2. Patients with a thyroid nodule. Thyroid cancers are usually nonfunctioning (cold) nodules.
3. Patients with hyperthyroidism. Scanning assists in differentiating Graves' disease (diffusely enlarged hyperfunctioning thyroid gland) from Plummer's disease (nodular hyperfunctioning gland).
4. Patients with metastatic tumors without a known primary site. A normal scan excludes the thyroid gland as a possible primary site.
5. Patients with a well-differentiated form of thyroid cancer. Areas of metastasis may show up on subsequent whole-body nuclear scans.

Another form of thyroid scan is called the *whole-body thyroid scan*. This scan is performed on patients who have previously had a thyroid cancer treated. Iodine-125 is injected intravenously, and the entire body is scanned to look for metastatic thyroid tissue. A hot spot indicates recurrent tumor. This test is routinely (every 1 to 2 years) performed on patients who have had a thyroid cancer larger than 1 cm.

Contraindications

- Patients who are allergic to iodine or shellfish
- Patients who are pregnant, unless the benefits outweigh the risks.

Potential complications

- Radiation-induced oncogenesis
  This complication is eliminated if technetium or low-radioactive iodine isomers are used instead of iodine-131.

Interfering factors

- Iodine-containing foods
- Recent administration of x-ray contrast agents
- Drugs that may affect test results include cough medicines, multiple vitamins, oral contraceptives (some), and thyroid drugs.

Procedure and patient care

Before

PT Explain the procedure to the patient.
- Check the patient for allergies to iodine.
PT Instruct the patient about medications that need to be restricted for weeks before the test (e.g., thyroid drugs, medications containing iodine).
- Obtain a history concerning previous contrast x-ray studies, nuclear scanning, or intake of any thyroid-suppressive or antithyroid drugs.
PT Tell the patient that fasting is usually not required. Check with the laboratory.

During

- Note the following procedural steps:
  1. A standard dose of radioactive technetium is usually given to the patient by mouth. The capsule is tasteless.
  2. Scanning is usually performed 24 hours later. If technetium is used, scanning may be performed 2 hours later.
  3. At the designated time, the patient is placed in a supine position and a detector is passed over the thyroid area.
  4. The radioactive counts are recorded and displayed.
- Note that this study is performed by a radiologic technologist in less than 30 minutes.
PT Tell the patient that no discomfort is associated with this study.

After

PT Assure the patient that the dose of radioactive technetium used in this test is minute and therefore harmless. No isolation and no special urine precautions are needed.

Abnormal findings

Adenoma
Toxic and nontoxic goiter
Cyst
Carcinoma
Lymphoma
Thyroiditis
Graves' disease
Plummer's disease
Metastasis
Hyperthyroidism
Hypothyroidism
Hashimoto's disease

notes

Type of test Blood

Normal findings

Adult: 0.4-5.6 milli-international units/L or 0.4-5.6 milli-international units/L (SI units)

Newborn: 3-20 milli-international units/L or 3-20 milli-international units/L (SI units)

Cord: 3-12 µU/ml or 3-12 mU/L

(Values vary between laboratories.)

Test explanation and related physiology

The TSH concentration aids in differentiating primary from secondary hypothyroidism. Pituitary TSH secretion is stimulated by hypothalamic thyroid-releasing hormone (TRH). Low levels of triiodothyronine and thyroxine (T_3, T_4) are the underlying stimuli for TRH and TSH. Therefore, a compensatory elevation of TRH and TSH occurs in patients with primary hypothyroid states such as surgical or radioactive thyroid ablation; patients with burned-out thyroiditis, thyroid agenesis, idiopathic hypothyroidism, or congenital cretinism; or patients taking antithyroid medications.

In secondary hypothyroidism the function of the hypothalamus or pituitary gland is faulty because of tumor, trauma, or infarction. Thus TRH and TSH cannot be secreted, and plasma levels of these hormones are near 0 despite low T_3 and T_4 levels.

The *TRH stimulation test* is sometimes used to stimulate low levels of TSH to identify primary from secondary hypothyroidism in cases in which TSH is low. However, this test is not commonly used because extremely low levels of TSH can be identified now with the use of immunoassays.

The TSH test is used as well to monitor exogenous thyroid replacement. The goal of thyroid replacement therapy is to provide an adequate amount of thyroid medication so that TSH secretion is in the low normal range, indicating a euthyroid state. Therefore, doses of medication are given to keep the TSH level less than 2. Even lower TSH levels are preferred if thyroid suppression is the clinical goal. This test is also done to detect primary hypothyroidism in newborns with low screening T_4 levels. TSH and T_4 levels are frequently measured to differentiate pituitary from thyroid dysfunction. A decreased T_4 and normal or

T

elevated TSH level can indicate a thyroid disorder. A decreased T_4 with a decreased TSH level can indicate a pituitary disorder.

Interfering factors

- Recent radioisotope administration may affect test results.
- Severe illness may cause decreased TSH levels.
- Drugs that may cause *increased* levels include antithyroid medications, lithium, potassium iodide, and TSH injection.
- Drugs that may cause *decreased* levels include aspirin, dopamine, heparin, steroids, and T_3.

Procedure and patient care

Before
- PT Explain the procedure to the patient.
- PT Tell the patient that no food or drink restrictions are necessary.

During
- Collect approximately 5 ml of venous blood in a red-top tube.
- Use a heel stick to obtain blood from newborns.

After
- Apply pressure to the venipuncture site.

Abnormal findings

▲   **Increased levels**

Primary hypothyroidism
   (thyroid dysfunction)
Thyroiditis
Thyroid agenesis
Congenital cretinism

▼   **Decreased levels**

Secondary
   hypothyroidism
   (pituitary dysfunction)
Hyperthyroidism
Pituitary hypofunction

notes

thyroid-stimulating hormone stimulation test (TSH stimulation test)

Type of test Blood

Normal findings Increased thyroid function with administration of exogenous TSH

Test explanation and related physiology

The TSH stimulation test is used to differentiate *primary* (or thyroidal) hypothyroidism from *secondary* (or hypothalamic-pituitary) hypothyroidism. Normal people and patients with hypothalamic-pituitary hypothyroidism can increase thyroid function when exogenous TSH is given. However, patients with primary thyroidal hypothyroidism do not; their thyroid gland is inadequate and cannot function, no matter how much stimulation it receives. Patients with less than a 10% increase in radioactive iodine uptake (RAIU) or less than a 1.5 mcg/dl rise in thyroxine (T_4) are considered to have a primary cause for their hypothyroid state. If the initially low uptake is caused by inadequate pituitary stimulation of an intrinsically normal thyroid gland, the RAIU should increase at least 10%, and the T_4 level should rise 1.5 mcg/dl or more. This is characteristic of secondary hypothyroidism.

Procedure and patient care

Before

PT Explain the procedure to the patient.
- Obtain baseline levels of RAIU or T_4 (see p. 924) as indicated.
PT Tell the patient that no fasting is required.

During
- Administer 5 to 10 units of TSH intramuscularly for 3 days.
- Repeat the levels of RAIU or T_4 as indicated.

After
- Apply pressure to the venipuncture site.

Abnormal findings

Primary (thyroidal) hypothyroidism
Secondary (hypothalamic-pituitary) hypothyroidism

thyroid-stimulating immunoglobulins ([TSI], Long-acting thyroid stimulator [LATS], Thyroid binding inhibitory immunoglobulin [TBII], Thyrotropin receptor antibody)

Type of test Blood

Normal findings

TSI <130% of basal activity
TBII <10%

Test explanation and related physiology

The nomenclature for various thyroid stimulator hormone receptor assays is confusing. The characterizations of these hormones demonstrate that they act very similarly but are thought to be different because of the different animal test systems used to identify the various antibodies. Thyroid-stimulating immuoglobulins (TSI) represent a group of immunoglobulin-G (IgG) antibodies directed against the thyroid cell receptor for thyroid-stimulating hormone (TSH). The autoimmune complexes then act to stimulate (or in some cases, inhibit) the release of thyroid hormones from the thyroid cells. These immunoglobulins, present in 90% of patients with Graves' disease, play a major role in the pathogenesis of that disease. In some cases TSIs are inhibitory and have been demonstrated in patients with Hashimoto's thyroiditis.

The use of these antibodies is helpful in the evaluation of patients for whom the diagnosis of Graves' disease is confused by conflicting data (such as subclinical Graves' hyperthyroidism or euthyroid patients with ophthalmopathy). In these cases, the antibodies help determine and support the diagnosis of Graves' disease.

The effect of these antibodies on the thyroid may be long lasting, and titers do not decrease until nearly 1 year after successful treatment of the thyroid disease. However, measurement of these antibodies may be helpful in identifying remission or relapse of Graves' disease after treatment. Because TSI can cross the placenta, they may be found in neonates whose mothers have Graves' disease. These infants experience hyperthyroidism for as long as 4 to 8 months. This syndrome must be identified and treated early.

Interfering factors

- Recent administration of radioactive iodine may affect test results.

Procedure and patient care

Before

PT Explain the procedure to the patient.

PT Tell the patient that no fasting or special preparation is required.

During

- Collect approximately 5 ml of venous blood in a red- or gold-top tube.
- Notify the laboratory if the patient has received radioactive iodine in the preceding 2 days.
- Handle the blood sample gently. Hemolysis may interfere with interpretation of test results.

After

- Apply pressure to the venipuncture site.

Abnormal findings

▲ **Increased levels**

Hyperthyroidism
Malignant exophthalmos
Graves' disease
Hashimoto's thyroiditis

notes

T

thyroid ultrasound (Thyroid echogram, Thyroid sonogram)

Type of test   Ultrasound

Normal findings   Normal size, shape, and position of the thyroid gland

Test explanation and related physiology

Ultrasound examination of the thyroid gland is valuable for distinguishing cystic from solid thyroid nodules. If the nodule is found to be purely cystic (fluid filled), the fluid can simply be aspirated (cysts are not cancerous), and surgery is avoided. If the nodule has a mixed or solid appearance, however, a tumor may be present, and surgery may be required for diagnosis and treatment.

This study may be repeated at intervals to determine the response of a thyroid mass to medical therapy. This test is also the procedure of choice for studying the thyroid gland of pregnant patients because no radioactive material is used.

Procedure and patient care

Before
- PT Explain the procedure to the patient.
- PT Tell the patient that breathing or swallowing will not be affected by the placement of a transducer on the neck.
- PT Inform the patient that a liberal amount of lubricant will be applied to the neck to ensure effective transmission and reception of sound waves.
- PT Tell the patient that no fasting or sedation is required.

During
- Note the following procedural steps:
  1. The patient is taken to the ultrasonography department (usually in the radiology department) and placed in the supine position with the neck hyperextended.
  2. Gel is applied to the patient's neck.
  3. A sound transducer is passed over the nodule.
  4. Photographs are taken of the image displayed.
- Note that an ultrasound technologist usually performs this study in approximately 15 minutes and that a radiologist evaluates the results.
- PT Tell the patient that no discomfort is associated with this study.

After
- Assist the patient in removing the lubricant from his or her neck.

Abnormal findings

Cyst
Tumor
Thyroid adenoma
Thyroid carcinoma
Goiter

notes

thyrotropin-releasing hormone test (TRH test, Thyrotropin-releasing factor test [TRF test])

Type of test   Blood

Normal findings

Baseline thyroid-stimulating hormone (TSH): <10 µU/ml
Stimulated TSH: more than double baseline

Test explanation and related physiology

The TRH test assesses the responsiveness of the anterior pituitary gland via its secretion of TSH to an IV injection of TRH. After the TRH injection, the normally functioning pituitary gland should secrete TSH. In hyperthyroidism, either slight or no increase in the TSH level is seen because pituitary TSH production is suppressed by the direct effect of excess circulating thyroxine and triiodothyronine (T_4, T_3) on the pituitary gland. A normal result is considered reliable evidence for excluding the diagnosis of thyrotoxicosis. Since the development of very sensitive radioimmunoassay for TSH, the TRH stimulation test is no longer required to diagnose hyperthyroidism. However, it still has a role in the evaluation of pituitary deficiency.

In addition to assessing the responsiveness of the anterior pituitary gland, this test aids in the detection of primary, secondary, and tertiary hypothyroidism. In primary hypothyroidism (thyroid gland failure), the increase in the TSH level is two or more times the normal result. With secondary hypothyroidism (anterior pituitary failure), no TSH response occurs. Tertiary hypothyroidism (hypothalamic failure) may be diagnosed by a delayed rise in the TSH level. Multiple injections of TRH may be needed to induce the appropriate TSH response in this case.

The TRH test also may be useful in differentiating primary depression from manic-depressive psychiatric illness and from secondary types of depression. In primary depression, the TSH response is blunted in most patients, whereas patients with other types of depression have a normal TRH-induced TSH response.

Interfering factors

- Pregnancy may increase the TSH response to TRH.
- Drugs that may modify the TSH response include antithyroid drugs, aspirin, corticosteroids, estrogens, levodopa, and T_4.

Procedure and patient care

Before
- PT Explain the procedure to the patient.
- PT Instruct the patient to discontinue thyroid preparations for 3 to 4 weeks before the TRH test.
- Assess the patient for medications currently being taken.
- PT Tell the patient that no fasting or sedation is required.

During
- Administer a 500-mg IV bolus of TRH.
- Obtain venous blood samples at intervals and measure for TSH levels.

After
- Apply pressure to the venipuncture site.
- Indicate on the laboratory slip if the patient is pregnant.
- List any medications that the patient is taking.

Abnormal findings

Hyperthyroidism
Hypothyroidism
Psychiatric primary depression
Acute starvation
Old age (especially in men)
Pregnancy

notes

T

thyroxine, free (FT₄)

Type of test Blood

Normal findings

0-4 days: 2-6 ng/dl or 26-77 pmol/L (SI units)
2 weeks-20 years: 0.8-2 ng/dl or 10-26 pmol/L (SI units)
Adult: 0.8-2.8 ng/dl or 10-36 pmol/L (SI units)

Test explanation and related physiology

This test is used to determine thyroid function, especially when the patient has concurrent clinical situations that may alter protein blood levels. Greater than normal levels indicate hyperthyroid states, and subnormal values are seen in hypothyroid states.

Thyroid hormone is made up of thyroxine (T_4) and triiodothyronine (T_3). More than 90% of thyroid hormone is made up of T_4. Ninety-nine percent of T_4 is bound to proteins (thyroid-binding globulin [TBG] and albumin). Only 1% to 5% of total T_4 is unbound or "free." The free T_4 is the metabolically active thyroid hormone. When measuring total T_4 (see p. 924), the bound and the unbound are measured. Abnormalities in protein levels can have a significant effect on the results of the total T_4. Pregnancy and hormone replacement therapy increase TBG and cause T_4 to be falsely elevated, suggesting that hyperthyroidism exists when in fact the patient is euthyroid. If the free T_4 is measured in these patients, it would be normal, indicating that free T_4 is a more accurate indicator of thyroid function than total T_4. Likewise, in cases in which TBG is reduced (e.g., hypoproteinemia), the total T_4 is likewise reduced, suggesting hypothyroidism. Measurement of free T_4 would indicate normal levels and thereby discount the abnormal total T_4 as merely a result of the reduced TBG and not as a result of hypothyroidism.

Interfering factors

- Neonates have higher levels than do older children and adults.
- Prior use of radioisotopes can alter test results because the method used to determine free T_4 levels is radioimmunoassay.
- Drugs that *increase* free T_4 levels include heparin, aspirin, danazol, and propranolol.
- Drugs that *decrease* free T_4 levels include furosemide, phenytoins, methadone, and rifampicin.

☒ Exogenously administered thyroxine causes elevated free T_4 results.

Procedure and patient care

Before

PT Explain the procedure to the patient.

- Evaluate the patient's medication history.

PT If indicated, instruct the patient to stop exogenous T_4 medication 1 month before testing.

PT Tell the patient that no fasting is required.

During

- Collect a venous blood specimen in a red-top tube.
- List on the laboratory slip any drugs that may affect test results.

After

- Apply pressure to the venipuncture site.

Abnormal findings

▲ **Increased levels**

Graves' disease
Plummer's disease
Toxic thyroid adenoma
Acute thyroiditis
Factitious hyperthyroidism
Struma ovarii

▼ **Decreased levels**

Cretinism
Surgical ablation
Myxedema
Pituitary insufficiency
Hypothalamic failure
Iodine insufficiency
Renal failure
Cushing's disease
Cirrhosis
Advanced cancer

notes

thyroxine, total (T₄, Thyroxine screen)

Type of test Blood

Normal findings

1-3 days: 11-22 mcg/dl
1-2 weeks: 10-16 mcg/dl
1-12 months: 8-16 mcg/dl
1-5 years: 7-15 mcg/dl
5-10 years: 6-13 mcg/dl
10-15 years: 5-12 mcg/dl
Adult male: 4-12 mcg/dl or 51-154 nmol/L (SI units)
Adult female: 5-12 mcg/dl or 64-154 nmol/L (SI units)
Adult >60 years: 5-11 mcg/dl or 64-142 nmol/L (SI units)

Possible critical values

Newborn: <7 mcg/dl
Adult: <2 mcg/dl if myxedema coma possible; >20 mcg/dl if
   thyroid storm possible

Test explanation and related physiology

The serum thyroxine (T_4) study is a direct measurement of
the total amount of T_4 present in a patient's blood. T_4 makes up
nearly all of what we call thyroid hormone. Greater than normal
levels indicate hyperthyroid states, and subnormal values are
seen in hypothyroid states. Newborns are screened by T_4 tests to
detect hypothyroidism. Mental retardation can be prevented by
early diagnosis.

This is a very reliable test of thyroid function; however, results
are affected by thyroid-binding globulin (TBG). Because T_4 is
bound by serum proteins such as TBG, any increase in these
proteins (as in pregnant women and patients taking oral contraceptives) will cause factitiously elevated levels of T_4 and, to some
extent, triiodothyronine (T_3). T_4 testing is also used to monitor
replacement and suppressive therapy.

Interfering factors

- T_4 levels may be increased after x-ray iodinated contrast
  studies.
- Pregnancy causes increased levels.
- Drugs that may cause *increased* levels include clofibrate,
  estrogens, heroin, methadone, and oral contraceptives.

✗ Drugs that may cause *decreased* levels include anabolic steroids, androgens, antithyroid drugs (e.g., propylthiouracil), lithium, phenytoin (Dilantin), and propranolol (Inderal).

Procedure and patient care

Before
PT Explain the procedure and tell the patient that no fasting is required.

PT If indicated, instruct the patient to stop exogenous T_4 medication 1 month before testing.

During

Adult
- Collect a venous blood specimen in a red-top tube.

Newborn
- Perform a heel stick to obtain blood.
- Thoroughly saturate the circles on the filter paper with blood.
- Note that prompt collection and processing are crucial to the early detection of hypothyroidism.
- Note that the optimal collection time is 2 to 4 days after birth.
- All newborns should be screened before discharge (regardless of age), because of the consequences of delayed diagnosis.

After
- Apply pressure to the venipuncture site.

Abnormal findings

▲ **Increased levels**
Graves' disease
Plummer's disease
Toxic thyroid adenoma
Acute thyroiditis
Familial dysalbuminemic
  hyperthyroxinemia
Factitious hyperthyroidism
Struma ovarii
Pregnancy
Hepatitis
Congenital hyperproteinemia

▼ **Decreased levels**
Cretinism
Surgical ablation
Myxedema
Pituitary insufficiency
Hypothalamic failure
Protein-depleted
  disease states
Iodine insufficiency
Renal failure
Cushing's syndrome
Cirrhosis

T

thyroxine-binding globulin (TBG, Thyroid-binding globulin)

Type of test Blood

Normal findings

Age	Male (mg/dl)	Female (mg/dl)
1-5 days	2.2-4.2	2.2-4.2
1-11 months	1.6-3.6	1.7-3.7
1-9 years	1.2-2.8	1.5-2.7
10-19 years	1.4-2.6	1.4-3.0
>20 years	1.7-3.6	1.7-3.6
Oral contraceptives	—	1.5-5.5
Pregnancy (third trimester)	—	4.7-5.9

Test explanation and related physiology

TBG is the major thyroid hormone protein carrier. When it is elevated, T_3 and T_4 are also elevated. This may give the false sense that the patient has hyperthyroidism when in fact the patient just has elevated TBGs. When total T_4 is elevated, one must ascertain whether that elevation is caused by an elevation in TBG or a real elevation in T_4 alone, which is associated with hyperthyroidism.

The most common causes of elevated TBGs are pregnancy, hormone replacement therapy, or use of oral contraceptives. Elevated TBGs are also present in some cases of porphyria and in infectious hepatitis. Decreased TBGs are commonly associated with other causes of hypoproteinemia (e.g., nephrotic syndrome, gastrointestinal malabsorption, and malnutrition).

Interfering factors

- Previous administration of diagnostic radioisotopes may confound test results because TBG is measured by radioimmunoassay.
- Drugs that *increase* TBG include estrogens, methadone, tamoxifen, and oral contraceptives.
- Drugs that *decrease* TBG include steroids, androgens, danazol, phenytoin, and propranolol.

Procedure and patient care

Before

- **PT** Explain the procedure to the patient.
- **PT** Tell the patient that no fasting is required.

During
- Collect approximately 5 to 7 ml of venous blood in a red-top tube.
- List on the laboratory slip any drugs that may affect test results.

After
- Apply pressure to the venipuncture site.

Abnormal findings

▲ **Increased levels**

Pregnancy
Estrogen replacement therapy
Estrogen-producing tumors
Infectious hepatitis
Genetic increased TBG
Acute intermittent porphyria

▼ **Decreased levels**

Protein-losing enteropathy
Protein-losing nephropathy
Malnutrition
Testosterone-producing tumors
Ovarian failure
Major stress

notes

T

thyroxine index, free (FTI, FT$_4$ index, FT$_4$I)

Type of test   Blood

Normal findings   0.8-2.4 ng/dl or 10-31 pmol/L (SI units)

Test explanation and related physiology

The FT$_4$I study measures the amount of free thyroxine (T$_4$), which is only 1% of the total T$_4$. Free T$_4$ is the unbound T$_4$ that enters the cell and is metabolically active. The diagnostic value of measuring the FT$_4$I is that it is not affected by thyroid-binding globulin (TBG) abnormalities; therefore, it correlates more closely with the true hormonal status than do total T$_4$ or tri-iodothyronine (T$_3$) determinations. To determine the FT$_4$I, T$_3$ uptake is measured and multiplied by the measured T$_4$ (see p. 924). The following mathematic computation,

$$FT_4I = \frac{T_4 \text{ (total)} \times T_3 \text{ uptake (\%)}}{100},$$

corrects the estimated total T$_4$ assay for the effects of TBG protein alterations. If TBG is increased, T$_3$ uptake decreases and corrects for the increased T$_4$ associated with increased TBG. However, when TBG is normal and T$_4$ is elevated, FT$_4$ will be increased, indicating true hyperthyroidism. Therefore, the FT$_4$I indicates the same information as the free T$_4$ radioimmunoassay (p. 922).

This index is useful in diagnosing hyperthyroidism and hypothyroidism, especially in patients with abnormalities in TBG levels. High FTI calculations suggest hyperthyroidism; low FTI values suggest hypothyroidism. The FTI study also aids in the evaluation of the thyroid status of pregnant women and patients who have abnormal TBG levels as a result of being treated with certain drugs (e.g., estrogen, phenytoin, salicylates).

Interfering factors

- Recent radionuclear scan

Procedure and patient care

Before

PT Explain the procedure to the patient.

- Obtain the T$_4$ value and T$_3$ uptake ratio.

During

- Multiply the T_3 uptake value by the T_4 value to obtain the FTI (see p. 928).

After

- Apply pressure to the venipuncture site.

Abnormal findings

▲   **Increased levels**

Graves' disease
Plummer's disease
Toxic thyroid adenoma
Acute thyroiditis
Factitious hyperthyroidism
Struma ovarii

▼   **Decreased levels**

Hypothyroid states
Cretinism
Surgical ablation
Myxedema
Pituitary insufficiency
Hypothalamic failure
Iodine insufficiency

notes

T

TORCH test

The term TORCH (toxoplasmosis, other, rubella, cytomegalovirus, herpes) has been applied to infections with recognized detrimental effects on the fetus. The effects on the fetus may be direct or indirect (e.g., precipitating abortion or premature labor). Included in the category of *other* are infections such as syphilis. All of these tests are discussed separately:

Toxoplasmosis, p. 931
Rubella, p. 812
Cytomegalovirus, p. 349
Herpesvirus, p. 524

notes

toxoplasmosis antibody titer

Type of test Blood

Normal findings

Titers <1:16 indicate no previous infection.
Titers 1:16-1:256 are usually prevalent in general population.
Titers >1:256 suggest recent infection.
Rising titers are of great significance.

Test explanation and related physiology

Toxoplasmosis is a protozoan disease caused by *Toxoplasma gondii*, which is found in poorly cooked or raw meat and in cat feces. Most often, humans are asymptomatic from the infection. When symptoms occur, this disease is characterized by central nervous system lesions, which may lead to blindness, brain damage, and death. The condition may occur congenitally or postnatally. Because approximately 25% to 50% of the adult population are asymptomatically affected with toxoplasmosis, the Centers for Disease Control and Prevention (CDC) recommend that patients who are pregnant be serologically tested for this disease.

The presence of antibodies before pregnancy indicates prior exposure and chronic asymptomatic infection. The presence of these antibodies probably ensures protection against congenital toxoplasmosis in the child. Fetal infection occurs if the mother acquires toxoplasmosis after conception and passes it to the fetus through the placenta. Repeat testing of pregnant patients with low or negative titers may be done before the twentieth week and before delivery to identify antibody converters and determine appropriate therapy (e.g., therapeutic abortion at 20 weeks, treatment during the remainder of the pregnancy, or treatment of the newborn).

Hydrocephaly, microcephaly, chronic retinitis, and convulsions are complications of congenital toxoplasmosis. Congenital toxoplasmosis is diagnosed when the antibody levels are persistently elevated or a rising titer is found in the infant 2 to 3 months after birth. Toxoplasmosis is an infection included in the acronym TORCH (toxoplasmosis, other, rubella, cytomegalovirus, herpes), which is associated with recognized detrimental effects on the fetus.

T

Procedure and patient care

Before

PT Explain the procedure to the patient.

During

- Collect approximately 5 ml of blood in a red-top tube.
- Indicate on the laboratory slip if the patient is pregnant or has been exposed to cats.

After

- Apply pressure to the venipuncture site.

Abnormal findings

Toxoplasmosis infection

notes

transesophageal echocardiography (TEE)

Type of test Endoscopy/ultrasound

Normal findings Normal position, size, and movement of the heart muscle, valves, and heart chambers

Test explanation and related physiology

TEE provides ultrasonic imaging of the heart from a retrocardiac vantage point, avoiding interference with the ultrasound by the interposed subcutaneous tissue, bony thorax, and lungs. In this procedure, a high-frequency ultrasound transducer placed in the esophagus by endoscopy provides better resolution than that of images obtained with routine transthoracic echocardiography (see p. 365). For TEE, the distal end of the endoscope is advanced into the esophagus. The transducer is positioned behind the heart (Figure 40). Controls on the handle of the endoscope permit the transducer to be rotated and flexed in both the anteroposterior and right-left lateral planes. TEE images have better resolution than those obtained by routine transthoracic echocardiography because of the higher-frequency sound waves and closer proximity of the transducer to the cardiac structures. (See p. 365 for a discussion of M-mode, two-dimensional, and color Doppler echocardiography.)

TEE is helpful in the evaluation of structures that are inaccessible or poorly visualized by the transthoracic probe approach. It is especially helpful in patients who are obese or have large lung-air spaces.

This test is performed for the following reasons:
1. To better visualize the mitral valve
2. To differentiate intracardiac from extracardiac masses and tumors
3. To better visualize the atrial septum (for atrial septal defects)
4. To diagnose thoracic aortic dissection
5. To better detect valvular vegetation indicative of endocarditis
6. To determine cardiac sources of arterial embolism
7. To detect coronary artery disease

TEE can also be used intraoperatively to monitor high-risk patients for ischemia. Ischemic muscle movement is much different from normal muscle movement; therefore, TEE is a

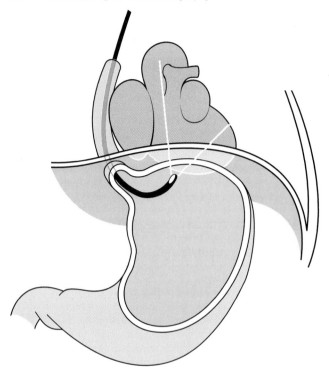

Figure 40 Transesophageal echocardiography. Diagram illustrates location of the transesophageal endoscope within the esophagus.

very sensitive indicator of myocardial ischemia. TEE can be used to monitor patients undergoing major abdominal, peripheral vascular, and carotid artery procedures who are at high risk for intraoperative ischemia because of coronary artery disease.

TEE is more sensitive than electrocardiography (ECG) for detecting ischemia. It is also used intraoperatively to evaluate surgical results of valvular or congenital heart disease. Furthermore, TEE is also the most sensitive technique for detecting air emboli, a serious complication of neurosurgery, performed with the patient in the upright position (cervical laminectomy).

Contraindications

- Patients with known upper esophageal pathology
- Patients with known esophageal varices
- Patients with Zenker's diverticulum
- Patients with esophageal abnormalities (e.g., stricture diverticula, scleroderma, esophagitis)
- Patients with bleeding disorders
- Patients who have had prior esophageal surgery
- Patients who cannot cooperate with the procedure

Potential complications

- Esophageal perforation or bleeding
- Cardiac arrhythmias

Procedure and patient care

Before

PT Explain the procedure to the patient.
PT Instruct the patient to fast for 4 to 6 hours before the test.
PT Tell the patient to remove all oral prostheses.
- Obtain IV access.

During

- Intravenous sedation is commonly provided with a short-acting benzodiazepine. Other sedation may be provided.
- Apply ECG leads and continually monitor heart rhythm.
- Apply a blood pressure cuff and monitor blood pressure periodically.
- Pulse oximetry is monitored to determine oxygen saturation in sedated patients.
- Note the following procedural steps:
  1. The pharynx is anesthetized with a local topical agent to depress the gag reflex.
  2. The patient is placed in the left lateral decubitus position.
  3. Intubation is carried out through the mouth and into the upper esophagus.
  4. The patient is asked to swallow, and the transducer is advanced into position behind the heart.
  5. The room is darkened, and the ultrasound images are displayed on a monitor. Views can be obtained of the ultrasound image after desired images are visualized.
- The procedure is performed by a cardiologist and/or a gastrointestinal endoscopist in approximately 20 minutes in the endoscopy suite. It also can be performed at the bedside.
- Very little discomfort is associated with this test.

T

After
- Naloxone or flumazenil may be administered to reverse the sedative effects of the narcotics.
- Observe the patient closely for approximately 1 hour after the procedure, until the effects of sedation have worn off.

Abnormal findings

Myocardial ischemia
Myocardial infarction
Valvular heart disease
Intracardiac thrombi
Cardiac valvular vegetation
Ventricular and atrial septal defects
Cardiomyopathy
Marked cardiac chamber dilation
Cardiac tumors

notes

triglycerides (TGs)

Type of test Blood

Normal findings
Adult/elderly
 Male: 40-160 mg/dl or 0.45-1.81 mmol/L (SI units)
 Female: 35-135 mg/dl or 0.40-1.52 mmol/L (SI units)

Child	Male	Female
0-5 years:	30-86 mg/dl	32-99 mg/dl
6-11 years:	31-108 mg/dl	35-114 mg/dl
12-15 years:	36-138 mg/dl	41-138 mg/dl
16-19 years:	40-163 mg/dl	40-128 mg/dl

Possible critical values >400 mg/dl

Test explanation and related physiology

TGs are a form of fat that exists within the bloodstream. They are transported by very-low-density lipoproteins (VLDLs) and low-density lipoproteins (LDLs). TGs are produced in the liver by using glycerol and other fatty acids as building blocks. A TG acts as a storage source for energy. When TG levels in the blood are in excess, TGs are deposited into the fatty tissues. TGs are a part of a lipid profile that also evaluates cholesterol (see p. 262) and lipoproteins (see p. 592). A lipid profile is performed to assess the risk of coronary and vascular disease.

Interfering factors

- Ingestion of fatty meals may cause elevated TG levels.
- Ingestion of alcohol may cause elevated levels.
- Pregnancy may cause increased levels.
- ℣ Drugs that may cause *increased* TG levels include cholestyramine, estrogens, and oral contraceptives.
- ℣ Drugs that may cause *decreased* levels include ascorbic acid, asparaginase, clofibrate, and colestipol.

Procedure and patient care

Before
ᴾᵀ Explain the procedure to the patient.
ᴾᵀ Instruct the patient to fast for 12 to 14 hours before the test. Only water is permitted.

T

PT Tell the patient not to drink alcohol for 24 hours before the test.

PT Inform the patient that dietary indiscretion for as much as 2 weeks before this test will influence results.

During

- Collect 5 to 10 ml of venous blood in a red-top tube.

After

- Apply pressure to the venipuncture site.
- Mark the patient's age and gender on the laboratory slip.

PT Instruct the patient with increased TG levels regarding diet, exercise, and appropriate weight.

Abnormal findings

▲ **Increased levels**

Glycogen storage disease
Hyperlipidemias
Hypothyroidism
High-carbohydrate diet
Poorly controlled diabetes
Risk of arteriosclerotic occlusive coronary disease and peripheral vascular disease
Nephrotic syndrome
Hypertension
Alcoholic cirrhosis
Pregnancy
Myocardial infarction

▼ **Decreased levels**

Malabsorption syndrome
Malnutrition
Hyperthyroidism

notes

triiodothyronine (T_3 radioimmunoassay [T_3 by RIA])

Type of test Blood

Normal findings

1-3 days: 100-740 ng/dl
1-11 months: 105-245 ng/dl
1-5 years: 105-270 ng/dl
6-10 years: 95-240 ng/dl
11-15 years: 80-215 ng/dl
16-20 years: 80-210 ng/dl
20-50 years: 75-220 ng/dl or 1.2-3.4 nmol/L (SI units)
>50 years: 40-180 ng/dl or 0.6-2.8 nmol/L (SI units)

Test explanation and related physiology

As with the thyroxine (T_4) test, the serum T_3 test is an accurate measure of thyroid function. T_3 is less stable than T_4 and occurs in minute quantities in the active form. Only about 7% to 10% of thyroid hormone is composed of T_3. Seventy percent of that T_3 is bound to proteins (thyroid-binding globulin [TBG] and albumin). This test is a measurement of total T_3 (i.e., the free and the bound T_3). Generally when the T_3 level is below normal, the patient is in a hypothyroid state.

Other severe nonthyroidal diseases can decrease T_3 levels by diminishing the conversion of T_4 to T_3 in the liver. This makes T_3 levels less useful in indicating hypothyroid states. Further, there is considerable overlap between hypothyroid states and normal thyroid function. Because of this, T_3 levels are mostly used just to assist in the diagnosis of hyperthyroid states. An elevated T_3 indicates hyperthyroidism, especially when the T_4 is also elevated. There is a rare form of hyperthyroidism called *T_3 toxicosis,* in which the T_4 is normal and the T_3 is elevated.

Interfering factors

- Radioisotope administration before the test may alter the results.
- T_3 values are increased in pregnancy.
- Drugs that may cause *increased* levels include estrogen, methadone, and oral contraceptives.
- Drugs that may cause *decreased* levels include anabolic steroids, androgens, phenytoin (Dilantin), propranolol (Inderal), reserpine, and salicylates (high dose).

Procedure and patient care

Before

PT Explain the procedure to the patient.

- Determine whether the patient is taking any exogenous T_3 medication, because this will affect test results.
- Withhold drugs that may affect results (with physician's approval).

PT Tell the patient that no fasting is required.

During

- Collect approximately 5 to 10 ml of venous blood in a red-top tube.
- List on the laboratory slip any medications the patient is currently taking.

After

- Apply pressure to the venipuncture site.

Abnormal findings

▲ **Increased levels**

Graves' disease
Plummer's disease
Toxic thyroid adenoma
Acute thyroiditis
Factitious hyperthyroidism
Struma ovarii
Pregnancy
Hepatitis
Congenital hyperproteinemia

▼ **Decreased levels**

Hypothyroidism
Cretinism
Thyroid surgical ablation
Myxedema
Pituitary insufficiency
Hypothalamic failure
Protein malnutrition and other protein-depleted states (e.g., nephrotic syndrome)
Iodine insufficiency
Renal failure
Cushing's syndrome
Cirrhosis
Liver diseases

notes

troponins (Cardiac-specific troponin T [cTnT]; Cardiac-specific troponin I [cTnI])

Type of test Blood

Normal findings

Cardiac troponin T: <0.2 ng/ml
Cardiac troponin I: <0.03 ng/ml

Test explanation and related physiology

Cardiac troponins are promising biochemical markers for cardiac disease. This test is used to assist in the evaluation of patients with suspected acute coronary ischemic syndromes. In addition to improving the diagnosis of acute ischemic disorders, troponins are also valuable for early risk stratification in patients with unstable angina. They can be used to predict the likelihood of future cardiac events.

Troponins are proteins that exist in skeletal and cardiac muscle that regulate the calcium-dependent interaction of myosin with actin for the muscle contractile apparatus. Cardiac troponins can be separated from skeletal troponins by the use of monoclonal antibodies, or enzyme-linked immunosorbent assay. There are two cardiac-specific troponins: cardiac troponin T (cTnT), and cardiac troponin I (cTnI).

Because of their extraordinarily high specificity for myocardial cell injury, cardiac troponins are very helpful in the evaluation of patients with chest pain. Their use is similar to that of creatine phosphokinase MB (CPK-MB). However, cardiac troponins have several advantages over CPK-MB. Cardiac troponins are more specific for cardiac muscle injury. CPK-MB can be elevated with severe skeletal muscle injury, brain or lung injury, or in renal failure. Cardiac troponins will nearly always be normal in noncardiac muscle diseases. Cardiac troponins become elevated sooner and remain elevated longer than CPK-MB. This expands the time window of opportunity for diagnosis and thrombolytic treatment of myocardial injury. Finally, cTnT and cTnI are more sensitive to muscle injury than CPK-MB. That is most important in evaluating patients with chest pain.

Cardiac troponins become elevated as early as 3 hours after myocardial injury. Levels of cTnI may remain elevated for 7 to 10 days after myocardial infarction, and cTnT levels may remain elevated for 10 to 14 days. Measurement of these troponins is

T

preferable to measurement of LDH (see p. 572) and its isoenzymes in patients who seek medical attention more than 24 to 48 hours after the onset of symptoms.

Troponins can be detected by monoclonal antibody immunoassay; by enzyme-linked immunosorbent assay; and most recently, by monoclonal "sandwich" antibody qualitative testing. The test results using the first two laboratory techniques listed are available after about 2 hours. The "sandwich" technique is performed at the bedside in about 20 minutes and is read visually much like a glucometer.

Cardiac troponins are used in the following cardiac clinical situations:

1. Evaluation of patient with unstable angina. These patients can be separated into two groups based on cardiac troponins. If cardiac troponins are normal, no myocardial injury has occurred, and there will be no lasting cardiac dysfunction. If cardiac troponins are elevated, muscle injury has occurred. Revascularization may be indicated because this latter group is at great risk for a subsequent cardiac event (infarction or sudden death).

2. Detection of reperfusion associated with coronary recanalization. A "washout" or second peak of cardiac troponin levels accurately indicates reperfusion by way of recanalization or coronary angioplasty.

3. Estimation of myocardial infarction size. Late (4 weeks) cardiac troponin levels are inversely related to left ventricular ejection fraction. These late elevations in cardiac troponins are due to degradation of the contractile apparatus.

4. Detection of perioperative myocardial infarction. The use of CPK-MB determinations in the diagnosis of myocardial infarction after surgery is difficult because of the frequent increase of this enzyme associated with skeletal muscle injury during surgery. Cardiac troponins are not affected by skeletal muscle injury.

Interfering factors

- Severe skeletal muscle injury may cause false elevation of cTnT.

Procedure and patient care

Before

PT Explain the procedure to the patient.

PT Discuss with the patient the need and reason for frequent venipuncture in diagnosing myocardial infarction.

PT Tell the patient that no food or fluid restrictions are necessary.

During

- Collect a venous blood sample in a yellow-top (serum separator) tube. This is usually done initially and 12 hours later followed by daily testing for 3 to 5 days and possibly weekly for 5 to 6 weeks.
- Rotate the venipuncture sites.
- Record the exact time and date of venipuncture on each laboratory slip. This aids in the interpretation of the temporal pattern of enzyme elevations.
- If a qualitative immunoassay is to be done at the bedside, whole blood is obtained in a micropipette and placed in the sample well of the testing device. A red or purple color in the "read" zone indicates that 0.2 ng/ml or more cardiac troponin is present in the patient's blood.

After

- Apply pressure or a pressure dressing to the venipuncture site.
- Observe the venipuncture site for bleeding.

Abnormal findings

▲   **Increased levels**

Myocardial injury
Myocardial infarction

T

notes

tuberculin test (PPD skin test)

Type of test Skin

Normal findings Negative; reaction <5 mm

Test explanation and related physiology

Although this test is used to detect tuberculosis (TB) infection, it is unable to indicate whether the infection is active or dormant. For this test, a *purified protein derivative (PPD)* of the tubercle bacillus is injected intradermally. If the patient is infected with TB (whether active or dormant), lymphocytes will recognize the PPD antigen and cause a local reaction; if the patient is not infected, no reaction will occur. If the test is negative and the physician strongly suspects TB, a "second-strength" PPD can be used. If this test is negative, the patient does not have TB. (See p. 946 for tuberculosis culture.) The PPD skin test usually becomes positive 6 weeks after infection. Once positive, the reaction usually persists for life.

The PPD test also can be used as part of a series of skin tests to assess the immune system. If the immune system is nonfunctioning because of poor nutrition or chronic illness (e.g., neoplasia, infection), the PPD test will be negative despite the patient having had an active or dormant TB infection. Other skin tests used to test immune function include *Candida,* mumps virus, and *Trichophyton,* organisms to which most people in the United States have been exposed.

Testing for TB is usually performed as part of the routine prenatal evaluation in pregnant women. Often this may be the mother's first contact with the health care system in several years.

When a patient known to have active TB receives a PPD test, the local reaction may be so severe as to cause a complete skin slough requiring surgical care. When these patients are eliminated from PPD testing, the test has no complications. The PPD test will not cause active TB because no live organisms exist in the test solution.

Contraindications

- Patients with known active TB
- Patients who have received *bacille Calmette-Guérin (BCG)* immunization against PPD, because these patients will

demonstrate a positive reaction to the PPD vaccination even though they have never had TB infection

Procedure and patient care

Before

PT Explain the procedure to the patient.

PT Assure the patient that she or he will not develop TB from this test.

- Assess the patient for previous history of TB. Report a positive history to the physician.
- Evaluate the patient's history for previous PPD results and BCG immunization.

During

- Prepare the patient's forearm with alcohol and allow it to dry.
- Intradermally inject the PPD. A skin wheal will occur.
- Circle the area with indelible ink.
- Record the time at which the PPD was injected.

After

- Read the results in 48 to 72 hours.
- Examine the test site for induration (hardening). Measure the area of induration (not redness) in millimeters.
- If the test is positive, ensure that the physician is notified and the patient treated appropriately.
- If the test is positive, check the patient's arm 4 to 5 days after the test to be certain that a severe skin reaction has not occurred.

Abnormal findings

Positive results
TB infection
Nontuberculous mycobacteria infections

Negative result
Possible immunoincompetence

notes

tuberculosis culture (TB culture, BACTEC method, Polymerase chain reaction)

Type of test   Microbiology culture

Normal findings   Negative for tuberculosis

Test explanation and related physiology

Diagnosis of TB can be made only by identification and culture of *Mycobacterium tuberculosis* in a specimen. Conventional culture techniques for growth, identification, and susceptibility of acid-fast mycobacteria take 4 to 6 weeks. Because a patient suspected of having TB cannot be isolated for that duration, the disease may spread to many other people while he or she waits for the diagnosis. With the resurgence and increasing incidence of TB in the U.S. population (especially among immunocompromised patients with acquired immunodeficiency syndrome), newer, more rapid culture techniques have been identified and are now being performed.

The *BACTEC* method is a culture technique in which the growth medium for culturing mycobacteria is supplanted with a substrate labeled with radioactive carbon (^{14}C). This substrate is used by mycobacteria; during metabolism, radioactive carbon dioxide ($^{14}CO_2$) is produced from the substrate. The $^{14}CO_2$ is detected and quantitated. This permits quick identification of mycobacterial growth.

Polymerase chain reaction culture methods have also recently been developed. With the addition of a deoxyribonucleic acid (DNA) polymerase, genetic chromosomal parts can be multiplied. This allows amplification of genomes, which then can be detected by genetic DNA probes. With the newer techniques already described, *M. tuberculosis* can be identified in as few as 36 to 48 hours. With this reduction in diagnostic time, treatment can be started earlier. Thus it is anticipated that the spread of tuberculosis will be greatly reduced. The average detection time, however, is longer for extrapulmonary specimens than for sputum specimens. The time for identification is greatly reduced when numerous mycobacteria are present. Generally, organisms in specimens from patients already receiving antituberculosis treatment take longer to grow.

After identification and growth of mycobacteria, antibiotic susceptibility testing is performed to identify the most effective antimycobacterial drugs. The culture specimen can be performed on sputum, body fluids, cerebrospinal fluid, and even biopsy tissue specimens.

When tuberculosis is suspected, a *sputum smear for acid-fast bacillus (AFB)* can be obtained. After taking up a dye such as fuchsin, *M. tuberculosis* is not decolorized by acid alcohol (i.e., it is acid-fast). It is seen under the microscope as a red, rod-shaped organism. If this bacillus is seen, the patient may have active TB. At least 5000 organisms must be present in each milliliter of specimen to be seen on a microscope smear. Other specimens such as cerebrospinal fluid, tissue, and synovial fluid may be used. Smears may be negative as much as 50% of the time, even with positive cultures. AFB is also used to monitor treatment for TB. If after adequate therapy (2 months), the sputum still contains AFB (even though the culture may be negative due to anti-TB drugs), treatment failure should be considered.

Interfering factors

✘ Antituberculosis drugs

Procedure and patient care

Before

PT Explain the procedure to the patient.

PT Tell the patient that no fasting is required.

During

- For *sputum* collection, it is best to induce sputum production with an ultrasonic or nebulizing device. Collect three to five early morning sputum specimens. All specimens must contain mycobacteria to make the diagnosis of TB.
- For *urine* collection, obtain three to five single, clean-voided specimens early in the morning.
- *Swabs, intestinal washings,* and *biopsy* specimens should be transported to the laboratory immediately for preparation.
- Follow the institution's policy for universal specimen handling.
- Once the specimen is received by the laboratory, a decontamination process is applied to it to kill all nonmycobacteria. The specimen is then cultured in the appropriate medium.
- With the rapid growth techniques, the specimen is evaluated every 24 hours.

- When culture growth is considered adequate, the organisms are stained for acid-fast bacillus and identified.
- With genetic probes, the *Mycobacterium* species is identified.
- At this point, if *M. tuberculosis* is present, the report will read "culture more positive for mycobacteria." If the species has been identified, this also will be reported.
- Drug-susceptibility testing then will be carried out and subsequently reported.

After

PT Instruct the patient as to appropriate isolation of sputum and other body fluids to avoid potential spread of suspected TB.

Abnormal findings

TB
Atypical mycobacterial nontuberculosis disease

notes

upper gastrointestinal x-ray study (Upper GI series, UGI)

Type of test X-ray with contrast dye

Normal findings Normal size, contour, patency, filling, positioning, and transit of barium through the lower esophagus, stomach, and upper duodenum

Test explanation and related physiology

The upper GI study consists of a series of x-ray films of the lower esophagus, stomach, and duodenum, usually using barium sulfate as the contrast medium. When there is concern for leakage of x-ray contrast through a perforation of the GI tract, however, Gastrografin (a water-soluble contrast) is used. This test can be performed in conjunction with a barium swallow or a small bowel series (see pp. 150 and 860), which can precede or succeed the upper GI study, respectively.

The purpose of this examination is to detect ulcerations, tumors, inflammations, or anatomic malpositions (e.g., hiatal hernia) within these organs. Obstruction of the upper GI tract is also easily detected.

In this test the patient is asked to drink barium. As the contrast descends, the lower esophagus is examined for position, patency, and filling defects (e.g., tumors, scarring, varices). As the contrast enters the stomach, the gastric wall is examined for benign or malignant ulcerations, filling defects (most often in cancer), and anatomic abnormalities (e.g., hiatal hernia). The patient is placed in a flat or head-down position, and the gastroesophageal area is examined for evidence of gastroesophageal reflux of barium.

As the contrast leaves the stomach, patency of the pyloric channel and the duodenum is evaluated. Benign peptic ulceration is the most common pathologic condition affecting these areas. Extrinsic compression caused by tumors, cysts, or enlarged pathologic organs (e.g., liver) near the stomach also can be identified by anatomic distortion of the outline of the upper GI tract. The small intestine can then be studied (see discussion of small bowel follow-through, p. 860).

Contraindications

- Patients with complete bowel obstructions

- Patients suspected of upper GI perforation
  Water-soluble Gastrografin should be used instead of barium.
- Patients with unstable vital signs
  These patients should be supervised during the time required
  for this test.
- Patients who are uncooperative, because of the necessity of
  frequent position changes

Potential complications

- Aspiration of barium
- Constipation or partial bowel obstruction caused by
  inspissated barium in the small bowel or colon

Interfering factors

- Previously administered barium may block visualization of the
  upper GI tract.
- Incapacitated patients cannot assume the multiple positions
  required for the study.
- Food and fluid in the stomach give the false impression of
  filling defects within the stomach, precluding adequate
  evaluation of the gastric mucosa.

Procedure and patient care

Before

PT Explain the procedure to the patient. Allow the patient to
verbalize concerns.

PT Instruct the patient to abstain from eating for at least
8 hours before the test. Usually keep the patient NPO after
midnight on the day of the test.

PT Assure the patient that the test will not cause any discomfort.

During

- Note the following procedural steps:
  1. The patient is asked to drink approximately 16 ounces of
     barium sulfate. This is a chalky substance usually
     suspended in milkshake form and drunk through a straw.
     Usually the drink is flavored to increase palatability.
  2. After drinking the barium, the patient is moved through
     several position changes (e.g., prone, supine, lateral) to
     promote filling of the entire upper GI tract.
  3. Films are taken at the discretion of the radiologist
     observing the flow of barium fluoroscopically.
  4. The flow of barium is followed through the lower
     esophagus, stomach, and duodenum.

5. Several films are taken throughout the course of the test.

6. In an *air-contrast upper GI study,* the patient is asked to swallow rapidly carbonated powder. This creates carbon dioxide in the stomach, providing air contrast to the barium within the stomach and increased visualization of the gastric mucosa.

- Note that a radiologist performs this procedure in approximately 30 minutes.

PT Tell the patient that he or she may be uncomfortable lying on the hard x-ray table and may experience the sensation of bloating or nausea during the test.

After

PT Inform the patient that if Gastrografin was used, he or she may have significant diarrhea. Gastrografin is an osmotic cathartic.

PT Instruct the patient to use a cathartic (e.g., milk of magnesia) if barium sulfate was used as the contrast medium. Water absorption may cause the barium to harden and create a fecal impaction if catharsis is not carried out.

PT Instruct the patient to watch his or her stools to ensure that all of the barium has been removed. The stools should return to normal color after completely expelling the barium, which may take as much as a day and a half.

Abnormal findings

Esophageal cancer
Esophageal varices
Hiatal hernia
Esophageal diverticula
Gastric cancer
Gastric inflammatory disease (e.g., Ménétrier's disease)
Benign gastric tumor (e.g., leiomyoma)
Extrinsic compression by pancreatic pseudocysts, cysts, pancreatic tumors, or hepatomegaly
Perforation of the esophagus, stomach, or duodenum
Congenital abnormalities (e.g., duodenal web, pancreatic rest, malrotation syndrome)
Gastric ulcer (benign and malignant)
Gastritis
Duodenal ulcer
Duodenal cancer
Duodenal diverticulum

U

urea nitrogen blood test (Blood urea nitrogen [BUN], Serum urea nitrogen)

Type of test Blood

Normal findings

Adult: 10-20 mg/dl or 3.6-7.1 mmol/L (SI units)
Elderly: may be slightly higher than those of adults
Child: 5-18 mg/dl
Infant: 5-18 mg/dl
Newborn: 3-12 mg/dl
Cord: 21-40 mg/dl

Possible critical values >100 mg/dl (indicates serious impairment of renal function)

Test explanation and related physiology

The BUN measures the amount of urea nitrogen in the blood. Urea is formed in the liver as the end product of protein metabolism. During ingestion, protein is broken down into amino acids. In the liver these amino acids are catabolized, and free ammonia is formed. The ammonia is combined to form urea, which is then deposited into the blood and transported to the kidneys for excretion. Therefore BUN is directly related to the metabolic function of the liver and the excretory function of the kidney. It serves as an index of the function of these organs. Patients who have elevated BUN levels are said to have azotemia.

Nearly all renal diseases cause an inadequate excretion of urea, which causes the blood concentration to rise above normal. If the disease is unilateral, however, the unaffected kidney can compensate for the diseased kidney, and BUN may not become elevated. BUN also increases in conditions other than primary renal disease. For example, when excess amounts of protein are available for hepatic catabolism (from a high-protein diet or gastrointestinal [GI] bleeding), large quantities of urea are made. BUN levels also may vary according to the state of hydration, with increased levels seen in dehydration and decreased levels seen in overhydration. Finally, one must be aware that the synthesis of urea depends on the liver. Patients with severe primary liver disease will have a decreased BUN. With combined liver and renal disease (as in hepatorenal syndrome), BUN can be normal not because renal excretory function is good but because poor hepatic functioning has resulted in decreased formation of urea.

BUN is interpreted in conjunction with the creatinine test (see p. 326). These tests are referred to as *renal function studies.*

The BUN/creatinine ratio is a good measurement of kidney and liver function. The normal adult range is 6 to 25, with 15.5 being the optimal adult value for this ratio.

Interfering factors

- Changes in protein intake may affect BUN levels.
- Advanced pregnancy may cause increased BUN levels.
- Overhydration and underhydration will affect BUN levels.
- Drugs that may cause *increased* BUN levels include allopurinol, aminoglycosides, cephalosporins, chloral hydrate, cisplatin, furosemide, guanethidine, indomethacin, methotrexate, methyldopa, nephrotoxic drugs (e.g., aspirin, amphotericin B, bacitracin, carbamazepine, colistin, gentamicin, methicillin, neomycin, penicillamine, polymyxin B, probenecid, vancomycin), propranolol, rifampin, spironolactone, tetracyclines, thiazide diuretics, and triamterene.
- Drugs that may cause *decreased* BUN levels include chloramphenicol and streptomycin.
- GI bleeding can cause *increased* BUN levels

Procedure and patient care

Before

PT Explain the procedure to the patient.
PT Tell the patient that no fasting is required.

During

- Collect approximately 5 ml of blood in a red-top tube.
- Avoid hemolysis.

After

- Apply pressure or a pressure dressing to the venipuncture site.

Abnormal findings

▲ **Increased levels**

Prerenal causes
Hypovolemia
Shock
Burns
Dehydration
Congestive heart failure
Myocardial infarction
GI bleeding
Excessive protein ingestion
Alimentary tube feeding
Excessive protein catabolism
Starvation
Sepsis

Renal causes
Renal disease
    (e.g., glomerulonephritis,
    pyelonephritis, acute
    tubular necrosis)
Renal failure
Nephrotoxic drugs

Postrenal azotemia
Ureteral obstruction
Bladder outlet obstruction

▼ **Decreased levels**

Liver failure
Overhydration caused
    by fluid overload or
    syndrome of
    inappropriate
    antidiuretic hormone
    (SIADH)
Negative nitrogen
    balance (e.g.,
    malnutrition
    or malabsorption)
Pregnancy
Nephrotic syndrome

notes

uric acid, blood and urine

Type of test Blood; urine

Normal findings

Blood

Adult

Male: 4.0-8.5 mg/dl or 0.24-0.51 mmol/L

Female: 2.7-7.3 mg/dl or 0.16-0.43 mmol/L

Elderly: values may be slightly increased

Child: 2.5-5.5 mg/dl or 0.12-0.32 mmol/L

Newborn: 2-6.2 mg/dl

Urine: 250-750 mg/24 hr or 1.48-4.43 mmol/day (SI units)

Possible critical values Blood: >12 mg/dl

Test explanation and related physiology

Uric acid is a nitrogenous compound that is a product of purine (a deoxyribonucleic acid [DNA] building block) catabolism. Uric acid is excreted to a large degree by the kidney and to a smaller degree by the intestinal tract. When uric acid levels are elevated (hyperuricemia), the patient may have gout. Causes of hyperuricemia can be overproduction or decreased excretion of uric acid (e.g., kidney failure). Overproduction of uric acid may occur in patients with a catabolic enzyme deficiency that stimulates purine metabolism, or in patients with cancer in whom purine and DNA turnover is great. Other causes of hyperuricemia may include alcoholism, leukemias, metastatic cancer, multiple myeloma, hyperlipoproteinemia, diabetes mellitus, renal failure, stress, lead poisoning, and dehydration caused by diuretic therapy. Ketoacids (as occur in diabetic or alcoholic ketoacidosis) may compete with uric acid for tubular excretion and may cause decreased uric acid excretion. Many causes of hyperuricemia are undefined and therefore labeled as *idiopathic*.

Elevated uric acid in the urine is called uricosuria. Uric acid can become supersaturated in the urine and crystallize to form kidney stones that can block the renal system. Urinary excretion of uric acid depends on uric acid levels in the blood, along with glomerular filtration and tubular secretion of uric acid into the urine. Uric acid is less well saturated in an acidic urine. As the urine pH rises, more uric acid can exist without crystallization and stone formation. Therefore, when a person is known to have high uric acid in the urine, the urine can be alkalinized by ingestion of a strong base to prevent stone formation.

Interfering factors

- Stress may cause increased uric acid levels.
- Recent use of x-ray contrast agents may cause decreased serum levels.
- Recent use of x-ray contrast agents may increase uric acid levels in the urine.
- ✘ Drugs that may cause *increased* serum levels include alcohol, ascorbic acid, aspirin (low dose), caffeine, cisplatin, diazoxide, diuretics, epinephrine, ethambutol, levodopa, methyldopa (Aldomet), nicotinic acid, phenothiazines, and theophylline.
- ✘ Drugs that may cause *decreased* serum levels include allopurinol, aspirin (high dose), azathioprine (Imuran), clofibrate, corticosteroids, estrogens, glucose infusions, guaifenesin, mannitol, probenecid, and warfarin.
- ✘ Drugs that may cause *increased* urine levels include ascorbic acid, calcitonin, citrate, dicumarol, estrogens, steroids, iodinated dyes, glyceryl, phenolsulfonphthalein, probenecid, salicylates, and outdated tetracycline.

Procedure and patient care

Before
PT Explain the procedure to the patient.
- Follow the institution's requirements regarding fasting. (Some recommend that the patient fast.)

During

Blood
- Collect approximately 5 to 7 ml of venous blood in a red-top tube.
- List on the laboratory slip any drugs that may affect test results.

Urine
PT Instruct the patient to begin the 24-hour urine collection after voiding. Discard the initial specimen and start the 24-hour timing at that point.
- Collect all the urine passed during the next 24 hours. A preservative may be used.
PT Show the patient where to store the urine container.

- Keep the specimen on ice or refrigerated during the entire 24 hours. (Note that some laboratories do not require refrigeration.)
- Indicate the starting time on the urine container and laboratory slip.
- Post the hours for the urine collection in a noticeable place to prevent accidental discarding of the specimen.

PT Instruct the patient to void before defecating so the urine is not contaminated by feces.

PT Remind the patient not to put toilet paper in the collection container.

PT Encourage the patient to drink fluids during the 24 hours.

PT Instruct the patient to collect the last specimen as close as possible to the end of the 24-hour period. Add this urine to the container.

After

Blood

- Apply pressure to the venipuncture site.

Urine

- Transport the urine specimen promptly to the laboratory.

Abnormal findings

▲ Increased blood levels (hyperuricemia)	▼ Decreased blood levels
Gout	Wilson's disease
Increased ingestion of purines	Fanconi's syndrome
Genetic inborn error in purine metabolism	Lead poisoning
Metastatic cancer	Yellow atrophy of the liver
Multiple myeloma	
Leukemias	
Cancer chemotherapy	
Hemolysis	
Rhabdomyolysis (e.g., heavy exercise, burns, crush injury, epileptic seizure, or myocardial infarction)	
Chronic renal disease	
Acidosis (ketotic or lactic)	
Hypothyroidism	

U

Toxemia of pregnancy
Hyperlipoproteinemia
Alcoholism
Shock or chronic blood
   volume depletion states
Idiopathic

▲   **Increased urine levels
    (uricosuria)**

Gout
Metastatic cancer
Multiple myeloma
Leukemias
Cancer chemotherapy
High purine diet
Lead toxicity

▼   **Decreased urine levels**

Kidney disease
Eclampsia
Chronic alcohol
   ingestion
Acidosis (ketotic or
   lactic)

notes

urinalysis (UA)

Type of test   Urine

Normal findings

Appearance: clear
Color: amber yellow
Odor: aromatic
pH: 4.6-8.0 (average 6.0)
Protein
   None or up to 8 mg/dl
   50-80 mg/24 hr (at rest)
   <250 mg/24 hr (exercise)
Specific gravity
   Adult: 1.005-1.030 (usually 1.010-1.025)
   Elderly: values decrease with age
   Newborn: 1.001-1.020
Leukocyte esterase: negative
Nitrites: negative
Ketones: negative
Crystals: negative
Casts: none present
Glucose (see urine glucose discussion, p. 487)
   Brand new specimen: negative
   24-hour specimen: 50-300 mg/day or 0.3-1.7 mmol/
   day (SI units)
White blood cells (WBCs): 0-4 per low-power field
WBC casts: negative
Red blood cells (RBCs): up to 2
RBC casts: none

Test explanation and related physiology

   A total urinalysis involves multiple routine tests on a urine specimen. This specimen is not necessarily a clean-catch specimen. However, if urinary tract infection is suspected, often a midstream clean-catch specimen is obtained. This urine is then split into two parts. One is sent for urinalysis, and the other is held in the laboratory refrigerator and cultured (see p. 972) if the urinalysis indicates infection. Routinely a urinalysis includes remarks about the color, appearance, and odor of the urine. The pH is determined. The urine is tested for the presence of proteins, glucose, ketones, blood, and leukocyte esterase. The urine

U

is examined microscopically for RBCs, WBCs, casts, crystals, and bacteria.

Examination of the urine sediment provides a significant amount of information about the urinary system. The test is done on a centrifuged urinary sediment. There are many different methods to prepare the sediment for microscopic review. As a result, normal values may vary significantly among laboratories. Reference ranges have been provided to recognize marked abnormalities.

Appearance and color

Urine appearance and color are noted as part of routine urinalysis. The appearance of a normal urine specimen should be clear. Cloudy urine may be caused by the presence of pus, RBCs, or bacteria; however, normal urine also may be cloudy because of ingestion of certain foods (e.g., large amounts of fat, ureates, or phosphates). The color of urine ranges from pale yellow to amber because of the pigment urochrome. The color indicates the concentration of the urine and varies with specific gravity. Dilute urine is straw colored, and concentrated urine is deep amber.

Abnormally colored urine may result from a pathologic condition or the ingestion of certain foods or medicines. For example, bleeding from the kidney produces dark red urine, whereas bleeding from the lower urinary tract produces bright red urine. Dark yellow urine may indicate the presence of urobilinogen or bilirubin. *Pseudomonas* organisms may produce green urine. Beets may cause red urine, and rhubarb can color the urine brown. Many frequently used drugs also may affect urine color (Table 23).

Odor

Determination of urine odor is a part of routine urinalysis. The aromatic odor of fresh, normal urine is caused by the presence of volatile acids. Urine of patients with diabetic ketoacidosis has the strong, sweet smell of acetone. In patients with a urinary tract infection, the urine may have a very foul odor. Patients with a fecal odor to their urine may have an enterobladder fistula.

pH

The analysis of the pH of a freshly voided urine specimen indicates the acid-base balance of the patient. An alkaline pH is obtained in a patient with alkalemia. Also, bacteria, urinary tract infection, or a diet high in citrus fruits or vegetables may cause

TABLE 23 Frequently used drugs that may affect urine color

Generic and brand names	Drug classification	Urine color
Cascara sagrada	Stimulant laxative	Red in alkaline urine; yellow-brown in acid urine
Chloroquine (Aralen)	Antimalarial	Rusty yellow or brown
Chlorzoxazone (Paraflex)	Skeletal muscle relaxant	Orange or purple-red
Docusate calcium (Doxidan, Surfak)	Laxative	Pink to red to red-brown
Furazolidone (Furoxone)	Antiinfective, antiprotozoal	Brown
Iron preparations (Ferotran, Imferon)	Hematinic	Dark brown or black on standing
Levodopa	Antiparkinsonian	Dark brown on standing
Methylene blue (Urolene Blue)	Antimethemoglobinemic	Blue-green
Methyldopa (Aldomet)	Antihypertensive	Darkening
Metronidazole (Flagyl)	Antiinfective	Darkening, reddish brown
Nitrofurantoin (Macrodantin, Nitrodan)	Antibacterial	Brown-yellow
Phenazopyridine (Pyridium)	Urinary tract analgesic	Orange to red
Phenolphthalein (Ex-Lax)	Contact laxative	Red or purplish pink in alkaline urine
Phenothiazines (e.g., prochlorperazine [Compazine])	Antipsychotic, neuroleptic, antiemetic	Red-brown
Phenytoin (Dilantin)	Anticonvulsant	Pink, red, red-brown
Riboflavin (vitamin B)	Vitamin	Intense yellow
Rifampin	Antibiotic	Red-orange
Sulfasalazine (Azulfidine)	Antibacterial	Orange-yellow in alkaline urine
Triamterene (Dyrenium)	Diuretic	Pale blue fluorescence

U

an increased urine pH. Certain medications (e.g., streptomycin, neomycin, kanamycin) are effective in treating urinary tract infections when the urine is alkaline. Acidic urine is generally obtained in patients with acidemia, which can result from metabolic or respiratory acidosis, starvation, dehydration, or a diet high in meat products or cranberries.

The urine pH is useful in identifying crystals in the urine and determining the predisposition to form a given type of stone. Acidic urine is associated with xanthine, cystine, uric acid, and calcium oxalate stones. To treat or prevent these urinary calculi, urine should be kept alkaline. Alkaline urine is associated with calcium carbonate, calcium phosphate, and magnesium phosphate stones; for these stones urine should be kept acidic.

Protein

Evaluation of protein is a sensitive indicator of kidney function. Normally protein is not present in the urine because the spaces in the normal glomerular filtrate membrane are too small to allow its passage. If the glomerular membrane is injured, as in glomerulonephritis, the spaces become much larger, and protein seeps out into the filtrate and then into the urine. If this persists at a significant rate, the patient can become hypoproteinemic because of the severe protein loss through the kidneys. This decreases the normal capillary oncotic pressure that holds fluid within the vasculature and causes severe interstitial edema. The combination of proteinuria and edema is known as the nephrotic syndrome.

Proteinuria is probably the most important indicator of renal disease. The urine of all pregnant women is routinely checked for proteinuria, which can be an indicator of preeclampsia. In addition to screening for nephrotic syndrome, urinary protein also screens for complications of diabetes mellitus, glomerulonephritis, amyloidosis, and multiple myeloma (see test for Bence Jones protein, p. 153).

Glucose

See discussion on pp. 487 to 489.

Specific gravity

The specific gravity is a measure of the concentration of particles, including wastes and electrolytes, in the urine. A high specific gravity indicates a concentrated urine; a low specific gravity indicates dilute urine. Specific gravity refers to the weight of the urine compared to that of distilled water (which has a specific gravity of 1.000). Particles in the urine give it weight or specific gravity.

The specific gravity is used to evaluate the concentrating and excretory power of the kidney. Renal disease tends to diminish the concentrating capability of the kidney. As a result, chronic renal diseases are associated with a low specific gravity. The specific gravity must be interpreted in light of the presence or absence of glycosuria and proteinuria. The specific gravity is also a measurement of the hydration status of the patient. An overhydrated patient will have a more dilute urine with a lower specific gravity. The specific gravity of the urine in a dehydrated patient can be expected to be abnormally high. The measurement of urine specific gravity is easier and more convenient than the measurement of osmolality (see p. 670). The specific gravity correlates roughly with osmolality. Knowledge of the specific gravity is needed for interpreting the results of most parts of the urinalysis. Specific gravity is usually evaluated by the use of a refractometer or a dipstick.

Leukocyte esterase (WBC esterase)

Leukocyte (WBC) esterase is a screening test used to detect leukocytes in the urine. When positive, this test indicates a urinary tract infection. This examination uses chemical testing with a leukocyte esterase dipstick; a shade of purple is considered positive. Some laboratories have established screening protocols in which a microscopic examination (see p. 972) is performed only if a leukocyte esterase test is positive.

Nitrites

Like the leukocyte esterase, the nitrite test is a screening test for the identification of urinary tract infections. This test is based on the principle that many bacteria produce an enzyme called *reductase,* which can reduce urinary nitrates to nitrites. Chemical testing is done with a dipstick containing a reagent that reacts with nitrites to produce a pink color, thus indirectly suggesting the presence of bacteria. A positive test result would indicate the need for a urine culture. Nitrite screening enhances the sensitivity of the leukocyte esterase test to detect urinary tract infections.

Ketones

Normally no ketones are present in the urine; however, a patient with poorly controlled diabetes who is hyperglycemic may have massive fatty acid catabolism. The purpose of this catabolism is to provide an energy source when glucose cannot be transferred into the cell because of an insufficiency of insulin. Ketones (beta-hydroxybutyric acid, acetoacetic acid, and acetone) are the end products of this fatty acid breakdown. As with glucose, ketones spill over into the urine when the blood levels of patients with diabetes are elevated. The excess production of ketones in the urine is usually associated with poorly controlled diabetes. This test for ketonuria is also important in evaluating ketoacidosis associated with alcoholism, fasting, starvation, high-protein diets, and isopropanol ingestion. Ketonuria may occur with acute febrile illnesses, especially in infants and children.

Crystals

Crystals found in urinary sediment on microscopic examination indicate that renal stone formulation is imminent, if not already present. Urea crystals occur in patients with high serum uric acid levels (gout). Phosphate and calcium oxalate crystals occur in the urine of patients with parathyroid abnormalities or malabsorption states. The type of crystal found varies with the disease and the pH of the urine (see prior discussion on urinary pH).

Casts

Casts are clumps of materials or cells. They are formed in the renal distal and collecting tubules where the material is maximally concentrated. These amorphous clumps of material and cells have the shape of the tubule, thus the term cast. Casts are most usually associated with some degree of proteinuria and stasis within the renal tubules. There are two kinds of casts: hyaline and cellular.

Hyaline casts are conglomerations of protein and indicate proteinuria. A few hyaline casts are normally found, especially after strenuous exercise.

Cellular casts, conglomerations of degenerated cells, are described in the following paragraphs.

Granular casts result from the disintegration of cellular material into granular particles within a WBC or epithelial cell cast. Granular casts are found after exercise and in patients with various renal diseases. The basic etiology is the same as their cellular component.

In some diseases the epithelial cells desquamate into the renal tubule. As the cell degenerates, fatty deposits within the cell coalesce and become incorporated with protein into *fatty casts*. These casts are all associated with the nephrotic syndrome/nephrosis. Free oval fat bodies may also be associated with fatty emboli that occur in patients with bone fractures.

Waxy casts may be cell casts, hyaline casts, or renal failure casts. Waxy casts probably represent further degeneration of granular casts. They occur when urine flow through the renal tubule is diminished, giving time for granular casts to degenerate. Waxy casts are found especially in patients with chronic renal diseases and are associated with chronic renal failure. They also occur in patients with diabetic nephropathy, malignant hypertension, and glomerulonephritis.

Epithelial cells can enter the urine anywhere along the process of urinary excretion. The presence of occasional epithelial cells is not remarkable. Large numbers, however, are abnormal and can conglomerate into *tubular (epithelial) casts*. These are most suggestive of glomerulonephritis.

Normally, few WBCs are found in urine sediment on microscopic examination. The presence of five or more WBCs in the urine indicates a urinary tract infection involving the bladder, kidney, or both. A clean-catch urine culture should be done for further evaluation. *WBC casts* are most commonly found in infections of the kidney, such as acute pyelonephritis.

Any disruption in the blood-urine barrier whether at the glomerular, tubular, or bladder level will cause RBCs to enter the urine. The bleeding can be microscopic or gross hematuria. *RBC casts* suggest glomerulonephritis. RBC casts are also seen in patients with acute necrosis, pyelonephritis, renal trauma, or renal tumor.

Interfering factors

- Certain foods affect urine color. Carrots may cause a dark yellow urine. Beets may cause a red urine. Rhubarb may cause a red or brown discoloration.
- Urine color darkens with prolonged standing.
- Some foods (e.g., asparagus) produce characteristic urine odors.
- When urine stands for a long time and begins to decompose, it has an ammonia-like smell.
- Urine pH becomes alkaline on standing because of the action of urea-splitting bacteria, producing ammonia.
- Urine pH of an uncovered specimen will become alkaline because carbon dioxide will vaporize from the urine and into the air.
- Dietary factors affect urine pH.
  An alkaline urine is observed in people who eat large quantities of citrus fruits, dairy products, and vegetables.

U

Acidic urine is observed with a diet high in meat and certain foods (e.g., cranberries).

- A transient proteinuria may be associated with severe emotional stress, excess exercise, and cold baths.
- Radiopaque contrast media received within the past 3 days may cause false-positive results for protein in the urine.
- Urine contaminated with vaginal secretions may cause proteinuria.
- Recent use of radiographic dyes in the urine increases specific gravity.
- False-positive leukocyte esterase results may occur in specimens contaminated with vaginal secretions (e.g., heavy menstrual discharge, *Trichomonas* infection, and parasites).
- False-negative leukocyte esterase results may occur in specimens containing high levels of protein or ascorbic acid.
- Special diets (carbohydrate-free, high-protein, high-fat) may cause ketonuria.
- Radiographic dyes may cause precipitation of urinary crystals.
- Vaginal discharge may contaminate the urine specimen and factitiously cause WBCs in the urine.
- Strenuous physical exercise may cause RBC casts.
- Traumatic urethral catheterization may cause RBCs in the urine.
- Many drugs affect urine color and appearance (see Table 23), including antibiotics and vitamins.
- Drugs that may cause acidic urine include ammonium chloride, chlorothiazide diuretics, and methenamine mandelate.
- Drugs that may cause alkaline urine include acetazolamide, potassium citrate, and sodium bicarbonate.
- Drugs that may cause *increased* protein levels include acetazolamide, aminoglycosides, amphotericin B, cephalosporins, colistin, griseofulvin, lithium, methicillin, nafcillin, nephrotoxic drugs (e.g., arsenicals, gold salts), oxacillin, penicillamine, penicillin G, phenazopyridine, polymyxin B, salicylates, sulfonamides, tolbutamide, and vancomycin.
- Drugs that may cause *increased* specific gravity include dextran and sucrose.
- Drugs that may cause false-positive results for ketones include isoniazid, isopropanol, levodopa, paraldehyde, phenazopyridine, and PSP dye.

Procedure and patient care

Before

PT Explain the procedure to the patient.

During

- Collect a fresh urine specimen in a urine container.
- If the urine specimen contains vaginal discharge or bleeding, a clean-catch or midstream specimen will be needed. This requires meticulous cleaning of the urinary meatus with an iodine preparation to reduce contamination of the specimen by external organisms. The cleansing agent then must be completely removed or it will contaminate the specimen. The *midstream collection* is obtained by:
  1. Having the patient begin to urinate in a bedpan, urinal, or toilet and then stop urinating (this washes the urine out of the distal urethra)
  2. Correctly positioning a sterile urine container into which the patient voids 3 to 4 ounces of urine
  3. Capping the container
  4. Allowing the patient to finish voiding
- For ketones, this test can be performed immediately after collection by placing a drop of urine on an Acetest tablet. If acetone is present, shades of lavender will appear at the designated time.
- With a Ketostix, dip the reagent into the urine specimen and remove it. Read the strip in 15 seconds by comparing it with the color chart.
- For urine specific gravity, a first-voided specimen is best obtained.
- For protein, again the first-voided specimen is best; however, occasionally a 24-hour urine collection (see p. 416) is preferred.

After

- Transport the urine specimen to the laboratory promptly.
- If the specimen cannot be processed immediately, refrigerate it.
- If a 24-hour urine collection is requested, the specimen should be refrigerated or preserved with formalin during the collection time.
- Casts will break up as urine is allowed to sit. Urine examinations for casts should be performed on fresh specimens.

Abnormal findings

Appearance and color

Bacteria
Pus
Red blood cells
Certain foods (e.g., beets, carrots)
Drug therapy (see Table 23)
Pathologic conditions (e.g.,
  bleeding from the kidney)

Dehydration
Overhydration
Diabetes insipidus
Fever
Excessive sweating
Jaundice

Odor

Infection
Ketonuria
Urinary tract infection
Rectal fistula

Maple syrup urine
  disease
Phenylketonuria
Hepatic failure

pH

▲ **Increased levels**

  Respiratory alkalosis
  Metabolic alkalosis
  Urea-splitting bacteria
  Vegetarian diet
  Renal failure with inability
    to form ammonia
  Gastric suction
  Vomiting
  Diuretic therapy
  Renal tubular acidosis
  Urinary tract infection

▼ **Decreased levels**

  Metabolic acidosis
  Diabetes mellitus
  Diarrhea
  Starvation
  Respiratory acidosis
  Emphysema
  Sleep
  Pyrexia

Protein

▲   **Increased levels**

Nephrotic syndrome
Diabetes mellitus
Multiple myeloma
Preeclampsia
Glomerulonephritis
Congestive heart failure
Malignant hypertension
Polycystic disease
Diabetic glomerulosclerosis
Amyloidosis
Systemic lupus erythematosus
Goodpasture's syndrome
Renal vein thrombosis
Heavy-metal poisoning
Galactosemia
Bacterial pyelonephritis
Nephrotoxic drug therapy
Bladder tumor

Specific gravity

▲   **Increased levels**

Dehydration
Pituitary tumor or trauma
   that causes syndrome of
   inappropriate antidiuretic
   hormone (SIADH)
Decrease in renal blood flow
   (as in heart failure, renal
   artery stenosis,
   or hypotension)
Glycosuria and proteinuria
Water restriction
Fever
Excessive sweating
Vomiting
Diarrhea
X-ray contrast dye

▼   **Decreased levels**

Overhydration
Diabetes insipidus
Renal failure
Diuresis
Hypothermia
Glomerulonephritis
Pyelonephritis

U

Leukocyte esterase

Possible urinary tract infection

Nitrites

Possible urinary tract infection

Ketones

Uncontrolled diabetes mellitus
Starvation
Excessive aspirin ingestion
Ketoacidosis of alcoholism
Febrile illnesses in infants and
  children
Weight reduction diets

Following anesthesia
Prolonged vomiting
Anorexia
Fasting
High-protein diets
Isopropanol ingestion
Dehydration

Crystals

Renal stone formation
Drug therapy
Urinary tract infection

Granular casts

Acute tubular necrosis
Urinary tract infection
Glomerulonephritis
Pyelonephritis
Nephrosclerosis

Chronic lead poisoning
Reaction after exercise
Stress
Renal transplant rejection

Fatty casts

Nephrotic syndrome
Diabetic nephropathy

Glomerulonephritis
Chronic renal disease

Epithelial casts

Glomerulonephritis
Eclampsia
Heavy-metal poisoning

Ethylene glycol intoxication
Acute renal allograft
  rejection

Waxy casts

Chronic renal disease
Chronic renal failure
Diabetic nephropathy
Malignant hypertension

Glomerulonephritis
Renal transplant rejection
Nephrotic syndrome

Hyaline casts

Proteinuria
Fever
Strenuous exercise
Stress

Glomerulonephritis
Pyelonephritis
Congestive heart failure
Chronic renal failure

Red blood cells and casts

▲ **Increased RBC levels**

Glomerulonephritis
Interstitial nephritis
Acute tubular necrosis
Pyelonephritis
Renal trauma
Renal tumor
Renal stones
Cystitis
Prostatitis
Traumatic bladder catheterization

▲ **Increased RBC cast levels**

Glomerulonephritis
Subacute bacterial endocarditis
Renal infarct
Goodpasture's syndrome
Vasculitis
Sickle cell anemia
Malignant hypertension
Systemic lupus erythematosus

White blood cells and casts

▲ **Increased WBC levels**

Bacterial infection in the urinary tract

▲ **Increased WBC cast levels**

Acute pyelonephritis
Glomerulonephritis
Lupus nephritis

notes

U

urine culture and sensitivity (c&s)

Type of test   Urine; microscopic

Normal findings

Negative: <10,000 bacteria per milliliter of urine
Positive: >100,000 bacteria per milliliter of urine

Test explanation and related physiology

Urine cultures and sensitivities are obtained to determine the presence of pathogenic bacteria in patients with suspected urinary tract infections. Most often, urinary tract infections are limited to the bladder. However, the kidneys, ureters, bladder, or urethra can be the source of infection. All cultures should be performed before antibiotic therapy is initiated; otherwise the antibiotic may interrupt the growth of the organism in the laboratory. Most organisms require approximately 24 hours to grow in the laboratory, and a preliminary report can be given at that time. Occasionally 48 to 72 hours are required for growth and identification of the organism. Cultures may be repeated after appropriate antibiotic therapy to assess for complete resolution of the infection (especially in urinary tract infections).

To save money in some institutions, urine cultures are done only if the urinalysis suggests a possible infection (e.g., increased number of white blood cells [WBCs], bacteria, high pH, positive leukocyte esterase). In these institutions urine is collected and "split." One half is sent for urinalysis, and the other is held in the laboratory refrigerator and evaluated only if the urinalysis indicates a possible infection.

An important part of any routine culture is to assess the sensitivity of any bacteria that are growing within the urine to various antibiotics. The physician can then more appropriately recommend the correct antibiotic therapy. Antibiotics that are safest, least expensive, and most effective for the treatment of specific bacteria are prescribed.

Interfering factors

- Contamination of the urine with stool, vaginal secretions, hands, or clothing will cause false positives.
- Drugs that may affect test results include antibiotics.

Procedure and patient care

Before

PT Explain to the patient the procedure for obtaining a clean-catch (midstream) urine collection.

- Hold antibiotics until after the urine specimen has been collected.
- Provide the patient with the necessary supplies for the collection.

During

- Note that a *clean-catch* or *midstream urine* collection is required for C&S testing. This requires meticulous cleansing of the urinary meatus with an iodine preparation to reduce contamination of the specimen by external organisms. Then the cleansing agent must be completely removed or it will contaminate the urine specimen. The midstream collection is obtained by:
  1. Having the patient begin to urinate in a bedpan, urinal, or toilet and then stop urinating (this washes the urine out of the distal urethra)
  2. Correctly positioning a sterile urine container, into which the patient voids 3 to 4 ounces of urine
  3. Capping the container
  4. Allowing the patient to finish voiding
- Note that *urinary catheterization* may be needed for patients unable to void. This procedure is not usually performed, however, because of the risk of inducing organisms and because of patient discomfort.
- For inpatients with an *indwelling urinary catheter,* obtain a specimen by attaching a small-gauge (e.g., No. 25) needle to a syringe and aseptically inserting the needle into the catheter at a point distal to the sleeve leading to the balloon. Urine is aspirated and then placed in a sterile urine container. (Usually the catheter tubing distal to the puncture site needs to be clamped for 15 to 30 minutes before the aspiration of urine to allow urine to fill the tubing. After the specimen is withdrawn, the clamp is removed.)
- Note that *suprapubic aspiration* of urine is a safe method of obtaining urine in neonates and infants. The abdomen is prepared with an antiseptic, and a 25-gauge needle is inserted into the suprapubic area 1 inch above the symphysis pubis. Urine is aspirated into the syringe and then transferred to a sterile urine container.

U

- Collect specimens from infants and young children in a disposable pouch called a *U bag*. This bag has an adhesive backing around the opening to attach to the child.
- Note that for patients with a *urinary diversion* (e.g., an ileal conduit), catheterization should be done through the stoma.
- Urine should *not* be collected from an ostomy pouch.
- Indicate on the laboratory slip any medications that may affect test results.

After

- Transport the specimen to the laboratory immediately (at least within 30 minutes). If this is not possible, the specimen may be refrigerated up to 2 hours.
- Notify the physician of any positive results so that appropriate antibiotic therapy can be initiated.

Abnormal findings

Urinary tract infection

notes

urine flow studies (Uroflowmetry, Urodynamic studies)

Type of test   Urodynamic

Normal findings   Depend on the patient's age, gender, and volume voided

Test explanation and related physiology

Uroflowmetry is the simplest of the urodynamic techniques, being noninvasive and requiring uncomplicated and relatively inexpensive equipment. This study measures the volume of urine expelled from the bladder per second. This test is indicated to investigate dysfunctional voiding or suspicious outflow tract obstruction. It is also done before and after any procedure designed to modify the function of the urologic outflow tract.

The urine flow depends greatly on the volume of urine voided. The flow rates are highest and most predictable in the urine volume range of 200 to 400 ml. When the bladder contains more than 400 ml of urine, the efficiency of the bladder muscle is greatly decreased. Nomograms of maximal flow versus voided volume may be used for accurate test result interpretation, taking into account the patient's gender and age. If the flow rates are abnormally low, the test should be repeated to check for accuracy.

Modern urine flowmeters provide a permanent graphic recording. If flowmeters are not available, the patient can time the urinary stream with a stopwatch and record the voided volume; from this, the average flow is calculated.

In some cases it is more valuable to analyze several voided volumes and flow rates rather than a single flow rate. If this is to be done, the patient is taught to use a flowmeter. A graph of flow versus volume can be plotted. Together with clinical observation, this provides very valuable information on the severity of outflow obstruction, the likelihood of urinary retention, and the state of compensation or decompensation of the detrusor muscle.

Procedure and patient care

Before

PT Explain the procedure to the patient.

PT Instruct the patient how to void into the urine flowmeter.

- Determine the number of flow rates that will be needed.

U

During

- Note that this test should be performed when the patient has a normal desire to void and in conditions suitable for privacy. The bladder should be adequately full. Essentially, all the patient must do is urinate into the flowmeter. Several different types of flowmeters are available.

PT Tell the patient that no discomfort is associated with this test.

- Note that the duration of this test is several seconds.

After

- Record the position of the patient, the method of filling the bladder (it should be natural), and whether this study was part of another evaluation.

Abnormal findings

Dysfunctional voiding
Urethral stricture
Prostate cancer
Prostatic hypertrophy

notes

uroporphyrinogen-1-synthase

Type of test Blood

Normal findings 1.27-2 mU/g of hemoglobin or
81.9-129.6 units/mol Hgb (SI units)

Test explanation and related physiology

Porphyria is a group of genetic disorders characterized by an
accumulation of porphyrin products, usually in the liver. This
group of disorders results from enzymatic deficiencies in synthesis of heme (a part of hemoglobin). Acute intermittent porphyria (AIP) is the most common form of the liver porphyrias; it is
caused by a deficiency in uroporphyrinogen-1-synthase (also
called porphobilinogen deaminase). This enzyme is necessary for
erythroid cells to make heme.

Most patients with AIP have no symptoms (latent phase) until
the acute phase is precipitated by medication or some other factor. The acute phase is highlighted by symptoms of abdominal
and muscular pain, nausea, vomiting, hypertension, mental confusion, sensory loss, and hemolysis.

This enzyme is significantly reduced during the acute and latent
phases of this disorder. It is important to identify this deficiency to
prevent acute bouts of porphyria. The acute phase can be prevented by avoiding factors that can precipitate the acute symptoms.

Procedure and patient care

Before

PT Tell the patient that no fasting is required.

During

- Collect 7 ml of peripheral venous blood in a purple-top tube.
- Because this test is based on the hemoglobin measurement,
  concurrently obtain a hemoglobin level on the patient.

After

- Indicate on the laboratory slip if the patient is having
  symptoms of acute porphyria.
- Apply pressure to the venipuncture site.

Abblormal findings

▼ **Decreased levels**

Acute intermittent porphyria

U

vanillylmandelic acid and catecholamines (VMA and epinephrine, norepinephrine, metanephrine, normetanephrine, dopamine)

Type of test Urine (24-hour)

Normal findings

VMA
Adult/elderly: <6.8 mg/24 hr or <35 μmol/24 hr (SI units)
Adolescent: 1-5 mg/24 hr
Child: 1-3 mg/24 hr
Infant: <2 mg/24 hr
Newborn: <1 mg/24 hr

Catecholamines
Free catecholamines
<100 mcg/24 hr or <590 nmol/day (SI units)
Epinephrine
Adult/elderly: <20 mcg/24 hr or <109 nmol/day (SI units)
Child
   0-1 years: 0-2.5 mcg/24 hr
   1-2 years: 0-3.5 mcg/24 hr
   2-4 years: 0-6 mcg/24 hr
   4-7 years: 0.2-10 mcg/24 hr
   7-10 years: 0.5-14 mcg/24 hr
Norepinephrine
Adult/elderly: <100 mcg/24 hr or <590 nmol/day (SI units)
Child
   0-1 years: 0-10 mcg/24 hr
   1-2 years: 0-17 mcg/24 hr
   2-4 years: 4-29 mcg/24 hr
   4-7 years: 8-45 mcg/24 hr
   7-10 years: 13-65 mcg/24 hr
Dopamine
Adult/elderly: 65-400 mcg/24 hr
Child
   0-1 years: 0-85 mcg/24 hr
   1-2 years: 10-140 mcg/24 hr
   2-4 years: 40-260 mcg/24 hr
   >4 years: 65-400 mcg/24 hr
Metanephrine
<1.3 mg/24 hr or <7 μmol/day (SI units)

Normetanephrine
15-80 mcg/24 hr or 89-473 nmol/day (SI units)

Test explanation and related physiology

This 24-hour urine test for VMA and catecholamines is performed primarily to diagnose hypertension secondary to pheochromocytoma. This test is also used to detect the presence of neuroblastomas and rare adrenal tumors.

A *pheochromocytoma* is an adrenal tumor that frequently secretes abnormally high levels of epinephrine and norepinephrine. These hormones cause episodic or persistent hypertension by causing peripheral arterial vasoconstriction. Dopamine is the precursor of epinephrine and norepinephrine. Metanephrine and normetanephrine are catabolic products of epinephrine and norepinephrine, respectively. VMA is the product of catabolism of both metanephrine and normetanephrine. In patients with pheochromocytoma, one or all of these substances will be present in excessive quantities in a 24-hour collection of urine.

A 24-hour urine test is preferable to a blood test because catecholamine secretion from the tumor may be episodic and could potentially be missed at any one time during the day. The urine provides the laboratory with a specimen that reflects catecholamine production over one whole day. It is best to perform testing when the symptoms (hypertension) of the potential adrenal tumor are significant. At that time, catecholamine production is greatest and will be more assuredly identified.

Interfering factors

- Increased levels of VMA may be caused by certain foods (e.g., tea, coffee, cocoa, vanilla, chocolate).
- Vigorous exercise, stress, and starvation may cause increased VMA levels.
- Falsely decreased levels of VMA may be caused by uremia, alkaline urine, and radiographic iodine contrast agents.
- Drugs that may cause *increased* VMA levels include caffeine, epinephrine, levodopa, lithium, and nitroglycerin.
- Drugs that may cause *decreased* VMA levels include clonidine, disulfiram (Antabuse), guanethidine, imipramine, monoamine oxidase inhibitors, phenothiazines, and reserpine.
- Drugs that may cause *increased* catecholamine levels include alcohol (ethyl), aminophylline, caffeine, chloral hydrate, clonidine (chronic therapy), contrast media (iodine containing), disulfiram, epinephrine, erythromycin, insulin,

V

methenamine, methyldopa, nicotinic acid (large doses), nitroglycerin, quinidine, riboflavin, and tetracyclines.

- Drugs that may cause *decreased* catecholamine levels include guanethidine, reserpine, and salicylates.

Procedure and patient care

Before

PT Explain the procedure to the patient.

PT Explain the dietary restrictions and the 24-hour urine collection procedure to the patient.

PT For 2 or 3 days before the 24-hour collection for VMA and throughout the collection, place the patient on a VMA-restricted diet. Generally, instruct the patient to avoid coffee, tea, bananas, chocolate, cocoa, licorice, citrus fruit, all foods and fluids containing vanilla, and aspirin. Obtain specific restrictions from the laboratory.

PT Inform the patient of the need to avoid taking antihypertensive medications and sometimes all medications during this period and possibly even longer.

During

- Collect the 24-hour urine specimen using a preservative.

PT Instruct the patient to begin the 24-hour urine collection after voiding. Discard the initial specimen and note the time; this is the starting time.

- Collect all urine passed during the next 24 hours. Refrigerate or keep on ice during the collection period.
- Post the hours for the urine collection in a prominent place to avoid accidental discarding of the specimen.

PT Remind the patient to void before defecating so that the urine is not contaminated by feces.

PT Instruct the patient not to put toilet paper in the collection container.

PT Encourage the patient to drink fluids during the 24 hours unless contraindicated for medical purposes.

- Collect the last specimen as close as possible to the end of the 24-hour period. Add this urine to the container.
- Indicate the time of the last specimen collected on the laboratory slip or urine container.
- Identify and minimize factors contributing to patient stress and anxiety. Excessive physical exercise and emotion may alter catecholamine test results by causing an increased secretion of epinephrine and norepinephrine.

After
- Send the specimen to the laboratory as soon as the test is completed.
- Allow the patient to have foods and drugs that have been restricted in preparation for the test.

Abnormal findings

▲   **Increased levels**

Pheochromocytomas
Neuroblastomas
Ganglioneuromas
Ganglioblastomas
Severe stress
Strenuous exercise
Acute anxiety

notes

vascular ultrasound studies (Venous/arterial Doppler ultrasound, Venous/arterial duplex scan)

Type of test Ultrasound

Normal findings

Venous

A normal Doppler venous signal with spontaneous respiration
Normal venous system without evidence of occlusion

Arterial

Normal arterial Doppler signal with systolic and diastolic
  components
No reduction in blood pressure in excess of 20 mm Hg
  compared with the normal extremity
A normal ankle-to-brachial arterial blood pressure index of 0.85
  or greater
No evidence of arterial occlusion

Test explanation and related physiology

Vascular ultrasound studies are used to identify occlusion of
the veins or arteries of an extremity. Venous patency is demonstrated with Doppler ultrasound by detecting moving red blood
cells (RBCs) within the vein. The Doppler transducer directs an
ultrasound beam at the vein. Moving RBCs scatter the frequency of the beam. The change in frequency of the sound wave
reflected back to the transducer is proportional to the velocity of
the blood flow. Venous Doppler studies are not accurate for
detection of venous occlusive disease of the lower calf.

Vascular duplex scanning is called *duplex* because it combines
the benefits of Doppler with B-mode scanning. With the use of
the transducer, a B-mode ultrasound grayscale image of the vessel is obtained. A pulsed Doppler probe within the transducer is
used to evaluate blood flow velocity and direction in the artery
and to measure the amplitude and waveform of the carotid arterial pulse. A computer combines that information and provides a
two-dimensional image of the vessel along with an image of
blood flow. With this technique, one is able to directly visualize
areas of vascular narrowing or occlusion. The degree of occlusion
is measured in percentage of the entire lumen that is occluded.

Color Doppler ultrasound (CDU) can be added to arterial
duplex scanning. CDU assigns color for direction of blood flow

within the vessel, and the intensity of that color is dependent on the mean computed velocity of blood traveling in the vessel. This allows visualization of stenotic areas based on slowing or reversal of direction of blood flow at a particular area of the artery. With the use of duplex scanning, an accurate representation of the vessel anatomy and patency can be obtained.

With a single-mode transducer, *venous* blood flow can be heard audibly and is augmented by an audio speaker as a swishing noise. If the vein is occluded, no swishing sounds are detected.

With single-mode *arterial* Doppler studies, peripheral arteriosclerotic occlusive disease of the extremities can be easily located. By slowly deflating blood pressure cuffs placed on the calf and ankle, systolic pressure in the arteries of the extremities can be accurately measured by detecting the first evidence of blood flow with the Doppler transducer. The extremely sensitive Doppler ultrasound detector can recognize the swishing sound of even the most minimal blood flow. Normally systolic blood pressure is slightly higher in the arteries of the arms than in the legs. If the difference in blood pressure exceeds 20 mm Hg, occlusive disease is believed to exist immediately proximal to the area tested. Lower extremity arterial bypass graft patency can also be assessed with Doppler ultrasound.

Interfering factors

- Venous or arterial occlusive disease proximal to the site of testing
- Cigarette smoking, because nicotine can cause constriction of the peripheral arteries and alter the results

Procedure and patient care

Before

PT Explain the procedure to the patient.
PT Inform the patient that this is a painless procedure.
- Remove all clothing from the extremity to be examined.
PT Instruct the patient to abstain from cigarette smoking for at least 30 minutes before the test.

During

- Note the following procedural steps:

Venous studies

1. A conductive gel is applied to the skin overlying the venous system of the extremity in multiple areas.
2. Usually, for the lower extremity, the deep venous system is identified in the ankle, calf, thigh, and groin.

V

3. The characteristic "swishing" sound of the blood flow indicates a patent venous system. Failure to detect this signal indicates venous occlusion.
4. Usually both the superficial and deep venous systems are evaluated.

Arterial studies

1. These are performed with the use of blood pressure cuffs, which are placed around the thigh, calf, and ankle.
2. A conductive paste is applied to the skin overlying the artery distal to the cuffs.
3. The proximal cuff is inflated to a level above systolic blood pressure in the normal extremity.
4. The Doppler ultrasound transducer is placed immediately distal to the inflated cuff.
5. The pressure in the cuff is slowly released.
6. The highest pressure at which blood flow is detected by the characteristic "swishing" Doppler signal is recorded as the blood pressure of that artery.
7. The test is repeated at each successive level.
8. When the ankle pressure is divided by the arm (brachial artery) pressure, this is known as the AB index. If the *AB index* is less than 0.85, significant arterial occlusive disease exists within the extremity.

- Note that these studies are usually performed in the vascular laboratory or radiology department and take approximately 30 minutes.

After

- Encourage the patient to verbalize his or her fears in terms of test results.
- Remove the transducer gel from the extremity.
- **PT** Inform the patient that the physician must interpret the studies and that results will be available in a few hours.

Abnormal findings

Venous occlusion, secondary to thrombosis or thrombophlebitis
Venous varicosities
Small or large vessel arterial occlusive disease
Spastic arterial disease (e.g., Raynaud's phenomenon)
Small vessel arterial occlusive disease (as in diabetes)
Embolic arterial occlusion
Arterial aneurysm

venography of lower extremities (Phlebography, Venogram)

Type of test X-ray with contrast dye

Normal findings No evidence of venous thrombosis or obstruction

Test explanation and related physiology

Venography is an x-ray study designed to identify and locate thrombi within the venous system of the lower extremities. During this study dye is injected into the venous system of the affected extremity. X-ray films are then taken at timed intervals to visualize the venous system. Obstruction to the flow of dye or a filling defect within the dye-filled vein indicates that thrombosis exists. A positive study accurately confirms the diagnosis of venous thrombosis; however, a normal study, although not as accurate, does make the diagnosis of venous thrombosis very unlikely. Often both extremities are studied, even though only one leg is suspected to contain deep-vein thrombosis. The normal extremity is used for comparison with the involved extremity. Unlike venous plethysmography (see p. 721), venography is accurate for thrombi in veins below the knee.

Contraindications

- Patients with severe edema of the legs, making venous access impossible
- Patients who are uncooperative
- Patients who are allergic to iodinated dye or shellfish
- Patients with renal failure, because the iodinated dye is nephrotoxic

Potential complications

- Allergic reaction to iodinated dyes
- Renal failure, especially in elderly people who are chronically dehydrated or may have a mild degree of renal failure
- Subcutaneous infiltration of the dye, causing cellulitis and pain
- Venous thrombophlebitis caused by the dye
- Bacteremia caused by a break in sterile technique
- Venous embolism caused by dislodgment of a deep-vein clot induced by the dye injection

V

- Hypoglycemia or acidosis may occur in patients who are taking metformin (Glucophage) and receive iodine dye.

Procedure and patient care

Before

PT Explain the procedure to the patient.

PT Obtain informed consent for this procedure.

- Assess the patient for allergies to iodinated dyes and shellfish.
- If needed, provide appropriate pain medication so the patient is able to lie still during the procedure.

PT Ensure that the patient is appropriately hydrated before testing. Injection of the iodinated contrast may cause renal failure, especially in the elderly.

During

- Note the following procedural steps:
  1. The patient is taken to the radiology department and placed in a supine position on the x-ray table.
  2. Catheterization of a superficial vein on the foot is performed. This may require a surgical cutdown.
  3. An iodinated, radiopaque dye is injected into the vein.
  4. X-ray films are taken to follow the course of the dye up the leg.
  5. Frequently a tourniquet is placed on the leg to prevent filling of the superficial saphenous vein. As a result, all of the dye goes to filling the deep venous system, which contains the most clinically significant thrombosis that can embolize.
- Note that a radiologist performs this study in approximately 30 to 90 minutes.

PT Tell the patient that the venous catheterization is only as uncomfortable as a cutaneous heel stick or a small incision in the foot.

PT The dye may cause the patient to feel a warm flush. (This is not as severe as that noted with arteriography.) Inform the patient that occasionally mild degrees of nausea, vomiting, or skin itching also may occur.

After

- Continue appropriate hydration of the patient to prevent dehydration caused by the diuretic action of the dye.
- Observe the puncture site for infection, cellulitis, or bleeding.
- Assess the patient's vital signs for signs of bacteremia (e.g., high temperature, tachycardia, chills).

- See p. xix for appropriate interventions concerning the care of patients with iodine allergy.

🏠 Home care responsibilities

- Monitor the puncture site for redness, swelling, or bleeding.
- Note that fever and chills may indicate bacteremia.
- Encourage the patient to drink fluids to prevent dehydration caused by the dye injection.

Abnormal findings

Obstructed venous systems
Acute deep-vein thrombosis

notes

viral cultures

Type of test Blood; urine; stool; throat; skin

Normal findings No virus isolated

Test explanation and related physiology

It is now recognized that viral infections are the most common infections affecting children and adults. Viruses are subdivided by the nuclear material they contain (RNA or DNA). Infections from viruses are often indistinguishable from bacterial infections. Definitive diagnosis of viral disease is made by culture of the virus (discussed here). Other methods used to identify viral disease include:

1. Serologic methods of identifying antibodies to a specific virus
2. Serologic methods of identifying antigen parts of a virus
3. Direct detection by electron microscopy
4. Indirect detection by nucleic acid probes

Ability to isolate a viral culture depends on many aspects of the culture process. The first is determining the correct specimen for culture. That depends on the organ involved and the type of virus suspected (Table 24). Timing is important. Viral load is always greatest in the early stages of the disease. Cultures obtained in the first few days after symptoms appear offer the best chance of identifying the infective culture. Using the correct culture medium is essential. In general, the culture medium used to grow the viral culture is a tissue/cell culture. Different viruses vary greatly in their ability to grow in specific cell cultures. Viral cultures take 3 to 7 days to be reported.

Interfering factors

- Inadequate specimen, timing, or choice of culture medium will cause false-negative tests.
- The use of a cotton swab or wooden applicator for specimen collection may destroy the virus.

Procedure and patient care

Before
PT Explain the method of collection of the specimen to the patient.
- Obtain a history regarding the timing of symptoms.
- Accurately record the source of the specimen.

TABLE 24 Specimen culture for common viruses and diseases

Common virus	Specimen	Disease
Adenovirus, influenza, respiratory syncytial, rhinovirus	Throat culture, bronchoscopic aspiration	Influenza, pneumonia, pharyngitis
Rubella, rubeola, coxsackie, varicella	Throat, skin vesicle	Skin rash, zoster
Arbovirus, enterovirus, herpes, cytomegalovirus	Throat culture, cerebrospinal fluid	Meningitis, encephalitis
Parvovirus, adenovirus	Stool Blood, sputum	Skin rash, arthropathy, upper respiratory infection
Influenza A, Epstein-Barr	Throat, blood	Flu syndrome, mononucleosis

During
- Use a closed specimen system to obtain and transport the specimen to the laboratory.
- Transport the specimen immediately to the laboratory. Viruses in specimens quickly lose their vitality.
- Place samples on ice if delivery to the laboratory is not immediate.
- Small volume specimens, such as tissue aspirates, are often best transported in a liquid medium. If bacterial cultures are to be performed, use sterile saline solution for transfer.
- If blood is the specimen, obtain 5 to 7 ml of blood in a lavender- or blue-top tube.

After
PT Explain that the patient may still be infectious and should minimize exposure to others.

Abnormal findings
Viral infectious disease (Table 24).

vitamin B$_{12}$ (Cyanocobalamin)

Type of test Blood

Normal findings 160-950 pg/ml or 118-701 pmol/L
(SI units)

Test explanation and related physiology

Vitamin B$_{12}$ is necessary for conversion of the inactive form of
folate to the active form. This function is most notable in the
formation and function of red blood cells (RBCs). Vitamin B$_{12}$
deficiency, like folic acid deficiency, causes anemia. The RBCs
formed in light of these deficiencies consist of large megaloblastic RBCs. These RBCs cannot conform to the size of small capillaries. Instead they fracture and hemolyze. The shortened life
span ultimately leads to anemia.

In the stomach, gastric acid detaches vitamin B$_{12}$ from its
binding proteins. Intrinsic factor (IF), necessary for vitamin B$_{12}$
absorption in the small intestine, is made in the stomach mucosa.
Without IF, vitamin B$_{12}$ cannot be absorbed. Deficiency of IF is
the most common cause of vitamin B$_{12}$ deficiency (pernicious
anemia [PA]). The next most common cause of vitamin B$_{12}$
deficiency is lack of gastric acid to separate the ingested vitamin
B$_{12}$ from its binding proteins. A third cause of vitamin B$_{12}$ deficiency is malabsorption caused by diseases of the small terminal
ileum.

Interfering factors

- Drugs known to *increase* vitamin B$_{12}$ levels include chloral
  hydrate.
- Drugs known to *decrease* vitamin B$_{12}$ levels include alcohol,
  aminoglycosides, ASA, anticonvulsants, colchicine, and oral
  contraceptives.

Procedure and patient care

Before
- **PT** Explain the procedure to the patient.
- **PT** Tell the patient that no fasting is usually required. (However,
  some laboratories prefer an 8-hour fast.)
- **PT** Instruct the patient not to consume alcoholic beverages before
  the test. Check the time period with the physician or laboratory.
- Draw the specimen before starting vitamin B$_{12}$ therapy.

During
- Collect approximately 5 to 10 ml of venous blood in a red-top tube.
- Indicate on the laboratory slip any medications that may affect test results.

After
- Apply pressure to the venipuncture site.
- Transport the blood immediately to the laboratory after collection.

Abnormal findings

▲ Increased levels	▼ Decreased levels
Leukemia	Pernicious anemia
Polycythemia vera	Malabsorption syndromes
Severe liver dysfunction	Inflammatory bowel disease
Myeloproliferative disease	Intestinal worm infestation
	Atrophic gastritis
	Zollinger-Ellison syndrome
	Large proximal gastrectomy
	Resection of terminal ileum
	Achlorhydria
	Pregnancy
	Vitamin C deficiency
	Folic acid deficiency

notes

V

West Nile virus testing

Type of test   Blood; CSF

Normal findings   Negative for West Nile antibody

Test explanation and related physiology

West Nile virus (WNV) is an RNA virus of the Flavivirus family. Reservoir hosts include birds (especially crows and jays) and farm animals (particularly horses). The vector is the common household mosquito, which carries the virus from the hosts to humans. Before 1999, this disease was mostly limited to the African continent. Now, every state in America has reported incidences of the disease.

Common symptoms of this infection are flulike and include fever, lethargy, headache, neck/body aches, and a skin rash. This disease can progress to encephalitis, aseptic meningitis, and an atypical form of Guillain-Barré acute flaccid paralysis.

Testing for WNV is indicated when the flulike symptoms occur in an area where the virus exists. In other areas, testing is only performed when the disease has progressed to one of the more complicated syndromes, as discussed above.

There are two categories of blood testing for WNV: front-line testing and confirmatory testing. Front-line testing measures immunoglobulin M (IgM) antibodies to flaviviruses. This antibody is measurable about 10 days after symptoms start in nearly all patients. If the front-line test for IgM is positive and the symptoms fulfill the Centers for Disease Control criteria, the diagnosis of WNV can be made and treatment altered. This is especially true if the person lives or has traveled to an area that is known to harbor WNV.

If the front-line testing is positive, confirmatory tests may be carried out (especially in areas where the WNV has not been known to exist). This testing is more important for public health officials and researchers. Confirmatory tests may include:

1. A second IgM serology on convalescing serum 3 to 4 weeks later. A fourfold rise would be confirmatory.
2. Direct detection of WNV RNA by nucleic acid amplification testing (Plague Reduction Neutralization test performed by the CDC)

Interfering factors

- Other flavivirus infections, such as St. Louis encephalitis virus, will cause elevations of serologic testing, especially when combined total IgM and IgG is tested.

Procedure and patient care

Before

PT Explain the procedure to the patient and family.

During

- Blood: Obtain 2 ml of venous blood in a red-top tube. CSF: At lumbar puncture (see p. 608) 1 to 2 ml is reserved in a sterile tube until bacteriologic specimens are found to be negative. Then the reserved specimen is sent out for testing.

After

- There is no treatment specific for WNV; however, these patients may need acute medical/nursing support for neurologic and respiratory sequelae.
PT Explain to patient and family that testing is only carried out at a few centers and the specimen must be sent out.
PT Explain that results may not be available for 2 weeks.

Abnormal findings

West Nile virus infections

notes

W

white blood cell count and differential count
(WBC and differential, Leukocyte count, Neutrophil count, Lymphocyte count, Monocyte count, Eosinophil count, Basophil count)

Type of test Blood

Normal findings

Total WBCs
Adult/child >2 years: 5000-10,000/mm^3 or 5-10 × 10^9/L (SI units)
Child ≤2 years: 6200-17,000/mm^3
Newborn: 9000-30,000/mm^3

Differential count

	(%)	*Absolute (per mm^3)*
Neutrophils	55-70	2500-8000
Lymphocytes	20-40	1000-4000
Monocytes	2-8	100-700
Eosinophils	1-4	50-500
Basophils	0.5-1	25-100

Possible critical values WBCs <2500 or >30,000/mm^3

Test explanation and related physiology

The WBC count has two components. The first is a count of the total number of WBCs (leukocytes) in 1 mm^3 of peripheral venous blood. The other component, the differential count, measures the percentage of each type of leukocyte present in the same specimen. An increase in the percentage of one type of leukocyte means a decrease in the percentage of another. Neutrophils and lymphocytes make up 75% to 90% of the total leukocytes. These leukocyte types may be identified easily by their morphology on a venous blood smear. The total leukocyte count has a wide range of normal values, but many diseases may induce abnormal values. An increased total WBC count (leukocytosis: WBC >10,000) usually indicates infection, inflammation, tissue necrosis, or leukemic neoplasia. Trauma or stress, either emotional or physical, may increase the WBC count. A decreased total WBC count (leukopenia: WBC <4000) occurs in many forms of bone marrow failure (e.g., after antineoplastic chemotherapy or radiation therapy, marrow infiltrative diseases, overwhelming infections, dietary deficiencies, and autoimmune diseases).

The major function of the WBCs is to fight infection and react against foreign bodies or tissues. Five types of WBCs may easily be identified on a routine blood smear. These cells, in order of frequency, include neutrophils, lymphocytes, monocytes, eosinophils, and basophils. All of these WBCs arise from the same "pluripotent" stem cell within the bone marrow, as do red blood cells (RBCs). Beyond this origin, however, each cell line differentiates separately. Most mature WBCs are deposited into the circulating blood.

White blood cells are divided into granulocytes and nongranulocytes. Granulocytes include neutrophils, basophils, and eosinophils. Granulocytes have multilobed nuclei and are sometimes referred to as polymorphonuclear leukocytes (PMNs or "polys").

Neutrophils are the most common PMN and are produced in 7 to 14 days and exist in the circulation for only 6 hours. The primary function of the neutrophil is phagocytosis (killing and digestion of bacterial microorganisms). Acute bacterial infections and trauma stimulate neutrophil production, resulting in an increased WBC count. Often when neutrophil production is significantly stimulated, early immature forms of neutrophils enter the circulation. These immature forms are called *band* or *stab* cells. This occurrence, referred to as a "shift to the left" in WBC production, is indicative of an ongoing acute bacterial infection.

Basophils (also called mast cells), and especially *eosinophils*, are involved in the allergic reaction. Parasitic infestations also are capable of stimulating the production of these cells. These cells are capable of phagocytosis of antigen-antibody complexes. As the allergic response diminishes, the eosinophil count decreases. Eosinophils and basophils do not respond to bacterial or viral infections.

Nongranulocytes (agranulocytes) include lymphocytes and monocytes (the count also includes histiocytes). They have no cytoplasmic granules and have small single rounded nuclei. *Lymphocytes* are divided into two types: T cells and B cells. T cells are primarily involved with cellular-type immune reactions, whereas B cells participate in humoral immunity (antibody production). The primary function of the lymphocytes is fighting chronic bacterial infection and acute viral infections. The differential count does not separate the T and B cells but rather counts the combination of the two.

Monocytes are phagocytic cells capable of fighting bacteria in a way very similar to that of neutrophils. However, monocytes can be produced more rapidly and can spend a longer time in the circulation than neutrophils.

The WBC and differential counts are routinely measured as part of the complete blood count (see p. 294). Serial WBC counts and differential counts have both diagnostic and prognostic value. For example, a persistent increase in the WBC count may indicate a worsening of an infectious process (e.g., appendicitis). A dramatic decrease in the WBC count below the normal range may indicate marrow failure. In patients receiving chemotherapy, a reduced WBC count may delay further chemotherapy.

The absolute count is calculated by multiplying the differential count (%) by the total WBC count. For example, the *absolute neutrophil count (ANC)* is helpful in determining the patient's real risk for infection. It is calculated by multiplying the WBC count by the percent of neutrophils and percent of bands, that is:

$$ANC = WBC \times (\% \text{ neutrophils} + \% \text{ bands})$$

If the ANC is less than 1000, the patient should be placed in protective isolation because he or she is severely immunocompromised and is at great risk for infection.

Interfering factors

- Physical activity and stress may cause an increase in WBC and differential values.
- Pregnancy (final month) and labor may cause increased WBC levels.
- Patients who have had a splenectomy have a persistent, mild elevation of WBC counts.
- Drugs that may cause *increased* WBC levels include adrenaline, allopurinol, aspirin, chloroform, epinephrine, heparin, quinine, steroids, and triamterene (Dyrenium).
- Drugs that may cause *decreased* WBC levels include antibiotics, anticonvulsants, antihistamines, antimetabolites, antithyroid drugs, arsenicals, barbiturates, chemotherapeutic agents, diuretics, and sulfonamides.

Procedure and patient care

Before

PT Explain the procedure to the patient.
PT Tell the patient that no fasting is required.

During

- Collect approximately 5 to 7 ml of venous blood in a lavender-top tube.

After

- Apply pressure to the venipuncture site.

Abnormal findings

▲ **Increased WBC count (leukocytosis)**

Infection
Leukemic neoplasia
Trauma
Stress
Tissue necrosis
Inflammation

▼ **Decreased WBC count (leukopenia)**

Drug toxicity (e.g., chloramphenicol)
Bone marrow failure
Overwhelming infections
Dietary deficiency
Autoimmune disease
Bone marrow infiltration (e.g., myelofibrosis)
Congenital marrow aplasia

▲▼ **Increased/decreased differential count**
See Table 25

notes

W

TABLE 25 Causes for abnormalities in the WBC and differential count

Type of WBC	Elevated	Decreased
Neutrophils	*Neutrophilia*	*Neutropenia*
	Physical or emotional stress	Aplastic anemia
	Acute suppurative infection	Dietary deficiency
	Myelocytic leukemia	Overwhelming bacterial infection (especially in the elderly)
	Trauma	
	Cushing's syndrome	Viral infections (e.g., hepatitis, influenza, measles)
	Inflammatory disorders (e.g., rheumatic fever, thyroiditis, rheumatoid arthritis)	Radiation therapy
		Addison's disease
	Metabolic disorders (e.g., ketoacidosis, gout, eclampsia)	Drug therapy: myelotoxic drugs (as in chemotherapy)
Lymphocytes	*Lymphocytosis*	*Lymphocytopenia*
	Chronic bacterial infection	Leukemia
	Viral infection (e.g., mumps, rubella)	Sepsis
		Immunodeficiency diseases
	Lymphocytic leukemia	Systemic lupus erythematosus
	Multiple myeloma	
	Infectious mononucleosis	Later stages of human immunodeficiency virus infection
	Radiation	Drug therapy: adrenocorticosteroids, antineoplastics
	Infectious hepatitis	Radiation therapy

TABLE 25 Causes for abnormalities in the WBC and differential count—cont'd

Type of WBC	Elevated	Decreased
Monocytes	*Monocytosis* Chronic inflammatory disorders Viral infections (e.g., infectious mononucleosis) Tuberculosis Chronic ulcerative colitis Parasites (e.g., malaria)	*Monocytopenia* Drug therapy: prednisone
Eosinophils	*Eosinophilia* Parasitic infections Allergic reactions Eczema Leukemia Autoimmune diseases	*Eosinopenia* Increased adrenosteroid production
Basophils	*Basophilia* Myeloproliferative disease (e.g., myelofibrosis, polycythemia rubra vera) Leukemia	*Basopenia* Acute allergic reactions Hyperthyroidism Stress reactions

W

white blood cell scan (WBC scan, Inflammatory scan)

Type of test Nuclear scan

Normal findings No signs of WBC localization outside the liver or spleen

Test explanation and related physiology

This test is based on the fact that WBCs are attracted to an area of infection or inflammation. When a patient is suspected of having had infection or inflammation, yet the site cannot be localized, the injection of radiolabeled WBCs may identify and localize the area of inflammation or infection. This is especially helpful in patients who have a fever of unknown origin, suspected occult intra-abdominal infection, or suspected (yet radiographically inapparent) osteomyelitis. The scan can differentiate infectious from noninfectious processes. For example, it is used to indicate whether an abnormal mass (e.g., a pancreatic pseudocyst) is infected.

Areas of noninfectious inflammation (e.g., inflammatory bowel disease) also take up radiolabeled WBCs.

This scan requires drawing blood from the patient, separating out the WBCs, labeling the WBCs with technetium or indium, and reinjecting them back into the patient. Imaging of the whole body 4 to 24 hours later may show an area of increased radioactivity suggestive of accumulation of the radiolabeled WBCs in an area of infection or inflammation.

The liver, spleen, and bone marrow normally tend to accumulate radiolabeled WBCs, thereby obscuring vision behind these organs.

Procedure and patient care

Before

PT Explain the procedure to the patient.

PT Assure the patient that he or she will not be exposed to large amounts of radioactivity, because only tracer doses of the isotope are used.

PT Tell the patient that no preparation or sedation is required.

During

- Note the following procedural steps:
  1. Approximately 40 to 50 ml of blood is withdrawn from the patient, and the WBCs are extracted from the rest of the blood cells. This is usually done by centrifugation. With leukopenia, the WBC count is so low that separating WBCs out from the other blood cellular components would be very difficult. In these instances, donor WBCs are used instead of autologous WBCs. Donor WBCs are also used for human immunodeficiency virus–positive patients to minimize the risk to laboratory workers.
  2. The WBCs are suspended in saline and tagged with ^{99m}technetium (^{99m}Tc) or ^{111}indium (^{111}In) lipid-soluble product. ^{99m}Tc is preferable to ^{111}In because its half-life is longer. Therefore it is cheaper and more readily available for the infrequent times this scan is requested.
  3. The tagged WBCs are reinjected into the patient.
  4. At 4, 24, and 48 hours after injection, a gamma ray detector/camera is placed over the body.
  5. The patient is placed in supine, lateral, and prone positions so that all surfaces of the body can be visualized.
  6. The radionuclide image is recorded on film.

After

PT Inform the patient that because only tracer doses of radioisotopes are used, no precautions need to be taken against radioactive exposure.

Abnormal findings

Infection (e.g., abscess or osteomyelitis)
Inflammation (e.g., inflammatory bowel disease, arthritis)

notes

W

wound culture and sensitivity (C&S)

Type of test Microscopic examination

Normal findings Negative

Test explanation and related physiology

Wound cultures are obtained to determine the presence of pathogens in patients with suspected wound infections. Wound infections are most often caused by pus-forming organisms.

All cultures should be performed before antibiotic therapy is initiated. Otherwise, the antibiotic may interrupt the growth of the organism in the laboratory. More often than not, however, the physician will want to institute antibiotic therapy before the culture results are reported. In these instances a *Gram stain* of the specimen smeared on a slide is most helpful and can be reported in less than 10 minutes. All forms of bacteria are grossly classified as gram-positive (blue staining) or gram-negative (red staining). Knowledge of the shape of the organism (e.g., spheric, rod shaped) also may be very helpful in the tentative identification of the infecting organism. With knowledge of the Gram stain results, the physician can institute a reasonable antibiotic regimen based on experience as to the organism's possible identity. Most organisms require approximately 24 hours to grow in the laboratory, and a preliminary report can be given at that time. Occasionally 48 to 72 hours are required for growth and identification of the organism. Cultures may be repeated after appropriate antibiotic therapy to assess for complete resolution of the infection.

Interfering factors

✔ Drugs that may alter test results include antibiotics.

Procedure and patient care

Before

PT Explain the procedure to the patient.

During

- Aseptically place a sterile cotton swab into the pus of the patient's wound, and then place the swab into a sterile, covered test tube. (Culturing specimens from the skin edge is much less accurate than culturing the suppurative material.)

- If an anaerobic organism is suspected, obtain an anaerobic culture tube from the microbiology laboratory.
- If wound cultures are to be obtained on a patient requiring wound irrigation, obtain the culture before the wound is irrigated.
- If any antibiotic ointment or solution has been previously applied, remove it with sterile water or saline before obtaining the culture.
- Handle all specimens as though they were capable of transmitting disease.
- Indicate on the laboratory slip any medications the patient may be taking that could affect test results.

After

- Transport the specimen to the laboratory immediately after testing (at least within 30 minutes).
- Notify the physician of any positive results so that appropriate antibiotic therapy can be initiated.

Abnormal findings

Wound infection

notes

W

D-xylose absorption test   (Xylose tolerance test)

Type of test Blood; urine

Normal findings

Age	60 min-plasma (mg/dl)	120 min-plasma (mg/dl)	Urine (g/5 hr) [%]
Child	>15-20	>20	>4, [16-32]
Adult	20-57	30-58	>3.5-4, [>14]

Test explanation and related physiology

D-Xylose is a monosaccharide that is easily absorbed by the normal intestine. In patients with malabsorption, intestinal D-xylose absorption is diminished, and as a result, blood levels and urine excretion are reduced. D-xylose is the monosaccharide chosen for the test because it is not metabolized by the body. Its serum levels directly reflect intestinal absorption.

This particular monosaccharide is used because absorption does not require pancreatic or biliary exocrine function. Its absorption is directly determined by the small intestine. This test is used to separate patients with diarrhea caused by maldigestion (pancreatic/biliary dysfunction) from those with diarrhea caused by malabsorption (sprue, Whipple's disease, Crohn's disease).

In this test the patient is asked to drink a fluid containing a prescribed amount of D-xylose. Blood and urine levels are subsequently evaluated. Excellent gastrointestinal absorption is documented by high blood levels and a good urine secretion of D-xylose. Poor intestinal absorption is marked by decreased blood levels and urine excretion.

Contraindications

- Patients with abnormal kidney function
- Patients who are dehydrated

Interfering factors

▮ Drugs that may affect test results include aspirin, atropine, and indomethacin.

Procedure and patient care

Before

PT Explain the procedure to the patient.

PT Instruct the adult patient to fast for 8 hours before testing.

PT Tell the pediatric patient or the parents that the patient should fast for at least 4 hours before testing.

During

- Collect approximately 7 ml of venous blood in a red-top tube before the patient ingests the D-xylose.
- Collect a first-voided morning urine specimen and send it to the laboratory.
- Ask the patient to drink 25 g of D-xylose dissolved in 8 ounces of water. Record the time of ingestion.
- Calibrate pediatric doses according to the patient's body weight.
- Repeat venipunctures to obtain blood in exactly 2 hours for an adult and 1 hour for a child.
- Collect urine for a designated time, usually 5 hours. Refrigerate the urine during the collection period.
- Observe the patient for nausea, vomiting, and diarrhea, which may occur as side effects of D-xylose.
- PT Instruct the patient to remain in a restful position. Intense physical activity may alter the digestive process and affect the test results.

After

- Apply pressure to the venipuncture site.
- PT Provide the patient with food or drink and inform the patient that normal activity may be resumed after completion of the study.

Abnormal findings

▼ **Decreased levels**

Sprue
Lymphatic obstruction
Enteropathy (e.g., radiation)
Crohn's disease
Whipple's disease
Small intestine bacterial overgrowth
Hookworm
Viral gastroenteritis
Giardia lamblia infestation
Short-bowel syndrome

X

Appendix A: List of tests by body system

Tests in this list are grouped by the following: cancer studies; cardiovascular, endocrine, gastrointestinal, hematologic, hepatobiliary, and immunologic systems; miscellaneous studies; and nervous, pulmonary, renal/urologic, reproductive, and skeletal systems.

CANCER STUDIES

Acid phosphatase, 7
Bence Jones protein, 153
Beta$_2$ microglobulin, 155
Bladder cancer markers, 167
Bone scan, 189
Breast cancer genetic testing, 472
Breast cancer tumor analysis, 197
Breast ductal lavage, 200
CA 15-3 and CA 27.29 tumor markers, 211
CA 19-9 tumor marker, 213
CA-125 tumor marker, 215
Carcinoembryonic antigen, 230
Cathepsin D, 197
Cervical biopsy, 251
Colon cancer genetic testing, 472
DNA ploidy status, 197

Estrogen receptor assay, 418
Gallium scan, 461
HER 2 protein, 198
Ki67 protein, 199
Lymphangiography, 623
Mammography, 637
Octreotide scan, 664
Oncoscint scan, 666
Ovarian cancer genetic testing, 472
P53 protein, 199
Papanicolaou smear, 674
Progesterone receptor assay, 748
Prostate-specific antigen, 755
Salivary gland nuclear imaging, 816
Sentinel lymph node biopsy, 833
S-phase fraction, 198
Sputum cytology, 874

CARDIOVASCULAR SYSTEM

Adenosine stress test, 241
Aldosterone, 32
Antimyocardial antibodies, 86
Antistreptolysin O titer, 102
Apolipoproteins, 110
Arteriography, 126
Aspartate aminotransferase, 143
Atrial natriuretic peptide, 657
Brain natriuretic peptide, 657
Cardiac catheterization, 232

Cardiac exercise stress testing, 239
Cardiac flow studies, 244
Cardiac nuclear scanning, 244
Cardiovascular disease genetic testing, 472
Carotid artery duplex scanning, 249
Catecholamines, 978
Chest x-ray, 254

Cholesterol, 262
CK-MB/CK relative index, 323
Computed tomography of the chest, 304
Creatine phosphokinase, 322
Cryoglobulin, 331
C-type natriuretic peptide, 657
Digital subtraction angiography, 126
Dipyridamole-thallium scan, 240
Dobutamine stress test, 241
Echocardiography, 365
Electrocardiography, 368
Electrophysiologic study, 387
Fibrinogen, 454
Holter monitoring, 533
Homocysteine, 535
Isonitrile scan, 244
Lactate dehydrogenase, 572
Lipoproteins, 592
Lipoprotein electrophoresis, 590
MUGA scan, 246

Myoglobin, 655
Natriuretic peptide, 657
Pericardiocentesis, 698
Plethysmography
    Arterial, 719
    Venous, 721
Positron emission tomography, 729
Renin assay
    Plasma, 800
    Renal vein, 801
Tilt-table testing, 387
Transesophageal echocardiography, 933
Transthoracic echocardiography, 365
Triglycerides, 937
Troponins, 941
Vanillylmandelic acid and catecholamines, 978
Vascular ultrasound studies, 982
Venography of lower extremities, 985

ENDOCRINE SYSTEM

Adrenal arteriography, 127
Adrenocorticotropic hormone, 12
    Stimulation test with cosyntropin, 15
    Stimulation test with metyrapone, 18
Aldosterone, 32
Androstenediones, 65
Antidiuretic hormone, 75
Antithyroglobulin antibody, 106
Antithyroid peroxidase antibody, 108
Blood glucose, 482
Calcitonin, 217
Calcium, 220
Catecholamines, 978
Chromosome karyotype, 273

Computed tomography of adrenals, 295
Cortisol
    Blood, 314
    Urine, 314
C-peptide, 317
Dehydroepiandrosterone, 65
Dehydroepiandrosterone sulfate, 65
Dexamethasone suppression test, 355
Diabetes mellitus autoantibody panel, 359
Erythropoietin, 404
Estriol excretion, 414
Estrogen fractions, 414
Follicle-stimulating hormone assay, 618

Free thyroxine, 922
Gastrin, 465
Glucagon, 480
Glucose
    Blood, 482
    Postprandial, 485
    Urine, 487
Glucose tolerance test, 492
Glutamic acid decarboxylase
    antibody, 359
Glycated proteins, 496
Glycosylated hemoglobin,
    496
Growth hormone, 499
    Stimulation test, 502
    Suppression test, 500
17-Hydroxycorticosteroids, 543
Insulin assay, 558
Insulin autoantibody, 359
Insulin-like growth factor
    binding proteins, 868
Islet cell antibody, 359
Ketones, 959
17-Ketosteroids, 569
Long-acting thyroid
    stimulator, 916
Luteinizing hormone assay,
    618
Metyrapone, 18
Osmolality, blood, 668
O'Sullivan test, 485, 493
Parathyroid hormone, 684
Parathyroid scan, 686

Pheochromocytoma
    suppression and provocative
    testing, 704
Phosphate, 706
Phosphorus, 706
Postprandial glucose, 485
Prolactin levels, 750
Renin assay
    Plasma, 800
    Renal vein, 801
Somatomedin C, 868
Testosterone, 890
Thyroid binding inhibitory
    immunoglobulins, 916
Thyroid scanning, 910
Thyroid-stimulating
    hormone, 913
    Stimulation test, 915
Thyroid-stimulating
    immunoglobulins, 916
Thyroid ultrasound, 918
Thyrotropin receptor
    antibody, 916
Thyrotropin-releasing hor-
    mone test, 920
Thyroxine, free, 922
Thyroxine, total, 924
Thyroxine-binding globulin,
    926
Thyroxine index, free, 928
TRH stimulation test, 913
Triiodothyronine, 939
Vanillylmandelic acid, 978

GASTROINTESTINAL SYSTEM

Abdominal ultrasound, 1
Anti-parietal cell antibody, 92
Barium enema, 146
Barium swallow, 150
Carcinoembryonic antigen, 230
Clostridial toxin assay, 275
Colonoscopy, 285
Computed tomography of
    abdomen, 295

Computed tomography arteri-
    ography, 295
Computed tomography
    colonoscopy, 295
Computed tomography por-
    togram, 307
Endomysial antibodies, 478
Esophageal function studies,
    406

Esophagogastroduodenoscopy, 410
Fecal fat, 428
Gastrin, 465
Gastroesophageal reflux scan, 467
Gastrointestinal bleeding scan, 469
Gliadin antibodies, 478
Helicobacter pylori antibodies test, 507
5-Hydroxyindoleacetic acid, 546
Lactose tolerance test, 577
Laparoscopy, 579
Meckel's diverticulum nuclear scan, 640
Obstruction series, 661
Paracentesis, 678

Prealbumin, 738
Protein, blood, 758
Schilling test, 821
Sialography, 845
Sigmoidoscopy, 849
Small bowel follow-through, 860
Stool culture, 876
Stool for occult blood, 878
Swallowing examination, 884
Transrectal ultrasonography, 752
Upper gastrointestinal x-ray study, 949
Urea nitrogen blood test, 952
Videofluoroscopy, 884
Virtual colonoscopy, 295
D-Xylose absorption test, 1004

HEMATOLOGIC SYSTEM

Activated clotting time, 9
Antithrombin III, 104
Basophils, 994
Bleeding time, 169
Blood smear, 174
Blood typing, 177
Bone marrow biopsy, 183
Clot retraction test, 277
Coagulating factors concentration, 279
Complete blood count and differential count, 294
Coombs' test
  Direct, 310
  Indirect, 312
D-Dimer test, 351
Delta-aminolevulinic acid, 353
2,3-Diphosphoglycerate, 361
Disseminated intravascular coagulation screening, 363
Eosinophils, 994
Erythropoietin, 404

Euglobulin lysis time, 422
Ferritin, 430
Fibrin monomers, 908
Fibrinogen, 454
Fibrinopeptide, 908
Folic acid, 456
Glucose-6-phosphate dehydrogenase, 490
Ham's test, 504
Haptoglobin, 505
Hematocrit, 511
Hemoglobin, 514
  Electrophoresis, 516
Iron level and total iron-binding capacity, 565
Leukoagglutinin test, 587
Lymphocytes, 994
Methemoglobin, 645
Monocytes, 994
Neutrophils, 994
Partial thromboplastin time, activated, 689

Plasminogen, 708
Platelet aggregation test, 710
Platelet antibody detection, 712
Platelet count, 714
Platelet volume, mean, 717
Porphyrins and porphobilinogens, 726
Protein C, 764
Protein S, 764
Prothrombin fragment, 908
Prothrombin time, 766
Red blood cell count, 782

Red blood cell indices, 785
Red blood cell survival study, 789
Red blood cells and casts, urine, 965
Reticulocyte count, 805
Sickle cell test, 847
Thrombosis indicators, 908
Uroporphyrinogen-1-synthase, 977
Vitamin B_{12}, 990
White blood cell count and differential count, 994

HEPATOBILIARY SYSTEM

Abdominal ultrasound, 1
Alanine aminotransferase, 28
Aldolase, 30
Alkaline phosphatase, 36
Alpha-fetoprotein, 47
Ammonia level, 52
Amylase
  Blood, 60
  Urine, 60
Aspartate aminotransferase, 143
Bilirubin, blood, 157
CA 19-9 tumor marker, 213
Cholesterol, 262
Computed tomography of the abdomen, 295
Endoscopic retrograde cholangiopancreatography, 394
Epstein-Barr virus titer, 399
Fecal fat, 428

Gallbladder nuclear scanning, 459
Gallium scan, 461
Gamma-glutamyl transpeptidase, 463
Hepatitis virus studies, 519
Lactate dehydrogenase, 572
Leucine aminopeptidase, 585
Lipase, 588
Liver biopsy, 595
Liver and pancreaticobiliary system ultrasonography, 1
Liver/spleen scanning, 599
5'-Nucleotidase, 659
Obstruction series, 661
Percutaneous transhepatic cholangiography, 394
Protein, blood, 758
Secretin-pancreozymin, 828
Sweat electrolytes test, 886

IMMUNOLOGIC SYSTEM

Agglutinins, febrile/cold, 21
AIDS serology, 23
Aldolase, 30
Allergy blood testing, 38
Allergy skin testing, 41

Anticardiolipin antibodies, 71
Anticentromere antibody test, 73
Antideoxyribonuclease-B titer, 74

Anti-DNA antibody test, 78
Anti-extractable nuclear anti-
    gens, 80
Antiglomerular basement
    membrane antibodies, 82
Anti-Jo-1 antibodies, 80
Antimitochondrial antibody,
    84
Antimyocardial antibodies, 86
Antineutrophil cytoplasmic
    antibody, 87
Antinuclear antibody, 89
Anti-parietal cell antibody, 92
Antiscleroderma antibody, 94
Anti-smooth muscle antibody,
    96
Anti-SS-A, anti-SS-B, and
    anti-SS-C antibody, 100
CD4/CD8 for HIV, 626
Complement assay, 292
Cryoglobulin, 331
Cutaneous immunofluores-
    cence biopsy, 333
Cytokines, 346
Diabetes mellitus autoanti-
    body panel, 360
Epstein-Barr virus titer, 399

Fungal antibody tests, 458
Glutamic decarboxylase anti-
    body, 360
HIV oral testing, 25
HIV urine testing, 25
HIV viral load, 529
Human lymphocyte antigen
    B27, 538
Human T-cell lymphotrophic
    virus I/II antibody, 542
Immunofixation electrophore-
    sis, 555
Immunoglobulin elec-
    trophoresis, 555
Insulin autoantibody, 360
Islet cell antibody, 360
Lyme disease test, 621
Lymphocyte immunopheno-
    typing, 626
Mononucleosis spot test, 649
Parvovirus B19 antibody,
    692
Protein electrophoresis, 758
Rabies-neutralizing antibody
    test, 781
Rheumatoid factor, 810
Rubeola antibody, 814

MISCELLANEOUS TESTS

Bioterrorism infectious agents
    testing, 161
Blood culture and sensitivity,
    172
Carbon dioxide content, 226
Carboxyhemoglobin, 228
Chloride, blood, 260
Cholinesterase, 266
C-reactive protein test, 319
Erythrocyte sedimentation
    rate, 402
Ethanol, 420
Forensic genetic testing, 472

Fungal antibody tests, 458
Glucose, blood, 482
Glucose, urine, 487
Magnesium, 630
Paternity genetic testing, 472
Positron emission tomogra-
    phy, 729
Potassium
    Blood, 733
    Urine, 736
Protein, blood, 758
Rubeola antibody, 814
Sexual assault testing, 836

Sialography, 845
Sleep studies, 856
Sodium
    Blood, 863
    Urine, 866
Substance abuse testing, 881
Tay-Sachs disease genetic
    testing, 474
Therapeutic drug monitoring,
    893

Throat and nose cultures,
    905
Toxicology screening, 881
Urine culture and sensitivity,
    972
Viral cultures, 988
West Nile virus testing, 992
White blood cell scan, 1000
Wound culture and sensitivity,
    1002

NERVOUS SYSTEM

Acetylcholine receptor anti-
    body, 5
Amyloid beta protein precur-
    sor, soluble, 63
Apolipoproteins, 110
Apolipoprotein E-4, 112
Caloric study, 224
Cerebral angiography, 127
Cerebrospinal fluid examina-
    tion, 602
Computed tomography of
    brain, 300
C-reactive protein test, 319
Digital subtraction angiogra-
    phy, 126
Electroencephalography, 373
Electromyography, 376

Electroneurography, 381
Electronystagmography, 384
Evoked potential studies, 424
Hexosaminidase, 527
Lumbar puncture, 602
Magnetic resonance angiogra-
    phy, 633
Magnetic resonance imaging,
    632
Magnetic resonance spec-
    troscopy, 633
Myelography, 651
Positron emission tomogra-
    phy, 729
Skull x-ray, 854
Spinal x-rays, 870
Tau protein, 63

PULMONARY SYSTEM

Acid-fast bacilli, 946
Alpha$_1$-antitrypsin, 45
Alpha$_1$-antitrypsin phenotyp-
    ing, 45
Angiotensin-converting
    enzyme, 67
Arterial blood gases, 117
Body plethysmography, 777
Bronchoscopy, 206
Carbon dioxide content, 226
Carboxyhemoglobin, 228

Chest x-ray, 254
Computed tomography of the
    chest, 304
Cystic fibrosis genetic testing,
    472
Gas dilution test, 777
Legionnaires' disease antibody
    test, 583
Lung biopsy, 611
Lung scan, 615
Mediastinoscopy, 643

Nose culture, 905
Oximetry, 672
Pleural biopsy, 723
Pulmonary angiography, 771
Pulmonary function tests, 774
SARS testing, 818
Sleep studies, 856
Sputum culture and
   sensitivity, 872

Sputum cytology, 874
Strept screen, 905
Thoracentesis and pleural
   fluid analysis, 897
Thoracoscopy, 903
Throat and nose cultures, 905
Tuberculin test, 944
Tuberculosis culture, 946
Urine pH, 959

RENAL/UROLOGIC SYSTEM

Acid phosphatase, 7
Aldosterone, 32
Amino acid profiles, 50
Anion gap, 69
Antidiuretic hormone, 75
Antistreptolysin O titer, 102
Beta$_2$ microglobulin, 155
Bilirubin, 157
Bladder cancer markers, 167
Captopril renal scan, 796
Carbon dioxide content, 226
Catecholamines, 978
Chloride, blood, 260
Computed tomography of
   kidney, 295
Creatinine, blood, 326
Creatinine clearance, 328
Crystals, 964
Cystography, 334
Cystometry, 336
Cystoscopy, 340
Epithelial casts, 965
Erythropoietin, 404
Fatty casts, 964
Granular casts, 964
Hyaline casts, 964
Intravenous pyelography, 560
Ketones, 963
Kidney sonogram, 1
Kidney, ureter, and bladder
   x-ray study, 661

Lactic acid, 575
Leukocyte esterase, 963
Microalbumin, 647
Nitrites, 963
Osmolality
   Blood, 668
   Urine, 670
Pelvic floor sphincter elec-
   tromyography, 379
Percent free PSA, 756
Potassium
   Blood, 733
   Urine, 736
Prostate/rectal sonogram,
   752
Prostate-specific antigen, 755
Protein, urine, 962
PSA velocity, 756
Renal angiography, 126
Renal biopsy, 792
Renal scanning, 796
Renin assay
   Plasma, 800
   Renal vein, 801
Retrograde pyelography, 807
Scrotal nuclear imaging, 824
Scrotal ultrasound, 826
Sodium
   Blood, 863
   Urine, 866
Testicular sonogram, 826

Urea nitrogen blood test, 952
Urethral pressure profile, 336
Uric acid, 955
Urinalysis, 959
Urine appearance and color, 960
Urine culture and sensitivity, 972
Urine flow studies, 975
Urine odor, 960
Urine pH, 960
Urine specific gravity, 962
Vanillylmandelic acid, 978
Waxy casts, 965
White blood cells and casts, 965

REPRODUCTIVE SYSTEM

Alpha-fetoprotein, 47
Amniocentesis, 54
Amniotic fluid index, 435
Antispermatozoal antibody, 98
Apt test, 115
Breast cancer genetic screening, 472
Breast cancer tumor analysis, 197
Breast scintography, 202
Breast sonogram, 204
CA 15-3 and CA 27.29 tumor markers, 211
CA-125 tumor marker, 215
Chlamydia, 257
Chorionic villus sampling, 269
Colposcopy, 289
Contraction stress test, 437
Cytomegalovirus, 349
Electromyography of the pelvic floor sphincter, 379
Endometrial biopsy, 391
Estriol excretion, 414
Estrogen fractions, 414
Fetal biophysical profile, 433
Fetal contraction stress test, 437
Fetal fibronectin, 441
Fetal hemoglobin, 443
Fetal nonstress test, 446
Fetal nuchal translucency, 695
Fetal oxygen saturation monitoring, 448
Fetal scalp blood pH, 448
Fetoscopy, 451
Follicle-stimulating hormone, 618
Gonorrhea culture, 840
Herpes genitalis, 524
Herpes simplex, 524
Human placental lactogen, 540
Hysterosalpingography, 548
Hysteroscopy, 550
IUD localization, 695
Lamellar body count, 55
Laparoscopy, 579
Luteinizing hormone assay, 618
Mammography, 637
Maternal triple screen, 47
Obstetric ultrasonography, 694
Oxytocin challenge test, 437
Papanicolaou smear, 674
Pelvic ultrasonography, 694
Phenylketonuria test, 702
Pregnancy tests, 740
Pregnanediol, 743
Progesterone assay, 746
Prolactin levels, 750
Rubella antibody test, 812

Semen analysis, 830
Sexual assault testing, 836
Sexually transmitted disease
    cultures, 840
Sims-Huhner test, 852

Syphilis detection test, 888
TORCH test, 930
Toxoplasmosis antibody titer,
    931

SKELETAL SYSTEM

Aldolase, 30
Alkaline phosphatase, 36
Arthrocentesis with synovial
    fluid analysis, 133
Arthrography, 137
Arthroscopy, 139
Bone densitometry, 179
Bone scan, 189
Bone turnover biochemical
    markers, 192
Bone x-ray, 195
Electromyography, 379

Human lymphocyte antigen
    B27, 538
Lactate dehydrogenase, 572
Magnetic resonance imaging,
    632
Myoglobin, 655
N-telopeptide, 192
Osteocalcin, 192
Pyridinium crosslinks, 192
Rheumatoid factor, 810
Spinal x-rays, 870
Uric acid, 955

Appendix B: List of tests by type

Tests in this list are grouped by the following types: blood, electrodiagnostic, endoscopy, fluid analysis, manometric, microscopic examinations, nuclear scans, other studies, sputum, stool, ultrasound, urine, and x-ray.

BLOOD TESTS

Acetylcholine receptor antibody, 5

Acid phosphatase, 7

Activated clotting time, 9

Adrenocorticotropic hormone, 12

    Stimulation test with cosyntropin, 15

    Stimulation test with metyrapone, 18

Agglutinins, febrile/cold, 21

AIDS serology, 23

Alanine aminotransferase, 28

Albumin, 758

Aldolase, 30

Aldosterone, 32

Alkaline phosphatase, 36

Allergy blood testing, 38

Alpha$_1$-antitrypsin, 45

Alpha$_1$, antitrypsin phenotyping, 45

Alpha-fetoprotein, 47

Amino acid profiles, 50

Ammonia level, 52

Amylase, 60

Androstenediones, 65

Angiotensin-converting enzyme, 67

Anion gap, 69

Anticardiolipin antibodies, 71

Anticentromere antibody test, 73

Antideoxyribonuclease-B titer, 74

Antidiuretic hormone, 75

Anti-DNA antibody test, 78

Anti-extractable nuclear antigens, 80

Antiglobulin, 310

Antiglomerular basement membrane antibodies, 82

Anti-Jo-1 antibodies, 80

Antimitochondrial antibody, 84

Antimyocardial antibodies, 86

Antineutrophil cytoplasmic antibody, 87

Antinuclear antibody, 89

Anti-parietal cell antibody, 92

Antiscleroderma antibody, 94

Anti-smooth muscle antibody, 96

Antispermatozoal antibody, 98

Anti-SS-A and anti-SS-B antibody, 100

Antistreptolysin O titer, 102

Antithrombin III, 104

Antithyroglobulin antibody, 106

Antithyroid perioxidase antibody, 108

Apolipoproteins, 110

Arterial blood gases, 117

Aspartate aminotransferase, 143

Atrial natriuretic peptide, 657

Basophils, 994
Beta$_2$ microglobulin, 155
Bilirubin, 157
Bioterrorism infectious agents, 161
Bleeding time, 169
Blood culture and sensitivity, 172
Blood gases, 117
Blood smear, 174
Blood typing, 177
Bone turnover biochemical markers, 192
Brain natriuretic peptide, 657
Breast cancer genetic screening, 472
CA 15-3 and CA 27.29 tumor markers, 211
CA 19-9 tumor marker, 213
CA-125 tumor marker, 215
Calcitonin, 217
Calcium, 220
Carbon dioxide content, 226
Carboxyhemoglobin, 228
Carcinoembryonic antigen, 230
CD4/CD8 for HIV, 626
Chlamydia, 257
Chloride, 260
Cholesterol, 262
Cholinesterase, 266
Chromosome karyotype, 273
CK-MB/CK relative index, 323
Clonidine suppression test, 704
Clot retraction test, 277
Coagulating factors concentration, 279
Complement assay, 292
Complete blood count, 294
Coombs' test
  Direct, 310
  Indirect, 312
Cortisol, 314
C-peptide, 317
C-reactive protein test, 319
Creatine phosphokinase, 322
Creatinine, 326
Creatinine clearance, 328
Cryoglobulin, 331
C-type natriuretic peptide, 657
Cytokines, 346
Cytomegalovirus, 349
Dehydroepiandrosterone, 65
Dehydroepiandrosterone S, 65
Dexamethasone suppression test, 355
Diabetes mellitus autoantibody panel, 359
Differential count, 294
D-Dimer test, 351
2,3-Diphosphoglycerate, 361
Disseminated intravascular coagulation screening, 363
Endomysial antibodies, 478
Eosinophils, 994
Epstein-Barr virus titer, 399
Erythrocyte sedimentation rate, 402
Erythropoietin, 404
Estriol excretion, 414
Ethanol, 420
Euglobulin lysis time, 422
Ferritin, 430
Fetal hemoglobin, 443
Fetal scalp blood pH, 448
Fibrin monomers, 408
Fibrinogen, 454
Fibrinopeptide, 408
Folic acid, 456
Follicle-stimulating hormone assay, 618
Free thyroxine, 922
Fungal antibody test, 458

Gamma-glutamyl transpeptidase, 463
Gastrin, 465
Genetic testing, 472
Gliadin antibodies, 478
Glucagon, 480
Glucagon stimulation test, 704
Glucose
    Blood, 482
    Postprandial, 485
Glucose-6-phosphate dehydrogenase, 490
Glucose tolerance test, 492
Glutamic acid decarboxylase antibody, 359
Glycated proteins, 496
Glycosylated hemoglobin, 496
Growth hormone, 499
Stimulation test, 502
Growth hormone suppression test, 500
Ham's test, 504
Haptoglobin, 505
Helicobacter pylori antibodies test, 507
Hematocrit, 511
Hemoglobin, 514
    Electrophoresis, 516
Hepatitis virus studies, 519
Herpes simplex, 524
Hexosaminidase, 527
HIV viral load, 529
HLA-B27 antigen, 538
Homocysteine, 535
Human lymphocyte antigen B27, 538
Human placental lactogen, 540
Human T-cell lymphotrophic virus I/II antibody, 542
Immunofixation electrophoresis, 553

Immunoglobulin electrophoresis, 555
Insulin assay, 558
Insulin autoantibody, 359
Insulin-like growth factor binding proteins, 868
Iron level and total iron-binding capacity, 565
Islet cell antibody, 359
Lactate dehydrogenase, 572
Lactic acid, 575
Lactose tolerance test, 577
Legionnaires' disease antibody test, 583
Leucine aminopeptidase, 585
Leukoagglutinin test, 587
Lipase, 588
Lipoproteins, 592
Lipoprotein electrophoresis, 590
Long-acting thyroid stimulator, 916
Luteinizing hormone assay, 618
Lyme disease test, 621
Lymphocytes, 994
Lymphocyte immunophenotyping, 626
Magnesium, 630
Maternal triple screen, 47
Methemoglobin, 645
Metyrapone, 18
Monocytes, 994
Mononucleosis spot test, 649
Myoglobin, 655
Natriuretic peptides, 657
Neutrophils, 994
N-telopeptide, 192
5'-Nucleotidase, 659
Osmolality, 668
O'Sullivan test, 485, 493
Osteocalcin, 192
Parathyroid hormone, 684

Partial thromboplastin time, activated, 689
Parvovirus B19 antibody, 692
Percent free PSA, 756
Phenylketonuria test, 702
Pheochromocytoma suppression and provocative testing, 704
Phosphate, 706
Phosphorus, 706
Plasminogen, 708
Platelet aggregation test, 710
Platelet antibody detection, 712
Platelet count, 714
Platelet volume, mean, 717
Potassium, 733
Prealbumin, 738
Pregnancy tests, 740
Progesterone assay, 746
Prolactin levels, 750
Prostate-specific antigen, 755
Protein, 758
Protein C, 764
Protein S, 764
Prothrombin fragment, 908
Prothrombin time, 766
PSA velocity, 755
Rabies-neutralizing antibody test, 781
Red blood cell count, 782
Red blood cell indices, 785
Renin assay
    Plasma, 800
    Renal vein, 801
Reticulocyte count, 805
Rheumatoid factor, 810
Rubella antibody test, 812
Rubeola antibody, 814
SARS, 818
Sexual assault testing, 836
Sexually transmitted disease cultures, 840

Sickle cell test, 847
Sodium, 863
Somatomedin C, 868
Substance abuse testing, 881
Syphilis detection test, 888
Testosterone, 890
Therapeutic drug monitoring, 893
Thrombosis indicators, 908
Thyroid-binding globulin, 926
Thyroid-binding inhibitory immunoglobulins, 916
Thyroid-stimulating hormone, 913
    Stimulation test, 913
Thyroid-stimulating immunoglobulins, 916
Thyrotropin receptor antibody, 916
Thyrotropin-releasing hormone test, 920
Thyroxine, free, 922
Thyroxine, total, 924
Thyroxine-binding globulin, 926
Thyroxine index, free, 928
Toxicology screening, 881
Toxoplasmosis antibody titer, 931
TRH stimulation test, 913
Triglycerides, 937
Triiodothyronine, 939
Troponins, 941
Urea nitrogen blood test, 952
Uric acid, 955
Uroporphyrinogen-1-synthase, 977
Viral cultures, 988
Vitamin B_{12}, 990
West Nile virus, 992
White blood cell count and differential count, 994
D-Xylose absorption test, 1004

ELECTRODIAGNOSTIC TESTS

Caloric study, 224
Cardiac exercise stress testing, 239
Contraction stress (fetal), 437
Electrocardiography, 368
Electroencephalography, 373
Electromyography, 376
Electromyography of the pelvic floor sphincter, 379
Electroneurography, 381
Electronystagmography, 384
Electrophysiologic study, 387

Evoked potential studies, 424
Fetal contraction stress test, 437
Fetal nonstress test, 446
Holter monitoring, 533
Nonstress (fetal), 446
Pelvic floor sphincter electromyography, 379
Signal-averaged electrocardiography, 370
Sleep studies, 856

ENDOSCOPY

Arthroscopy, 139
Bronchoscopy, 206
Colonoscopy, 285
Colposcopy, 289
Cystoscopy, 340
Endoscopic retrograde cholangiopancreatography, 394
Esophagogastroduodenoscopy, 410

Fetoscopy, 451
Gastroscopy, 410
Hysteroscopy, 550
Laparoscopy, 579
Mediastinoscopy, 642
Sigmoidoscopy, 849
Thoracoscopy, 903
Transesophageal echocardiography, 933

FLUID ANALYSIS

Amniocentesis, 54
Amyloid beta protein precursor, soluble, 63
Antispermatozoal antibody, 98
Arthrocentesis with synovial fluid analysis, 133
Beta$_2$ microglobulin, 155
Breast ductal lavage, 200
Fetal fibronectin, 441
Genetic testing, 472
HIV oral testing, 25
Lumbar puncture and cerebrospinal fluid examination, 602

Paracentesis, 678
Pericardiocentesis, 698
SARS, 818
Secretin-pancreozymin, 828
Semen analysis, 830
Sexual assault testing, 836
Sims-Huhner test, 852
Substance abuse testing, 881
Sweat electrolytes test, 886
Tau protein, 63
Thoracentesis and pleural fluid analysis, 897
West Nile virus, 992

MANOMETRIC TESTS

Cystometry, 336
Electrophysiologic study, 387
Esophageal function studies, 406
Plethysmography, arterial, 719
  Venous, 721
Urethral pressure profile, 336

MICROSCOPIC EXAMINATIONS

Antiglomerular basement
  membrane antibodies, 82
Bioterrorism infectious
  agents, 161
Bone marrow biopsy, 183
Breast cancer tumor analysis,
  197
Cathepsin D, 198
Cervical biopsy, 251
Chlamydia, 257
Cutaneous immunofluores-
  cence biopsy, 333
DNA ploidy status, 198
Endometrial biopsy, 391
Estrogen receptor assay, 418
Gonorrhea culture, 840
Helicobacter pylori antibodies
  test, 507
HER 2 protein, 198
Herpes genitalis, 524
Herpes simplex, 524
Liver biopsy, 595
Ki67 protein, 199
Lung biopsy, 611
Nose culture, 905
p53 protein, 199
Papanicolaou smear, 674
Pleural biopsy, 723
Progesterone receptor assay,
  748
Renal biopsy, 792
Sexually transmitted disease
  cultures, 840
S-phase fraction, 198
Strept screen, 905
Throat and nose cultures, 905
Tuberculosis culture, 946
Urine culture and sensitivity,
  972
Viral cultures, 988
Wound culture and sensitivity,
  1002

NUCLEAR SCANS

Bone scan, 189
Breast scintigraphy, 202
Cardiac exercise stress testing,
  239
Cardiac flow studies, 244
Cardiac nuclear scanning, 244
Gallbladder nuclear scanning,
  459
Gallium scan, 461
Gastroesophageal reflux scan,
  467
Gastrointestinal bleeding scan,
  469
Isonitrile scan, 244
Liver/spleen scanning, 599
Lung scan, 615
Meckel's diverticulum nuclear
  scan, 640
MUGA scan, 246
Octreotide scan, 664
Oncoscint scan, 666
Parathyroid scan, 686
Positron emission tomogra-
  phy, 729
Red blood cell survival study,
  789

Renal scanning, 796
Salivary gland nuclear imaging, 816
Scrotal nuclear imaging, 824

Sentinel lymph node biopsy, 833
Thallium scan, 244
Thyroid scanning, 910
White blood cell scan, 1000

OTHER STUDIES

Allergy skin testing, 41
Bioterrorism infectious agents testing, 161
Body plethysmography, 777
Chorionic villus sampling, 269
Colposcopy, 289
Ethanol, 420
Fetal nonstress test, 446
Fetal oxygen saturation monitoring, 448
Gas dilution test, 777
Genetic testing, 472
Helicobacter pylori antibodies test, 507

Magnetic resonance angiography, 633
Magnetic resonance imaging, 632
Magnetic resonance spectroscopy, 633
Oximetry, 672
Pulmonary function tests, 774
Sleep studies, 856
Substance abuse testing, 881
Tilt-table testing, 387
TORCH test, 930
Tuberculin test, 944
Urine flow studies, 975
Viral cultures, 988

SPUTUM TESTS

Acid-fast bacilli, 946
Bioterrorism infectious agents, 161

Culture and sensitivity, 872
Cytology, 874

STOOL TESTS

Apt test, 115
Bioterrorism infectious agents, 161
Clostridial toxin assay, 275
Culture, 876

Fecal fat, 428
Occult blood, 878
Ova and parasites, 876
Viral cultures, 988

ULTRASOUND TESTS

Abdominal ultrasound, 1
Amniotic fluid index, 435
Breast sonogram, 204

Carotid artery duplex scanning, 249
Echocardiography, 365

Fetal biophysical profile, 433
Fetal nuchal translucency, 695
IUD localization, 695
Kidney sonogram, 1
Liver and pancreaticobiliary
  system ultrasonography, 1
Obstetric ultrasonography,
  694
Pelvic ultrasonography, 694
Prostate/rectal sonogram,
  752

Scrotal ultrasound, 826
Testicular ultrasound, 826
Thyroid ultrasound, 918
Transesophageal echocardiog-
  raphy, 933
Transthoracic echocardiogra-
  phy, 365
Transrectal ultrasonography,
  752
Vascular ultrasound studies,
  982

URINE TESTS

Adrenocorticotropic hormone
  stimulation test with
  metyrapone, 18
Aldosterone, 32
Amino acid profiles, 50
Amylase, 60
Appearance and color, 960
Bence Jones protein, 153
Beta$_2$ microglobulin, 155
Bladder cancer markers 167
Bone turnover biochemical
  markers, 192
Calcium, 220
Cortisol, 314
Creatinine clearance, 328
Crystals, 964
Culture and sensitivity, 972
Delta-aminolevulinic acid,
  353
Dexamethasone suppression
  test, 355
Epithelial casts, 965
Estriol excretion, 414
Estrogen fractions, 414
Ethanol, 420
Fatty casts, 964
Flow studies, 975
Glucose, 482
Glucose tolerance test, 492

Granular casts, 964
HIV urine testing, 25
Hyaline casts, 964
17-Hydroxycorticosteroids,
  543
5-Hydroxyindoleacetic acid,
  546
Immunofixation electrophore-
  sis, 553
Ketones, 963
17-Ketosteroids, 569
Leucine aminopeptidase, 585
Leukocyte esterase, 963
Metyrapone, 18
Microalbumin, 647
N-telopeptide, 192
Nitrites, 963
Odor, 960
Osmolality, 670
pH, 960
Phenylketonuria test, 702
Porphyrins and porphobilino-
  gens, 726
Potassium, 733
Prealbumin, 738
Pregnancy tests, 740
Pregnanediol, 743
Protein, 962
Pyridinium, 192

Red blood cells and casts, 965
Schilling test, 821
Sodium, 866
Specific gravity, 962
Substance abuse testing, 881
Toxicology screening, 881
Uric acid, 955
Urinalysis, 959
Urine culture and sensitivity, 972

Vanillylmandelic acid and catecholamines, 978
Viral cultures, 988
Waxy casts, 965
White blood cells and casts, 965
D-Xylose absorption test, 1004

X-RAY EXAMINATIONS

Adrenal angiography, 126
Arteriography, 126
Arthrography, 137
Barium enema, 146
Barium swallow, 150
Bone densitometry, 179
Bone x-ray, 195
Cardiac catheterization, 232
Cerebral angiography, 127
Chest x-ray, 254
Computed tomography
    Of abdomen, 295
    Of adrenals, 295
    Of brain, 300
    Of chest, 304
    Of kidney, 295
Computed tomography arteriography, 295
Computed tomography colonoscopy, 295
Computed tomography portogram, 307
Cystography, 334
Digital subtraction angiography, 126
Hysterosalpingography, 548
Intravenous pyelography, 560

Kidney, ureter, and bladder x-ray study, 661
Lymphangiography, 623
Magnetic resonance imaging, 632
Mammography, 637
Myelography, 651
Obstruction series, 661
Percutaneous transhepatic cholangiography, 394
Positron emission tomography, 729
Pulmonary angiography, 771
Renal angiography, 126
Retrograde pyelography, 807
Sialography, 845
Skull x-ray, 854
Small bowel follow-through, 860
Swallowing examination, 884
Spinal x-rays, 870
Upper gastrointestinal x-ray study, 949
Venography of lower extremities, 985
Videofluoroscopy, 884
Virtual colonoscopy, 295

Appendix C: Disease and organ panels

Note: These panels may be modified or expanded in different clinical settings.

Anemia

Complete blood count, (CBC), 294
Red blood cell (RBC) indices, 785
Reticulocyte count, 805
Microcytic: ESR, 402; iron panel, 565
Normocytic: ESR, 402; hemolysis profile, 1026
Macrocytic: Vit B_{12}, 990; folate, 456; TSH, 913

Arthritis

Antinuclear antibody (ANA), 89
C-reactive protein, 319
ESR (sedimentation rate), 402
Rheumatoid factor, 810
Uric acid, 955

Basic metabolic panel

Blood urea nitrogen (BUN), 952
Calcium, 220
Carbon dioxide, 226
Chloride, 260
Creatinine, 326
Glucose, 482
Potassium, 733
Sodium, 863

Bone/joint

Albumin, 758
Alkaline phosphatase, 36
Calcium, 220
Osteocalcin, 192
Phosphorus, 706
Protein, total, 758
Uric acid, 955

Cardiac injury

Creatine kinase (CK), 322
CK-MB, 322
Myoglobin, 655
Troponin I, 941

Coagulation screening

Bleeding time, 169
Partial thromboplastin time (PTT), 689
Platelet count, 714
Prothrombin time (PT), 766

Coma

Alcohol, 420
Ammonia, 52
Anion gap, 69
Arterial blood gases, 117
Basic metabolic panel, 1025
Calcium (total and ionized), 220
Lactic acid, 575
Osmolality (serum), 668
Salicylate, 895
Toxicology screen, 881

Comprehensive metabolic panel

Albumin, 758
Bilirubin, 157
Blood urea nitrogen (BUN), 952
Calcium, 220
Carbon dioxide, 226
Chloride, 260
Creatinine, 326
Glucose, 482
Phosphatase, alkaline, 36

Potassium, 733
Protein, total, 758
Sodium, 863
Transferase, aspartate amino
(AST) (SGOT), 143

DIC

Complete blood count
(CBC), 294
Fibrinogen, 454
Fibrin split products, 908
Partial thromboplastin time
(PTT), 689
Platelet count, 714
Prothrombin time (PT),
766

Diabetes mellitus management

Anion gap, 69
Basic metabolic panel,
1025
Hemoglobin A_{1c}, 496
Lipid profile, 262

Electrolyte panel

Carbon dioxide, 226
Chloride, 260
Potassium, 733
Sodium, 863

General health

Complete blood count
(CBC), 294
Comprehensive metabolic
panel, 1025
Gamma-glutamyl transferase
(GGT), 463
Lipid profile, 262
Lactic dehydrogenase (LD),
572
Thyroid-stimulating hormone
(TSH), 913
Uric acid, 955

Hemolysis profile

Antiglobulin, 310
Bilirubin, 157
Complete blood count
(CBC), 294
Haptoglobin, 505
Hemoglobin, free (serum,
514; and urine, 959)
Lactic dehydrogenase (LD),
572
Reticulocyte count, 805

Hepatic function

Albumin, 758
Alkaline phosphatase, 36
Alanine aminotransferase
(ALT)/serum glutamic-
pyruvic transaminase
(SGPT), 28
Asparate aminotransferase
(AST)/serum glutamic-
oxaloacetic transaminase
(SGOT), 143
Bilirubin, direct and total,
157
Gamma-glutamyl transferase
(GGT), 463
Protein, total, 758
Prothrombin time (PT), 766

Hepatitis, acute

Hepatitis A antibody IgM,
519
Hepatitis B core antibody
IgM, 522
Hepatitis B surface antigen,
520
Hepatitis C antibody, 522

HIV

HIV antibody (ELISA) with
Western blot confirmation,
23

Complete blood count (CBC), 294
CD4 and CD8, 626

Hypertension

Basic metabolic panel, 1025
Cortisol, urinary free, 314
Metanephrines, urinary, 978
Renin, 800
Thyroid screening panel, 1028
Urinalysis, 959

Lipid panel

HDL cholesterol, 592
Total cholesterol, 262
Triglycerides, 937
Low-density lipoprotein (LDL) – calculated, 592
Very low-density lipoprotein (VLDL) – calculated, 592

Obstetric

Complete blood count (CBC), 294
Hepatitis B surface antigen, 520
Rubella antibody, 812
Syphilis test (RPR, VDRL), 888
Blood type, 177, and screen, 312

Pancreatic

Amylase, 60
Calcium (total and ionized), 220
Glucose, 482
Lipase, 588
Triglycerides, 937

Parathyroid

Albumin, 758
Alkaline phophatase, 36
Calcium (total and ionized), 220

Calcium, urinary, 220
Creatinine, 326
Magnesium, 630
Phosphorus, 706
PTH, 684
Protein, total, 758

Prenatal

ABO and Rh typing, 177
Antibody screen, 312
Blood urea nitrogen (BUN), 952
Complete blood count (CBC), 294
Cervical cultures for GC, chlamydia, group B streptococci, 840
Creatinine, 326
Cytomegalovirus (CMV), 349
Glucose, 482
Hepatitis B surface antigen, 519
Herpes simplex I and II, 524
Pap smear, 674
Rubella titer, 812
Thyroxine, free, 922
Toxoplasmosis antibody, 931
Uric acid, 955
Urinalysis, 959
Urine culture, 972
VDRL, 888

Renal

Albumin, 758
Basic metabolic panel, 1025
Complete blood count (CBC), 294
Calcium, 220
Creatinine clearance, 328
Creatinine, 24-hour urine, 328
Magnesium, 630
Phosphorus, 706

Protein, total, 758
Protein, urine, 962
Protein, 24-hour urine, 959

Thyroid screening panel

Thyroxine (free T_4), 922
Thyroid-stimulating hormone
  (TSH), 915

TORCH antibody panel

Cytomegalovirus antibody,
  349
Herpes simplex antibody, 524
Rubella antibody, 812
Toxoplasmosis antibody, 931

Toxicology screening (urine)

Amphetamines, 881
Barbiturates, 881
Benzodiazepines, 881
Cocaine metabolites, 881
Marijuana metabolites, 881
Methadone, 881
Methaqualone, 881
Opiate metabolites, 881
Phencyclidine, 881
Propoxyphene, 881

Appendix D: Symbols and units of measurement

<	less than
≤	less than or equal to
>	greater than
≥	greater than or equal to
c (prefix)	centi (10^{-2})
C	celsius
cg	centigram
cm	centimeter
cm H_2O	centimeter of water
cu	cubic
d (prefix)	deci (10^{-1})
dl	deciliter (100 ml)
fL	femtoliter
fmol	femtomole
g	gram
hr	hour
IU	international unit
ImU	international milliunit
IµU	international microunit
k (prefix)	kilo (10^3)
kat	katal
kg	kilogram (1000 grams)
L	liter
m (prefix)	milli (10^{-3})
m	meter
m^2	square meter
m^3	cubic meter
mcg	microgram
mEq	milliequivalent
mEq/L	milliequivalent per liter
mg	milligram (1/1000 gram)
min	minute
ml	milliliter
mm	millimeter (1/10 centimeter)
mm^3	cubic millimeter
mM	millimole
mm Hg	millimeter of mercury
mm H_2O	millimeter of water
mol	mole
mmol	millimole

mOsm	milliosmole
mμ	millimicron
mU	milliunit
mV	millivolt
μ (prefix)	micro (10^{-6})
$μ^3$	cubic micron
μkat	microkatal
μl	microliter
μm	micrometer
$μm^3$	cubic micrometer
μmol	micromole
μU	microunit
n (prefix)	nano (10^{-9})
ng	nanogram
nkat	nanokatal
nm	nanometer
nmol	nanomole
p (prefix)	pico (10^{-12})
Pa	pascal
pg	picogram
pl	picoliter
pm	picometer
pmol	picomole
sec	second
SI units	International System of Units
U	unit
yr	year

bibliography

Ball EM, et al: Diagnosis and treatment of sleep apnea within the community: the Walla Walla project, *Arch Intern Med* 157(4):419-424, 1997.

Barrick B, Vogel S: Application of laboratory diagnostics in HIV testing, *Nursing Clin North Am* 31(1):41-45, 1996.

Blum WF, et al: A specific radioimmunoassay for the growth hormone (GH)-dependent somatomedin-binding protein: its use for diagnosis of GH deficiency, *J Clin Endocrinol Metab* 70:1292-1298, 1990.

Braunwald E, et al, eds.: *Harrison's principles of internal medicine,* ed 15, New York, 2001, McGraw-Hill.

Brooks MJ, et al: The infectious etiology of peptic ulcer disease: diagnosis and implications for therapy, *Primary Care* 23(3):443-454, 1996.

Byers T, et al: American Cancer Society guidelines for screening and surveillance for early detection of colorectal polyps and cancer: update 1997, *Cancer* 47(3):154-160, 1997.

Carnaille B, et al: Scintiscans and carcinoid tumors, *Surgery* 116(6):1118-1122, 1994.

Catalona WJ, et al: Use of the percentage of free prostate-specific antigen to enhance differentiation of prostate cancer from benign prostatic disease, *JAMA* 279(19):1542-1547, 1998.

Clifford EJ, et al: Scintimammography in the diagnosis of breast cancer, *Am J Surg* 172:483-486, 1996.

Collinson PO: The need for a point of care testing: an evidence-based appraisal, *Scand J Clin Lab Invest Suppl (UCR)* 230:67-73, 1999.

Couch FJ, et al: BRCA 1 mutations in women attending clinics that evaluate the risk of breast cancer, *N Engl J Med* 336(20):1409-1415, 1997.

Coudrey L: The troponins, *Arch Intern Med* 158:1173-1179, 1998.

Dalence CR, et al: Amniotic fluid lamellar body count: a rapid and reliable fetal lung maturity test, *Obstet Gynecol* 86(2):235-239, 1995.

De Veciana M, et al: Postprandial versus preprandial blood glucose monitoring in women with gestational diabetes mellitus requiring insulin therapy, *N Engl J Med* 333(19):1237-1241, 1995.

Frank AP, et al: Anonymous HIV testing using home collection and telemedicine counseling, *Arch Intern Med* 157(3):309-313, 1997.

Giannitsis E, Katus HA: Strategies for clinical assessment of patients with suspected acute coronary syndromes, *Scand J Clin Lab Invest Suppl (UCR)* 230:36-42, 1999.

Greenberg LR, Moore TR, Murphy H: Gestational diabetes mellitus: antenatal variables as predictors of postpartum glucose intolerance, *Gest Diabetes* 86(1):97-101, 1995.

Henry JB: *Clinical diagnosis and management by laboratory methods,* ed 20, Philadelphia, 2001, WB Saunders.

Kikuchi S, et al: Serum anti-*Helicobacter pylori* antibody and gastric carcinoma among young adults, *Cancer* 75(12):2789-2792, 1995.

Knight EL, et al: Atrial natriuretic peptide and the development of congestive heart failure in the oldest old: a seven-year prospective study, *J Am Geriatr Soc* 47:407-411, 1999.

Leitch AM, et al: American Cancer Society guidelines for the early detection of breast cancer: update 1997, *Cancer* 47(3):150-153, 1997.

Lensing AW, et al: A comparison of compression ultrasound with color Doppler ultrasound for diagnosis of symptomless postoperative deep vein thrombosis, *Arch Intern Med* 157(7):758-762, 1997.

Maack T: Role of atrial natriuretic factor in volume control, *Kidney International* 49:1732-1737, 1996.

Mellors JW, et al: Plasma viral load and CD4+ lymphocytes as prognostic markers of HIV-1 infection, *Ann Intern Med* 126:946-954, 1997.

Merrigan T, Bartlett J, Bolognesi D: *Textbook of AIDS medicine*, ed 2, Baltimore, 1999, Williams & Wilkins.

Midka NK, Stratton CW: Laboratory test in critical care, *Crit Care Clin* 14(1):15-34, 1998.

Miller KE: Sexually transmitted diseases, *Primary Care* 24(1):179-193, 1997.

Murphy MJ, Berding CB: Use of measurements of myoglobin and cardiac troponins in the diagnosis of acute myocardial infarction, *Crit Care Nurse* 19(1):58-66, 1999.

Pagana KD, Pagana TJ: *Mosby's manual of diagnostic and laboratory tests*, ed 2, St Louis, 2002, Mosby.

Plebani M, Zaninotto M: Cardiac markers: present and future, *Int J Clin Lab Res* 29(2):56-63, 1999.

Polascik TJ, Oesterling JE, Partin AW: Prostate-specific antigen: a decade of discovery—what we have learned and where we are going, *J Urol*, 162(Aug):293-306, 1999.

Potter SR, Reckwitz T, Partin AW: The use of percent free PSA for early detection of prostate cancer, *J Androl* 20(4):449-453, 1999.

Rao JK, et al: The role of antineutrophil cytoplasmic antibody (c-ANCA) testing in the diagnosis of Wegener granulomatosis, *Ann Intern Med* 123(12):925-932, 1995.

Rice MS, MacDonald DC: Appropriate roles of cardiac troponins in evaluating patients with chest pain, *J Am Board Fam Pract*, 12(3):214-218, May-June 1999.

Ridker PM: Evaluating novel cardiovascular risk factors: can we better predict heart attacks? *Ann Intern Med*, 130(11):933-937, 1999.

Rosen CJ, Tenenhouse A: Biochemical markers of bone turnover, *Postgrad Med*, 104(4):101-114, 1998.

Sutinen J: Etiology of central nervous system infections in the Philippines and the role of serum C-reactive protein in excluding acute bacterial meningitis, *Int J Infect Dis* 3(2):88-93, Winter 1998-1999.

Taillefer R, et al: Technetium-99m sestamibi prone scintimammography to detect primary breast cancer and axillary lymph node involvement, *J Nuclear Med* 36(10):1758-1765, 1995.

Tonin P, et al: Frequency of recurrent BRCA 1 and BRCA 2 mutations in Ashkenazi Jewish breast cancer families, *Nat Med* 2(11):1179-1183, 1996.

Urnovitz HB, et al: Urine antibody tests: new insights into the dynamics of HIV-1 infection, *Clin Chem* 45(9):1602-1613, 1999.

Warren CJ: What is hemocysteine? *AJN* 99(10):39-41, 1999.

index

A

A1AT (alpha$_1$-antitrypsin), 45-46

AAT alpha$_1$-antitrypsin phenotyping, 45-46

Abdomen, computed tomography of, 295-299

Abdominal aorta ultrasound, 1, 4

Abdominal paracentesis, 678-683, 679f

Abdominal scintigraphy, 469-471

Abdominal sonogram, 1-4, 2f

Abdominal ultrasound, 1-4, 2f

Abdominal x-ray
cross-table lateral, 661-662
erect, 661
supine, 661, 662

ABEPs (auditory brain stem-evoked potentials), 424-427

ABGs (blood gases), 117-125, 119t

ABO system, 177-178

Absolute neutrophil count (ANC), 996

Absorptiometry
bone, 179
dual-energy x-ray, 179-180
dual-photon, 179-180
single x-ray, 180

ACA (anticardiolipin antibodies), 71-72

ACE (angiotensin-converting enzyme), 67-68

Acetaminophen monitoring data, 894t

Acetoacetic acid, 963-964

Acetone, 963-964

Acetylcholine (ACh), 5

Acetylcholine receptor antibody (AChR Ab), 5-6

Acetylcholine receptor-binding antibody, 5

Acetylcholine receptor-blocking antibody, 5

Acetylcholine receptor-modulating antibody, 5

Acetylcholinesterase, 266-268

ACh (acetylcholine), 5

AChR Ab (acetylcholine receptor antibody), 5-6

Acid clearing test, 407, 408f

Acid perfusion test, 407

Acid phosphatase, 7-8

Acid reflux with pH probe, 407, 408f

Acid serum test for paroxysmal nocturnal hemoglobinuria, 504

Acid-base balance, 733

Acid-base disturbances, 120t

Acid-fast bacillus (AFB) smears
pericardial fluid, 700
sputum, 947
synovial fluid, 134

aCL (anticardiolipin) antibodies, 71-72

Acquired immunodeficiency syndrome (AIDS) serology, 23-27, 841t

Acquired immunodeficiency syndrome (AIDS) T-lymphocyte cell markers, 626-629

ACT (activated clotting time), 9-11

ACTH (adrenocorticotropic hormone), 12-14

NOTE: Page numbers designated *f* and *t* refer to figures and tables, respectively.

1035

ACTH (adrenocorticotropic hormone) stimulation test
with cosyntropin, 15-17
with metyrapone, 18-20
ACTH (adrenocorticotropic hormone) suppression test, 355-358
Activated clotting time (ACT), 9-11
Activated coagulation time, 9-11
Activated PTT (APTT), 689-691
AD (androstenedione), 65-66
ADB (anti-DNase-B), 74, 102
Adenosine, 241
ADH (antidiuretic hormone), 75-77
ADH (antidiuretic hormone) stimulation test, water deprivation, 75-76
ADH (antidiuretic hormone) suppression test, 76
ADNase-B, 74
Adrenal angiography, 132
Adrenal arteriography, 127
Adrenal gland, computed tomography of, 299
Adrenocorticotropic hormone (ACTH), 12-14
Adrenocorticotropic hormone (ACTH) stimulation test
with cosyntropin, 15-17
with metyrapone, 18-20
Adrenocorticotropic hormone (ACTH) suppression test, 355-358
AFB (acid-fast bacillus) smears
pericardial fluid, 700
sputum, 947
synovial fluid analysis, 134
AFI (amniotic fluid index), 435
AFP (alpha-fetoprotein), 47-49
AG (anion gap), 69-70

AGBM (antiglomerulase basement membrane antibodies), 82-83
Age-adjusted PSA levels, 756
Agglutination inhibition test (AIT), 740-741
sperm agglutination and inhibition, 98-99
Agglutinins, febrile/cold, 21-22
Agranulocytes, 995
AIDS screen, 23-27
AIDS serology, 23-27, 841t
AIDS T-lymphocyte cell markers, 626-629
Air-contrast barium enema, 146
Air-contrast myelography, 651
Air-contrast upper GI study, 951
Airflow assessment, 774-780
Airflow monitors, 856
AIT (agglutination inhibition test), 740-741
sperm agglutination and inhibition, 98-99
ALA (aminolevulinic acid), 353-354, 726
Alanine aminotransferase (ALT), 28-29
Alanine aminotransferase (ALT)/AST ratio, 28
Albumin, 758-759, 760t
blood, 758-763
glycated, 497
macroaggregated, 615
microalbumin, 647-648
pericardial fluid, 665
prealbumin, 738-739
serum, 758-763
Albumin gradient
paracentesis, 680
thoracentesis, 899
Aldolase, 30-31
Aldosterone, 32-35, 733
Aldosterone stimulation test, 33

Aldosterone suppression test, 33
Alkaline phosphatase (ALP), 36-37
  isoenzymes of, 36
  peritoneal fluid, 680
Allergy blood testing, 38-40
Allergy skin testing, 41-44
ALP (alkaline phosphatase), 36-37
  isoenzymes of, 36
  peritoneal fluid, 680
Alpha$_1$-antitrypsin (A1AT), 45-46
Alpha$_1$-globulin, 759, 762
Alpha$_2$-globulin, 759, 760t, 762
Alpha-antitrypsin (AAT) phenotyping, 45-46
Alpha-fetoprotein (AFP), 47-49
ALT (alanine aminotransferase), 28-29
ALT/AST ratio, 28
AMA (antimitochondrial antibody), 84-85
AMA (antimyocardial antibodies), 86
Ambulatory electrocardiography, 533-534
Ambulatory monitoring, 533-534
Amikacin monitoring data, 894t
Amino acid profiles, 50-51
Amino acid screen, 50-51
Aminolevulinic acid (ALA), 353-354, 726
Aminophylline monitoring data, 894t
Amipaque (metrizamide), 651
Amitriptyline monitoring data, 894t
Ammonia level, 52-53
  peritoneal fluid, 680

Amniocentesis, 54-59, 58f
Amnioscopy, 449
Amniotic fluid analysis, 54-59, 58f
  genetic testing, 476
Amniotic fluid index (AFI), 435
Amniotic fluid volume, 54, 57, 434
Amobarbital monitoring data, 894t
Amylase, 60-62
  peritoneal, 680
  pleural, 899
Amylase/creatinine clearance ratio, 61
Amyloid beta protein precursor, soluble (sBPP), 63-64
ANA (antinuclear antibody), 89-91
  anticentromere, 73
  anti-DNA, 78
  anti-extractable nuclear antigens, 80-81
  antiscleroderma, 94-95
  anti-SS-A, anti-SS-B, and anti-SS-C, 100-101
  autoimmune disease and, 89t
  immunofluorescent staining patterns, 90f
  pleural fluid, 900
  Ro, La, and SS-C antibodies, 100-101
  Scl-70 antibody, 94-95
Anal canal culture, 842, 842f
Anatomic abnormalities, 55-56
ANC (absolute neutrophil count), 996
ANCA (antineutrophil cytoplasmic antibody), 87-88
Androstenedione (AD), 65-66
Androstenediones, 65-66
Anemia, categorization of according to RBC indices, 786t

Anemia panel, 1025
Angiocardiography, 232-238
Angiography, 126-132
  adrenal, 132
  bronchial, 771-773
  cerebral, 127
  coronary, 232-238
  CT, 295-299
  lymphangiography, 623-625
  magnetic resonance, 633
  pulmonary, 771-773
  renal, 126, 130f
Angioplasty, 237
  transluminal coronary, 233
Angiotensin-converting
    enzyme (ACE), 67-68
Anion gap (AG), 69-70
Anisocytosis, 787
Anoscopy, 849-851
ANP (atrial natriuretic
    peptide), 657-658
Anthrax, 161-164, 162t
Anti-acetylcholine receptor
    antibody, 5-6
Antibiotic-associated colitis
    assay, 275-276
Antibody(ies)
  acetylcholine receptor, 5-6
  AChR-binding, 5
  AChR-blocking, 5
  AChR-modulating, 5
  anti-acetylcholine receptor
    antibody, 5-6
  anticardiolipin, 71-72
  anticentromere, 73
  anticytoplasmic, 96-97
  antideoxyribonucleic acid,
    78-79
  anti-DNA, 78-79
  antifungal, 458
  antiglomerular basement
    membrane, 82-83
  anti-*H. pylori* IgG,
    507-510
  antimicrosomal, 108-109
  antimitochondrial, 84-85
  antimyocardial, 86

Antibody(ies)—cont'd
  antineutrophil cytoplasmic,
    87-88
  antinuclear, 89-91
    anticentromere, 73
    anti-DNA, 78
    anti-extractable nuclear
      antigens, 80-81
    antiscleroderma, 94-95
    anti-SS-A, anti-SS-B, and
      anti-SS-C, 100-101
    autoimmune disease and,
      89t
    immunofluorescent
      staining patterns, 90f
    pleural fluid, 900
    Ro, La, and SS-C
      antibodies, 100-101
    Scl-70 antibody, 94-95
  anti-parietal cell, 92-93
  antiphospholipid, 71
  antiplatelet antibody
    detection, 712-713
  anti-smooth muscle, 96-97
  anti-SS-A, 100-101
  anti-SS-B, 100-101
  anti-SS-C, 100-101
  antithyroglobulin, 106-107
  antithyroid microsomal,
    108-109
  antithyroid peroxidase,
    108-109
  autoantibodies
    diabetes mellitus panel,
      359-360
    insulin, 359-360
    thyroid, 106-107, 108-109
  blood antibody screening,
    312-313
  centromere, 73
  diabetes mellitus
    autoantibody panel,
    359-360
  DNA, 78-79
  to double-stranded DNA,
    78-79
  endomysial, 478-479

Antibody(ies)—cont'd
  to extractable nuclear
    antigens, 80-81
  fluorescent treponemal
    antibody test, 888-889
  fungal, 458
  gliadin, 478-479
  glomerular basement
    membrane, 82-83
  glutamic acid decarboxylase,
    359-360
  Goodpasture's, 82-83
  H. pylori, 507-510
  HAV-Ab/IgG, 519-520,
    521t
  HAV-Ab/IgM, 519, 521t
  HBcAb, 521t, 522
  HBeAb, 521t, 522
  HBsAb, 520, 521t
  HBVc-Ab, 521t
  HBVc-Ab/IgM, 521t
  HCV-Ab/IgG, 521t
  HDV-Ab, 521t
  HDV-Ab/IgM, 521t
  heterophil antibody test,
    649-650
  HIV, 23-27
  human T-cell lymphotrophic
    virus I/II, 542
  IgE test, 38-40
  insulin autoantibody,
    359-360
  islet cell, 359-360
  La, 100-101
  Legionnaire's disease
    antibody test, 583-584
  microsomal, 108-109
  monoclonal antibody
    immunoassay, 942
  monoclonal "sandwich"
    antibody qualitative
    testing, 942
  parvovirus B19, 692-693
  platelet antibody detection,
    712-713
  platelet-associated IgG,
    712-713

Antibody(ies)—cont'd
  rabies-neutralizing antibody
    test, 781
  RhoGAM, 444
  Ro, 100-101
  rubella antibody test,
    812-813
  rubeola, 814-815
  scleroderma, 94-95
  Sjögren's, 100-101
  skin biopsy, 333
  sperm, 98-99
  SS-C, 100-101
  thyroglobulin, 106-107
  thyroid antimicrosomal,
    108-109
  thyrotropin receptor, 916-917
  TORCH panel, 1028
  toxoplasmosis antibody titer,
    931-932
  viral capsid antigen-
    antibodies, 399
  viral capsid antigen-antibody
    IgG, 399, 400t
  viral capsid antigen-antibody
    IgM, 399, 400t
  Western blot test, 23-27
Anticardiolipin antibodies
  (aCL antibodies, ACA),
  71-72
Anticentromere antibody test,
  73
Anticytoplasmic antibodies,
  anti-smooth muscle,
  96-97
Antideoxyribonuclease-B titer,
  74, 102
Antideoxyribonucleic acid
  antibodies, 78-79
Antidiuretic hormone (ADH),
  75-77
Antidiuretic hormone (ADH)
  stimulation test, water
  deprivation, 75-76
Antidiuretic hormone (ADH)
  suppression test, 76
Anti-DNA antibody test, 78-79

Anti-DNase-B (ADB), 74, 102
Anti-double-stranded DNA,
    78-79
Anti-ds-DNA, 78-79
Anti-ENAs (anti-extractable
    nuclear antigens),
    80-81
Anti-extractable nuclear
    antigens (anti-ENAs),
    80-81
Antifungal antibodies, 458
Anti-GBM antibody, 82-83
Antigens
    anti-extractable nuclear
        antigens, 80-81
    Australian, 519-523
    bladder tumor, 167-168
    cancer antigen 15-3, 211-212
    cancer antigen 19-9, 213-214
    cancer antigen 27.29,
        211-212
    cancer antigen-125, 215-216
    carcinoembryonic antigen,
        230-231
    early antigen, 399-400
    early antigen-D, 399-400,
        400t
    EBV nuclear antigen, 399
    EBV nuclear antigen-IgG,
        399, 400t
    HDV, 521t
    hepatitis B core antigen
        (HBcAg), 521t, 522
    hepatitis B e-antigen
        (HBeAg), 521t, 522
    hepatitis B surface antigen
        (HBsAg), 520, 521t
    hepatitis-associated, 519-523
    histocompatibility A, 538-539
    human leukocyte A, 538-539
    human lymphocyte B27,
        538-539
    p24, 23-27
    platelet, 712
    platelet-specific, 712
    prostate-specific antigen,
        755-757

Antigens—cont'd
    prostate-specific membrane
        antigen, 756
    viral capsid antigen-
        antibodies, 399
    viral capsid antigen-antibody
        IgG, 399, 400t
    viral capsid antigen-antibody
        IgM, 399, 400t
    white blood cell, 538-539
Antiglobulin test, direct,
    310-311
Antiglomerular basement
    membrane antibodies
    (anti-GBM antibody),
    82-83
Anti-*Helicobacter pylori*
    immunoglobulin G
    (IgG) antibody, 507-510
Antihemophilic factor (factor
    VIII), 280t, 283t
Antihistidyl transfer synthase
    (anti-Jo-1), 80-81
Anti-Jo-1 (antihistidyl transfer
    synthase), 80-81
Anti-La (SS-B) antibody,
    100-101
Antimicrosomal antibody,
    108-109
Antimitochondrial antibody
    (AMA), 84-85
Antimyocardial antibodies
    (AMA), 86
Antineutrophil cytoplasmic
    antibody (ANCA),
    87-88
Antinuclear antibody (ANA),
    89-91
    anticentromere, 73
    anti-DNA, 78
    anti-extractable nuclear
        antigens, 80-81
    antiscleroderma, 94-95
    anti-SS-A, anti-SS-B, and
        anti-SS-C, 100-101
    autoimmune disease and,
        89t

Antinuclear antibody—cont'd
immunofluorescent staining
patterns, 90f
pleural fluid, 900
Ro, La, and SS-C antibodies,
100-101
Scl-70 antibody, 94-95
Antinuclear ribonucleoprotein
(anti-RNP), 80-81
Antinuclear Smith (anti-SM),
80-81
Anti-parietal cell antibody
(APCA), 92-93
Antiphospholipid antibodies,
71
Antiplatelet antibody
detection, 712-713
Antiretroviral therapy, 529, 531t
Antiribonucleoprotein
(anti-RNP), 80-81
Anti-RNP
(antiribonucleoprotein),
80-81
Anti-Ro (SS-A) antibody,
100-101
Antiscleroderma antibody,
94-95
Anti-SM (anti-Smith), 80-81
Anti-Smith (anti-SM), 80-81
Anti-smooth muscle antibody
(ASMA), 96-97
Antisperm antibodies, 98-99
Antispermatozoal antibody,
98-99
Anti-SS-A (Ro) antibody,
100-101
Anti-SS-B (La) antibody,
100-101
Anti-SS-C antibody, 100-101
Antistreptolysin O titer (ASO
titer), 102-103
Antithrombin III (AT-III),
104-105
Antithyroglobulin antibody,
106-107
Antithyroid microsomal
antibody, 108-109

Antithyroid peroxidase
antibody (anti-TPO),
108-109
Anti-TPO (antithyroid
peroxidase) antibody,
108-109
Antitrypsin
alpha₁-antitrypsin, 45-46
alpha₁-antitrypsin
phenotyping, 45-46
Antral or duodenal biopsy
specimen, 507-510
Anus, culture of, 840-844
Aortic artery pressure, 234t
APCA (anti-parietal cell
antibody), 92-93
Apo A-I (apolipoprotein A-I),
110-114
Apo A-I/Apo B ratio, 110
Apo B (apolipoprotein B),
110-114
Apo E (apolipoprotein E),
110-114
Apolipoprotein A-I (Apo A-I),
110-114
Apolipoprotein A-I (Apo
A-I)/Apo B ratio, 110
Apolipoprotein B (Apo B),
110-114
Apolipoprotein E (Apo E),
110-114
Apolipoproteins, 110-114
Apt test, 115-116
APTT (partial thromboplastin
time, activated),
689-691
Argentaffin-staining
(enteroendocrine) cells,
546
Arginine stimulation test, 480
Arginine test, 502-503
Arterial blood gases, 117-125,
119t
Arterial Doppler ultrasound,
982-984
Arterial plethysmography,
719-720

Arteriography, 126-132
  adrenal, 127
  brain, 132
  CT, 295-299
  kidney, 132
  lower extremity, 127, 132
  pulmonary, 771-773
Arthritis panel, 1025
Arthrocentesis with synovial
      fluid analysis, 133-136
Arthrography (arthrogram),
      137-138
Arthroscopy, 139-142, 139f
Ascitic fluid cytology, 678-683
ASMA (anti-smooth muscle
      antibody), 96-97
ASO (antistreptolysin O) titer,
      102-103
Aspartate aminotransferase
      (AST), 143-145
  ALT/AST ratio, 28
Aspermia, 830
Aspiration
  bone marrow, 183-188,
      186f
  bronchoscopic, 989t
  endotracheal, 873
  joint, 133-136
  suprapubic, of urine, 973
  transbronchial needle, 612,
      613f
  transtracheal, 873
Aspiration scan, 467-468
AST (aspartate
      aminotransferase),
      143-145
  ALT/AST ratio, 28
AT-III (antithrombin III),
      104-105
Atrial natriuretic peptide
      (ANP), 657-658
Audiovisual recordings, 857
Auditory brain stem-evoked
      potentials (ABEPs),
      424-427
Augmented limb leads, 368
Australian antigen, 519-523

Autoantibodies
  diabetes mellitus panel,
      359-360
  insulin, 359-360
  thyroid, 106-107,
      108-109
Autoimmune disease, 89t

B
B cells, 626
B_2M (beta-$_2$ microglobulin),
      155-156
Bacillus anthracis, 161-164,
      162t
BACTEC method, 946-948
Bacteria, peritoneal, 681
Bacterial cultures
  peritoneal fluid, 681
  pleural fluid, 900
  synovial fluid, 134
Band cells, 995
Barium enema, 146-149
  scout films, 662
  small bowel enema, 860,
      862
Barium swallow, 150-152
Base excess, arterial, 117-125
Base excess/deficit, 121
Basic metabolic panel, 1025
Basophil count, 994-999
Basophils, 995, 999t
Bence Jones protein, 153-154
Bernstein test, 407, 408f
Beta amyloid protein
      precursor, soluble
      (sBPP), 63-64
Beta globulin, 759, 760t, 762
Beta-$_2$ microglobulin (B_2M),
      155-156
Beta-hydroxybutyric acid,
      963-964
Bethesda system for reporting
      cervical and vaginal
      cytologic diagnoses,
      674
BGP (bone Gla protein),
      192-194

Bicarbonate (HCO₃)
  arterial, 117-125, 119t
  fetal scalp blood, 448
  serum, 226
Bile ducts
  ERCP of, 394-398
  ultrasound of, 4
Biliary tract
  computed tomography of, 299
  ultrasound of, 1-4, 2f
Biliary tract radionuclide scan, 459-460
Bilirubin, 157-160, 158f
Biophysical profile (BPP), 433-436
Biopsy
  antral or duodenal, 507-510
  bone marrow, 183-188
  cervical, 251-253
  chorionic villus, 269-272
  cone, 251-253
  cutaneous immunofluorescence, 333
  endometrial, 391-393
  kidney, 792-795, 793f
  liver, 595-598, 595f
  lung, 611-614, 613f
  lymph node, 161-166
  needle
    percutaneous, 612
    transbronchial, 613f
  pleural, 723-725
  renal, 792-795, 793f
  sentinel lymph node, 833-835
  skin, 161-166
  stereotactic, 638
  tuberculosis, 947
Bioterrorism infectious agents testing, 161-166, 162t-163t
Bladder, cystoscopic examination of, 340, 340f
Bladder cancer markers, 167-168

Bladder tumor antigen (BTA), 167-168
Bladder x-ray, 661
Bleeding, gastrointestinal, 469-471
Bleeding time, 169-171
"Blind" stick liver biopsy, 596
Blood
  cerebrospinal fluid, 603-604
  occult, xviii, 878-880
  serum cardiac enzymes, 322f
  swallowed, 115-116
Blood albumin, 758-763
Blood alcohol, 420-421
Blood antibody screening, 312-313
Blood chromosome analysis, 273-274
Blood collection, 820
  color-coded test tubes, xiv
  order of draw, xiv
Blood count, complete (CBC), 294
Blood creatinine, 326-327
Blood culture, xvi
Blood culture and sensitivity, 172-173
Blood EtOH, 420-421
Blood gases (ABGs), 117-125, 119t
Blood indices, 785-788
Blood pH, fetal scalp, 448-450
Blood pressure
  cuff pressure test, 721-722
  normal values, 234t
Blood protein, 758-763
Blood smear, 174-176
Blood sugar, 482-484
  2-hour postprandial, 485-486
Blood testing
  color-coded test tubes, xiv
  multiphasic screening machines, xiii
  order of draw, xiv
  preparation and procedures, xiii-xvi

Blood testing—cont'd
  puncture sites, xvi
  tourniquet application, xiv
Blood tests, 1016-1019
  acetylcholine receptor
      antibody, 5-6
  acid phosphatase, 7-8
  acid serum test for
      paroxysmal nocturnal
      hemoglobinuria, 504
  activated clotting time, 9-11
  adrenocorticotropic
      hormone, 12-14
  adrenocorticotropic hormone
      stimulation test with
      cosyntropin, 15-17
  adrenocorticotropic
      hormone stimulation
      test with metyrapone,
      18-20
  agglutination inhibition test,
      740-741
  agglutinins, febrile/cold,
      21-22
  AIDS serology, 23-27
  alanine aminotransferase,
      28-29
  aldolase, 30-31
  aldosterone, 32-35
  alkaline phosphatase, 36-37
  allergy blood testing, 38-40
  alpha$_1$-antitrypsin, 45-46
  alpha-antitrypsin
      phenotyping, 45-46
  alpha-fetoprotein, 47-49
  amino acid profiles, 50-51
  ammonia level, 52-53
  amylase, 60-62
  androstenediones, 65-66
  angiotensin-converting
      enzyme, 67-68
  anion gap, 69-70
  anticardiolipin antibodies,
      71-72
  anticentromere antibody, 73
  antideoxyribonuclease-B
      titer, 74

Blood tests—cont'd
  antidiuretic hormone, 75-77
  anti-DNA antibody, 78-79
  anti-extractable nuclear
      antigens, 80-81
  antiglomerular basement
      membrane antibodies,
      82-83
  anti-Jo-1, 80-81
  antimitochondrial antibody,
      84-85
  antimyocardial antibodies,
      86
  antineutrophil cytoplasmic
      antibody, 87-88
  antinuclear antibody, 89-91
  anti-parietal cell antibody,
      92-93
  antiscleroderma antibody,
      94-95
  anti-smooth muscle
      antibody, 96-97
  antispermatozoal antibody,
      98-99
  anti-SS-A (Ro), anti-SS-B
      (La), and anti-SS-C,
      100-101
  antistreptolysin O titer,
      102-103
  antithrombin III, 104-105
  antithyroglobulin antibody,
      106-107
  antithyroid peroxidase
      antibody, 108-109
  apolipoproteins, 110-114
  arterial blood gases,
      117-125, 119t
  aspartate aminotransferase,
      143-145
  atrial natriuretic peptide,
      657-658
  basophils, 994-999
  beta-$_2$ microglobulin,
      155-156
  bilirubin, 157-160
  bioterrorism infectious
      agents, 161-166

Blood tests—cont'd
  bleeding time, 169-171
  blood culture, xvi
  blood culture and sensitivity,
      172-173
  blood gases, 117-125
  blood smear, 174-176
  blood typing, 177-178, 177t
  bone turnover biochemical
      markers, 192-194
  brain natriuretic peptide,
      657-658
  breast cancer genetic testing,
      472-473
  CA 15-3 and CA 27.29
      tumor markers, 211-212
  CA 19-9 tumor marker,
      213-214
  CA-125 tumor marker,
      215-216
  calcitonin, 217-219
  calcium, 220-223
  carbon dioxide content,
      226-227
  carboxyhemoglobin, 228-229
  carcinoembryonic antigen,
      230-231
  CD4/CD8 ratio, 626-629
  Chem-7 and Chem-12, xiii
  Chlamydia, 257-259
  chloride, 260-261
  cholesterol, 262-265
  cholinesterase, 266-268
  chromosome karyotype,
      273-274
  clonidine suppression test,
      704-705
  clot retraction test, 277-278
  coagulating factors
      concentration, 279-284
  complement assay, 292-293
  complete blood count, 294
  Coombs' test
      direct, 310-311
      indirect, 312-313
  cortisol, 314-316
  C-peptide, 317-318

Blood tests—cont'd
  CPK-MB/CPK relative
      index, 323
  C-reactive protein test,
      319-321
  creatine phosphokinase,
      322-325
  creatinine, 326-327
  creatinine clearance, 328-330
  cryoglobulin, 331-332
  C-type natriuretic peptide,
      657-658
  cytokines, 346-348
  cytomegalovirus, 349-350
  D-dimer, 351-352
  dehydroepiandrosterone,
      65-66
  dehydroepiandrosterone
      sulfate, 65-66
  dexamethasone suppression
      test, 355-358
  diabetes mellitus
      autoantibody panel,
      359-360
  differential count, 294
  2,3-diphosphoglycerate,
      361-362
  disseminated intravascular
      coagulation screening,
      363, 364t
  endomysial antibodies,
      478-479
  eosinophils, 994-999
  Epstein-Barr virus titer,
      399-400
  erythrocyte sedimentation
      rate, 402-403
  erythropoietin, 404-405
  estriol excretion, 414-417
  estrogen fractions, 414-417
  ethanol, 420-421
  euglobulin lysis time,
      422-423
  ferritin, 430-432
  fetal hemoglobin testing,
      443-445
  fetal scalp blood pH, 448-450

Blood tests—cont'd
fibrin monomers, 908-909
fibrinogen, 454-455
fibrinopeptide A, 908-909
folic acid, 456-457
follicle-stimulating hormone
assay, 618-620
free thyroxine, 922-923
fungal antibody test, 458
gamma-glutamyl
transpeptidase, 463-464
gastrin, 465-466
genetic testing, 476
gliadin antibodies, 478-479
glucagon, 480-481
glucagon stimulation test,
704-705
glucose, 482-484
postprandial, 485-486
glucose tolerance test,
492-495, 493f
glucose-6-phosphate
dehydrogenase, 490-491
glutamic acid decarboxylase
antibody, 359-360
glycosylated hemoglobin,
496-498
growth hormone, 499-501
growth hormone stimulation
test, 502-503
growth hormone
suppression testing,
500, 501
H. pylori antibodies test,
507-510
Ham's test, 504
haptoglobin, 505-506
hematocrit, 511-513, 512f
hemoglobin, 514-515
hemoglobin electrophoresis,
516-518
hepatitis virus studies,
519-523
herpes simplex, 524-526
hexosaminidase, 527-528
HIV viral load, 529-532,
530t, 531t

Blood tests—cont'd
HLA-B27 antigen, 538-539
homocysteine, 535-537
human lymphocyte antigen
B27, 538-539
human placental lactogen,
540-541
human T-cell lymphotrophic
virus I/II antibody, 542
immunofixation
electrophoresis, 553-554
immunoglobulin
electrophoresis, 555-557
insulin assay, 558-559
insulin autoantibody, 359-360
insulin-like growth factor,
868-869
iron level and total iron-
binding capacity,
565-568
Islet cell antibody, 359-360
lactate dehydrogenase,
572-574
lactic acid, 575-576
lactose tolerance test,
577-578
Legionnaires' disease
antibody test, 583-584
leucine aminopeptidase,
585-586
leukoagglutinin, 587
lipase, 588-589
lipoprotein electrophoresis,
590-591
lipoproteins, 592-594
long-acting thyroid
stimulator, 916-917
luteinizing hormone,
618-620
Lyme disease test, 621-622
lymphocyte
immunophenotyping,
626-629
lymphocytes, 994-999
magnesium, 630-631
maternal triple screen test,
47-48

Blood tests—cont'd
methemoglobin, 645-646
metyrapone, 18-20
monocytes, 994-999
mononucleosis spot test,
649-650
myoglobin, 655-656
natriuretic peptides,
657-658
neutrophils, 994-999
5′-nucleotidase, 659-660
osmolality, 668-669
osteocalcin, 192-194
O'Sullivan test, 485-486,
492-495
parathyroid hormone,
684-685
partial thromboplastin time,
activated, 689-691
parvovirus B19 antibody,
692-693
percent free PSA, 756
phenylketonuria test, 702-703
pheochromocytoma
suppression and
provocation testing,
704-705
phosphate, 706-707
phosphorus, 706-707
plasminogen, 708-709
platelet aggregation test,
710-711
platelet antibody detection,
712-713
platelet count, 714-716
platelet volume, mean,
717-718
potassium, 733-735
prealbumin, 738-739
pregnancy tests, 740-742
progesterone assay, 746-747
prolactin levels, 750-751
prostate-specific antigen,
755-757
protein, 758-763
protein C, 764-765
protein S, 764-765

Blood tests—cont'd
prothrombin fragment,
908-909
prothrombin time, 766-770
PSA velocity, 756
rabies-neutralizing antibody
test, 781
red blood cell count, 782-784
red blood cell indices,
785-788
renal vein assays, 801
renin assay, plasma, 800-804
reticulocyte count, 805-806
rheumatoid factor, 810-811
rubella antibody test,
812-813
rubeola antibody, 814-815
SARS viral testing,
818-820
sexual assault testing,
836-839
sexually transmitted disease
cultures, 840-844
sickle cell test, 847-848
sodium, 863-865
somatomedin C, 868-869
substance abuse testing,
881-883
syphilis detection test,
888-889
N-telopeptide, 192-194
testosterone, 890-892
therapeutic drug
monitoring, 893-896,
894t-895t
thrombosis indicators,
908-909
thyroid-binding globulin,
926-927
thyroid-binding inhibitory
immunoglobulin,
916-917
thyroid-stimulating
hormone, 913-914
thyroid-stimulating
hormone stimulation
test, 915

Blood tests—cont'd
  thyroid-stimulating
    immunoglobulins,
    916-917
  thyrotropin receptor
    antibody, 916-917
  thyrotropin-releasing
    hormone test, 920-921
  thyroxine, free, 922-923
  thyroxine, total, 924-925
  thyroxine index, free,
    928-929
  thyroxine-binding globulin,
    926-927
  toxicology screening, 881-883
  toxoplasmosis antibody titer,
    931-932
  TRH stimulation test,
    913-914
  triglycerides, 937-938
  triiodothyronine, 939-940
  troponins, 941-943
  urea nitrogen, 952-954
  uric acid, 955-958
  uroporphyrinogen-
    1-synthase, 977
  viral cultures, 988-989, 989t
  vitamin B_{12}, 990-991
  West Nile virus testing,
    992-993
  white blood cell count and
    differential count,
    994-999, 998t-999t
  D-xylose absorption test,
    1004-1005
Blood typing, 177-178, 177t
Blood urea nitrogen (BUN),
  952-954
Blood-clotting factors, 279-284
BMC (bone mineral content),
  179-182
BMD (bone mineral density),
  179-182
B-mode ultrasound
  carotid artery duplex
    scanning, 249
  venous/arterial, 982-984

BNP (brain natriuretic
  peptide), 657-658
Body plethysmography, 777
Bone absorptiometry, 179-182
Bone densitometry, 179-182
Bone G1a protein (BGP),
  192-194
Bone marrow aspiration,
  183-188, 186f
Bone marrow biopsy, 183-188
Bone marrow examination,
  183-188
Bone mineral content (BMC),
  179-182
Bone mineral density (BMD),
  179-182
Bone scan, 189-191
Bone turnover biochemical
  markers, 192-194
Bone x-ray, 195-196
Bone/joint panel, 1025
Botulism infection, 161, 162t
BPP (beta amyloid protein
  precursor), soluble,
  63-64
BPP (biophysical profile),
  433-436
Brain arteriography, 132
Brain imaging
  computed tomography,
    300-303
  PET scan, 729-732
Brain natriuretic peptide
  (BNP), 657-658
BRCA (BReast CAncer) gene
  testing, 472-473
Breast, MRI of, 633
Breast cancer
  Gail or Claus risk models,
    200
  genetic testing, 472-473
  predictors, 197-199
  tumor analysis, 197-199
Breast ductal lavage, 200-201
Breast scan, 202-203
Breast scintigraphy, 202-203
Breast sonogram, 204-205

Breast stimulation technique, 438

Breath tests
drug testing, 881-883
ethanol, 420-421
H. pylori, 507-510
inhalation tests, 779
pulmonary function tests, 774-780

Bronchial angiography, 771-773

Bronchial provocation studies, 779

Bronchoscopic aspiration, 989t

Bronchoscopy, 206-210, 208f
fiberoptic, 207-209
flexible, 206
sputum collection, 873

Brucellosis/*Brucella abortus, suis, melitensis,* or *canis,* 163t, 165

BTA (bladder tumor antigen), 167-168

Buccal swabs, 476

BUN (blood urea nitrogen), 952-954

Butabarbital monitoring data, 894t

C

c erbB2 protein, 197-199

C1 esterase, 292

C3 and C4 complement, 292-293

Ca (calcium), 220-223

CA 15-3 tumor marker, 211-212

CA 19-9 tumor marker, 213-214

CA 27.29 tumor marker, 211-212

CA-125 tumor marker, 215-216

Calcitonin, 217-219

Calcium (Ca) (factor IV), 220-223, 283t

Calcium infusion test, 217-218, 466

Calcium pyrophosphate dihydrate crystals, 134

Caloric study, 224-225

Campylobacter pylori, 507-510

Campylobacter-like organism (CLO) test, 507-510

C-ANCA, 87

Cancer antigen 15-3, 211-212

Cancer antigen 19-9, 213-214

Cancer antigen 27.29, 211-212

Cancer antigen-125, 215-216

Cancer studies, 1006

Candida, 841t

Captopril renal scan, 799, 802

Captopril renography/ scintigraphy, 797

Captopril scan, 797

Carbamazepine monitoring data, 894t

Carbon dioxide (CO_2) content, 226-227
arterial, 118-120

Carbon dioxide (CO_2) monitor, 856

Carbon dioxide partial pressure (Pco_2)
arterial, 117-125, 119t
fetal scalp blood, 448

Carbon monoxide, 228-229

Carboxyhemoglobin (COHb), 228-229

Carcinoembryonic antigen (CEA), 230-231
peritoneal fluid, 681
pleural fluid, 900

Carcinoid nuclear scan, 664-665

Cardiac catheterization, 232-238, 235f

Cardiac echo, 365-367

Cardiac enzymes, serum, 322f

Cardiac exercise stress testing, 239-243

Cardiac flow studies, 244-248

Cardiac index (CI), 234t

Cardiac injury panel, 1025

Cardiac mapping, 387-390

Cardiac monitoring, 234t
Cardiac nuclear scanning, 244-248
Cardiac output (CO), 234t
Cardiac scan, 244-248
Cardiac stress testing, 366
Cardiac-specific troponin I (cTnI), 941-943
Cardiac-specific troponin T (cTnT), 941-943
Cardiolipin antibodies, 71-72
Cardiovascular disease genetic testing, 472, 473-474
Cardiovascular system tests, 1006-1007
Carotid artery duplex scanning, 249-250
Carotid ultrasound, 249-250
Casts, urinary, 964-965, 970-971
CAT scan, of abdomen, 295-299
Catecholamines, 978-981
Cathepsin D, 197-199
Catheterization
  cardiac, 232-238, 235f
  pericardial, 698-701, 699f
  ureteral, 341, 341f
  urinary, xvii, 973
CATT (computerized axial transverse tomography), 300-303
CBC (complete blood count), 294
CBF (cerebral blood flow), 300-301
CC (creatinine clearance), 328-330
CD4 marker, 626-629
CD4 percentage, 626-629
CD4/CD8 ratio, 626-629
CD8 (T-suppressor) cells, 626-629
CDU (color Doppler ultrasound)
  carotid artery, 249
  venous/arterial, 982-983

CEA (carcinoembryonic antigen), 230-231
  peritoneal fluid, 681
  pleural fluid, 900
Cell analysis, chorionic villus sampling, 269-272, 271f
Cell counts
  absolute neutrophil count, 996
  basophils, 994-999
  complete blood count, 294
  differential count, 294
  eosinophils, 994-999
  erythrocytes, 782-784
  hematocrit, 511-513, 512f
  hemoglobin, 514-515
  lamellar bodies, 55
  leukocytes, 994-999
  lymphocytes, 994-999
  mean corpuscular hemoglobin, 785, 786-787, 788
  mean corpuscular hemoglobin concentration, 785, 787, 788
  mean corpuscular volume, 785-786, 788
  mean platelet volume, 717-718
  monocytes, 994-999
  neutrophils, 994-999
  pericardial fluid, 665
  peritoneal fluid, 680
  platelets, 714-716
  pleural fluid, 898
  red blood cell, 782-784
  red blood cell indices, 785-788
  reticulocytes, 805-806
  synovial fluid analysis, 134
  thrombocytes, 714-716
  total CD4 cell count, 626
  white blood cell count, 994-999, 998t-999t
  white blood cell differential count, 994-999, 998t-999t

Cellular casts, 964
Cellularity, bone marrow,
      184-185
Central venous pressure, 234t
Centromere antibody, 73
Cerebral angiography, 127
Cerebral blood flow (CBF),
      300-301
Cerebrospinal fluid (CSF)
      analysis
   amyloid beta protein
         precursor, soluble, 63-64
   lumbar puncture and,
         599-601
   viral culture, 989t
   West Nile virus testing,
         992-993
Cervical biopsy, 251-253
Cervical block, 252
Cervical culture, 840-844
   Chlamydia, 258
   herpes simplex, 525
Cervical cytology, liquid-based,
      675
Cervical mucus sperm
      penetration test,
      852-853
Cervical x-ray studies, 870-871
Cervix, culture of, 840-844
CH 50, 292
Chem-7 panel, xiii
Chem-12 panel, xiii
Chemical stress testing, 239, 240
Chest CT scan, 304-306
Chest impedance, 856
Chest radiography, 254-256
Chest x-ray (CXR), 254-256
   lung scan, 615
Chlamydia, 257-259, 841t
Chloramphenicol monitoring
      data, 894t
Chloride (Cl)
   blood, 260-261
   cerebrospinal fluid, 605
   sweat test, 886
Chlorpromazine, prolactin
      stimulation test with, 750

Cholangiography
   IV, 394
   percutaneous transhepatic,
         394-395
Cholangiopancreatography,
      endoscopic retrograde,
      394-398, 397f
Cholecystography, oral, 394
Cholescintigraphy, 459-460
Cholesterol, 262-265, 263t
Cholesterol crystals, 134
Cholesterol to HDL ratio,
      263t
Cholinesterase (CHS), 266-268
Cholinesterase RBC, 266-268
Chorionic villus biopsy (CVB),
      269-272
Chorionic villus sampling
      (CVS), 269-272, 271f
   genetic testing, 476
Christmas factor (factor IX),
      281t, 283t
Chromosomal aberrations, 55
Chromosome karyotype,
      273-274
Chromosome studies, 273-274
CHS (cholinesterase), 266-268
Chylomicrons, 591
CI (cardiac index), 234t
Cimetidine, 712
CK (creatine kinase), 322-325
Cl (chloride)
   blood, 260-261
   cerebrospinal fluid, 605
   sweat test, 886
Claus breast cancer risk
      models, 200
Clean-catch urine specimens,
      xvi, 973
CLO (*Campylobacter*-like
      organism) test, 507-510
Clonidine suppression test
      (CST), 704-705
Closed lung biopsy, 611
Clostridial toxin assay, 275-276
Clostridium botulinum, 161,
      162t

Clostridium difficile, 275-276

Clot retraction test, 277-278

CMG (cystometrogram), 336-339

CMV (cytomegalovirus), 349-350

CNP (C-type natriuretic peptide), 657-658

CO (cardiac output), 234t

CO_2 (carbon dioxide) combining power, 226-227

CO_2 (carbon dioxide) content, 226-227
  arterial, 118-120

CO_2 (carbon dioxide) monitor, 856

Coagulating factors, 279-284

Coagulating factors concentration, 279-284, 283t

Coagulation factor excess or deficiency, 280t-281t

Coagulation screening, 1025

Coccygeal x-ray studies, 870-871

COHb (carboxyhemoglobin), 228-229

Cold agglutinins, 21-22

Colitis
  antibiotic-associated colitis assay, 275-276
  pseudomembranous colitis toxic assay, 275-276

Colon cancer genetic testing, 472, 473

Colonoscopy, 285-288
  CT, 295-299
  virtual, 295-299

Color Doppler echocardiography, 365

Color Doppler ultrasound (CDU)
  carotid artery duplex scanning, 249
  venous/arterial, 982-983

Color-coded test tubes, xiv

Colposcopy, 289-291, 289f

Coma panel, 1025

Complement assay, 292-293
  pleural fluid, 900
  synovial fluid analysis, 134

Complete blood count (CBC), 294

Composite urine specimens, xvii

Comprehensive metabolic panel, 1025-1026

Computed tomography (CT)
  of abdomen, 295-299
  of brain, 300-303
  of chest, 304-306
  liver biopsy with, 596
  quantitative, 180

Computed tomography (CT) angiography, 295-299

Computed tomography (CT) arteriography, 295-299

Computed tomography (CT) colonoscopy, 295-299

Computed tomography (CT) portogram, 307-309

Computerized axial transverse tomography (CATT), 300-303

Conduction velocity, 382

Cone biopsy, 251-253

Conization, 251-253

Conjugated (direct) bilirubin, 157

Conjunctival smear, 258

Connecting peptide insulin, 317-318

Contraction stress test (CST), 437-440

Contrast dye, x-ray with
  arteriography, 126-132
  arthrography, 137-138
  barium enema, 146-149
  barium swallow, 150-152
  cardiac catheterization, 232-238, 235f
  computed tomography of the abdomen, 295-299

Contrast dye, x-ray with—cont'd
  computed tomography of the brain, 300-303
  computed tomography of the chest, 304-306
  cystography, 334-335
  hysterosalpingography, 548-549
  intravenous pyelography, 560-564
  lymphangiography, 623-625, 625f
  mammography, 651-654
  pulmonary angiography, 771-773
  retrograde pyelography, 807-809
  small bowel follow-through, 860-862
  swallowing examination, 884-885
  upper gastrointestinal x-ray study, 949-951
  venography of lower extremities, 985-987
Coombs' test
  direct, 310-311
  indirect, 312-313
Coproporphyrin, 726
Coronary angiography, 232-238
Coronary angioplasty, transluminal, 233
Corticotropin, 12-14
Cortisol, blood and urine, 314-316
Cortisol stimulation test, 15-17
Cortisol suppression test, 355-358
Cosyntropin, ACTH stimulation test with, 15-17
Coumarin ingestion, 767
CP (creatine phosphokinase), 322-325
C-peptide, 317-318
CPK (creatine phosphokinase), 322-325
CPK (creatine phosphokinase) isoenzymes, 323
CPK (creatine phosphokinase)-MB/CPK relative index, 323
Craniocaudal view, 639
C-reactive protein (CRP)
  cerebrospinal fluid, 606
  high sensitive assay (hs-CRP), 319-320
C-reactive protein (CRP) test, 319-321
Creatine kinase (CK), 322-325
Creatine phosphokinase (CPK), 322-325
Creatine phosphokinase (CPK) isoenzymes, 323
Creatine phosphokinase (CPK)-MB/CPK relative index, 323
Creatinine
  blood, 326-327
  serum, 326-327
Creatinine clearance (CC), 328-330
Cross-table lateral abdominal x-ray, 661-662
CRP (C-reactive protein)
  cerebrospinal fluid, 606
  high sensitive assay (hs-CRP), 319-320
CRP (C-reactive protein) test, 319-321
Cryoglobulin, 331-332
Crystals
  synovial fluid, 134
  urinary, 964, 970
C&S (culture and sensitivity)
  sputum, 872-873
  stool, 876-877
  urine, xvi, 972-974
  wound, 1002-1003
CSF (cerebrospinal fluid) analysis
  amyloid beta protein precursor, soluble, 63-64

CSF (cerebrospinal fluid)
analysis—cont'd
lumbar puncture and,
599-601
prealbumin, 738-739
CST (clonidine suppression
test), 704-705
CST (contraction stress test),
437-440
CT (computed tomography)
of abdomen, 295-299
of brain, 300-303
of chest, 304-306
liver biopsy with, 596
quantitative, 180
CT (computed tomography)
angiography, 295-299
CT (computed tomography)
arteriography, 295-299
CT (computed tomography)
colonoscopy, 295-299
CT (computed tomography)
portogram, 307-309
cTnI (cardiac-specific
troponin I), 941-943
cTnT (cardiac-specific
troponin T), 941-943
C-type natriuretic peptide
(CNP), 657-658
Cuff pressure test, 721-722
Culture(s)
anal, 840-844, 842f
bacterial
peritoneal fluid, 681
pleural fluid, 900
synovial fluid, 134
blood, 172-173
cerebrospinal fluid, 603
cervical, 840-844
Chlamydia, 258
herpes simplex, 525
fungal, 900
peritoneal fluid, 681
pleural fluid, 900
synovial fluid, 134
M. tuberculosis, 900
microbiology, 946-948

Culture(s)—cont'd
nasal, 906
nasopharyngeal, 906
oropharyngeal, 843
pericardial fluid, 700
polymerase chain reaction,
946-948
rectal, 842, 842f, 843f
sputum, 872-873
stool, 876-877
throat and nose, 905-907
tuberculosis, 946-948
urethral, 840-844, 843f
viral, 988-989
Culture and sensitivity (C&S)
sputum, 872-873
stool, 876-877
urine, xvi, 972-974
wound, 1002-1003
Cutaneous
immunofluorescence
biopsy, 333
CVB (chorionic villus biopsy),
269-272
CVS (chorionic villus
sampling), 269-272,
271f
genetic testing, 476
CXR (chest x-ray), 254-256
lung scan, 615
Cyanocobalamin, 990-991
Cystic fibrosis genetic testing,
472, 474-475
Cystography, 334-335
Cystometrogram (CMG),
336-339
Cystometry, 336-339
Cystoscopy, 340-345, 340f,
341f
Cystourethrography, 334-335
Cytogenetics, 273-274
Cytokines, 346-348
Cytologic test for cancer,
674-677
Cytology
ascitic fluid, 678-683
cerebrospinal fluid, 605-606

Cytology—cont'd
  liquid-based cervical, 675
  pericardial fluid, 665
  peritoneal fluid, 681
  pleural fluid, 900
  seminal, 830-832
  sputum, 874-875
Cytomegalovirus (CMV),
    349-350

D

Dane particle, 520-522
D-dimer test, 351-352
Dead space, 777
Decubitus chest x-ray, 254
Dehydroepiandrosterone
    (DHEA), 65-66
Dehydroepiandrosterone
    sulfate (DHEA S),
    65-66
Delta hepatitis, 523
Delta-ALA, 353-354
Delta-aminolevulinic acid,
    353-354
Densitometry, dual energy,
    179
Density coefficient, 295
DeRitis ratio, 28
Desipramine monitoring data,
    894t
Detuned ELISA, 24
Detuned HIV antibody,
    23-27
DEXA (dual-energy x-ray
    absorptiometry),
    179-180
Dexamethasone suppression
    test (DST), 355-358
DHEA (dehydro-
    epiandrosterone), 65-66
DHEA S (dehydro-
    epiandrosterone
    sulfate), 65-66
Diabetes mellitus, gestational,
    485-486
Diabetes mellitus autoantibody
    panel, 359-360

Diabetes mellitus management
    panel, 1026
Diabetic control index,
    496-498
Diaper test, 703
DIC (disseminated
    intravascular
    coagulation), 364f
DIC (disseminated intravascular
    coagulation) panel,
    1026
DIC (disseminated intravascular
    coagulation) screening,
    363, 364t
Diethylenetriamine pentaacetic
    acid (DTPA)
  renal scan, 796-799
  ventilation scan, 615-616
diff (differential count), 294
Differential count (diff),
    294
Differentiation, bilirubin,
    158-159
Diffusing capacity of the lung
    (D_L), 779
Digital subtraction
    angiography (DSA),
    126
Digitoxin monitoring data,
    894t
Digoxin monitoring data,
    894t
2,3-Diphosphoglycerate (2,
    3-DPG), 361-362
Dipyridamole (Persantine),
    240
Direct antiglobulin test,
    310-311
Direct bilirubin, 157
Direct Coombs' test,
    310-311
Direct lateral (90 degree) view,
    639
DISIDA scanning, 459-460
Disodium monomethane
    arsonate (DSMA)
    renal scan, 797

Disopyramide monitoring data, 894t

Disseminated intravascular coagulation (DIC), 364f

Disseminated intravascular coagulation (DIC) panel, 1026

Disseminated intravascular coagulation (DIC) screening, 363, 364t

Distal latency, 381

Diuretic renal scan, 798

D_L (diffusing capacity of the lung), 779

DNA antibody, 78-79

DNA evidence collection, 839

DNA ploidy status, 197-199

Dobutamine, 241

Dopamine, 978-981

Doppler ultrasound
  carotid artery duplex scanning, 249
  venous/arterial, 982-984

Double lumen endotracheal tube, 613

Double tracer subtraction test (DTST), 687, 688

Double-stimulated GH test, 502

Double-stranded DNA, antibodies to, 78-79

Double-voided (urine) specimen, 488

Downey test, 115-116

DPA (dual-photon absorptiometry), 179-180

2,3-DPG (2, 3-diphosphoglycerate), 361-362

Dreiling tube, 828

Drug monitoring, therapeutic, 893-896, 894t-895t

Drug screening, 881-883

Drug testing, urine, 881-883

Drug-induced thrombo-cytopenia, 712-713

DSA (digital subtraction angiography), 126

DSMA (disodium monomethane arsonate) renal scan, 796-799

DST (dexamethasone suppression test), 355-358

DTPA (diethylenetriamine pentaacetic acid)
  renal scan, 796-799
  ventilation scan, 615-616

DTST (double tracer subtraction test), 687, 688

Dual energy densitometry, 179

Dual-energy x-ray absorptiometry (DEXA), 179-180

Dual-photon absorptiometry (DPA), 179-180

Duodenal biopsy specimen, 507-510

Duplex scanning
  carotid artery, 249-250
  venous/arterial, 982-984

Dynamic CT scanning, 296

E

E_1 (estrone), 415

E_2 (estradiol), 414, 415

E_2 (estradiol) receptor, 418-419

E_3 (estriol), 414, 415

E_3 (estriol) excretion, 414-417

EA (early antigen), 399-400

EA-D (early antigen-D), 399-400, 400t

Ear oximetry, 672-673

Early antigen (EA), 399-400

Early antigen-D (EA-D), 399-400, 400t

EBNA (EBV nuclear antigen), 399

EBNA-IgG (EBV nuclear antigen-IgG), 399, 400t

Ebola virus, 162t

EBV (Epstein-Barr virus) titer, 399-400
ECG (electrocardiography), 368-372, 369f
  ambulatory, 533-534
  signal-averaged (SAECG), 370
  sleep studies, 856
  stress testing, 239-243
Echo stress testing, 239-243
Echocardiography, 365-367
  transesophageal, 366, 933-936, 934f
Echography (echogram)
  abdominal, 1-4, 2f
  obstetric, 694-697
  thyroid, 918-919
EDV (end-diastolic volume), 234t
EEG (electro-encephalography), 373-375
  sleep studies, 856
EF (ejection fraction), 234t, 245, 460
  gated, 246
EGD (esophago-gastroduodenoscopy), 410-413
EIA (enzyme immunoassay)
  AIDS serology, 23
  antiglomerular basement membrane antibodies, 82
  homocysteine, 536
Ejection fraction (EF), 234t, 245, 460
  gated, 246
EKG (electrocardiography), 368-372, 369f
  ambulatory, 533-534
  sleep studies, 856
  stress testing, 239-243
Electrocardiography (ECG, EKG), 368-372, 369f
  ambulatory, 533-534
  signal-averaged (SAECG), 370

Electrocardiography (ECG, EKG)—cont'd
  sleep studies, 856
  stress testing, 239-243
Electrodiagnostic tests, 1020
  caloric study, 224-225
  cardiac exercise stress testing, 239-243
  contraction stress test, 437-440
  electrocardiography, 368-372, 369f
  electroencephalography, 373-375
  electromyography, 376-378
  electromyography of the pelvic floor sphincter, 379-380
  electroneurography, 381-383
  electronystagmography, 384-386
  electrophysiologic study, 387-390
  evoked potential studies, 424-427
  fetal contraction stress test, 437-440
  fetal nonstress test, 446-447
  Holter monitoring, 533-534
  nonstress test, 446-447
  pelvic floor sphincter electromyography, 379-380
  signal-averaged ECG, 370
  sleep studies, 856-859
Electroencephalography (EEG), 373-375
  sleep studies, 856
Electrolyte panel, 1026
Electrolytes, 260
  sweat test, 886-887
Electromyography (EMG), 376-378
  of pelvic floor sphincter, 379-380
  sleep studies, 856

Electromyoneurography, 376, 381

Electroneurography (ENG), 381-383

Electronystagmography, 384-386

Electro-oculography, 856

Electrophoresis
gama globulin, 555-557
hemoglobin, 516-518
immunofixation, 553-554, 556, 761
immunoglobulin, 555-557
lipoprotein, 590-591
protein, 758-763, 760t

Electrophysiologic study (EPS), 387-390

Electroretinography, 425

ELISA (enzyme-linked immunosorbent assay)
detuned, 24
H. pylori antibodies test, 508-509
for HIV antibody, 23-27
SARS viral testing, 818
troponins, 942

EMG (electromyography), 376-378
of pelvic floor sphincter, 379-380
sleep studies, 856

End-diastolic left ventricular pressure, 234t

End-diastolic volume (EDV), 234t

Endocervical biopsy, 251-253

Endocervical curettage, 251-253

Endocervical mucus sample, 852

Endocrine system tests, 1007-1008

Endometrial biopsy, 391-393

Endomysial antibodies, 478-479

Endoscopic retrograde cholangiopancreatograp hy (ERCP), 394-398, 397f

Endoscopy, 1020
arthroscopy, 139-142, 139f
bronchoscopy, 206-210, 208f
colonoscopy, 285-288
colposcopy, 289-291, 289f
cystoscopy, 340-345, 340f, 341f
endoscopic retrograde cholangiopancreatography, 394-398, 397f
esophagogastroduodenoscopy, 410-413
fetoscopy, 451-453, 452f
gastroscopy, 410-413
hysteroscopy, 550-552, 551f
laparoscopy, 579-582, 579f
mediastinoscopy, 642-644
pelvic, 579-582, 579f
sigmoidoscopy, 849-851
thoracoscopy, 903-904
transesophageal echocardiography, 933-936, 934f
upper gastrointestinal, 410-413

Endoscopy, preparation and procedures, xxii-xxiii

Endotracheal aspiration, 873

Endotracheal tube, double lumen, 613

Endourology, 340-345

End-systolic volume (ESV), 234t

Enemas
barium, 146-149
small bowel, 860, 862

ENG (electroneurography), 381-383

Enteroendocrine (argentaffin-staining) cells, 546

Enteroscopy, 410

Enzyme immunoassay (EIA)
AIDS serology, 23
antiglomerular basement membrane antibodies, 82
homocysteine, 536

Enzyme-linked immunosorbent assay (ELISA)
detuned, 24
H. pylori antibodies test, 508-509
for HIV antibody, 23-27
SARS viral testing, 818
troponins, 942
Enzymes
alkaline phosphatase isoenzymes, 36
creatine phosphokinase isoenzymes, 323
pancreatic, 828-829
serum cardiac, 322f
Eosinophil count, 994-999
Eosinophils, 995, 999t
EP (evoked potential) studies, 424-427
Epinephrine, 978-981
Epithelial casts, 965, 970
EPO (erythropoietin), 404-405
EPS (electrophysiologic study), 387-390
Epstein-Barr virus nuclear antigen (EBNA), 399
Epstein-Barr virus nuclear antigen-IgG (EBNA-IgG), 399, 400t
Epstein-Barr virus (EBV) titer, 399-400, 400t
ER (estrogen receptor) assay (ERA), 418-419
ERA (estrogen receptor assay), 418-419
ERCP (endoscopic retrograde cholangiopancreato-graphy), 394-398, 397f
Erect abdominal x-ray, 661
ERV (expiratory reserve volume), 776, 776f
Erythrocyte count, 782-784
Erythrocyte indices, 785-788

Erythrocyte sedimentation rate (ESR), 402-403
Erythrocytes, 361-362
Erythropoietin (EPO), 404-405
Esophageal function studies, 406-409, 408f
barium swallow, 150-152
swallowing examination, 884-885
Esophageal manometry, 406-409
Esophageal motility studies, 406-409
Esophageal pH probe, 857
Esophagogastroduodenoscopy (EGD), 410-413
ESR (erythrocyte sedimentation rate), 402-403
Estradiol (E_2), 414, 415
Estradiol (E_2) receptor, 418-419
Estriol (E_3), 414, 415
Estriol (E_3) excretion, 414-417
Estrogen, total, 414
Estrogen fractions, 414-417
Estrogen receptor assay (ER assay, ERA), 418-419
Estrone (E_1), 415
ESV (end-systolic volume), 234t
Ethanol, 420-421
Ethosuximide monitoring data, 894t
Ethyl alcohol, 420-421
EUG (excretory urography), 560-564
Euglobulin clot lysis, 422-423
Euglobulin lysis time, 422-423
Event recorders, 533-534
Evoked brain potentials, 424-427
Evoked potential (EP) studies, 424-427
Evoked responses, 424-427

Excretory urography (EUG), 560-564

Exercise stress testing, 239-240

Exercise testing, 239-243

Expiratory reserve volume (ERV), 776, 776f

Extrahepatic ducts ultrasound, 2

Exudates
peritoneal, 678, 683
pleural, 897, 902

F

F1+2 (prothrombin fragment), 908-909

Factor assay, 279-284

Factor I (fibrinogen), 279, 280t, 283t, 454-455

Factors, coagulating, 279-284

Fallopian tubes, computed tomography of, 299

Fasting blood sugar (FBS), 482-484

Fat, fecal, 428-429

Fat absorption, 428-429

Fat retention coefficient, 429

Fatty casts, 964, 970

FBS (fasting blood sugar), 482-484

FDG (fluorodeoxyglucose) positron emission tomography, 729-732

FDPs (fibrin degradation products), 908-909

Fe (iron level), 565-568

Febrile/cold agglutinins, 21-22

Fecal fat, 428-429

$FEF_{200-1200}$ (forced expiratory $flow_{200-1200}$), 777

Ferning, 852

Ferritin, 430-432, 565

Fetal activity determination, 446-447

Fetal activity study, 433-436

Fetal biophysical profile, 433-436

Fetal body movements, 434

Fetal breathing movements, 433-434

Fetal contraction stress test, 437-440

Fetal distress, 56

Fetal fibronectin (fFN), 441-442

Fetal heart rate reactivity, 433

Fetal hemoglobin stool test, qualitative, 115-116

Fetal hemoglobin testing, 443-445

Fetal maturity status, 54-55

Fetal nonstress test, 446-447

Fetal nuchal translucency (FNT), 694-697

Fetal oxygen saturation monitoring ($FSpo_2$), 448-450

Fetal scalp blood pH, 448-450

Fetal status affected by Rh isoimmunization, 55

Fetal tone, 434

α-Fetoprotein, 47-49

Fetoscopy, 451-453, 452f

Fetus, sex of, 55

FEV_1 (forced expiratory volume in 1 second), 775

fFN (fetal fibronectin), 441-442

Fiberoptic bronchoscopy, 207-209
flexible, 206
sputum collection, 873

Fibrin clot dissolution, secondary, 282f

Fibrin clot formation, secondary, 282f

Fibrin degradation fragment, 351-352

Fibrin degradation products (FDPs), 908-909

Fibrin monomers, 908-909

Fibrin split products (FSPs), 908-909

Fibrin stabilizing factor (factor XIII), 283t
Fibrinogen (factor I), 279, 280t, 283t, 454-455
Fibrinolysin, 708-709
Fibrinolysis/euglobulin lysis, 282f, 422-423
Fibrinopeptide A (FPA), 908-909
Fibronectin, fetal, 441-442
First morning specimen, xvi
Flexible fiberoptic bronchoscopy, 206
Flow cytometric method for fetal hemoglobin testing, 443-444
Flowmeters, urine, 975
Fluid analysis, 1020
  amniocentesis, 54-59, 58f
  amyloid beta protein precursor, soluble, 63-64
  antispermatozoal antibody, 98-99
  arthrocentesis with synovial fluid analysis, 133-136
  beta-$_2$ microglobulin, 155-156
  breast ductal lavage, 200-201
  fetal fibronectin, 441-442
  genetic testing, 472-477
  HIV antibody test, 23-27
  Lumbar puncture and cerebrospinal fluid examination, 602-610
  paracentesis, 678-683, 679f
  pericardiocentesis, 698-701, 699f
  peritoneal, 678-683
  pleural tap, 897-902
  SARS viral testing, 818-820
  secretin-pancreozymin, 828-829
  semen analysis, 830-832
  sexual assault testing, 836-839
  Sims-Huhner test, 852-853

Fluid analysis—cont'd
  substance abuse testing, 881-883
  sweat electrolytes test, 886-887
  synovial, 133-136
  tau protein, 63
  Thoracentesis and pleural fluid analysis, 897-902
  West Nile virus testing, 992-993
Fluorescent treponemal antibody (FTA) absorption (FTA-ABS) test, 888
Fluorescent treponemal antibody (FTA) test, 888-889
Fluorodeoxyglucose (FDG) positron emission tomography, 729-732
FNT (fetal nuchal translucency), 694-697
Folate, 456-457
Folic acid, 456-457
Follicle-stimulating hormone (FSH) assay, 618-620
Forced expiratory flow$_{200-1200}$ (FEF$_{200-1200}$), 777
Forced expiratory volume in 1 second (FEV$_1$), 775
Forced midexpiratory flow, 775
Forced vital capacity (FVC), 775
Forensic genetic testing, 472, 475-476
FPA (fibrinopeptide A), 908-909
%FPSA (percent free PSA), 756
Fractionation, bilirubin, 158-159
Fragment D-dimer, 351-352
Francisella tularensis, 163t, 165

FRC (functional residual capacity), 776f, 777
Free catecholamines, 978
Free thyroxine (FT$_4$), 922-923
Free thyroxine index (FT$_4$I, FTI), 928-929
Free urinary cortisol, 314-316
Fructosamine, glycated, 497
FRV (functional residual volume), 776, 776f
FSH (follicle-stimulating hormone) assay, 618-620
FSpo$_2$ (fetal oxygen saturation monitoring), 448-450
FSPs (fibrin split products), 908-909
FT$_4$ (free thyroxine), 922-923
FT$_4$ index (free thyroxine index), 922-923
FT$_4$I (free thyroxine index), 928-929
FTA (fluorescent treponemal antibody) absorption (FTA-ABS) test, 888
FTA (fluorescent treponemal antibody) test, 888-889
FTA-ABS (FTA absorption) test, 888
FTI (free thyroxine index), 928-929
Function tests
    esophageal, 406-409, 408f
    liver, 1026
    pulmonary, 774-780
    renal, 326
Functional antithrombin III assay, 104-105
Functional residual capacity (FRC), 776f, 777
Functional residual volume (FRV), 776, 776f
Fungal antibody tests, 458
Fungal cultures
    pericardial fluid, 700
    peritoneal fluid, 681

Fungal cultures—cont'd
    pleural fluid, 900
    synovial fluid, 134
FVC (forced vital capacity), 775

G
G-6-PD (glucose-6-phosphate dehydrogenase) screen, 490-491
GAD Ab (glutamic acid decarboxylase antibody), 359-360
Gadolinium (Magnevist), 635
Gail or Claus breast cancer risk models, 200
Gallbladder
    computed tomography of, 299
    ultrasound of, 2, 2f, 4
Gallbladder nuclear scanning, 459-460
Gallium scan, 461-462
Gama globulin electrophoresis, 555-557
Gamma globulin, 759, 760t, 763
Gamma-glutamyl transferase (GGT), 463-464
Gamma-glutamyl transpeptidase (GGTP), 463-464
Gardnerella vaginalis, 841t
Gas dilution tests, 777
Gas exchange/diffusing capacity of the lung (D$_L$), 779
Gastric tests, ethanol, 420-421
Gastrin, 465-466
Gastrin stimulation tests, 465
Gastroesophageal (GE) reflux scan, 467-468
Gastrointestinal (GI) bleeding scan, 469-471
Gastrointestinal (GI) scintigraphy, 469-471
Gastrointestinal (GI) system tests, 1008-1009

Gastroscopy, 410-413
Gated pool ejection fraction, 246
Gated pool imaging, 246
GBM (glomerular basement membrane) antibody, 82-83
GDM (gestational diabetes mellitus), 485-486
GE (gastroesophageal) reflux scan, 467-468
General health panel, 1026
Genetic and chromosomal aberrations, 55
Genetic testing, 472-477
Genotype testing, HCV, 522-523
Gentamicin monitoring data, 894t
Gestational diabetes mellitus (GDM), 485-486
GGT (gamma-glutamyl transferase), 463-464
GGTP (gamma-glutamyl transpeptidase), 463-464
γ-GTP (gamma-glutamyl transpeptidase), 463-464
GH (growth hormone), 499-501
GH (growth hormone) provocation test, 502-503
GH (growth hormone) stimulation test, 502-503
GH (growth hormone) suppression testing, 500, 501
GHb (glycohemoglobin), 496-498
GHB (glycosylated hemoglobin), 496-498
GI (gastrointestinal) bleeding scan, 469-471
GI (gastrointestinal) scintigraphy, 469-471

GI (gastrointestinal) system tests, 1008-1009
GI (gastrointestinal) tract, computed tomography of, 299
Gliadin antibodies, 478-479
Globulins, 759
    serum, 758-763
Glomerular basement membrane (GBM) antibody, 82-83
Glucagon, 480-481
Glucagon provocative test, 705
Glucagon stimulation test, 704-705
Glucagonoma, 480
Glucose
    blood, 482-484
    cerebrospinal fluid, 605
    pericardial fluid, 665
    peritoneal fluid, 680
    pleural, 899
    postprandial, 485-486
    urine, 487-489
Glucose screen for gestational diabetes mellitus, 1-hour, 485-486
Glucose tolerance test (GTT), 492-495, 493f
Glucose-6-phosphate dehydrogenase (G-6-PD), 490-491
Glucose-6-phosphate dehydrogenase (G-6-PD) screen, 490-491
Glutamic acid decarboxylase (GAD) antibody, 359-360
Glutamine, 606
Glutethimide monitoring data, 894t
Glycated albumin, 497
Glycated fructosamine, 497
Glycated proteins, 496-497
Glycohemoglobin (GHb), 496-498

Glycolated hemoglobin, 496-498
Glycosylated hemoglobin (GHb, GHB), 496-498
Gonorrhea, 841t
Goodpasture's antibody, 82-83
Gram stain
  pericardial fluid, 700
  peritoneal fluid, 681
  pleural fluid, 900
  sputum, 872-873
Granular casts, 964, 970
Growth factors, 346
Growth hormone (GH), 499-501
Growth hormone (GH) provocation test, 502-503
Growth hormone (GH) stimulation test, 502-503
Growth hormone (GH) suppression testing, 500, 501
GTT (glucose tolerance test), 492-495, 493f
Guthrie test, 702-703
Gynecologic video laparoscopy, 579-582, 579f

H

H. pylori antibodies test, 507-510
H. pylori breath test, 507-510
H. pylori serologic testing, 508
H. pylori stool test, 507-510
HAA (hepatitis-associated antigen), 519-523
Hageman factor (factor XII), 281t, 283t
Hair tests, 881-882
Ham's test, 504
Hantavirus, 162t
Haptoglobin, 505-506
HAV (hepatitis A virus), 519-520

HAV-Ab/IgG (hepatitis A virus-antibody/IgG), 519-520, 521t
HAV-Ab/IgM (hepatitis A virus-antibody/IgM), 519, 521t
Hb (hemoglobin), 514-515
  contents, 518t
  electrophoresis, 516-518
  fetal testing, 443-445
  glycolated, 496-498
  glycosylated, 496-498
  hyperchromic, 785, 787
  hypochromic, 785, 786t, 787
  mean corpuscular, 785, 786-787, 788
  mean corpuscular concentration, 785, 787, 788
  normochromic, 785, 787
  qualitative fetal stool test, 115-116
Hb (hemoglobin) A_1, 516, 518t
Hb (hemoglobin) A_{1c}, 496-498
Hb (hemoglobin) A_2, 516, 518t
Hb (hemoglobin) C, 517, 518t
Hb (hemoglobin) F, 516, 518t
Hb (hemoglobin) H, 518t
Hb (hemoglobin) M, 645-646
Hb (hemoglobin) S, 517, 518t
Hb (hemoglobin) S test, 847-848
HBcAb (hepatitis B core antibody), 521t, 522
HBcAg (hepatitis B core antigen), 521t, 522
HBeAb (hepatitis B e-antibody), 521t, 522
HBeAg (hepatitis B e-antigen), 521t, 522
HBsAb (hepatitis B surface antibody), 520, 521t

HBsAg (hepatitis B surface antigen), 520, 521t
HBV (hepatitis B virus), 520-522
HBVc-Ab (hepatitis B virus core antibody) total, 521t
HBVc-Ab/IgM (hepatitis B virus core antibody/IgM), 521t
HCG (human chorionic gonadotropin), 740-742
HCO_3 (bicarbonate)
  arterial, 117-125, 119t
  fetal scalp blood, 448
  serum, 226
Hct (hematocrit), 511-513, 512f
HCT (human calcitonin), 217-219
HCV (hepatitis C virus), 522
HCV (hepatitis C virus) genotype testing, 522-523
HCV-Ab/IgG (hepatitis C virus-antibody/IgG), 521t
Hcy (homocysteine), 535-537
HDL (high-density lipoprotein), 590, 592-594
  cholesterol to HDL ratio, 263t
HDL-C (high-density lipoprotein cholesterol), 592-594
HDV (hepatitis D virus), 523
HDV-Ab (hepatitis D virus-antibody) total, 521t
HDV-Ab/IgM (hepatitis D virus-antibody/IgM), 521t
Heart rate reactivity, fetal, 433
Heart scan, 244-248
  PET, 729-732

Heart sonogram, 365-367
Helical/spiral CT scan
  of abdomen, 295-299
  of brain, 300-303
  of chest, 304-306
  of urinary system, 561
Helicobacter pylori antibodies test, 507-510
Helicobacter pylori breath test, 507-510
Helicobacter pylori serologic testing, 508
Helicobacter pylori stool test, 507-510
Hematocrit (Hct), 511-513, 512f
Hematologic system tests, 1009-1010
Hemoccult slide test, 879
Hemoglobin (Hb, Hgb), 514-515
  contents, 518t
  electrophoresis, 516-518
  fetal testing, 443-445
  glycolated, 496-498
  glycosylated, 496-498
  hyperchromic, 785, 787
  hypochromic, 785, 786t, 787
  mean corpuscular, 785, 786-787, 788
  mean corpuscular concentration, 785, 787, 788
  normochromic, 785, 787
  qualitative fetal stool test, 115-116
Hemoglobin (Hb, Hgb) A_1, 516, 518t
Hemoglobin (Hb, Hgb) A_{1c}, 496-498
Hemoglobin (Hb, Hgb) A_2, 516, 518t
Hemoglobin (Hb, Hgb) C, 517, 518t
Hemoglobin (Hb, Hgb) F, 516, 518t

Hemoglobin (Hb, Hgb) H, 518t
Hemoglobin (Hb, Hgb) M, 645-646
Hemoglobin (Hb, Hgb) S, 517, 518t
Hemoglobin (Hb, Hgb) S test, 847-848
Hemoglobinuria, paroxysmal nocturnal, 504
Hemolysis panel, 1026
Hemorrhagic fever, 164
Hemostasis, 279
  secondary, 282f
Heparin, 689-691
Heparin cofactor, 104-105
Hepatic function panel, 1026
Hepatitis
  acute panel, 1026
  infectious, 519-520
  serum, 520-522
Hepatitis A virus (HAV), 519-520
Hepatitis A virus (HAV)-Ab/IgG, 519-520, 521t
Hepatitis A virus (HAV)-Ab/IgM, 519, 521t
Hepatitis B core antibody, 521t, 522
Hepatitis B core antigen, 521t, 522
Hepatitis B e-antibody (HBeAb), 521t, 522
Hepatitis B e-antigen (HBeAg), 521t, 522
Hepatitis B surface antibody (HBsAb), 520, 521t
Hepatitis B surface antigen (HBsAg), 520, 521t
Hepatitis B virus (HBV), 520-522
Hepatitis B virus core antibody (HBVc-Ab), 521t
Hepatitis B virus core antibody/IgM (HBVc-Ab/IgM), 521t

Hepatitis C virus (HCV), 522
Hepatitis C virus antibody/IgG (HCV-Ab/IgG), 521t
Hepatitis C virus (HCV) genotype testing, 522-523
Hepatitis D virus (HDV), 523
Hepatitis D virus (HDV) antibody (HDV-Ab), 521t
Hepatitis D virus (HDV) antibody/IgM (HDV-Ab/IgM), 521t
Hepatitis D virus (HDV) antigen (HDV Ag), 521t
Hepatitis E virus (HEV), 523
Hepatitis testing, 521t
  sexually transmitted disease cultures, 841t
Hepatitis virus studies, 519-523
Hepatitis-associated antigen (HAA), 519-523
Hepatobiliary imaging, 459-460
Hepatobiliary scintigraphy, 459-460
Hepatobiliary system tests, 1010
Hepatocellular liver disease, 766
HER 2 protein, 197-199
Hereditary metabolic disorders, 55
Herpes genitalis, 524-526, 841t
Herpes simplex, 524-526
Herpes simplex virus type 1 (HSV 1), 524
Herpes simplex virus type 2 (HSV 2), 524-526
Herpes virus type 2, 524-526
Heterophil antibody test, 649-650
HEV (hepatitis E virus), 523
Hex A (hexosaminidase A), 527-528

Hexosaminidase, 527-528
Hexosaminidase A (Hex A), 527-528
Hexosaminidase A and B, 527-528
Hgb (hemoglobin), 514-515
  contents, 518t
  electrophoresis, 516-518
  fetal testing, 443-445
  glycolated, 496-498
  glycosylated, 496-498
  hyperchromic, 785, 787
  hypochromic, 785, 786t, 787
  mean corpuscular, 785, 786-787, 788
  mean corpuscular concentration, 785, 787, 788
  normochromic, 785, 787
  qualitative fetal stool test, 115-116
Hgb (hemoglobin) A_1, 516, 518t
Hgb (hemoglobin) A_{1c}, 496-498
Hgb (hemoglobin) A_2, 516, 518t
Hgb (hemoglobin) C, 517, 518t
Hgb (hemoglobin) F, 516, 518t
Hgb (hemoglobin) H, 518t
Hgb (hemoglobin) M, 645-646
Hgb (hemoglobin) S, 517, 518t
Hgb (hemoglobin) S test, 847-848
HGH (human growth hormone), 499-501
5-HIAA (5-hydroxy-indoleacetic acid), 546-547
HIDA scanning, 459-460
High sensitive assay for CRP (hs-CRP), 319-320

High-density lipoprotein (HDL), 590, 592-594
  cholesterol to HDL ratio, 263t
High-density lipoprotein cholesterol (HDL-C), 592-594
Histamine challenge test, 779
Histocompatibility A antigen, 538-539
HIV (human immunodeficiency virus) antibody test, 23-27
HIV (human immunodeficiency virus) panel, 1026-1027
HIV (human immunodeficiency virus) RNA, 529-532, 530t, 531t
HIV (human immunodeficiency virus) viral load, 529-532, 530t, 531t
HLA-B27 antigen (human lymphocyte antigen B27), 538-539
Holter monitoring, 533-534
Home care
  AIDS serology, 27
  amniocentesis, 59
  arteriography, 131
  arthrocentesis with synovial fluid analysis, 136
  arthroscopy, 142
  barium enema, 149
  barium swallow, 152
  bone marrow biopsy, 188
  bone scan, 191
  bronchoscopy, 209
  cardiac catheterization, 238
  chorionic villus sampling, 271
  colonoscopy, 288
  cystoscopy, 345
  endometrial biopsy, 392
  endoscopic retrograde chol-angiopancreatography, 397

Home care—cont'd
  esophagogastroduodeno-
      scopy, 413
  fetoscopy, 453
  HIV viral load, 532
  intravenous pyelography, 564
  laparoscopy, 582
  liver biopsy, 598
  lumbar puncture and
      cerebrospinal fluid
      examination, 610
  lymphocyte immuno-
      phenotyping, 629
  mediastinoscopy, 643
  myelography, 654
  pericardiocentesis, 701
  pleural biopsy, 725
  prothrombin time, 769
  renal biopsy, 795
  retrograde pyelography, 809
  sigmoidoscopy, 851
  venography of lower
      extremities, 987
Homocysteine (Hcy), 535-537
Hot spots, 189
hPL (human placental
    lactogen), 540-541
HSV 1 (herpes simplex virus
    type 1), 524
HSV 2 (herpes simplex virus
    type 2), 524-526
HTLV (human T-cell
    lymphotrophic virus)
    I/II antibody, 542
Human calcitonin (HCT),
    217-219
Human chorionic
    gonadotropin (HCG),
    740-742
Human growth hormone
    (HGH), 499-501
Human immunodeficiency
    virus (HIV) antibody
    test, 23-27
Human immunodeficiency
    virus (HIV) panel,
    1026-1027

Human immunodeficiency
    virus (HIV) RNA,
    529-532, 530t, 531t
Human immunodeficiency
    virus (HIV) viral load,
    529-532, 530t, 531t
Human leukocyte A antigen,
    538-539
Human lymphocyte antigen
    B27 (HLA-B27),
    538-539
Human placental lactogen
    (hPL), 540-541
Human T-cell lymphotrophic
    virus (HTLV) I/II
    antibody, 542
Hyaline casts, 964, 971
Hybrid capture DNA test, 675
17-Hydrocorticosteroids
    (17-OCHS), 543-545
Hydrocortisone, 314-316
5-Hydroxyindoleacetic acid
    (5-HIAA), 546-547
Hyperchromic hemoglobin,
    785, 787
Hyperkalemia, 733, 735
Hypertension, renovascular, 801f
Hypertension panel, 1027
Hyperventilation, 375
Hypochromic hemoglobin,
    785, 786t, 787
Hypokalemia, 733, 735
Hysterogram, 548-549
Hysterosalpingography,
    548-549
Hysteroscopy, 550-552, 551f

I
IAA (insulin autoantibody),
    359-360
IC (inspiratory capacity), 776,
    776f
ICA (islet cell antibody),
    359-360
IDA (iminodiacetic acid
    analogue) gallbladder
    scanning, 459-460

Idiopathic thrombocytopenia purpura (ITP), 712
IF (intrinsic factor), Schilling test with, 821, 822-823
IFA (immunofluorescence assay), 818
IFE (immunofixation electrophoresis), 553-554, 556, 761
IgA (immunoglobulin A), 555, 556
IgD (immunoglobulin D), 555
IgE (immunoglobulin E), 555
  antibody test, 38-40
  electrophoresis, 555, 557
IGF BP (insulin-like growth factor binding proteins), 868-869
IGF-1 (insulin-like growth factor), 499-500, 868-869
IgG (immunoglobulin G), 555
  anti-*H. pylori* IgG antibody, 507-510
  electrophoresis, 555, 557
  HAV-Ab/IgG, 519-520, 521t
  HCV-Ab/IgG, 521t
  platelet-associated IgG antibodies, 712-713
IgM (immunoglobulin M), 555
  electrophoresis, 555, 557
  HAV-Ab/IgM, 519, 521t
  HBVc-Ab/IgM, 521t
  HDV-Ab/IgM, 521t
Imaging
  hepatobiliary, 459-460
  magnetic resonance, 632-636
  nuclear magnetic resonance, 632-636
  testicular, 824-825
IMC (immunochromatography), 508-509
Iminodiacetic acid analogue (IDA) gallbladder scanning, 459-460

Imipramine monitoring data, 894t
Immunochromatography (IMC), 508-509
Immunoelectrophoresis, 153
Immunofixation, 153
Immunofixation electrophoresis (IFE), 553-554, 556, 761
Immunofluorescence antinuclear antibody patterns, 90f
  cutaneous biopsy, 333
  skin biopsy, 333
Immunofluorescence assay (IFA), 818
Immunoglobulin A (IgA), 555, 556
Immunoglobulin D (IgD), 555
Immunoglobulin E (IgE), 555
  antibody test, 38-40
  electrophoresis, 555, 557
Immunoglobulin G (IgG), 555
  anti-*H. pylori* IgG antibody, 507-510
  electrophoresis, 555, 557
  HAV-Ab/IgG, 519-520, 521t
  HCV-Ab/IgG, 521t
  platelet-associated IgG antibodies, 712-713
Immunoglobulin M (IgM), 555
  electrophoresis, 555, 557
  HAV-Ab/IgM, 519, 521t
  HBVc-Ab/IgM, 521t
  HDV-Ab/IgM, 521t
Immunoglobulins, 555
  electrophoresis, 555-557
  thyroid binding inhibitory, 916-917
  thyroid-stimulating, 916-917
Immunohistopathology, skin, 333

Immunologic antithrombin III, 104-105

Immunologic pregnancy tests, 740-741

Immunologic system tests, 1010-1011

Immunophenotyping, lymphocyte, 626-629

Immunoscintigraphy, 666-667

^{111}In (^{111}indium) white blood cell scan, 1001

Indirect bilirubin, 157

Indirect Coombs' test, 312-313

^{111}Indium (^{111}In) white blood cell scan, 1001

Indwelling pericardial catheter, 700, 701

Indwelling urinary catheter, xvii, 973

Indwelling venous catheter, xiv

Infectious agents, bioterrorism, 161-166

Infectious hepatitis, 519-520

Infertility screen, 98-99

Inflammatory scan, 1000-1001

Inhalation tests, 779

Inhibin A, 48

Inorganic phosphate, 706

INR (international normalized ratio), 766-770, 768t

Inspiratory capacity (IC), 776, 776f

Inspiratory reserve volume (IRV), 776, 776f

Insulin assay, 558-559

Insulin autoantibody (IAA), 359-360

Insulin C-peptide, 317-318

Insulin tolerance test (ITT), 502-503

Insulin-like growth factor (IGF-1), 499-500, 868-869

Insulin-like growth factor binding proteins (IGF BP), 868-869

Interferon, 346

Interleukins, 346

Intermediate density lipoproteins, 591

International normalized ratio (INR), 766-770, 768t

Intestinal washings, 947

Intradermal allergy test, 41, 43

Intravenous pyelography (IVP), 560-564
scout films, 662

Intravenous urography (IUG, IVU), 560-564

Intrinsic factor (IF), Schilling test with, 821, 822-823

Iodine-131 (^{131}I) hippurate scan, 797

Iodine-131 (^{131}I) scan, 797

Ionized calcium, 220-223

Iontophoresis, pilocarpine, 886-887

Iontophoretic sweat test, 886-887

Iron, serum, 565-566

Iron level (Fe), 565-568

Iron-binding capacity, total (TIBC), 565-568

IRV (inspiratory reserve volume), 776, 776f

Islet cell antibody (ICA), 359-360

Isoenzymes
alkaline phosphatase, 36
creatine phosphokinase, 323

Isoimmunization, Rh, 55

Isonitrile scan, 244-248

Isonitrile stress test, 247

Isosulfan blue dye, 833, 834

ITP (idiopathic thrombocytopenic purpura), 712

ITT (insulin tolerance test), 502-503

IUG (intravenous urography), 560-564

IV cholangiography (IVC), 394

IVC (IV cholangiography), 394
IVP (intravenous pyelography), 560-564
  scout films, 662
IVU (intravenous urography), 560-564
Ivy bleeding time test, 169-171

J
Jaundice, 157
Joint aspiration, 133-136

K
K (potassium)
  blood, 733-735
  urine, 736-737
Kanamycin monitoring data, 894t
Karyotype, 273-274
Karyotyping, 273
Kernicterus, 157
Ketones, 963-964, 970
17-Ketosteroids (17-KS), 569-571
Ki67 protein, 197-199
Kidney(s)
  computed tomography of, 299
  ultrasound of, 1, 2f, 4
Kidney, ureter, and bladder (KUB) x-ray, 661
Kidney arteriography, 132
Kidney biopsy, 792-795, 793f
Kidney scan, 796-799
Kleihauer-Betke test, 443-445
Krypton gas ventilation scan, 615-616
17-KS (17-ketosteroids), 569-571
KUB (kidney, ureter, and bladder) x-ray, 661

L
La antibody, 100-101
Lactate, 575-576
Lactate dehydrogenase, 572-574
  cerebrospinal fluid, 605
  peritoneal fluid, 680
Lactic acid, 575-576
  cerebrospinal fluid, 605
Lactic dehydrogenase (LDH), 572-574
  cerebrospinal fluid, 605
  pericardial fluid, 665
  pleural, 899
Lactose tolerance test, 577-578
Lamellar body count, 55
LAP (leucine aminopeptidase), 585-586
Laparoscopy, 579-582, 579f
Large loop excision of the transformation zone (LLETZ), 251-253
Lasix renal scan, 798
Lateral chest x-ray, 254
LATS (long-acting thyroid stimulator), 916-917
LDH (lactic dehydrogenase), 572-574
  cerebrospinal fluid, 605
  pericardial fluid, 665
  pleural, 899
LDL (low-density lipoprotein), 590, 591, 592-594
LDL-C (low-density lipoprotein cholesterol), 592-594
Leads, ECG, 368
Lecithin/sphingomyelin (L/S) ratio, 54
LEEP (loop electrosurgical excision procedure) cervical biopsy, 251-253
Legionnaire's disease antibody test, 583-584
LES (lower esophageal sphincter) pressure, 406, 408f
Leucine aminopeptidase (LAP), 585-586
Leukoagglutinin test, 587
Leukocyte count, 994-999

Leukocyte esterase, 963, 970
Leukocytes,
        polymorphonuclear,
        995
Levodopa, prolactin
        suppression test with,
        750
LH (luteinizing hormone)
        assay, 618-620
Lidocaine monitoring data, 894t
Limb leads, 368
Lipase, 588-589
Lipid fractionation, 590-591
Lipid panel, 1027
Lipid profile testing, 262
Lipoprotein (a) [Lp(a)],
        110-114
Lipoproteins, 592-594
    apolipoproteins, 110-114
    electrophoresis, 590-591
    high-density, 263t, 590,
        592-594
    intermediate density, 591
    low-density, 590, 591,
        592-594
    phenotyping, 590-591
    very low-density, 590, 591,
        592-594
Liquid-based cervical cytology,
        675
Lithium monitoring data, 894t
Liver
    computed tomography of,
        299
    ultrasound of, 2, 2f, 4
Liver biopsy, 595-598, 595f
Liver function tests, 1026
Liver scanning, 599-601
Liver/spleen scanning, 599-601
LLETZ (large loop excision of
        the transformation
        zone), 251-253
Long-acting thyroid stimulator
        (LATS), 916-917
Loop electrosurgical excision
        procedure (LEEP),
        251-253

Lordotic chest x-ray, 254
Low-density lipoprotein (LDL),
        590, 591, 592-594
Low-density lipoprotein
        cholesterol (LDL-C),
        592-594
Lower esophageal sphincter
        (LES) pressure, 406,
        408f
Lower extremities
    arteriography of, 127, 132
    venography of, 985-987
LP (lumbar puncture),
        599-601, 608f
Lp(a) [lipoprotein (a)], 110-114
L/S (lecithin/sphingomyelin)
        ratio, 54
Lumbar puncture (LP),
        599-601, 608f
Lumbar x-ray studies, 870-871
Lung biopsy, 611-614, 613f
Lung perfusion scan, 615, 617
Lung scan, 615-617
Lung tissue, microscopic
        examination of, 82-83
Lung volumes and capacities,
        776f
Lupus anticoagulant, 71
Luteinizing hormone (LH),
        618-620
Lutropin, 618-620
Lyme disease test, 621-622
Lymph node biopsy, 161-166
Lymphangiography
        (lymphangiogram),
        623-625, 625f
Lymphocyte count, 994-999
Lymphocyte immuno-
        phenotyping, 626-629
Lymphocytes, 995, 998t
Lymphography, 623-625
Lymphoscintigraphy, 833-835

M
MA (microalbumin), 647-648
Macroaggregated albumin
        (MAA) lung scan, 615

Macrocytic red blood cells, 785, 786, 786t
Magnesium, 630-631
Magnetic field studies, 632-636
Magnetic resonance angiography (MRA), 633
Magnetic resonance imaging (MRI), 632-636
  liver biopsy with, 596
Magnetic resonance spectroscopy (MRS), 633-634
Magnevist (gadolinium), 635
Magnified spot view, 639
Male bladder, cystoscopic examination of, 340, 340f
Mammography (mammogram), 637-639
  scintimammography, 202-203
  ultrasound, 204-205
Mammotomy, 638
Manometric tests, 1021
  cystometry, 336-339
  electrophysiologic study, 387-390
  esophageal function studies, 406-409, 408f
  plethysmography
    arterial, 719-720
    venous, 721-722
  urethral pressure profile, 336-339
Mapping, cardiac, 387-390
Mast cells, 995
Maternal quadruple test, 48
Maternal triple screen test, 47-48
Maternal-fetal platelet antigen incompatibility, 712
Maturation index (MI), 675
Maximal breathing capacity, 775
Maximal midexpiratory flow (MMEF), 775

Maximal volume ventilation (MVV), 775-776
MCH (mean corpuscular hemoglobin), 785, 786-787, 788
MCHC (mean corpuscular hemoglobin concentration), 785, 787, 788
MCV (mean corpuscular volume), 785-786, 788
M/E (myeloid to erythroid cells) ratio, 185
Mean corpuscular hemoglobin (MCH), 785, 786-787, 788
Mean corpuscular hemoglobin concentration (MCHC), 785, 787, 788
Mean corpuscular volume (MCV), 785-786, 788
Mean platelet volume (MPV), 717-718
Meckel's diverticulum nuclear scan, 640-641
Meconiuum staining, 56
Mediastinoscopy, 642-644
Mediolateral view, 639
Meprobamate monitoring data, 895t
Metabolic disorders, hereditary, 55
Metanephrine, 978-981
Methacholine challenge test, 779
Methemoglobin, 645-646
Methionine loading, 536
Methotrexate monitoring data, 895t
Methyprylon monitoring data, 895t
Metrizamide (Amipaque), 651
Metyrapone, ACTH stimulation test with, 18-20
MI (maturation index), 675

Micral Urine Test Strip, 647, 648

Microalbumin (MA), 647-648

Microbiology culture, 946-948

Microcytic red blood cells, 785, 786, 786t

Microglobulin, beta-$_2$, 155-156

Microscopic examinations, 1021
  antiglomerular basement membrane antibodies, 82-83
  antral biopsy, 507-510
  bioterrorism infectious agents, 161-166
  bone marrow biopsy, 183-188
  breast cancer tumor analysis, 197-199
  cathepsin D, 197-199
  cervical biopsy, 251-253
  Chlamydia, 257-259
  cutaneous immunofluorescence biopsy, 333
  DNA ploidy status, 197-199
  duodenal biopsy, 507-510
  endometrial biopsy, 391-393
  estrogen receptor assay, 418-419
  gonorrhea culture, 841t
  H. pylori antibodies test, 507-510
  HER 2 protein, 197-199
  herpes genitalis, 524-526, 841t
  herpes simplex, 524-526
  Ki67 protein, 197-199
  liver biopsy, 595-598, 595f
  lung biopsy, 611-614, 613f
  of lung tissue, 82-83
  nose culture, 905-907
  p53 protein, 197-199
  Papanicolaou smear, 674-677
  pleural biopsy, 723-725
  progesterone receptor assay, 748-749

Microscopic examinations—cont'd
  renal biopsy, 792-795, 793f
  of renal tissue, 82-83
  sexually transmitted disease cultures, 840-844
  of skin tissue, 333
  S-phase fraction, 197-199
  strept screen, 905
  throat and nose cultures, 905-907
  tuberculosis culture, 946-948
  urine culture and sensitivity, 972-974
  viral cultures, 988-989
  wound culture and sensitivity, 1002-1003

Microsomal antibody, 108-109

Midstream urine specimens, xvi, 967, 973

Minute ventilation, 777

Minute volume (MV), 777

MMEF (maximal midexpiratory flow), 775

M-mode echocardiography, 365

Monilia, 841t

Monoclonal antibody immunoassay, 942

Monoclonal "sandwich" antibody qualitative testing, 942

Monocyte count, 994-999

Monocytes, 996, 999t

Mononuclear heterophil test, 649-650

Mononucleosis spot test, 649-650

Monospot heterophil test, 399, 400t

Monospot test, 649-650

Morphine sulfate, gallbladder nuclear scanning with, 459

Motility studies, esophageal, 406-409

MPV (mean platelet volume), 717-718

MRA (magnetic resonance angiography), 633

MRI (magnetic resonance imaging), 632-636
  liver biopsy with, 596

MRS (magnetic resonance spectroscopy), 633-634

MSLT (multiple sleep latency tests), 857, 858

MUGA (multigated acquisition) scan, 246

Multigated acquistion (MUGA) scan, 246

Multiphasic screening machines, xiii

Multiphasic testing, chloride, 260

Multiple sleep latency tests (MSLT), 857, 858

Multiple wake test (MWT), 856-859

MV (minute volume), 777

MVV (maximal volume ventilation), 775-776

MWT (multiple wake test), 857, 858

Mycobacterium tuberculosis culture, 900

Myelography (myelogram), 651-654

Myeloid to erythroid cells (M/E) ratio, 185

Myocardial infarction, 322f

Myocardial infarction scan, 245

Myocardial perfusion scan, 245

Myocardial scan, 244-248

Myoglobin, 655-656

N

Na (sodium)
  blood, 863-865
  sweat test, 886
  urine, 866-867

NANB (non-A/non-B) hepatitis, 522

Nasal culture, 906

Nasopharyngeal culture, 906

Nasopharyngeal swab, 819

Nasopharyngeal wash/aspirate, 819

Native double-stranded DNA, 78-79

Natriuretic peptides, 657-658

Natural killer cells, 626

Needle aspiration, transbronchial, 612, 613f

Needle biopsy
  percutaneous, 612
  transbronchial, 613f

Neonatal thrombocytopenia, 712

Nephrotomography, 561

Nerve conduction studies, 381-383

Nervous system tests, 1012

neu protein, 197-199

Neural tube defects, 267

Neuroendocrine nuclear scan, 664-665

Neutrophil count, 994-999

Neutrophils, 995, 998t

Newborn, physiologic jaundice of the, 157

^{99m}Tc (^{99m}technetium) white blood cell scan, 1001

90 degree view, 639

Nipple stimulation technique, 438, 439

Nitrites, urinary, 963, 970

NMP22 (nuclear matrix protein 22), 167-168

NMRI (nuclear magnetic resonance imaging), 632-636

Nocturnal hemoglobinuria, paroxysmal, 504

Nomograms
  activated clotting time, 10
  urine flow, 975

Non-A/non-B (NANB) hepatitis, 522
Nongranulocytes, 995
Nonstress test (NST), 446-447
Norepinephrine, 978-981
Normetanephrine, 978-981
Normochromic hemoglobin, 785, 786t, 787
Normocytic red blood cells, 785, 786t
Nortriptyline monitoring data, 895t
Nose culture, 905-907
NST (nonstress test), 446-447
N-telopeptide (NTx), 192-194
NTx (N-telopeptide), 192-194
Nuclear antigens
    anti-extractable, 80-81
    EBV nuclear antigen, 399
    EBV nuclear antigen-IgG, 399, 400t
Nuclear imaging
    of kidney, 796-799
    parotid gland, 816-817
    salivary gland, 816-817
    scrotal, 824-825
Nuclear magnetic resonance imaging (NMRI), 632-636
Nuclear matrix protein 22 (NMP22), 167-168
Nucleal scanning, preparation and procedures, xx-xxi
Nuclear scans, 1021-1022
    bone scan, 189-191
    breast scintigraphy, 202-203
    carcinoid, 664-665
    cardiac, 244-248
    cardiac exercise stress testing, 239-243
    cardiac flow studies, 244-248
    gallbladder, 459-460
    gallium, 461-462
    gastroesophageal reflux scan, 467-468

Nuclear scans—cont'd
    gastrointestinal bleeding scan, 469-471
    isonitrile scan, 244-248
    kidney, 796-799
    liver/spleen scanning, 599-601
    lung scan, 615-617
    Meckel's diverticulum, 640-641
    MUGA scan, 246
    neuroendocrine, 664-665
    octreotide, 664-665
    oncoscint scan, 666-667
    parathyroid scan, 686-688
    positron emission tomography, 729-732
    red blood cell survival study, 789-791
    renal, 796-799
    salivary gland nuclear imaging, 816-817
    Schilling test, 821-823
    scrotal nuclear imaging, 824-825
    sentinel lymph node biopsy, 833-835
    thallium, 244-248
    thyroid, 910-912
    white blood cell scan, 1000-1001
Nuclear stress testing, 239-243
Nuclear ventriculography, 246
5'-Nucleotidase, 659-660

O
O$_2$ (oxygen) content, arterial, 117-125
O$_2$ (oxygen) saturation, 672-673
    arterial, 117-125
    fetal monitoring, 448-450
OB (occult blood), stool for, xviii, 878-880
Oblique chest x-ray, 254
Obstetric echography, 694-697
Obstetric panel, 1027

Obstetric ultrasonography, 694-697

Obstruction series, 661-663

Obstructive biliary disease, 766

Occlusion cuff, 721

Occult blood (OB), stool for, xviii, 878-880

OCG (oral cholecystography), 394

17-OCHS (17-hydrocorticosteroids), 543-545

OCT (oxytocin challenge test), 437-440

Octreotide scan, 664-665

Oculovestibular reflex study, 224-225

OGTT (oral glucose tolerance test), 492-495

Oil-based myelography, 651

Oligoclonal gamma globulin bands, 605

Oligospermia, 830

Omnipaque, 651

Omni-Sal, 25

OMT (oral mucosal transudate), 25

Oncologic PET scan, 729-732

Oncoscint scan, 666-667

1-day bowel preparation, 286

1-hour glucose screen for gestational diabetes mellitus, 485-486

O&P (ova and parasites), stool for, 876-877

Open lung biopsy, 611, 612

Open pleural biopsy, 723

Oral cholecystography (OCG), 394

Oral glucose tolerance test (OGTT), 492-495

Oral HIV antibody test, 25

Oral mucosal transudate (OMT), 25

Orapette, 25

OraSure, 25

Order of draw for blood collection, xiv

Oropharyngeal culture, 819, 843

Oropharyngeal swab, 819

Osmolality
blood, 668-669
urine, 670-671

Osmolar gap
blood, 668
urine, 670

Osteocalc, 192-194

Osteocalcin, 192-194

O'Sullivan test, 485-486, 492-495

Ova and parasites (O&P), stool for, 876-877

Ovarian cancer genetic testing, 472-473

Ovaries, computed tomography of, 299

Oximetry, 672-673, 673f
pulse, 121, 672-673, 856

Oxygen (O_2) content, arterial, 117-125

Oxygen partial pressure (Po_2), 117-125
fetal scalp blood, 448

Oxygen (O_2) saturation, 672-673
arterial, 117-125
fetal monitoring, 448-450

Oxytocin challenge test (OCT), 437-440

P

P (phosphorus), 706-707

P wave, 369

p24 antigen capture assay, 23-27

p53 protein, 197-199

PA (posteroanterior) chest x-ray, 254

PAB (prealbumin), 738-739

Pacer stress testing, 239

Pacing, 241

Packed cell volume (PCV), 511-513, 512f

Packed red blood cell volume, 511-513, 512f

P-ANCA (perinuclear anti-neutrophil cytoplasmic antibody), 87

Pancreas
computed tomography of, 299
ultrasound of, 2, 2f, 4

Pancreatic ducts, ERCP of, 394-398

Pancreatic enzymes, 828-829

Pancreatic panel, 1027

Pancreatobiliary ultrasound, 1-4, 2f

Pancreozymin, 828-829

Pantopaque, 651

PAP (prostatic acid phosphatase), 7-8

Pap (Papanicolaou) smear, 674-677, 677f

Pap (Papanicolaou) test, 674-677, 677f

Papanicolaou (Pap) smear, 674-677, 677f

Paracentesis, 678-683, 679f

Parathormone, 684-685

Parathyroid hormone (PTH), 684-685

Parathyroid panel, 1027

Parathyroid scan, 686-688

Parathyroid scintigraphy, 686-688

Parenchymal (hepatocellular) liver disease, 766-767

Parentage analysis, 472, 475

Parotid gland nuclear imaging, 816-817

Paroxysmal nocturnal hemoglobinuria (PNH), 504

Partial pressure of carbon dioxide (P_{CO_2})
arterial, 117-125, 119t
fetal scalp blood, 448

Partial pressure of oxygen (P_{O_2})
arterial, 117-125
fetal scalp blood, 448

Partial thromboplastin time (PTT), 689-691

Partial thromboplastin time (PTT), activated (APTT), 689-691

Parvovirus B19 antibody, 692-693

Paternity investigations
genetic testing, 472, 475
human lymphocyte antigen B27, 538

P_{CO_2} (partial pressure of carbon dioxide)
arterial, 117-125, 119t
fetal scalp blood, 448

PCV (packed cell volume), 511-513, 512f

Peak expiratory flow rate (PEFR), 777

Peak inspiratory flow rate (PIFR), 777

Peak level, therapeutic drug monitoring, 893, 896

PEFR (peak expiratory flow rate), 777

Pelvic endoscopy, 579-582, 579f

Pelvic floor sphincter electromyography or EMG, 379-380

Pelvic ultrasonography, 694-697

Pelvic ultrasonography in pregnancy, 694-697

Pentagastrin stimulation, 217

Percent free PSA (%FPSA), 756

Percutaneous needle biopsy, 612

Percutaneous transhepatic cholangiography (PTHC), 394-395

Perfusion scans
lung, 615, 617
renal, 796

Pericardiocentesis, 698-701, 699f
Peripheral blood smear, 174-176
Peritoneal fluid analysis, 678-683
Peritoneal tap, 678-683
Persantine (dipyridamole), 240
PET (positron emission tomography), 729-732
PFTs (pulmonary function tests), 774-780
PG (phosphatidylglycerol), 55
PgR (progesterone receptor) assay (PRA), 748-749
pH
  arterial, 117-125, 119t
    esophageal probe, 857
    fetal scalp blood, 448-450
    pleural fluid, 900
    urinary, 960-961, 968
pH probe, acid reflux with, 407, 408f
Phenistix test, 703
Phenobarbital monitoring data, 895t
Phenotyping
  alpha-antitrypsin, 45-46
  lipoprotein, 590-591
  lymphocyte immunophenotyping, 626-629
Phenylalanine screening, 702-703
Phenylketonuria (PKU) test, 702-703
Phenytoin monitoring data, 895t
Pheochromocytoma, 979
Pheochromocytoma suppression and provocation testing, 704-705
Phlebography, 985-987
Phosphate (PO_4), 706-707
Phosphatidylglycerol (PG), 55

Phosphorus (P), 706-707
Photodiagnostic tests, 672-673, 673f
Photostimulation, 375
Physiologic jaundice of the newborn, 157
PIFR (peak inspiratory flow rate), 777
Pilocarpine iontophoresis, 886-887
PKU (phenylketonuria) test, 702-703
PL (placental lactogen), human, 540-541
Placental lactogen (PL), human, 540-541
Plague infections, 162t, 164
Plasma renin activity (PRA), 800-804
Plasma renin assay, 800-804
Plasma renin concentration (PRC), 800-804
Plasma thromboplastin antecedent (factor XI), 283t
Plasminogen, 708-709
Platelet aggregation test, 710-711
Platelet antibody detection, 712-713
Platelet antigen, maternal-fetal incompatibility, 712
Platelet count, 714-716
Platelet volume, mean, 717-718
Platelet-associated IgG antibodies, 712-713
Platelet-specific antigens, 712
Plethysmography
  arterial, 719-720
  venous, 721-722
Pleural biopsy, 723-725
Pleural fluid analysis, 897-902
Pleural tap, 897-902
PMNs (polymorphonuclear leukocytes), 995
PNH (paroxysmal nocturnal hemoglobinuria), 504

Po$_2$ (partial pressure of
oxygen)
arterial, 117-125, 119t
fetal scalp blood, 448
PO$_4$ (phosphate), 706-707
Polymerase chain reaction,
reverse transcription,
818
Polymerase chain reaction
culture, 946-948
Polymorphonuclear leukocytes
(PMNs, "polys"), 995
Polynucleated cells ("polys"),
294
Polys (polymorphonuclear
leukocytes), 995
Polys (polynucleated cells),
294
Polysomnography (PSG),
856-859
Pontiac fever, 583
Porphobilinogens, 726-728
Porphyrins, 726-728
Portogram, CT, 307-309
Positron emission tomography
(PET), 729-732
Postcoital cervical mucus test,
852-853
Postcoital test, 852-853
Posteroanterior (PA) chest
x-ray, 254
Postprandial blood sugar,
2-hour, 485-486
Postprandial glucose (PPG),
2-hour, 485-486
Posttransfusion purpura, 712
Potassium (K)
blood, 733-735
urine, 736-737
PPD (purified protein
derivative) skin test,
944-945
PPG (postprandial glucose),
2-hour, 485-486
PR (progesterone receptor)
assay (PRA), 748-749
PR interval, 369

PRA (plasma renin activity),
800-804
PRA (progesterone receptor
assay), 748-749
PRC (plasma renin
concentration),
800-804
Prealbumin (PAB), 738-739
Pregnancy tests, 740-742
Pregnanediol, 743-745
Pregnant uterus
ultrasonography,
694-697
Prenatal panel, 1027
Preoperative mammogram
localization, 638
Prick-puncture allergy test, 41,
43
Primidone monitoring data,
895t
PRLs (prolactin levels),
750-751
Proaccelerin (factor V), 280t,
283t
Procainamide monitoring data,
895t
Proconvertin (factor VII),
280t, 283t
Proctoscopy, 849-851
Progesterone assay, 746-747
Progesterone receptor (PR,
PgR) assay (PRA),
748-749
Proinsulin C-peptide,
317-318
Prolactin levels (PRLs),
750-751
Prolactin stimulation tests, 750
Prolactin suppression tests,
750
Prolonged/rapid DST, 355-358
Propranolol monitoring data,
895t
Prostate
computed tomography of,
299
ultrasound of, 752-754

Prostate/rectal sonogram, 752-754, 753f
Prostate-specific antigen (PSA), 755-757
Prostate-specific antigen (PSA) density, 756
Prostate-specific antigen (PSA) velocity, 756
Prostate-specific membrane antigen, 756
Prostatic acid phosphatase (PAP), 7-8
Protein
  blood, 758-763
  cerebrospinal fluid, 604-605
  pericardial fluid, 665
  total, 758-763
  urinary, 962, 969
Protein C, 764-765
Protein content, 899
Protein count, 680
Protein electrophoresis, 153, 758-763, 760t
Protein S, 764-765
Prothrombin (factor II), 279-284, 280t, 283t
Prothrombin fragment (F1+2), 908-909
Prothrombin time (PT), 766-770
Pro-time, 766-770
PSA (prostate-specific antigen), 755-757
PSA (prostate-specific antigen) density, 756
PSA (prostate-specific antigen) velocity, 756
Pseudocholinesterase, 266-268
Pseudomembranous colitis toxic assay, 275-276
PSG (polysomnography), 856-859
PT (prothrombin time), 766-770
PTH (parathyroid hormone), 684-685

PTHC (percutaneous transhepatic cholangiography), 394-395
PTT (partial thromboplastin time), 689-691
PTT (partial thromboplastin time), activated, 689-691
Pulmonary angiography, 771-773
Pulmonary arteriography, 771-773
Pulmonary artery pressure, 234t
Pulmonary function tests (PFTs), 774-780
Pulmonary scintiphotography, 615-617
Pulmonary system tests, 1012-1013
Pulmonary wedge pressure, 234t
Pulse oximetry, 121, 672-673
  sleep studies, 856
Punch biopsy, 251-253
Puncture sites, xvi
Purified protein derivative (PPD) skin test, 944-945
PYD (pyridinium) crosslinks, 192-194
Pyelography
  intravenous, 560-564
  retrograde, 807-809
Pyridinium (PYD) crosslinks, 192-194

Q
Q wave, 369
QCT (quantitative computed tomography), 180
QRS complex, 369
Quadruple test, maternal, 48
Qualitative fetal hemoglobin stool test, 115-116
Quantitative computed tomography (QCT), 180

Quantitative fibrinogen, 454-455
Quantitative stool fat determination, 428-429
Queckenstedt-Stookey test, 609
Quinidine monitoring data, 895t
Quinidine-like drugs, 712

R
R factor, 69-70
R wave, 369
Rabies-neutralizing antibody test, 781
Rack urine samples, 795
Radioallergosorbent test (RAST), 38-40
Radiography, chest, 254-256
Radioimmunoassay (RIA) pregnancy tests, 741
T_3, 939-940
Radionuclide renal imaging, 796-799
Radionuclide scans, biliary tract, 459-460
Radioreceptor assay (RRA), 741
Radiorenography, 796-799
Random urine specimens, xvi
Rapid DST, 355-358
Rapid immunologic tests, 905
Rapid plasma reagin (RPR), 888-889
Rapid stimulation test, 15-16
Rapid urease test, 507-510
RAST (radioallergosorbent test), 38-40
RBC (red blood cell) casts, 965, 971
RBC (red blood cell) count, 782-784
  pericardial fluid, 665
  synovial fluid, 134
RBC (red blood cell) smear, 174-176

RBCs (red blood cells)
  color abnormalities, 175
  distribution width, 785, 787, 788
  indices, 785-788
  intracellular structure, 175-176
  macrocytic, 785, 786, 786t
  microcytic, 785, 786, 786t
  morphology, 174-176
  normocytic, 785, 786t
  shape abnormalities, 175
  size abnormalities, 174-175
  survival study, 789-791
  urinary, 971
RDW (red cell distribution width), 785, 787, 788
Reagin, 888
Recording cuff, 721
Rectal culture
  female, 842, 842f
  male, 842, 843f
Rectal EMG procedure, 379-380
Rectal ultrasound, 752-754, 753f
Red blood cell (RBC) casts, 965, 971
Red blood cell (RBC) count, 782-784
  pericardial fluid, 665
  synovial fluid, 134
Red blood cell (RBC) smear, 174-176
Red blood cells (RBCs)
  color abnormalities, 175
  distribution width, 785, 787, 788
  indices, 785-788
  intracellular structure, 175-176
  macrocytic, 785, 786, 786t
  microcytic, 785, 786, 786t
  morphology, 174-176
  normocytic, 785, 786t
  packed, 511-513, 512f
  shape abnormalities, 175

Red blood cells (RBCs)—
    cont'd
  size abnormalities, 174-175
  survival study, 789-791
  urinary, 971
Red cell cholinesterase,
    266-268
Red cell distribution width
    (RDW), 785, 787, 788
Reductase, 963
Reflectance meters, 484
Reflexes, oculovestibular,
    224-225
Renal angiography, 126, 130f
Renal biopsy, 792-795, 793f
Renal blood flow (perfusion)
    scan, 796, 799
Renal function scan, 797, 799
Renal function studies, 326,
    953
Renal hypertension scan, 797
Renal obstruction scan,
    797-798
Renal panel, 1027-1028
Renal perfusion scan, 796, 799
Renal scanning, 796-799
Renal structural scan, 797, 799
Renal tissue, microscopic
    examination of, 82-83
Renal vein assays, 801
Renal/urologic system tests,
    1013-1014
Renin assay, plasma, 800-804
Renin stimulation test, 801-802
Renography (renogram), 797
Renovascular hypertension,
    801f
Reproductive system tests,
    1014-1015
Residual level, therapeutic
    drug monitoring, 893,
    896
Residual volume (RV), 776,
    776f
Retic count, 805-806
Reticulocyte count, 805-806
Reticulocyte index, 805

Retrograde pyelography,
    807-809
Retroperitoneum, computed
    tomography of, 299
Reverse transcription-
    polymerase chain
    reaction (RT-PCR),
    818
RF (rheumatoid factor),
    810-811
  pleural fluid, 900
Rh factors, 178
Rh isoimmunization, 55
Rheumatoid factor (RF),
    810-811
  pleural fluid, 900
RhIG (RhoGAM) antibodies,
    444
RhoGAM (RhIG) antibodies,
    444
RIA (radioimmunoassay)
  pregnancy tests, 741
  T_3, 939-940
RPR (rapid plasma reagin),
    888-889
RRA (radioreceptor assay)
  pregnancy tests, 741
RT-PCR (reverse transcription-
    polymerase chain
    reaction) SARS viral
    testing, 818
Rubella antibody test, 812-813
Rubeola antibody, 814-815
RV (residual volume), 776,
    776f

S
S wave, 369
SACE (serum angiotensin-
    converting enzyme),
    67-68
Sacral x-ray studies, 870-871
SAECG (signal-averaged
    ECG), 370
Salicylate monitoring data,
    895t
Saliva HIV antibody, 23-27

Saliva testing, 881
Salivary gland nuclear imaging, 816-817
"Sandwich" antibody qualitative testing, 942
SARS (severe acute respiratory syndrome) viral testing, 818-820
SBF (small bowel follow-through), 860-862
sBPP (amyloid beta protein precursor, soluble), 63-64
Scalp blood pH, fetal, 448-450
Schilling test, 821-823
Scintigraphy
    abdominal, 469-471
    breast, 202-203
    captopril, 797
    cholescintigraphy, 459-460
    GI, 469-471
    hepatobiliary, 459-460
    immunoscintigraphy, 666-667
    lymphoscintigraphy, 833-835
    parathyroid, 686-688
Scintimammography, 202-203
Scintiphotography, pulmonary, 615-617
Scl-70 antibody, 94-95
Scleroderma antibody, 94-95
Scout films, 662
Screening
    AIDS screen, 23-27
    amino acid screen, 50-51
    blood antibody, 312-313
    coagulation, 1025
    disseminated intravascular coagulation, 363, 364t
    drug, 881-883
    infertility screen, 98-99
    maternal triple screen test, 47-48
    multiphasic machines, xiii
    phenylalanine, 702-703
    strept screen, 905
    sweat test, 887

Screening—cont'd
    thyroid, 1028
    thyroxine, 924-925
    toxicology, 881-883, 1028
Scrotal nuclear imaging, 824-825
Scrotal scan, 824-825
Scrotal ultrasound, 826-827
Secretin test, 466
Secretin-pancreozymin, 828-829
Sed rate test, 402-403
Segmented cells ("segs"), 294
Segs (segmented cells), 294
Semen analysis, 830-832
Semen examination, 830-832
Seminal cytology, 830-832
Sentinel lymph node biopsy (SLNB), 833-835
Serial urine samples, 795
Serine protease inhibitor, 104-105
Serologic tests
    AIDS, 23-27
    Epstein-Barr virus, 399-400, 400t
    H. pylori, 508
    herpes simplex, 525
    syphilis, 606
    for syphilis (STS), 888-889
SERs (somatosensory-evoked responses), 424-427
Serum albumin, 758-763
Serum angiotensin-converting enzyme (SACE), 67-68
Serum bicarbonate, 226
Serum calcium, 220-223
Serum cardiac enzymes, 322f
Serum cortisol, 314-316
Serum creatinine, 326-327
Serum globulin, 758-763
Serum glutamic-oxaloacetic transaminase (SGOT), 143-145
Serum glutamic-pyruvic transaminase (SGPT), 28-29

Serum hepatitis, 520-522
Serum iron, 565-566
Serum osmolality, 668-669
Serum tests
  acid serum test for
    paroxysmal nocturnal
    hemoglobinuria, 504
  glucose tolerance test, 492,
    493f
  iron, 565-566
  pregnancy tests, 741
Serum total testosterone level,
    890-892
Serum urea nitrogen, 952-954
Sestamibi breast scan, 202-203
Sestamibi cardiac scan, 244-248
Severe acute respiratory
    syndrome (SARS) viral
    testing, 818-820
Sex of fetus, 55
Sexual assault testing, 836-839
Sexually transmitted disease
    (STD) cultures,
    840-844, 841t
SGOT (serum glutamic-
    oxaloacetic
    transaminase), 143-145
SGPT (serum glutamic-pyruvic
    transaminase), 28-29
SH (somatotropin hormone),
    499-501
Sialography, 845-846
Sickle cell preparation, 847-848
Sickle cell test, 847-848
Sickledex, 847-848
Sigmoidoscopy, 849-851
Signal-averaged ECG
    (SAECG), 370
Sims-Huhner test, 852-853
Single tracer double phase
    (STDP) test, 686, 687
Single x-ray absorptiometry, 180
Sjögren's antibodies, 100-101
Skeletal system tests, 1015
Skin biopsy
  bioterrorism infectious
    agents, 161-166

Skin biopsy—cont'd
  immunofluorescence, 333
Skin biopsy antibodies, 333
Skin immunohistopathology,
    333
Skin tests
  allergy, 41-44
  tuberculin, 944-945
  viral cultures, 988-989, 989t
Skin tissue, microscopic
    examination of, 333
Skull x-ray, 854-855
Sleep studies, 856-859
SLNB (sentinel lymph node
    biopsy), 833-835
Small bowel enema, 860, 862
Small bowel follow-through
    (SBF), 860-862
Smallpox, 163t, 164-165
Smears
  acid-fast bacillus
    pericardial fluid, 700
    sputum, 947
    synovial fluid, 134
  blood, 174-176
  conjunctival, 258
  Papanicolaou, 674-677,
    677f
Sodium (Na)
  blood, 863-865
  sweat test, 886
  urine, 866-867
Sodium resorption, 733
Sodium-depleted upright
    plasma renin assay, 800
Sodium-repleted upright
    plasma renin assay, 800
Soluble amyloid beta protein
    precursor (sBPP),
    63-64
Somatomedin C, 499-500,
    868-869
Somatosensory-evoked
    responses (SERs),
    424-427
Somatotropin hormone (SH),
    499-501

Sonograms
  abdominal, 1-4, 2f
  breast, 204-205
  heart, 365-367
  prostate/rectal, 752-754
  thyroid, 918-919
Sound sensors, 857
Specific gravity, urine,
    962-963, 969
Spectroscopy, magnetic
    resonance, 633-634
Sperm agglutination and
    inhibition, 98-99
Sperm antibodies, 98-99
Sperm count, 830-832
Sperm examination, 830-832
Sperm specimens, 99
S-phase fraction, 197-199
Spinal x-rays, 870-871
Spinnbarkeit, 852
Spirometry, 778-779
Spleen, computed tomography
    of, 299
Spleen scanning, 599-601
Splenic sequestration study,
    789-791
Spot tests, mononucleosis,
    649-650
Sputum cytology, 874-875
Sputum tests, 1022
  acid-fast bacillus smear,
    947
  bioterrorism infectious
    agents, 161-166
  culture and sensitivity,
    872-873
  cytology, 874-875
ST segment, 370
Stab cells, 995
Stable factor (factor VII),
    280t, 283t
STD (sexually transmitted
    disease) cultures,
    840-844, 841t
STDP (single tracer double
    phase) test, 686, 687
Stereotactic biopsy, 638

Stool testing, preparation and
    procedures, xviii-ix
Stool tests, 1022
  Apt test, 115-116
  bioterrorism infectious
    agents, 161-166
  clostridial toxin assay,
    275-276
  culture, 876-877
  culture and sensitivity,
    876-877
  fecal fat, 428-429
  H. pylori, 507-510
  occult blood, 878-880
  ova and parasites, 876-877
  swallowed blood, 115-116
  viral cultures, 988-989,
    989t
Strept screen, 905
Stress testing, 239-243
  cardiac, 366
  exercise, 239-240
  fetal contraction, 437-440
  isonitrile, 247
  thallium, 247
Stroke volume (SV), 234t
Structural renal scan, 799
STS (serologic test for
    syphilis), 888-889
Stuart factor (factor X), 281t,
    283t
Subarachnoid space pressure,
    603
Substance abuse testing,
    881-883
Sulfonamides, 712
Supine abdominal x-ray, 661,
    662
Suprapubic aspiration of urine,
    973
SV (stroke volume), 234t
Swabs
  buccal, 476
  nasopharyngeal or
    oropharyngeal, 819
  tuberculosis, 947
Swallow, barium, 150-152

Swallowed blood, stool for, 115-116
Swallowing examination, 884-885
Swallowing pattern, 406, 408f
Sweat electrolytes test, 886-887
Sweat tests, drug testing, 881
Synovial fluid analysis, 133-136
Syphilis, 606, 841t
Syphilis detection test, 888-889
Systolic left ventricular pressure, 234t

T
T cells, 626
T wave, 369, 370
T_3 (triiodothyronine), 939-940
T_3 (triiodothyronine) radioimmunoassay, 939-940
T_3 (triiodothyronine) toxicosis, 939
T_4 (thyroxine) free, 922-923 total, 924-925
T_4 (thyroxine) index, free, 928-929
T_4 (thyroxine) screen, 924-925
Tablet test, 879
Tape test, 877
Tartrate-resistant acid phosphatase (TRAP), 7-8
tau protein, 63
Tay-Sachs disease genetic testing, 472, 474
TB (tuberculosis) culture, 946-948
TBG (thyroxine-binding globulin), 926-927
TBII (thyroid binding inhibitory immunoglobulin), 916-917
TBPA (thyroxine-binding prealbumin), 738-739

Tc (technetium) sentinel lymph node biopsy, 833, 834
^{99m}Tc (^{99m}technetium) white blood cell scan, 1001
Tc-diethylenetriamine pentaacetic acid (Tc-DTPA) renal scan, 796-799 ventilation scan, 615-616
Tc-disodium monometha-narsonate (Tc-DSMA) renal scan, 797
Tc-macroaggregated albumin (Tc-MAA) lung scan, 615
TDM (therapeutic drug monitoring), 893-896
Technetium (Tc), 834 sentinel lymph node biopsy, 833
Tc-DSMA renal scan, 797
Tc-DTPA renal scan, 796-799
Tc-DTPA ventilation scan, 615-616
Tc-MAA lung scan, 615
Technetium-99m (^{99m}Tc) white blood cell scan, 1001
TEE (transesophageal echocardiography), 366, 933-936, 934f
N-Telopeptide (NTx), 192-194
Terrorism infectious agents testing, 161-166
Testes, ultrasound of, 826-827
Testicular imaging, 824-825
Testosterone, 890-892
Testosterone stimulation tests, 890
TGs (triglycerides), 590, 937-938 pleural, 899
Thallium exercise stress test, 247
Thallium scan, 244-248

Theophylline monitoring data, 895t

Therapeutic drug monitoring (TDM), 893-896, 894t-895t

"Thin prep" Pap smear, 675

Thoracentesis, 897-902, 898f

Thoracic x-ray studies, 870-871

Thoracoscopy, 903-904
lung biopsy, 613

Thoracotomy, video-assisted, 903

Thorascopic lung biopsy, 613-614

3-day fecal collection, xviii

Throat and nose cultures, 905-907
viral, 988-989, 989t

Thrombocyte count, 714-716

Thrombocythemia, 714

Thrombocytopenia, 714
drug-induced, 712-713
neonatal, 712

Thrombocytosis, 714

Thromboplastin (factor III), 283t

Thrombosis indicators, 908-909

Thyretin, 738-739

Thyrocalcitonin, 217-219

Thyroglobulin antibody, 106-107

Thyroid antimicrosomal antibody, 108-109

Thyroid antithyroglobulin antibody, 106-107

Thyroid autoantibody, 106-107, 108-109

Thyroid echogram, 918-919

Thyroid peroxidase antibody (TPO-Ab), 108-109

Thyroid scanning, 910-912

Thyroid scintiscan, 910-912

Thyroid screening, 1028

Thyroid sonogram, 918-919

Thyroid ultrasound, 918-919

Thyroid-binding globulin, 926-927

Thyroid-binding inhibitory immunoglobulin (TBII), 916-917

Thyroid-releasing hormone (TRH) stimulation test, 913-914

Thyroid-stimulating hormone (TSH), 913-914

Thyroid-stimulating hormone (TSH) stimulation test, 915

Thyroid-stimulating immunoglobulins (TSI), 916-917

Thyrotropin, 913-914

Thyrotropin receptor antibody, 916-917

Thyrotropin-releasing factor (TRF) test, 920-921

Thyrotropin-releasing hormone (TRH) test, 920-921

Thyroxine (T_4)
free, 922-923
total, 924-925

Thyroxine (T_4) index, free, 928-929

Thyroxine (T_4) screen, 924-925

Thyroxine-binding globulin (TBG), 926-927

Thyroxine-binding prealbumin (TBPA), 738-739

TIBC (total iron-binding capacity), 565-568

Tidal volume (TV, V_T), 776, 776f

Tilt-table testing, 387, 389

Tissue examination, microscopic
antiglomerular basement membrane antibodies, 82-83
bioterrorism infectious agents, 161-166

Tissue examination,
microscopic—cont'd
bone marrow biopsy,
183-188
endometrial biopsy, 391-393
liver biopsy, 595-598, 595f
lung biopsy, 611-614
lung tissue, 82-83
pleural biopsy, 723-725
renal biopsy, 792-795, 793f
renal tissue, 82-83
Tissue factor (factor III), 283t
TLC (total lung capacity),
776f, 777
T-lymphocyte cells, 626-629
Tobramycin monitoring data,
895t
Toluidine blue dye test, 837
Tomography
computed tomography (CT)
of abdomen, 295-299
of brain, 300-303
of chest, 304-306
computed tomography (CT)
portogram, 307-309
nephrotomography, 561
positron emission
tomography, 729-732
quantitative computed
tomography, 180
TORCH test, 930, 1028
cytomegalovirus, 349-350
herpes simplex, 524-526
rubella antibody test,
812-813
toxoplasmosis antibody titer,
931-932
Total/ionized calcium,
220-223
Total CD4 cell count, 626
Total cholesterol, 263t
Total estrogen, 414
Total hexosaminidase, 527-528
Total iron-binding capacity
(TIBC), 565-568
Total lung capacity (TLC),
776f, 777

Total protein, 758-763
Total testosterone serum level,
890-892
Total thyroxine, 924-925
Tourniquet application, xiv
Toxicology screening,
881-883, 1028
Toxoplasmosis antibody titer,
931-932
TPO-Ab (thyroid peroxidase
antibody), 108-109
Transbronchial brushing, 612
Transbronchial lung biopsy,
612, 613f
Transbronchial needle
aspiration, 612, 613f
Transbronchial needle biopsy,
613f
Transesophageal
echocardiography
(TEE), 366, 933-936,
934f
Transferrin, 565-568
Transferrin saturation (TS),
565-568
Transhepatic cholangiography,
percutaneous, 394-395
Transluminal coronary
angioplasty, 233
Transthoracic
echocardiography
(TTE), 365-367
Transthyretin, 738-739
Transtracheal aspiration, 873
Transudates
peritoneal, 678, 683
pleural, 897, 902
Transurethral renal biopsy, 792
TRAP (tartrate-resistant acid
phosphatase), 7-8
TRF (thyrotropin-releasing
factor) test, 920-921
TRH, prolactin stimulation
test with, 750
TRH (thyroid-releasing
hormone) stimulation
test, 913-914

TRH (thyrotropin-releasing hormone) test, 920-921
Trichomoniasis, 841t
Triglycerides (TGs), 590, 937-938
pleural, 899
Triiodothyronine (T_3), 939-940
Triiodothyronine (T_3) radioimmunoassay, 939-940
Triiodothyronine (T_3) toxicosis, 939
Triple renal study, 798
Triple screen test, maternal, 47-48
Triple-lumen catheter, xiv
Troponin I, cardiac-specific (cTnI), 941-943
Troponin T, cardiac-specific (cTnT), 941-943
Troponins, 941-943
True cholinesterase, 266
TS (transferrin saturation), 565-568
TSH (thyroid-stimulating hormone), 913-914
TSH (thyroid-stimulating hormone) stimulation test, 915
TSI (thyroid-stimulating immunoglobulins), 916-917
T-suppressor (CD8) cells, 626-629
TTE (transthoracic echocardiography), 365-367
Tuberculin test, 944-945
Tuberculosis (TB) culture, 946-948
Tubular (epithelial) casts, 965
Tularemia, 163t, 165
Tumor analysis
breast cancer, 197-199
progesterone receptor assay, 748-749

Tumor markers
CA 15-3 and CA 27.29, 211-212
CA 19-9, 213-214
CA-125, 215-216
cerebrospinal fluid, 606
cytokines, 346-348
TV (tidal volume), 776, 776f
12-lead ECG, 368
24-hour urine tests, xvii
creatinine clearance, 328-330
17-hydroxycorticosteroids, 543-545
5-hydroxyindoleacetic acid, 546-547
17-ketosteroids, 569-571
leucine aminopeptidase, 585-586
porphyrins and porphobilinogens, 726-728
potassium, 736-737
prealbumin, 738-739
pregnanediol, 743-745
preparation and procedures, xvii
Schilling test, 821-823
sodium, 866-867
vanillylmandelic acid and catecholamines, 978-981
2-day bowel preparation, 286
Two-dimensional echocardiography, 365
2-hour postprandial blood sugar, 485-486
2-hour postprandial glucose (PPG), 485-486

U
U bags, xvii-xviii, 974
U wave, 370
UA (urinalysis), 959-971
UGI (upper gastrointestinal) studies, 949-951
air-contrast, 951
endoscopy, 410-413

Ultrasound, 1022-1023
  abdominal, 1-4, 2f
  amniotic fluid index, 435
  bilary tree, 1-4, 2f
  breast, 204-205
  carotid, 249-250
  color Doppler, 982-983
  echocardiography, 365-367
  fetal biophysical profile, 433-436
  fetal nuchal translucency, 695
  of gallbladder, 1-4, 2f
  of kidney, 1-4, 2f
  of liver, 1-4, 2f
  mammography, 204-205
  obstetric, 694-697
  of pancreas, 1-4, 2f
  of pancreatobiliary system, 1-4, 2f
  pelvic, 694-697
  prostate, 752-754, 753f
  rectal, 752-754, 753f
  scrotal, 826-827
  of testes, 826-827
  thyroid, 918-919
  transesophageal echocardiography, 933-936, 934f
  transthoracic echocardiography, 365-367
  transrectal ultrasonography, 752-754
  vaginal, 694-697
  vascular studies, 982-984
Ultrasound absorption, 180
Ultrasound studies, preparation and procedures, xxi-xxii
Umbilical artery velocity, 435
Unconjugated (indirect) bilirubin, 157
UPP (urethral pressure profile), 336-339
Upper gastrointestinal (UGI) studies, 949-951
  air-contrast, 951
  endoscopy, 410-413
Upper GI series, 949-951

Upright plasma renin assay, sodium-depleted, 800
  sodium-repleted, 800
Urea nitrogen blood test, 952-954
Urease, rapid testing, 507-510
Ureter x-ray, 661
Ureteral catheterization through cystoscope, 341, 341f
Urethral culture, 840-844, 843f
  Chlamydia, 258
  herpes simplex, 525
Urethral pressure measurements, 336-339
Urethral pressure profile (UPP), 336-339
Uric acid, blood and urine, 955-958
Urinalysis (UA), 959-971
Urinary catheter, indwelling, xvii, 973
Urinary catheterization, xvii, 973
Urinary diversion, 974
Urine
  appearance, 960, 968
  cellular casts, 964
  color, 960, 961t, 968
  epithelial casts, 965, 970
  fatty casts, 964, 970
  granular casts, 964, 970
  hyaline casts, 964, 971
  odor, 960, 968
  pH, 960-961, 968
  RBC casts, 965, 971
  specific gravity, 962-963, 969
  waxy casts, 965, 970
  WBC casts, 965, 971
Urine drug testing, 881-883
Urine flow studies, 975-976
Urine flowmeters, 975
Urine glucose, 487-489

Urine osmolality, 670-671
Urine sugar, 487-489
Urine testing
 clean catch specimens, xvi,
  973
 composite specimens, xvii
 culture and sensitivity, xvi
 first morning specimen, xvi
 preparation and procedures,
  xvi-xviii
Urine tests, 1023-1024
 adrenocorticotropic
  hormone stimulation
  test with metyrapone,
  18-20
 agglutination inhibition test,
  740-741
 aldosterone, 32-35
 amino acid profiles, 50-51
 amylase, 60-62, 61
 Bence Jones protein,
  153-154
 beta-$_2$ microglobulin,
  155-156
 bioterrorism infectious
  agents, 161-166
 bladder cancer markers,
  167-168
 bone turnover biochemical
  markers, 192-194
 calcium, 220-223
 cortisol, 314-316
 creatinine clearance, 328-330
 crystals, 964
 delta-aminolevulinic acid,
  353-354
 dexamethasone suppression
  test, 355-358
 double-voided specimen,
  488
 epithelial casts, 965
 estriol excretion, 414-417
 estrogen fractions, 414-417
 ethanol, 420-421
 fatty casts, 964
 flow studies, 975-976
 glucose, 487-489

Urine tests—cont'd
 glucose tolerance test,
  492-495
 granular casts, 964
 HIV, 23-27
 Hyaline casts, 964
 17-hydroxycorticosteroids,
  543-545
 5-hydroxyindoleacetic acid,
  546-547
 immunofixation
  electrophoresis, 553-554
 ketones, 963-964
 17-ketosteroids, 569-571
 leucine aminopeptidase,
  585-586
 leukocyte esterase, 963
 metyrapone, 18-20
 microalbumin, 647-648
 N-telopeptide, 192
 nitrates, 963
 odor, 960
 osmolality, 670-671
 ph, 960
 phenylketonuria test, 702-703
 porphyrins and
  porphobilinogens,
  726-728
 potassium, 736-737
 prealbumin, 738-739
 pregnancy tests, 740-742
 pregnanediol, 743-745
 protein, 962, 969
 pyridinium, 192-194
 random specimens, xvi
 red blood cells and casts,
  959-971
 Schilling test, 821-823
 sodium, 866-867
 specific gravity, 962-963
 substance abuse testing,
  881-883
 N-telopeptide, 192-194
 toxicology screening,
  881-883, 1028
 uric acid, 955-958
 urinalysis, 959-971

Urine tests—cont'd
  vanillylmandelic acid and
      catecholamines, 978-981
  waxy cast, 965
  white blood cells and casts,
      959-971
  viral cultures, 988-989
  D-xylose absorption test,
      1004-1005
Urodynamic studies, 975-976
Uroflowmetry, 975-976
Urography
  excretory, 560-564
  intravenous, 560-564
Urologic system tests,
    1013-1014
Uroporphyrin, 726
Uroporphyrinogen-1-synthase,
    977
Uterosalpingography, 548-549
Uterotubography, 548-549
Uterus, computed tomography
    of, 299

V
Vaginal ultrasound, 694-697
Valproic acid monitoring data,
    895t
Vanillylmandelic acid (VMA),
    978-981
Variola virus, 163t
Vascular ultrasound studies,
    982-984
Vasopressin, 75-77
VAT (video-assisted
    thoracotomy), 903
VC (vital capacity), 776f, 777
VCA-IgG (viral capsid antigen-
    antibody IgG), 399, 400t
VCA-IgM (viral capsid
    antigen-antibody IgM),
    399, 400t
VCAs (viral capsid antigen-
    antibodies), 399
VDRL (Venereal Disease
    Research Laboratory)
    test, 888-889

Venereal Disease Research
    Laboratory (VDRL)
    test, 888-889
Venography (venogram) of
    lower extremities,
    985-987
Venous plethysmography,
    721-722
Venous/arterial Doppler
    ultrasound, 982-984
Venous/arterial duplex scan,
    982-984
Ventilation, maximal volume,
    775-776
Ventilation scan, 615-616, 617
Ventilation/perfusion (V/Q)
    scanning (VPS),
    615-617
Ventriculography, 232-238
VERs (visual-evoked
    responses), 425, 426
Very low-density lipoprotein
    (VLDL), 590, 591,
    592-594
Video laparoscopy,
    gynecologic, 579-582,
    579f
Video-assisted thoracotomy
    (VAT), 903
Videofluoroscopy swallowing
    examination, 884-885
Viral capsid antigen-antibodies
    (VCAs), 399
Viral capsid antigen-antibody
    IgG (VCA-IgG), 399,
    400t
Viral capsid antigen-antibody
    IgM (VCA-IgM), 399,
    400t
Viral cultures, 988-989, 989t
Virtual colonoscopy, 295-299
VisoV (volume of isoflow),
    778
Visual-evoked potentials,
    424-427
Visual-evoked responses
    (VERs), 425, 426

Vital capacity (VC), 776f, 777
Vitamin B$_{12}$, 990-991
Vitamin B$_{12}$ absorption test, 821-823
VLDL (very low-density lipoprotein), 590, 591, 592-594
VMA (vanillylmandelic acid), 978-981
Voiding cystography, 334-335
Voiding cystourethrography, 334-335
Volume of isoflow (VisoV), 778
Volume-adjusted PSA levels, 755
von Willebrand factor, 280t, 284
VPS (ventilation/perfusion scanning), 615-617
V/Q (ventilation/perfusion) scan, 615-617
V$_T$ (tidal volume), 776, 776f

W

Wassermann test, 888
Water deprivation ADH stimulation test, 75-76
Water load test (ADH suppression test), 76
Water-soluble myelography, 651
Waxy casts, 965, 970
WBC (white blood cell) antigens, 538-539
WBC (white blood cell) casts, 965, 971
WBC (white blood cell) count, 994-999, 998t-999t
    pericardial fluid, 665
    synovial fluid, 134
WBC (white blood cell) differential count, 994-999, 998t-999t
    synovial fluid, 134
WBC (white blood cell) esterase, 963

WBC (white blood cell) scan, 1000-1001
WBCs (white blood cells), urinary, 971
West Nile virus (WNV) testing, 992-993
Western blot test antibody, 23-27
White blood cell (WBC) antigens, 538-539
White blood cell (WBC) casts, 965, 971
White blood cell (WBC) count, 994-999, 998t-999t
    pericardial fluid, 665
    synovial fluid, 134
White blood cell (WBC) differential count, 994-999, 998t-999t
    synovial fluid, 134
White blood cell (WBC) esterase, 963
White blood cell (WBC) scan, 1000-1001
White blood cells (WBCs), urinary, 971
Whole-blood clot retraction test, 277-278
Whole-body thyroid scan, 910
WNV (West Nile virus) testing, 992-993
Wound culture and sensitivity, 1002-1003

X

Xenon CT scan of the brain, 300-301, 303
X-ray studies
    abdominal
        cross-table lateral, 661-662
        erect, 661
        supine, 661, 662
    adrenal angiography, 132
    arteriography, 126-132
    arthrography, 137-138
    barium enema, 146-149
    barium swallow, 150-152

	Hcy	Homocysteine
	HDL	High-density lipoprotein
	5-HIAA	Hydroxyindoleacetic acid
	HIDA	Hepatic iminodiacetic acid
	HIV	Human immunodeficiency virus
	HLA-B27	Human lymphocyte antigen B27
	HTLV	Human T-cell lymphotrophic virus
I	IAA	Insulin autoantibody
	ICA	Islet cell antibody
	Ig	Immunoglobulin
	INR	International normalization ratio
	IV-GTT	Intravenous glucose tolerance test
	IVP	Intravenous pyelography
	IVU, IUG	Intravenous urography
K	KS	Ketosteroid
	KUB	Kidney, ureter, and bladder x-ray study
L	LAP	Leucine aminopeptidase
	LATS	Long-acting thyroid stimulator
	LDH	Lactic dehydrogenase
	LDL	Low-density lipoprotein
	LFTs	Liver function tests
	LH	Luteinizing hormone
	LP	Lumbar puncture
	L/S ratio	Lecithin/sphingomyelin ratio
	LS spine	Lumbosacral spine
M	MA	Microalbumin
	MCH	Mean corpuscular hemoglobin
	MCHC	Mean corpuscular hemoglobin concentration
	MCV	Mean corpuscular volume
	M/E ratio	Myeloid/erythroid ratio
	MPV	Mean platelet volume
	MRI	Magnetic resonance imaging
	MUGA	Multigated acquisition cardiac scan
N	NST	Nonstress test
	NT_x	N-telopeptide
O	O&P	Ova and parasites
	OB	Occult blood
	OCT	Oxytocin challenge test
	OGTT	Oral glucose tolerance test
	17-OHCS	17-Hydroxycorticosteroids
P	PAB	Prealbumin
	PAP	Prostatic acid phosphatase
	Pco_2	Partial pressure of carbon dioxide
	PET	Positron emission tomography
	PFTs	Pulmonary function tests
	pH	Hydrogen ion concentration
	PKU	Phenylketonuria
	PMN	Polymorphonuclear
	PNH	Paroxysmal nocturnal hemoglobinuria
	Po_2	Partial pressure of oxygen
	Po_4	Phosphate

X-ray studies—cont'd
bone, 195-196
bone densitometry, 179-182
cardiac catheterization,
    232-238, 235f
cerebral angiography, 127
cervical studies, 870-871
chest x-ray, 254-256
coccygeal studies, 870-871
computed tomography of
    the abdomen, 295-299
computed tomography of
    adrenals, 295
computed tomography of
    the brain, 300-303
computed tomography of
    the chest, 304-306
computed tomography of
    kidney, 295
computed tomography
    portogram, 307-309
cystography, 334-335
digital subtraction
    angiography, 126
dual-energy x-ray
    absorptiometry, 179-180
hysterosalpingography,
    548-549
intravenous pyelography,
    560-564
KUB (kidney, ureter, and
    bladder) x-ray, 661
lumbar studies, 870-871
lymphangiography, 623-625,
    625f
magnetic resonance imaging
    (MRI), 632-636
mammography, 637-639,
    651-654
myelography, 651-654
obstruction series, 661-663

X-ray studies—cont'd
percutaneous transhepatic
    cholangiography,
    394-395
positron emission
    tomography, 729-732
pulmonary angiography,
    771-773
quantitative computed
    tomography, 180
renal angiography, 126,
    130f
retrograde pyelography,
    807-809
sacral studies, 870-871
sialography, 845-846
single x-ray absorptiometry,
    180
skull x-ray, 854-855
small bowel follow-through,
    860-862
spinal x-rays, 870-871
swallowing examination,
    884-885
thoracic studies, 870-871
upper gastrointestinal x-ray
    study, 949-951
venography of lower
    extremities, 985-987
videofluoroscopy, 884-885
virtual colonoscopy, 295-299
x-ray studies, preparation
    and procedures, xiv-xx
D-Xylose absorption test,
    1004-1005
Xylose tolerance test,
    1004-1005

Y
Yellow fever, 162t, 164
Yersinia pestis, 162t, 164